◄◄ Introduction to CV Exams: Vol II ►►

CV Review Book - Vol. 2:

Invasive Basics

6th Edition

by

J. Wesley Todd, BS, RCIS, RCES
Director, Cardiac Self Assessment
Spokane, WA 99216

DO NOT COPY!
Copyright © 2018

ISBN 978-1-7326393-1-7

Self Published by:
Cardiac Self Assessment
1605 South Clinton Rd.
Spokane, WA 99216-0420
phone (509) 926-0344
Email w.t@westodd.com
Web Site http://www.westodd.com

ABOUT THIS SERIES

This book represents only one volume of a much larger series of 5 books. This vol. 1 combines material from the basic sciences, cardiovascular anatomy, physiology, and pathology. This book has been revised each time the author has taken one of the exams.

This book will serve those studying for all the cardiovascular registry exams for staff working in the cath lab, electrophysiology lab, ultrasound and vascular labs. Everyone needs knowledge of A&P, pathology, patient care, asepsis, BLS, and invasive lab protocols. Thus, volume 1 can be used to prepare for any of the CCI exams cardiovascular specialty exams or the ARRT exams (CI and VI). Those preparing for these cardiovascular invasive registries (RCIS, CI or VI) will also need additional books: Vol. 2, 3, 4 and 5 shown below:

INVASIVE REGISTRY - STUDY MATERIAL

Vol. #	Ch #	Chapter Content	Published	ISBN
Vol. I		Invasive CV Basics (this book)	2018	978-1-7326393-0-0
		A. CV Science		
		B. CV Anatomy & Physiology		
		C. CV Pathology		
Vol. II		CV Diagnostic Techniques	2018	978-1-7326393-1-7
Vol. III		Hemodynamics	2018	978-1-7326393-2-4
Vol. IV		Interventions	2018	978-1-7326393-3-1
Vol V		Registry Practice Exams	2018	978-1-7326393-4-8

All 5 the above books and CD are available as a bundled set. See: www.westodd.com

DISCLAIMER

The author and the many reviewers have made every effort to insure the current accuracy of the material in this book. Where possible, recognized authorities are referenced and quoted. Due to the fast-moving nature of the cardiovascular field, and the changing nature of accepted practice, we cannot accept any responsibility for the errors or omissions or for the consequences from application of the information in this book. Although we have made every effort toward accuracy, you should always check with hospital standards and company literature such as drug package inserts, before applying the information in this book.

We have tried to include information that we believe will be on the national CV Invasive Registry examinations. But, since the examination agencies frequently update and change their test questions and formats, the questions included here will be similar but not identical to the ones you find on your national exam.

All rights reserved. No part of this book may be used or reproduced in any manner without written permission of the author.

Prior Editions Copyright 1996, 1997, 2002, 2005, 2011 ©, 6th Current Edition Copyright 2018

PREFACE to 6th Edition:

This edition of Todd's CV Review Books has been revised to include the new question formats given by CCI. CCI calls these new types of questions "innovative items." The exams are no longer just four item multiple choice questions, as in the past. New formats include matching, drag and drop, multiple response (checkbox) and hot spot questions. Although we have always used these formats in our Todd CV Review CDs & USBs we have modified many questions in this new edition to match these "innovative" formats.

Hundreds of new questions have been added. This 6th edition now includes new structural heart information and new devices like TAVR and Impella, and new diagnostic techniques like CTffr. Our new interactive CD & USB program will be available in 2019 to match the questions in this book and the current registry exams.
Wesley Todd, BS, RCIS, RCES 2018
Director, Cardiac Self Assessment

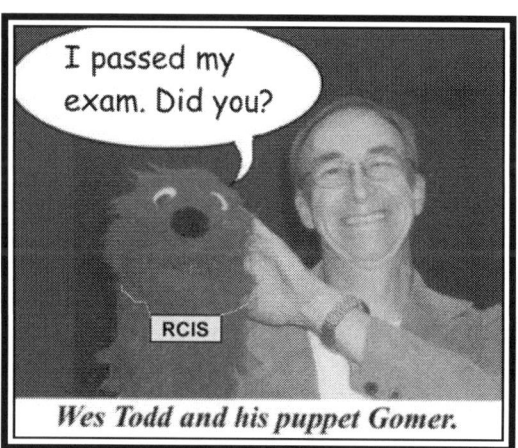
Wes Todd and his puppet Gomer.

PREFACE to 5th Edition:

This edition of Todd's CV Review Books keeps pace with the field and changes in the national exams. In 2010 CCI eliminated the CV Science exam, and merged it with the registry exam. The RCIS exam was increased by 60 basic science questions, making the exam longer. Now, there is only one exam and everyone's invasive exam will include this basic material. This is essential background knowledge common to all invasive professionals. Because of this, we changed the name of this book from "CV Science", to "Invasive Basics." This volume will include anatomy, physiology, pathology and other basic skills common to the Cath lab, EP Lab, and Vascular Radiology Lab. As such, this volume contains core knowledge for all the invasive cardiovascular specialties.

CCI also changed the blueprint and weighting on the registry exams. The categories within the exam are now based on job skills and duties, determined by an extensive survey of working nurses and techs. These skills are grouped into categories such as, "Conducting Intra-Procedural Activities" and "Performing Therapeutic Procedures". Categories such as statistics and math were removed. That does NOT mean there are no math questions on the exam, only that the math questions should relate directly to the field, such as hemodynamic calculations. This should make the exam more relevant. Changes coming to the 2013 RCIS include removal of Pediatric cath, ergonovine, and Foley catheterization.

Several hundred new questions have been added and others removed, to keep pace with advancing medical technology and invasive job descriptions.

Wesley Todd, BS, RCIS   6/23/13

PREFACE to 4th Edition:

This edition of Todd's CV Review Books is designed keep pace with the latest changes in exams and the tremendous increase in cardiovascular technology. In 2000 CCI did a task analysis of the CV field, which resulted in changes in the CV exams. This material is based on the latest 2002 updates. New exams increasingly weight patient care and pharmacology skills and knowledge. In addition CCI's Science matrix has decreased emphasis on the CV specialties, with increased emphasis on basic concepts. For example, physical principles were removed - including ultrasound physics and pressure measurement. These specialized topics have been shifted into the specialty exams: RCS, RVS, and RCIS. CCI is also preparing to give EP and Vascular Interventions examinations sometime in the near future.

The 2002-2003 RCIS and CIT exams place increased weight on Patient Care, Pharmacology, Equipment, and Interventions.

What's new? Todd's CV Review CD 2nd Edition will be updated to include all this new material and continuing education material. We now offer online classes for cardiology professionals who need a systematic review of this material. These are based on Todd's CV Review CD.   Wesley Todd, BS, RCIS   5/23/02

PREFACE to 1st Edition:

In my 23 years of teaching CVTs at the Spokane Community College I coached hundreds of CVT students through the national registry exams. With this experience I wrote this introduction to prepare them for the CV examinations. This book has hundreds of registry-quality multiple-choice test questions, answers, rationales, and reference material. It will also help **you** prepare for your national exam.

The students in our JRC-CVT approved CVT program have been tested with and helped refine many of the questions in this book. They have done very well on the RCVT examination. The RCVT exam has been in existence since 1973, when I first took it. I took the CCI/RCVT exam again in 1990, 1993, 1996, 1997 and 2002 and have ranked first in the country. In 1990 I started selling Self Assessment questions and answers by mail. Applicants taking the Science and RCVT exams around the country found it so helpful that I have refined it and expanded the number of questions and put them in this book.

Noninvasive (Echo) and Vascular technologists studying for the Basic CV Science Exam in preparation for their RCVT specialty exam also need this book. Although originally designed for those taking the Invasive RCVT exam, this book combines concepts of basic physical science that all branches of cardiovascular medicine need.

This book has become more than a review for the exam. It may also be used as a self study book and in-service education manual for working Cardiovascular Professionals of all types. Wesley Todd, BS, RCIS 1997, Director, Cardiac Self Assessment

INTRODUCTION

Volume II contains the background essential to all the CV invasisve registry exams taken by allied health and nursing staff. It is specifically designed for the Cardiovascular Invasive Exams (RCIS & CI).

I have organized this book around current exam content/matrix for the national CV exams, and designed it to be similar to the exam you will take. The content of each exam is detailed in this "Introduction to CV Exams." To prepare you for your exam, this book includes thousands of questions, answers, explanations, and references. It is up to you to match appropriate material from these volumes with the content of your exam. For example, RCIS and vascular candidates do not need the in depth EGM and action potential knowledge that EP candidates do.

GOALS OF THIS BOOK

Studying this book will improve your chances of passing the exam, but cannot replace formal education or clinical experience. This is not a "crash course." Neither can we cover all items that will appear on the exam. CCI's test bank includes more than 4000 test items, many more than in this book. If you have no formal training in your specialty, you will need extensive textbook study, tutoring, and clinical experience to gain the theoretical base necessary. These exams are difficult. Approximately 60-75% of the candidates pass these exams the first time. My experience shows that using this book to prepare for the exam can raise your exam score by as much as 20%.

This book will help you achieve your goal of passing the CV exams by helping you:
- evaluate your current Cardiovascular knowledge
- gain insight into your strengths and weaknesses
- form a directed plan of study to prepare for your exam
- gain confidence and reduce anxiety at test taking
- gain familiarity with the types of test items commonly used on these exams
- strengthen your test taking skills
- strengthen your problem-solving skills.
- Direct your study into recognized Cardiovascular references and textbooks.

References for each question are included.

© First Edition Copyright 1996
© 3rd Edition Copyright 1997
© 4th Edition Copyright 2002
© 5th Edition Copyright 2013
© 6th Edition Copyright 2018

REVIEWERS AND CONTRIBUTORS INCLUDE:

6th Edition Contributors:

Al Bennett, RCIS
Director Invasive Cardiology School
Carnegie Institute
550 Stephenson Hwy, Suite 100
Troy, Mi 48083

Todd Ginapp, RN, EMT-P, RCIS, FSICP
Memorial Herman SE Hospital
Cardiology Manager
Houston, TX

Jay Andrews, Technical services

Additional previous contributors:
Connie Marshall, RT(R), RCIS, M.A.
Anthony Williams, MSM, RN, RCIS
Sabrina Black, BS, RDCS, FASE
Patrick Hoier, BS, RCSA, RCIS, FSICP
Polly Keller MBA, RRT, RCIS
Kristy Schultz, M.Ed., RTRM, RCIS
Dan Sullivan, BSN, RN
Al Bennett, RCIS
Allan Mirehouse, RCIS
Christie Hodge, RCIS
Robert Howard, RCIS
Syed Mustafa Khundmiri, BS, RCIS
Esma Campbell RT, RCIS
Scott (William) Corson, RCIS
Lois Schaffer, MEd, RT®, RCIS
Marsha Holton, CCRN, RCIS, FSICP
Stephanie Ranck, BA, RCIS
Jeff Davis, RRT, RCIS, BS
Vicki Lemaster, BS, TR(R)(CV)
Richard Merschen, MS, RT(R)(CV)
Chuck Williams, BS, RCSA, RPA/RA, RCIS, RT(R)(CV)(CI), CPFT, CCT,

These knowledgeable reviewers have encouraged me and made suggestions throughout the years of book development.   Although they have all proofed, critiqued, and edited my work I have not always taken their suggestions. And, they are not responsible for errors in the text. Full responsibility for the contents and accuracy of the book rests with the author.

Special thanks to all the others who have received advanced copies and made suggestions, whose names I have forgotten.

NO COPIES PLEASE - Copyright 2018

Contact W. Todd   (509) 926-0344 ©

Copyright infringement is punishable by up to $150,000 fine and/or imprisonment.
Educational exceptions must be in writing and signed by the author.
Please report any suspected illegal copies to the author. You will be kept anonymous.

Wes Todd's Invasive Cardiovascular Study materials available:

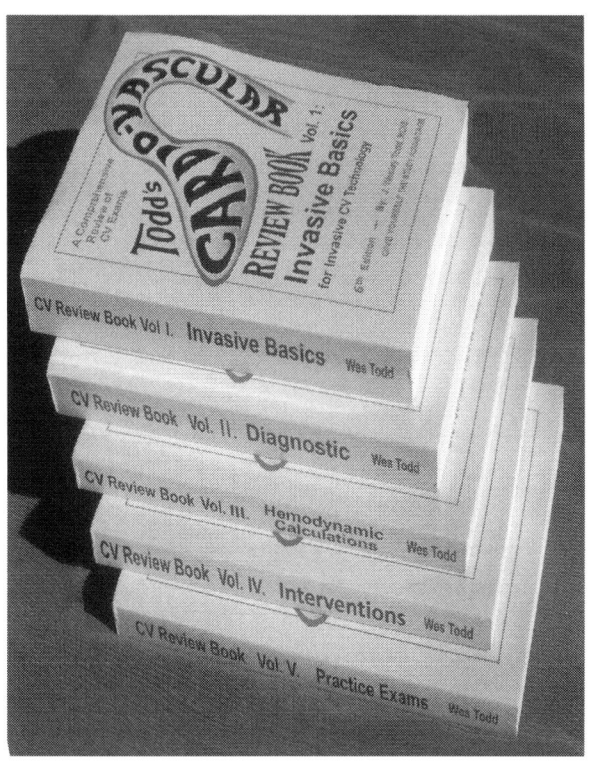

Todd's 5 Volume set

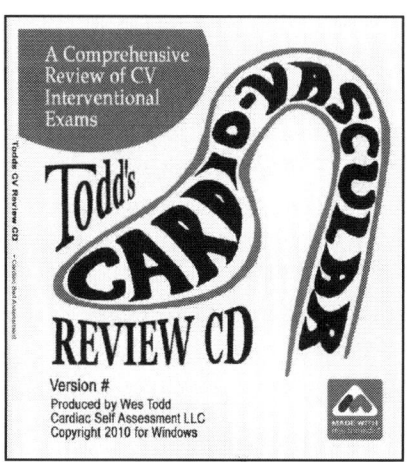

Todd's CV Review CD

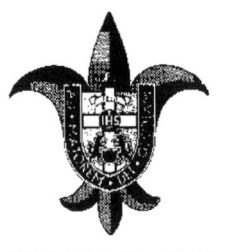

Forward:

The J. Gerard Mudd Cardiac Catheterization Laboratory

Morton J. Kern, M.D., Director

SAINT LOUIS UNIVERSITY

May 11, 1999

Dear Reader:

More than 1.5 million cardiac catheterizations are performed annually in the United States. The expansion of catheterization laboratory technology requires high levels of competency of both physicians and non-physician practitioners alike. For the non-physician staff, many laboratories have adopted the unified cardiovascular credentials (RCIS) as a means of determining this competency.

As a teacher of cardiac catheterization to cardiology trainees and technical staff, I know there is a need to have clear, concise, and comprehensive teaching materials available. This goal is accomplished, in large part, by Mr. Wes Todd's cardiac self-assessment review series. Mr. Todd's review text provides comprehensive information and assistance to cardiovascular professionals. Regardless of their backgrounds in Nursing, Radiology, or Cardiovascular Technology, the materials are of great help in solidifying concepts and practice. For the cardiovascular professional, credentialing examinations demonstrate competency through the award of the RCIS (Registered Cardiovascular Invasive Specialist) credential validates their position as a qualified multi-discipline team member. The value of such training is self-evident.

The review books are written in a clear, straightforward manner. Numerous illustrations make some difficult concepts simple and some add diverting humor to ease the plight of an overburdened student. An added bonus with the review books is a section of practice examinations which provide a comprehensive self-assessment for the reader.

Mr. Todd has created an invaluable resource to those professionals working in catheterization laboratories and especially for those who wish to demonstrate competency through the successful completion of a registry examination. The material compiled in the review and the examination books is a valuable up-to-date resource for registry examination preparation. The practice of intravascular cardiac catheterization and interventional techniques will be advanced by an educated technical and nursing staff using these materials.

Morton J. Kern, MD
Professor of Medicine
Director, J.G. Mudd Cardiac Catheterization Laboratory

Chapters in 5 Volumes of Todd CV Review Books

Vol. I. A. Basics (This Book   )
- A1. General Math & Units
- A2. Patient Care
- A3. Instrumentation
- A4.. Sterilization and Asepsis

Vol. I. B: Anatomy & Physiology
- B1: Embryology and Fetal Circ.
- B2: Blood and Acid Base
- B3: Cardiac Anatomy
- B4: Coronary Anatomy and Physiol.
- B5: Autonomic CNS & CV Reflexes
- B6: Hemodynamics and Pressures
- B7: Contractility and Frank Starling
- B8: Vascular Anatomy
- B9: Vascular Physiology

Vol. I. C: Pathology
- C1: Acquired Valvular Disease
- C2: Pericardial and Myocardial
- C3: Coronary Artery Disease & M.I.
- C4: Heart Failure and Shock
- C5: Congenital Heart Disease
- C6: Vascular Disease

Vol. II. D: Diagnostic Tech.
- D1: Catheters
- D2: Catheterization Equipment: Other
- D3: Indications, Risks, and Complications
- D4: Catheterization Protocol
- D5: Vascular Access, Scrub, & Hemostasis
- D6: Right Heart Catheterization
- D7: Coronary Arteriography
- D8: Left Heart Cath
- D9: Pediatric Cath.Techniques
- D10. Vascular Angiography
- D11. ECGs & Arrhythmias
- D12. Blocks & 12 lead ECGs
- D13. X-Ray

Vol. III. E: Hemodynamics
- E1: Pressure Introduction
- E2: Reading Pressures
- E3: Pressure Recording Systems
- E4: Pressure Pathology I
- E5: Valvular and other Pressure Pathology II
- E6: Fick CO and Shunt
- E7: Indicator Dilution CO
- E8: Quantitative LV Angiography
- E9: Vascular Resistance
- E10: Valve Area
- E11: Coronary Hemodynamics

Vol IV F: Interventions
- F1: PCI, PTCA
- F2: Stents & Other devices
- F3: Adjunct Devices
- F4. ACLS I
- F5. ACLS II
- F6. Cardiac Meds. I
- F7. Cardiac Meds. II
- F8. Cardiac Pacemakers
- F9. Balloon Pump I
- F10. Balloon Pump & LVAD
- F11. Surgery and Artificial Valves
- F12. Vascular Interventions
- F13. Congenital Interventions

Vol. V. Practice Exams
1. Post Test Vol I
2. Post Test Vol II
3. Post Test Vol III
4. Post Test Vol IV
5. RCIS Mock Exam I
6. RCIS Mock Exam II
7. RCIS Mock Exam III

CARDIOVASCULAR REVIEW BOOK
6th Edition

◄◄◄◄ ►►►►

CARDIOVASCULAR INVASIVE DIAGNOSIS: Volume # II

Invasive Diagnostic Techniques

	Introduction............... Page #	I
1:	Catheters.................................	1
2:	Catheterization Equipment: Other..........	41
3:	Indications, Risks, and Complications......	75
4:	Catheterization Protocol..................	117
5:	Vascular Access, Scrub, & Hemostasis.....	141
6:	Right Heart Catheterization...............	197
7:	Coronary Arteriography	233
8:	Left Heart Catheterization	283
9:	Pediatric Catheterization Techniques	328
10.	Vascular Angiography....................	391
11.	ECG & arrhythmias	423
12.	ECG: Blocks and 12 Lead	465
13.	X-Ray................................	493
	Commonly used formulas.................	537

Vol. 2 Post-Test .... In Vol. V, Practice Tests

Catheters

INDEX: D1:   Recent exams have very few catheter questions

1. Catheter construction & qualities
   a. General Catheter   .   .   .   p. 1   Review
   b. Construction & Plastics   .   .   p. 2   Review
   c. Qualities of catheters .   .   .   p. 6   Review
2. Catheter sizing   .   .   .   .   p. 8   Know
3. Catheter general types & configurations
   a. Right heart Catheters .   .   .   p. 12   Know
   b. Angio- flood (LV & Aortic) Catheters   p. 16   Know
   c. Angio- selective CORONARY Catheters   p. 19   Know
   d. Peripheral Catheters   .   .   .   p. 28   Review
   e. Transseptal Catheters .   .   .   p. 31   Review
4. Catheter care and handling   .   .   p. 33   Know
5. Chapter Outline: Catheters   .   .   p. 36
6. Catheters to know

Construction and Qualities of Catheters

GENERAL CATHETER

1. Identify the catheter component labeled #4 on the diagram.
   a. Hub
   b. Body
   c. Primary bend (1°)
   d. Secondary bend (2°)

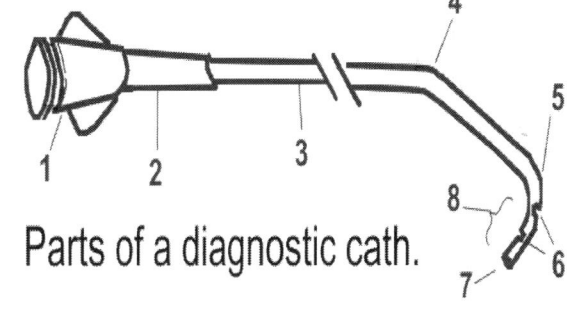

Parts of a diagnostic cath.

ANSWER d. Secondary bend (2°). **BE ABLE TO CORRECTLY MATCH ALL ANSWERS BELOW:**
   1. **HUB:** A plastic or metal connector attached to the body of a catheter for syringe or manifold attachment. **Hubs usually have the French size and other information stamped on them.**
   2. **HEAT SHRINK, reinforcing sleeve:** Some catheters use heat shrinkable tubing as a reinforcement sleeve. It strengthens the proximal end against kinking or pressure bursting. During injection, catheter pressure is greatest near the hub, and least at the tip. The hub end is where catheters may rupture and where reinforcement helps. Note the hub reinforcement in the diagram.
   3. **BODY:** The tubing that runs the length of the catheter usually incorporating a

wire braid.
4. **SECONDARY BEND:** the second bend from the tip end.
5. **PRIMARY BEND:** The bend nearest the tip end.
6. **SIDE-HOLES:** round holes punched into the side of the catheter to allow broader and safer dye dispersion. They reduce catheter kickback during the injection. They need to be symmetrical so the dye injection doesn't kick the tip to one side.
7. **END-HOLE:** Hole at the distal tip of a catheter allows a guide wire to pass through the catheter to provide tip guidance and to stiffen the catheter for more support.
8. **TIP**: Many catheters especially guiding catheters have soft tips to reduce vessel dissection and trauma.

See: Pepine chapter on "Catheters . . . equipment."

CONSTRUCTION AND PLASTICS

2. Interventional guiding catheters with large side-holes are sometimes used in order to:
a. Disperse angiographic contrast more evenly
b. Utilize a second guide wire (Kissing wire technique)
c. Prevent occlusion of the coronary ostium and resulting ischemia
d. Reduce guider trauma and dissection at the coronary ostium

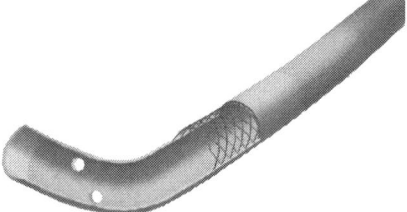

ANSWER c. Prevent occlusion of the coronary ostium by the catheter tip, because the side-holes allow blood flow through the catheter tip into the coronary system. Side-holes in a guider allows you to monitor the aortic pressure accurately. Since the sidehole will admit aortic pressure, it will not appear damped. But, it can be a false sense of security. Now, you are monitoring the aortic pressure, not coronary. The guider can still occlude the ostium. You just won't see it on the pressure monitor.

Guiding catheter side-holes.
after Cordis.com

You may purchase guiders with side-holes or cut your own. This may be done with a special needle with no bevel by drilling into the side of the catheter. Do not continue drilling through the other back wall. Two opposing holes would weaken the catheter at that point. Do not drill through the wire braid portion. Cutting your own side-holes is rarely done in modern labs. **See:** Tilkian and Daily, chapter on "Tools for Catheterization."

3. Don't use guiding catheters with side-holes unless you must. Check the 4 disadvantages of using multiple side-hole coronary guiding catheters.
a. Decreased contrast opacification of target vessel
b. Decreased backup support

c. Decreased blood flow to target vessel
d. **Decreased coronary pressure monitoring**
e. **Possible kinking of catheter at a side-hole**
f. **Increased chance of ostial dissection**

ANSWERS: a, b, d & e. The only advantage to side-holes is #c, they help with passive blood flow to the target vessel. This is important when you "deep throat" the guider in a widowmaker ostial lesion, because you cut off blood flow to that artery. Side-holes do nothing to prevent ostial dissection, and they prevent you for monitoring coronary pressure. With side-holes, you monitor aortic pressure.

   Freed says: "When damping is due to the presence of a small coronary artery or an ostial obstruction, the guiding catheter should be replaced with a sidehole catheter, side-holes allow passive entry of aortic blood into the guiding catheter and the coronary artery. If a sidehole catheter is not available, side-holes can be created with a sidehole cutter of the beveled end of the vascular access needle. Potential problems with sidehole catheters include suboptimal opacification (contrast escapes through the side-holes); decreased backup support due to weakness of the catheter shaft; and kinking at the side-holes, particularly in giant lumen guides. When sidehole guides are used for ostial lesions, the presence of side-holes will permit passive perfusion, but does not decrease the chance of guiding catheter injury to the vessel ostium."
See: Freed, Grines, & Safian, "The New Manual of Interventional Cardiology"

4. Flood catheters with side-holes (e.g., Pigtails) provide better angiographic injection dynamics than single end-hole catheters. The chief DISADVANTAGE of multiple side-holes in flood catheters is that they:
a. Hang up on guide wires and valves
b. Traumatize the vessel wall
c. **Tend to clot unless flushed frequently**
d. Mixed LV & AO pressure waveform

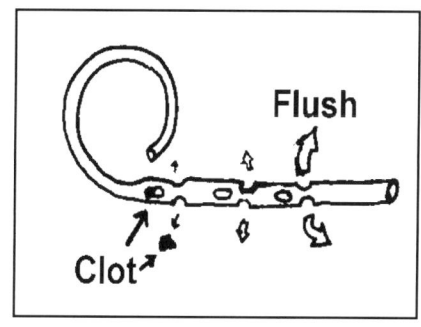

ANSWER c. Tend to clot unless flushed frequently. Pigtail catheters are especially prone to clotting, because of their many holes. A normal hand flush only exits the proximal holes and the distal holes remain full of blood. Judkins said, "A pigtail catheter should have no more than four side-holes...the extra ports serve no purpose and provide sites for accumulation of formed blood elements.

   Unless flushed frequently and forcefully these side-holes provide an eddy location for blood to stagnate and clot. Then these small clots can embolize during pressure injection and produce a stoke.

   When the pigtail holes straddle the AO valve, you can get a weird mixed LV & AO pressure waveform. When measuring LV pressure be sure all the sideholes are in the LV.
See: Johnsrude, chapter on "Equipment."

5. This diagram shows the construction of a typical PTCA guiding catheter. What material is labeled at #2 on the diagram?
a. Polyurethane (PU)
b. Hypothrombogenic coating
c. Teflon
d. Braided steel or Kevlar fiber

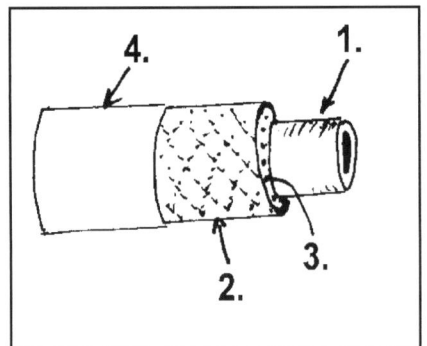

ANSWER a. Polyurethane. **BE ABLE TO CORRECTLY MATCH ALL ANSWERS BELOW:**
1. **TEFLON:** This smooth slippery plastic forms the inner lumen or core of the catheter. It makes it easier to slide the balloon catheter through the lumen.
2. **POLYURETHANE** polymer forms the body of the catheter in which the wire or fiber braid is imbedded. Many new guiders include stiff and strong Nylon within the thermoplastic.
3. **BRAID:** Flattened stainless steel wires are imbedded within the plastic jacket to make the catheter strong and torquable.
4. **COATING:** The slippery hypothrombogenic surface that coats many catheters may include silicone, heparin, hydrophilics, etc.

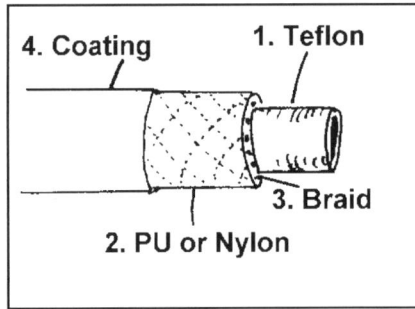

Guider construction

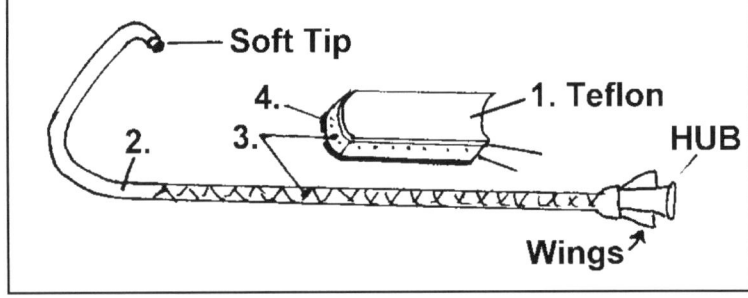

Guider cath construction

See: Tilkian and Daily, chapter on "Tools for Catheterization."

6. Which type of plastic has the least memory and torque control, and is so soft that it is used in construction of most balloon floatation catheters?
a. Polyurethane (PU)
b. Teflon
c. Polyethylene (PE)
d. Poly Vinyl Chloride (PVC)

ANSWER d. Polyvinyl Chloride (PVC). Balloon floatation catheters need to be soft and float with the current. PVC is like a

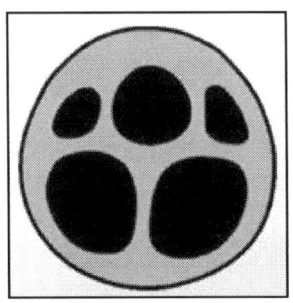

Figure 8 Cross section TD Swan after Edwards.com

"wet noodle" in the warm blood stream. It has almost no torque control or memory. Most balloon floatation catheters will admit a small guidewire to stiffen them if necessary. Since, PVC's bursting pressure is much lower than other plastics (250 PSI) they are never pressure injected.

These catheters often have multiple holes extruded for different functions of the catheter. The Edwards thermodilution catheter cross section shows the large holes for proximal and distal pressures and smaller holes for balloon and TD wires.
See: Tilkian and Daily, chapter on "Tools for Catheterization."

7. **Which type of catheter plastics have the GREATEST strength, stiffness and torque control?**
   a. **Polyester (PES) & polystyrene (PS)**
   b. **Polyurethane (PU) & polyethylene (PE)**
   c. **Polyvinyl chloride (PVC) & elastomeric copolymer (EC)**
   d. **Nylon & Teflon (PTFE)**

ANSWER d. Nylon & Teflon (PTFE). These catheters are strong and have a high melting point. Teflon sheaths and nylon walled catheters are thin and strong with good memory. PTFE is the chemical abbreviation for the registered trademark Teflon®. PE is slippery (supermarket bags). Polyurethane is softer and more flexible (car bumpers etc.). PVC is the softest. **See:** Tilkian and Daily, chapter on "Tools for Catheterization."

8. **Teflon (PTFE) is often used in the construction of sheaths and dilators. One danger with Teflon is that it:**
   a. **Is difficult to sterilize in high temperature autoclaves**
   b. **Has a rough surface which traumatize vessels**
   c. **Is more thrombogenic**
   d. **Has hard, sharp tips**

ANSWER d. Has dangerously hard and sharp tips. The sharp tips require a leading guide wire when advanced. PTFE makes good dilators which need to retain their point and be slippery enough to pass through scar tissue. Most sheaths are Teflon (PTFE) because it is ideal for the needed thin and slippery walls.

Teflon is NOT rough. It is slippery, and therefore atraumatic and nonthrombogenic. It makes an excellent inner lining for guider catheters, sheaths, and dilators. But, being strong and thin walled it tends to pierce tissue and kink easily. This material can withstand high temperature autoclaves. That's why they put Teflon coatings on many frying pans. See: Johnsrude, chapter on "Equipment."

9. **Polyurethane (PU) catheters should be used with a ____ guide wire.**
   a. **Stainless steel**
   b. **Teflon coated**
   c. **Heparin coated**
   d. **Platinum coated**

ANSWER b. Teflon coated. Polyurethane (PU) catheter surfaces feel "rubbery." And stainless steel wires often "stick" within their lumen. Teflon coated or lubricious wires are now commonly used with all Polyurethane (PU)catheters. Judkins said, "Teflon-coated safety guidewires can be inserted or withdrawn through polyurethane catheters with ease. This effortless handling markedly reduces the chance of damaging the guidewire and shortens procedure time. Use of coated guides is an integral part of the no-compromise-for-safety approach of this technique." Currently many other types of catheter materials are used besides polyurethane. **See:** in King, Judkins' chapter on "Coronary Arteriography and Left Ventriculography: Judkins Technique."

QUALITIES OF CATHETERS

10. **The ability to twist a catheter hub resulting in a corresponding twist at the catheter tip is termed:**
   a. Memory
   b. Torque control
   c. Extrusion
   d. Lamination process

ANSWER b. Torque control. Most catheters require twisting to direct the bend into the desired anatomic structures. The test of good torque control is to twist the catheter after it is bent completely in half (E.g., 180° bend around your arm). A 90° twist at the hub should produce a 90° twist at the tip. Steel braided catheters have the best torque control and increased bursting pressure.

These catheter walls are braided like a "May Pole" over an inner core of extruded plastic tubing. Then another layer of plastic is added to embed these wires. Like steel reinforcing in concrete it makes it very strong - especially for twisting or torque control. However, diagnostic catheter distal bends and tip do not usually incorporate these wires. Braiding in the tip of diagnostic catheters would make the tip too stiff and inflexible. Many interventional guiding catheter tips do contain braid for extra backup support.

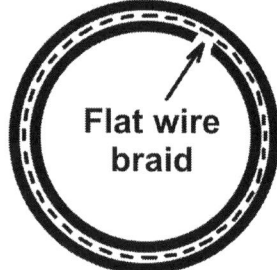

See: King, Interventional Cardiology, "Equipment for PCI"

11. **Identify 3 catheters that have a braided steel mesh laminated within the plastic.**
   a. Pigtail & Grollman
   b. Swan-Ganz & Foley
   c. Judkins & Amplatz
   d. Guider catheters

ANSWERS: a, c, & d.
a. Pigtail & Grollman - YES
b. Swan-Ganz & Foley - NO

c. Judkins & Amplatz - YES
d. Guider catheters - YES

Swan-Ganz & Foley catheters are not braided. Wire braiding is so effective at increasing strength and torque control that most arterial catheters now use this construction process. However, right heart balloon catheters (Swan-Ganz) need to be soft (like spaghetti) to follow venous flow antegrade. The Foley is a soft rubber urethral catheter. Almost all arterial catheters contain a laminated wire braid for torque control. Some arterial nylon catheters do not contain a braid.
See: Tilkian and Daily, chapter on "Tools for Catheterization."

12. Match the various desirable catheter characteristic with its number on the diagram.
  a. Torque control
  b. Pushability
  c. Backup support
  d. Trackability
  e. Memory
  f. Soft tip

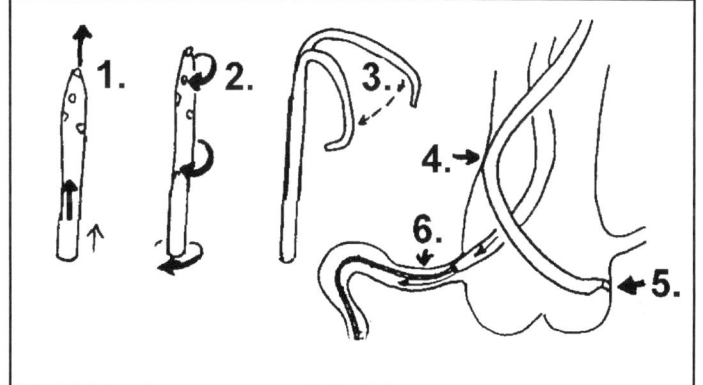

Qualities of a catheter

BE ABLE TO CORRECTLY MATCH ALL ANSWERS BELOW:
  1. **PUSHABILITY:** Ability to directly transmit push-pull forces from the end of the catheter to the tip. This is important in pushing a balloon catheter through a guider or through tortuous anatomy.
  2. **TORQUE CONTROL:** The ability to directly transmit rotational forces from the end of the catheter to the tip. "One good turn deserves another (1:1)."
  3. **MEMORY:** Ability to recover and maintain a specific configuration after insertion and guidewire removal. When the bend is opened with a guide wire or during passage up the aorta, a catheter with good memory will return to its original shape. It "remembers" its bend configuration, and always wants to returns to it. This allows it to "seek" the vessel for which it was designed.
  4. **BACKUP SUPPORT:** Ability to remain in position despite resistance. This is essential in a good Angioplasty guider catheter. When a balloon catheter is advanced through a guider catheter against resistance, it may buckle and back the guider out of the orifice. This is termed "power failure." Backup support prevents this. A buttress configuration as shown in the diagram "arches" off the opposite aortic wall to help push the tip into the left coronary artery.
  5. **SOFTNESS AND SOFT TIPS:** Ability to easily bend and to be shaped. Many

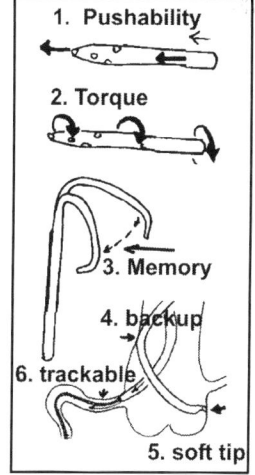

Catheter Qualities

diagnostic and guider catheters are capped with a soft rubber end-hole tip. When force is applied to this catheter tip, as it is in the diagram, the soft tip bends against the artery wall and distributes the pressure over a wider surface. This helps prevent dissection of the intima.

6. **TRACKABILITY:** Ability to follow a guidewire along its course through the vascular anatomy. This is especially important in balloon PTCA catheters that must pass through tortuous bends and tight stenoses. It depends on proper size, flexibility, and pushability.

See: Pepine chapter on "Catheters . . . equipment."

13. Most cardiac catheters cannot be reused. After being used in a patient what type of "Single Use Devices" may be resterilized by 3rd party reprocessor companies and then reused on other patients?
a. PTCA balloon catheters
b. Polyurethane (PU) catheters
c. Teflon Guider catheters
d. Diagnostic EP electrodes

ANSWER d. Diagnostic EP electrodes. With current concerns over blood transmitted diseases, the only catheters now commonly reused are the diagnostic EP pacing and sensing electrodes. This is a controversial medico-legal issue, because catheter manufacturers place "For Single Use Only" disclaimers on all catheters. Doubtless, this is to protect them from legal repercussions.

Since they have no lumen (technically not a catheter) EP electrodes are much easier to inspect, clean and sterilize. The FDA requires that each item reprocessed and resterilized be tracked, forms submitted, and strict quality control procedures followed. Equipment that is approved for reprocessing reuse includes: EP diagnostic catheters, EP cables, and femoral compression devices. Of course, most equipment that has NOT been used (i.e., expired or accidentally opened) CAN be resterilized and reprocessed. If any tubular catheter is used on a patient or otherwise contaminated with blood, then they can NOT be reprocessed or reused.

CATHETER SIZING

14. If a 1 mm ID catheter will transmit contrast at a rate of 1 ml/sec at 500 PSI, how much will a 2 mm ID catheter theoretically transmit at the same pressure according to Poiseuille's law?
a. 2 ml/sec
b. 4 ml/sec
c. 8 ml/sec
d. 16 ml/sec

ANSWER d. 16 ml/sec. According to Poiseuille's law as the radius is doubled the flow increases as the fourth power of this change. 2 to the 4th power is 2 x 2 x 2 x 2 = 16. 16 x 1 ml/sec = 16 ml/sec.

Catheter radius is obviously the most important factor in limiting flow though catheters. That is why most flood catheters have a large lumen and selective catheters tend to have a smaller lumen. However, as you see from the formula many other factors come in to play, such as contrast viscosity, pressure, length of catheter, turbulent flow through side-holes, etc. **See**: Berne & Levy, chapter on "Hemodynamics"

15. Femoral pigtail catheters for LV angiography are usually ___ cm long.
   a. 80
   b. 100
   c. 110
   d. 140

ANSWER c. 110. Femoral pigtail catheters are 110 cm long. It's a long way from the leg up-over the arch and across the aortic valve into the LV. In tall patients the LV may not be reached by the standard 100 cm diagnostic catheter. Consequently, most manufacturers have added 10 cm to the standard femoral LV pigtail length.
See: Pepine chapter on "Catheters . . . equipment."

16. How is the curve of Judkins right coronary catheters measured?
   a. Across the shortest diameter of the ellipse
   b. Across the longest diameter of the ellipse
   c. From primary to secondary curves
   d. From secondary to tertiary curves

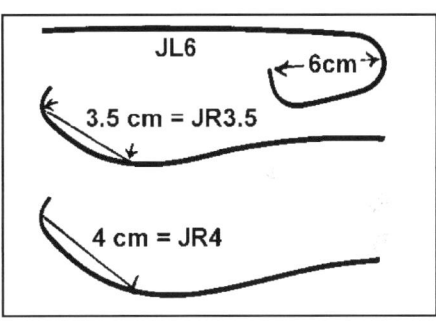

ANSWER c. From primary to secondary curves. The Judkins coronary catheter bend size is measured between the steepest portions of the primary and secondary curves. Note where the Judkins (JL6 cm) left coronary catheter is measured compared to the Judkins (JR) catheters. Again, The *longer bends are for more dilated aortas or more inferiorly directed coronary ostia.*
See: Grossman, chapter on "Cardiac Ventriculography."

Judkins Rt. Coronary bend

17. Determine the bend size of the Judkins catheter labeled at #3. Use the reduced cm. scale provided.
   a. 2.5 cm
   b. 3.5 cm
   c. 5 cm
   d. 6 cm

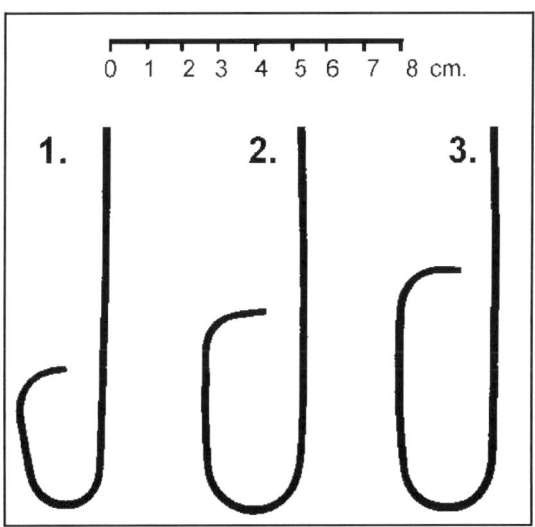

bend size measurement.
Note reduced Scale

ANSWER d. 6 cm. The Judkins Left coronary catheter is easy to measure. Note, that this diagram is reduced to ½ scale. Take a cm ruler (scale provided) and measure vertically the longest diameter across the ellipse (between the 2 bends.) MEASURE THE BENDS OF THE OTHER LABELED Judkins Left Coronary catheters.
1. 3.5 cm bend
2. 5. cm bend
3. 6 cm bend
The longer bends are for more dilated aortas.
See: Tilkian and Daily, chapter on "Tools for Catheterization."

18. **What is the normal LEFT Judkins femoral coronary diagnostic catheter for an average sized American adult?**
a. JR3.5
b. JR4
c. JL3.5
d. JL4
e. JL5

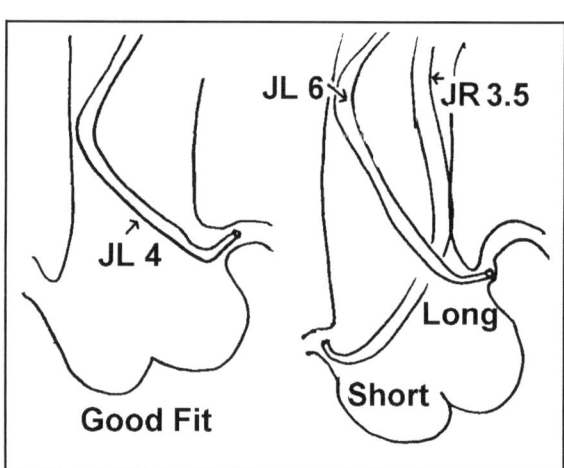

JL cath bend sizes in the AO

ANSWER d. JL4 = Judkins Left coronary bend size #4 is for an average sized aorta (4 cm bend diameter). Smaller bends are for smaller aortas or for superior angulation of the tip. Note in the diagram how the JR 3.5 catheter angles superiorly. *For Judkins coronary catheters small bends angle superiorly, large bends angle more inferiorly.* Note how the longer JL6 poorly engages the superiorly directed coronary artery. It should be changed to a JL3.5. Also, larger bends are used for larger aortas that affect the secondary bend angle. Coronary catheters from the radial approach often use smaller bends.
See: Tilkian and Daily, chapter on "Tools for Catheterization."

19. **In sizing catheter outside diameter, 1 French size is equal to:**
a. .25 mm
b. .33 mm
c. .40 mm
d. .50 mm
e. .66 mm

ANSWER b. .33 mm. = 1/3 mm = 1 Fr. This has been standardized due to the importance of catheter diameter in PTCA. Cardiologist's size the coronary lesions in reference to the catheter diameter. (A stenosis the same diameter as a 6 Fr. catheter is just 2 mm. in diameter) It is interesting that the French size in mm. is also equal to the circumference of any round or oval instrument. © = π D) See: Tilkian and Daily, chapter on "Tools for Catheterization."

20. What French size is a catheter with an outer diameter of 2.66 mm?
   a. 5 F
   b. 6 F
   c. 7 F
   d. 8 F

ANSWER d. 8 F. The way to remember this is that a 6 Fr. catheter is 2 mm in diameter. Other sizes are proportional. So to calculate this, set up a ratio.

$$\frac{2mm}{6\ Fr} = \frac{2.66mm}{x} \quad \quad \text{Solving } x = 8\ Fr.$$

See: Tilkian and Daily, chapter on "Tools for Catheterization."

21. The outside diameter of a 5.5 Fr. catheter is:
   a. 1.5 mm
   b. 1.66 mm
   c. 1.83 mm
   d. 2.00 mm
   e. 2.17 mm

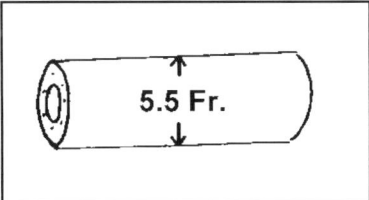

5.5 French O.D. Cath.

ANSWER c. 1.83 mm. This can be solved using the ratio method above.

$$\frac{2\ mm's}{6\ Fr.} = \frac{x}{5.5\ Fr.} \ ; \quad x = 1.83\ mm$$

Or remember the fact that each Fr. size is 1/3 of a mm.
5 Fr = 1.66 mm and 6 Fr = 2 mm, so half way between 5 and 6 Fr. would be half way between 1.66 and 2.0 mm, or 1.83 mm. As wall thickness diminishes, lumen diameters increase. Similarly, you can multiply the Fr. size by 0.33 to get the mm diameter. 5.5 x 0.33=1.82 mm
See: Tilkian and Daily, chapter on "Tools for Catheterization."

22. The TIP inner diameter on standard diagnostic coronary catheters is:
   a. Fr. size / 3 mm.
   b. Fr. size x .013 in.
   c. .038 inch
   d. .063 inch
   e. Depends on wall thickness

ANSWER c. .038 inch   All coronary diagnostic catheters are designed to be used with the standard .035-.038 inch guide wires that make a snug fit through the catheter tip. Tip ID does NOT depend on the catheter French size or wall thickness. Large PTCA guider catheters (non-diagnostic) are designed to be used with .063

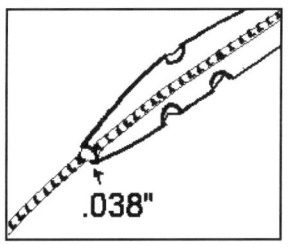

Diagnostic catheter tip diameter

inch guide wires.
See: Tilkian and Daily, chapter on "Tools for Catheterization."

23. Disadvantages of using guiding catheters, as compared to long sheaths in vascular interventions include: (Which 2 are true about guiders?)
   a. Larger arteriotomy required for guiders (use standard introducer sheath)
   b. No hemostatic side valve in guiders (requires Tuohy-Borst adaptor)
   c. No wire braid in guiders (less torque control)
   d. Fewer bend sizes in guiders (harder to fit to anatomy)

ANSWERS: a & b. These are true disadvantages of guiders. Advantages to guiders is that they have a wire braid and many more sizes are available. Schneider says: "Guiding catheters offer many more shapes and sizes than are available with guiding sheaths, but there are some significant disadvantages. Guiding catheters do not have a dilator or obturator to facilitate smooth passage... they are usually introduced through... a standard, hemostatic access sheath. This generally means that the arteriotomy is slightly larger than would otherwise be necessary. After passage into the artery, they often require another device, such as a selective catheter, to act as an obturator for passage into the desired side branch location. There is no end valve for hemostasis. A Tuohy-Borst adaptor must be used to make a guiding catheter hemostatic and allow it to be flushed. It is likely that when a broad array of guiding sheaths becomes available, guiding catheters will be used only rarely."
See: Schneider, chapter on "Access for Endovascular Therapy" p 193

24. When using a 5F selective catheter through a 90 cm 5F sheath in vascular procedures:
   a. It will not be possible to pass a 5F catheter - too tight
   b. It will not be possible to flush fluids through the sheath - too tight
   c. A Touhy borst adapter is required to prevent bleed back
   d. A .038 guidewire must be kept in place to prevent bleed back

ANSWER b. It is too tight to flush. Schneider says: "If a catheter is place through the sheath that is labeled the same as the sheath size (i.e., a 5 Fr catheter in a 5 Fr sheath) it will not be possible to administer contrast or heparinized saline through the sidearm since the catheter completely fills the sheath." This is especially ture of long sheaths.
See: Schneider, chapter on "Access for Endovascular Therapy" p. 191

CATHETER TYPES & CONFIGURATIONS

RIGHT HEART CATHETERS

25. Check the names of the 2 right heart end-hole catheters shown. (Select 2 below.)
a. Judkins Right
b. Amplatz
c. Swan Ganz
d. Brockenbrough
e. Cournand

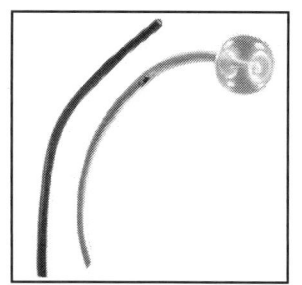

ANSWERS: c & e. Swan Ganz & Cournand. Both are single end hole catheters, good for measuring wedge pressures. The Swan Ganz is a balloon flow-directed catheter often used for thermodilution cardiac output. The Cournand is a woven Dacron catheter also used in EP studies as a quadrapolar electrode catheter. The JR and Amplatz are coronary selective catheters. Brockenbrough is for transseptal technique intended to enter the LA via the Fossa Ovale. **See:** Grossman, chapter on "Percutaneous Approach", **Keywords:** RHC = Lehman, Cournand

26. This is the "Swan-Ganz Guide-wire Thermodilution catheter" Identify the port (tail) labeled at #2 on the diagram.

a. Distal port (for PA pressure)
b. Balloon port (air filled rubber balloon)
c. Thermistor connector (goes to CO computer)
d. Guide-wire port
e. Proximal port (for cool water)

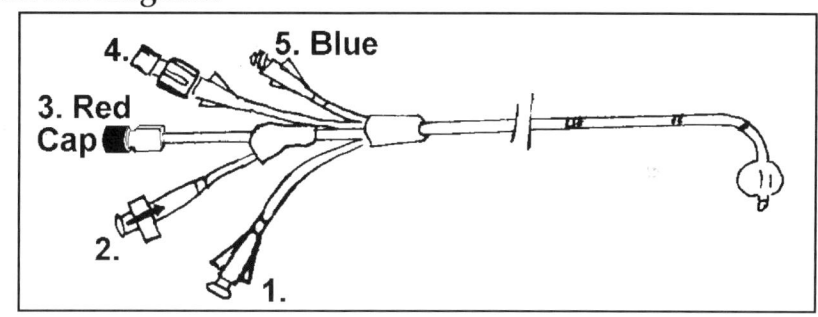

"Tails" of Swan-Ganz Thermodilution Guide-wire Catheter

ANSWER b. Balloon port (air filled rubber balloon).
BE ABLE TO CORRECTLY MATCH ALL ANSWERS BELOW:
1. **DISTAL PORT** (for measuring pressure) Is a simple white female Luer Lock (LL) connector marked "Distal." Attach a 3-way stopcock and connect to pressure transducer. Flush with heparinized saline to keep it from clotting when not in use.
2. **BALLOON PORT** (An air filled rubber balloon is usually 1.5 cc)
This is a female LL with a plastic sliding open-closed stopcock, open to inflate, close to lock in the air and keep balloon inflated.
3. **THERMISTOR CONNECTOR** (goes to CO computer) Usually a white 3 pin computer connector covered with a red cap. The thermistor measures the temperature of the blood in the PA. When the cold saline is injected through the proximal port, it flows

with the blood into the PA which cools the thermistor. This senses the blood flow and CO

4. **GUIDE WIRE PORT** accepts an .025 Teflon coated guide wire. This catheter lumen ends near the thermistor. So it does not exit the catheter. But it stiffens the catheter enough that it can negotiate large RA and the tricuspid valve in tricuspid regurgitation. This port has a locking guidewire adapter to prevent wire movement within the catheter.

5. **PROXIMAL PORT** (for cool/ice water) Is blue for the cold color of ICE. Iced saline is flushed into the RA to measure thermodilution Cardiac Output. Attach a 3-way stopcock and flush with heparinized saline to keep it from clotting when not in use. This port is usually placed in the RA, so the cool saline must flow through the RV into the PA where the thermistor tip rests. Most labs have switched from iced saline to room temperature saline. This RA port is 30 cm from tip.

See: Tilkian and Daily, chapter on "Tools for Catheterization."

27. In a quadruple-lumen Swan-Ganz thermodilution catheter where is the proximal injection port located?
  a. At the tip of the catheter
  b. 15 cm from the tip
  c. 30 cm from the tip
  d. 40 cm from the tip

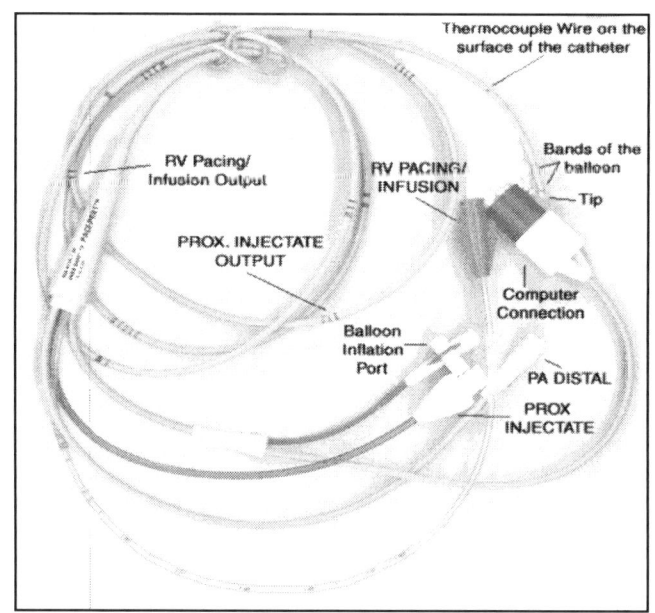

5 port Swan-Ganz catheter

ANSWER c. 30 cm from the tip is where the cold injectate emerges. When properly placed, this proximal port is in the RA and the thermistor is in the Rt or Lt. PA. The thermistor is 4 cm from the tip, so injected saline bolus travels 26 cm before the cooled blood is sensed. In the diagram, note the 3 bands at the prox. Injectate Output. Darovic says, "The most commonly used catheter for adults is the quadruple-lumen thermo-dilution catheter.... The proximal (RA) port opens to a lumen that terminates 30 cm from the tip of the catheter. The RA port may be used to monitor RA pressure, administer IV fluids,... and receive the injectate solution for cardiac output studies." See: Darovic, chapter on Pulmonary Artery Pressure Monitoring, Keywords: Swan injectate port at 30 cm

28. Which type of catheter is necessary for optimal WEDGE pressures?
  a. End-hole only
  b. 2 Side-holes + end-hole
  c. Multiple side holes with distal balloon
  d. Thermodilution Swan-Ganz

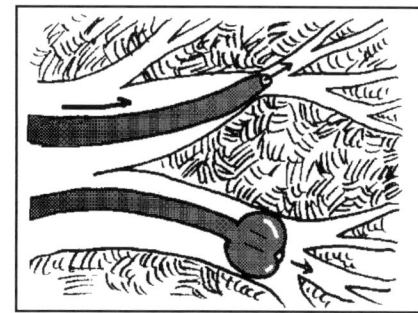

ANSWER a. End-hole only catheters are the best wedge catheters. The one end-hole then looks through the capillary bed and only measures distal pressure (Pulmonary capillary wedge = LA pressure).

Most wedge pressures are now taken with balloon floatation catheter with the balloon inflated. But a balloon is not necessary. In fact, where an accurate wedge waveform is critical, as in mitral disease, a stiff single-end-hole catheter is much more accurate (most like LA). A single end-hole catheters can be pushed out as far as it will go until it ends "wedged" into the capillary bed. It's really wedged in small arteries, not capillaries. The resulting wedge pressure gives a better LA pressure.

PA end-hole Wedge and balloon cath wedge

Side-holes may allow the PA pressure to enter and contaminate the wedge. However, multipurpose and birds eye 2 side-hole + end-hole catheters can be used to obtain adequate wedge pressures if precautions are taken. This is because the distal side-holes are quite close to the tip and are usually covered by arteriolar tissue.
See: Tilkian and Daily, chapter on "Tools for Catheterization."

29. **Your bilateral heart cath patient has left bundle branch block (LBBB) on the ECG. Which type of catheter should you insert first?**
   a. **Pigtail catheter in RFA**
   b. **JR4 catheter in RFA**
   c. **Temporary pacing electrode in RFV**
   d. **Swan Ganz pacing and wedge catheter in RFV**
   e. **Thermodilution Swan Ganz in subclavian vein**

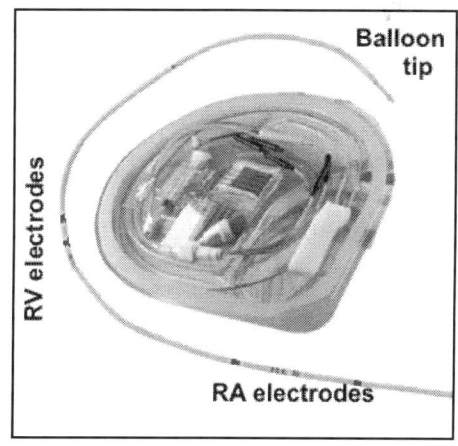

ANSWER d. A Swan Ganz pacing and wedge catheter in RFV allows both wedge pressure measurement and RV pacing when needed. LBBB can deteriorate into complete heart block if the RBB is irritated with your right heart catheter. Here a pacing catheter with open lumen should be used as the right heart catheter. Watson & Gorski say, "Catheter manipulation in the RV may produce transient RBB block. For patients with pre-existing LBB block, this would result in complete heart block (CHB). In patients with pre-existing RBB undergoing a left heart catheterization, CHB rarely occurs as the left bundle extends only a limited distance before its bifurcation."

Swan with pacing, TD & pressures

There are several types of pacing catheters which allow pressure measurement and RV pacing, some with balloon tips and some that are torquable. Swan Ganz balloon tipped thermodilution pacing catheters will float into the right heart via a vein. Arrow makes a Bipolar Pacing and Double Wedge Pressure Catheter.

Torquable pacing catheters like the Zukor, Myler, Gorlin or Baim Turi have an open lumen for pressure monitoring and are torque directed like standard arterial catheters.
See: Grossman, chapter on "Cardiac Ventriculography."

30. For ease and speed, which catheter below would be the usual first choice to catheterize the right heart to obtain hemodynamic measurements?
a. Balloon Swan-Ganz
b. Balloon Berman
c. Woven Dacron Cournand
d. Multipurpose

ANSWER a. A balloon floatation Swan-Ganz is usually inserted into the femoral vein. Then the balloon will be inflated in the RA and floated into the RV and PA while recording pressures.
  Grossman says, "When right heart catheterization is being performed only for measurement of right atrial, right ventricular, pulmonary artery, and pulmonary capillary wedge pressured, any of the end-hole catheters is adequate. Classic woven Dacron right heart catheters (e.g., Goodale-Lubin and Cournand) have now been replaced by flow-directed balloon flotation catheters.".
See: Grossman, chapter on "Brachial Approach."

31. Which of the following flow directed, balloon tipped, pediatric flood angiographic catheters can also measure wedge pressures?
a. Reverse Berman
b. Fogarty
c. Swan Ganz
d. Dotter

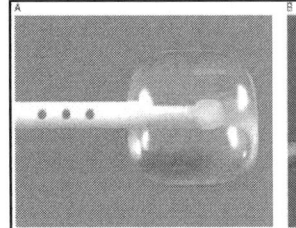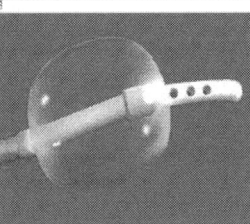

1. Berman   2. Reverse Berman.
from Arrowintl.com

ANSWER a. Reverse Berman. This is a PVC balloon floatation catheter with side-holes distal to the balloon tip. It is usually the Rt. ht. angiographic catheter of choice in infants and children. The reverse Berman distal-side-hole version can measure wedge pressure when a pulmonary artery branch is occluded by inflating the balloon.
See: Tilkian chapter on "Equipment."

ANGIO FLOOD (LV & AORTIC) CATHETERS

32. Identify the pigtail angiographic catheter labeled at #4 on the diagram.
   a. Standard straight pigtail
   b. Micro pigtail
   c. Grollman PA
   d. Angled pigtail
   e. Halo ventriculography

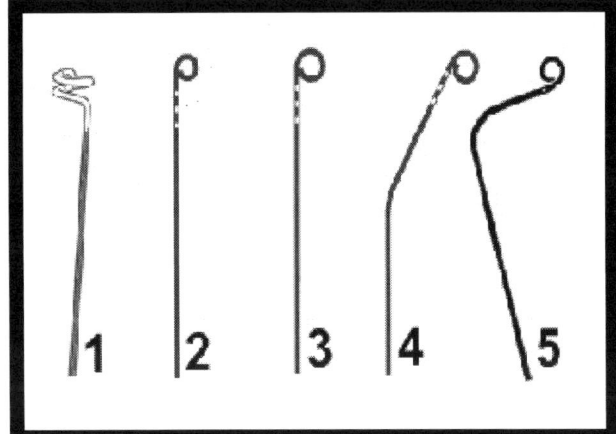
Pigtail catheters

ANSWER d. is an angled pigtail catheter.
BE ABLE TO CORRECTLY MATCH ALL ANSWERS BELOW:
1. HALO VENTRICULOGRAPHY: A spiral tip pigtail with side-holes pointed inward causes less ectopy in LV grams. See Kern chapter on Art. Access
2. MICRO PIGTAIL: smaller diameter tighter tail for smaller vessels.
3. PIGTAIL STANDARD STRAIGHT: The pigtail catheter is the most commonly used LV gram catheter. With up to 12 side-holes it evenly disperses the contrast within the LV.
4. ANGLED PIGTAIL: The 145-155 degree angle is 7 cm from the tip. This angle lifts the catheter off the inferior LV wall for a more centrally located LV gram. Also, it is useful for dilated aortas.
5. GROLLMAN PA: is an angled pigtail catheter with the curve generally on the reverse side. It is designed for RV and selective PA angiography by the femoral approach. There were recent recalls of this catheter for tip separation.
See: Johnsrude, chapter on "Equipment."

33. Which of the following flood catheters from the femoral approach will give the least recoil, staining, PVC and kickback problems during a high flow pressure injection?
   a. Multipurpose II/Amplatz
   b. Tiger/Jacky
   c. Newton/Mani
   d. Pigtail/Berman

ANSWER d. Pigtail/Berman catheters have many side-holes to prevent kickback during flood injections. The Berman angiographic catheter is commonly used because it has no end-hole, is softer, and has the added balloon floatation feature.
-A. MULTIPURPOSE: ANGIOGRAPHIC. MP catheters should not be injected at rates over 10 ml/sec. M2 has 2 sideholes. Amplatz is an end hole coronary catheter.
-B. Tiger and Jacky are radial coronary catheters with few sideholes.
-C. Newton/Mani, are selective end-hole headhunter catheters.
-D. PIGTAIL/Berman: Flood catheters must have many side-holes.

With up to 12 side-holes a pigtail evenly disperses the contrast within the LV, although, with high pressure injection the pigtail straightens and may slightly recoil. The Berman catheter is a large-lumen, balloon-tipped angiographic catheter with no end hole and with side holes placed proximal to the balloon."

See: Grossman, chapter on "Cardiac Ventriculography."

34. This LV--AO pullback tracing shows what problem associated with pigtail catheters.
a. False LV-AO gradient
b. Reverse gradient
c. Incomplete pullback
d. Falsely high mean recording
e. Pigtail entrapment in Chordae-tendinea

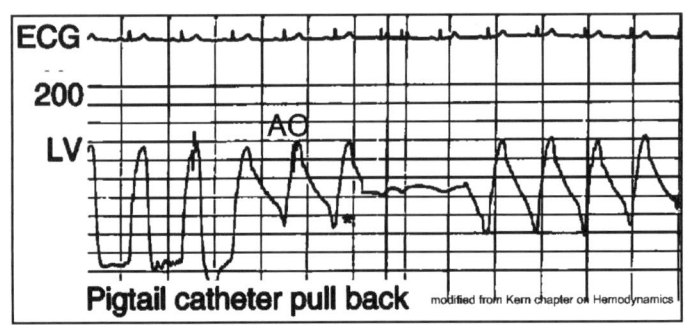

ANSWER c. Incomplete pullback, because of the falsely low diastolic arterial pressure. This is mixed LV & AO with the catheter tip is still recording some LV pressure. Note the sinusoidal shape of the aortic downslope with a dip in late diastole. See: Kern chapter on Hemodynamics

35. Identify the type of multipurpose catheter labeled #2 in the diagram.
a. B-1 MP
b. B-2 MP
c. A-1 MP
d. A-2 MP

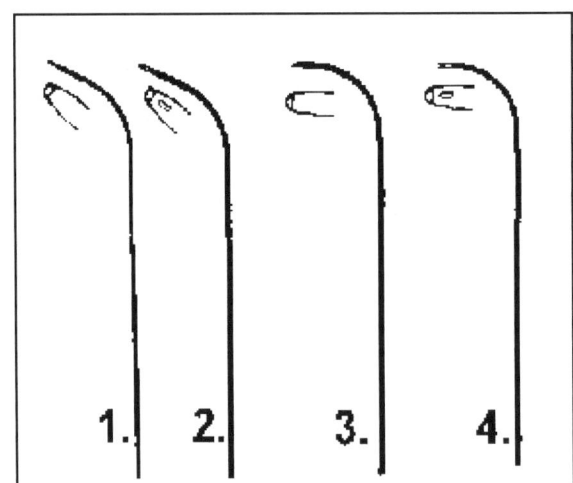

ANSWER d. A-2 Multipurpose (MP).
BE ABLE TO CORRECTLY MATCH ALL ANSWERS BELOW:
1. A-1 MP: Polyurethane (PU) with incorporated wire braid. The A bend is like a hockey stick with a straight tip. The 1 refers to one end-hole only.
2. A-2 MP: Same as A-1 except it has 2 side-holes and an end-hole.
3. B-1 MP: Polyurethane (PU) with incorporated wire braid. The B bend is a gradual 90° curve up to the tip. The 1 refers to one end-hole only.
4. B-2 MP: The same as B-1 except has 2 side-holes and end-hole.
See: Tilkian and Daily, chapter on "Tools for Catheterization."

36. When doing angiographic flood injections with 4 F or 5 F catheters the injector pressure should not exceed:
a. 500 psi
b. 1200 psi
c. 2000 psi
d. 3500 psi

Answer: b. 1200 psi. Cordis catheters list 1200 as the maximum burst pressure for their 4 & 5 F catheters. Beyond this limit the catheter may rupture near the hub and spray (sticky) contrast around the room. The highest pressure is near the hub, and the lowest pressure is at the tip of the catheter. If a catheter becomes kinked and your injector is set to 1200 max, a sensor in the injector will limit the pressure to 1200 psi and stop the injection to prevent rupture. Larger catheter sizes allow for larger injection pressures. Micro-catheters require lower injection pressures, around 900 psi. Refer to your catheter specification brochure. See: Cordis.com catheter brochure. Keywords: limit 5 F injection to 1200 psi

CORONARY CATHETERS

37. The internal mammary catheter (IMA) looks similar to what other catheter?
a. Multipurpose
b. Arani - double loop
c. Judkins Left Coronary
d. Judkins Right Coronary

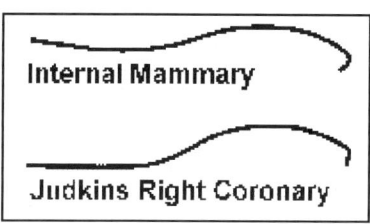

ANSWER d. IMA is like a JR catheter with a more angulated primary bend. The catheter is placed in the subclavia artery beyond the LIMA takeoff. Then with the guidewire removed, the catheter is carefully withdrawn until it hooks into the LIMA artery.
See: Grossman, chapter on "Coronary Arteriography."

38. Which catheter is designed to do a complete LV and coronary angiography study from the femoral artery without exchanging catheters?
a. Amplatz
b. Multipurpose
c. Judkins
d. Castillo
e. Jacki

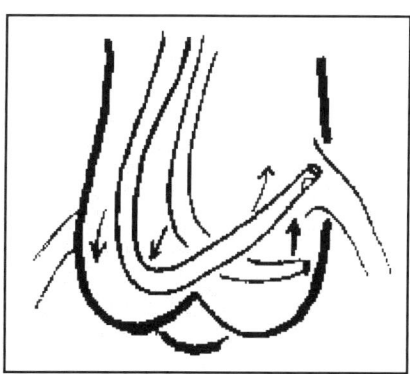

ANSWER b. Multipurpose catheter technique for doing both LV and coronary arteriography using the percutaneous femoral approach. This uses the standard A-2 Multipurpose catheter. Catheter manipulation is similar to using the Sones catheter. Slight advances of

the catheter in the coronary cusps forms a "J" with the catheter and the tip rises to enter the coronary artery. The Tiger/Jacki are Radial artery catheters that do the same thing.

The standard A2 - MP has 2 side-holes and has a 1 ½ inch small diameter unreinforced soft tip. This makes the catheter J very easily. By impinging it on the aortic valve cusps it is "J'd" and then hooked back until the coronary ostium is engaged.

The incorrect answers (distractors), Amplatz, Judkins, and Castillo are selective end-hole only coronary arteriography catheters unsuitable for LV flood angiography.
See: Tilkian and Daily, chapter on "Tools for Catheterization."

39. Which radial approach catheters are "universal" and designed specifically to inject both RCA & LCA?
   a. Radi & UltraRadial
   b. Multipurpose A & B
   c. Judkins & Amplatz
   d. Tiger & Jacky

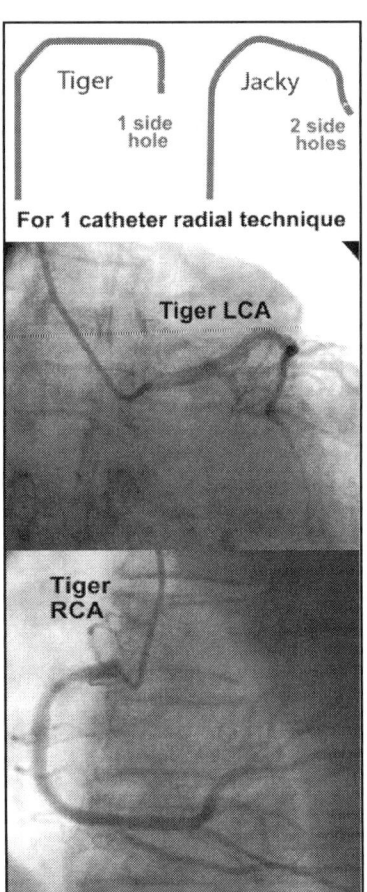

ANSWER d. Tiger & Jacky are sometimes called "universal radial catheters" - 1 catheter for both RCA & LCA.

Dicardiology.com says: "Although a JL 4 and JR 4 catheter can be used for left and right coronary artery cannulation, there are catheters on the market by various vendors designed specifically for radial artery access. Examples of radial-specific catheters are the Jacky Radial Catheter (Terumo), the Tiger Radial TIG Catheter (Terumo), and Sarah Radial (Terumo). The Ultimate 1 and 2 (Merit Medical) can also be used to cannulate either coronary ostia. These catheters have the common characteristic of a primary and secondary curve. A radial-specific catheter enables angiography of both right and left coronaries with a clockwise and counterclockwise rotation of one catheter. Eliminating catheter exchange can result in less total procedure time as well as fluoroscopy time and less incidence of radial artery spasm." See: https://www.dicardiology.com/article/choosing-tools-transradial-procedures

40. Identify the diagnostic femoral coronary catheter labeled at # 4 on the diagram.
  a. Amplatz Rt.
  b. JR4
  c. Amplatz Lt.
  d. Judkins Lt.

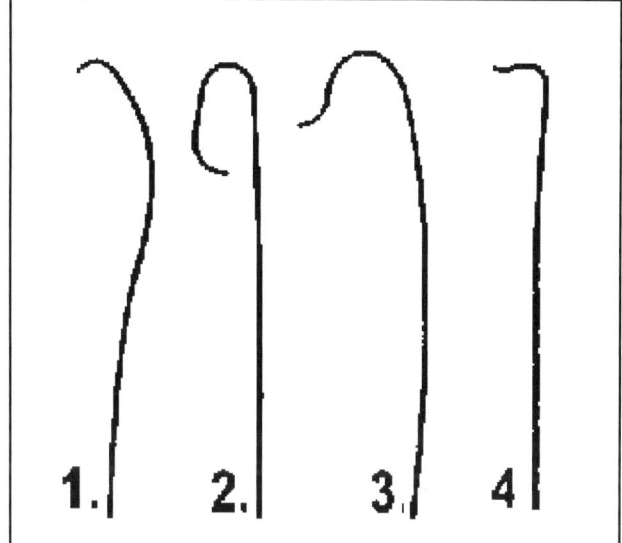

ANSWER a. Amplatz Rt. coronary catheter has a smaller duckbill shape than the left. Match all answers below. BE ABLE TO CORRECTLY MATCH ALL ANSWERS BELOW:

-1. JUDKINS RT: A Polyurethane (PU) single end-hole braided steel catheter. It has a blunt reduced diameter tip with a 90° bend allowing it to enter the coronary ostium. The secondary bend is a gradual 30° that provides backup support from the opposing aortic wall.

-2. JUDKINS LT: A Polyurethane (PU) single end-hole braided steel catheter. It has a blunt reduced diameter tip with a 90° bend allowing it to enter the coronary ostium. The secondary bend is 180° which provides backup support from the opposing aortic wall.

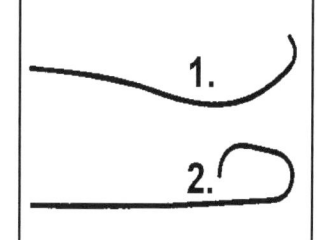

-3. AMPLATZ LT: This is a Polyurethane (PU) end-hole braided steel catheter. It is usually the second choice if a Judkins Left coronary is unsuccessful. It's duck bill shape is shaped to fit the sinus of Valsalva. The curve comes in 2-3 sizes all of which are larger than the Amplatz Rt. curve.

-4. AMPLATZ RT: This is a Polyurethane (PU) end-hole braided steel catheter. It is usually the second choice if a Judkins right coronary catheter is unsuccessful. It's duck bill shape is shaped to fit the sinus of Valsalva. The curve comes in 2-3 sizes all of which are smaller than the Amplatz left curves. The "AR" resembles the Amplatz Lt. except with a tighter curve radius.

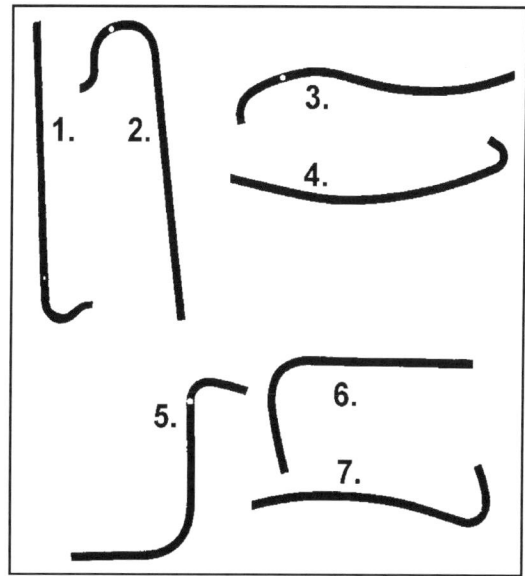

Just like the Judkins Left coronary, the Left Amplatz (duck bill) has a larger bend because it must reach further across the aortic root. The Rt. and Lt. Amplatz catheters are usually displayed together (as shown). Then it is easy to distinguish the Larger bends as Lt. Amplatz and the smaller as Rt. Amplatz.
See: Grossman, chapter on "Coronary Arteriography."

41. Identify the right coronary PCI guider catheter labeled at #5 on the diagram.
  a. Internal Mammary
  b. El Gamal
  c. Arani (Double Loop)
  d. Left Amplatz
  e. Rt. Amplatz

ANSWER c. Arani (Double Loop)
BE ABLE TO CORRECTLY MATCH ALL ANSWERS BELOW:
1. Rt. Amplatz
2. Left Amplatz
3. JR4
4. Internal Mammary
5. Arani (Double loop)
6. El Gamal
7. Hockey Stick
See: Pepine, chapter on "Intro. to Coronary Angioplasty."

42. Identify the left coronary PTCA guider catheter labeled at #4 on the diagram.
  a. Judkins Femoral Left
  b. Judkins Femoral Left short tip
  c. Voda Left
  d. Amplatz Left
  e. A-1 Multipurpose

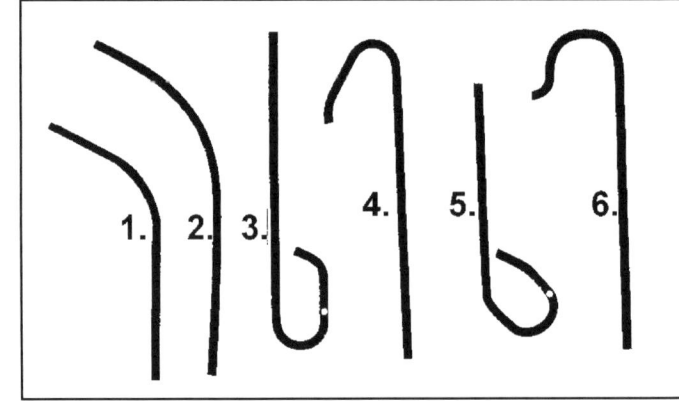

ANSWER b. Judkins Femoral Left short tip. Match all below.
BE ABLE TO CORRECTLY MATCH ALL ANSWERS BELOW:
1. A-1 MULTIPURPOSE
2. B-1 MULTIPURPOSE
3. JUDKINS FEMORAL LEFT
4. JUDKINS FEMORAL LEFT SHORT TIP
5. VODA LEFT
6. AMPLATZ LEFT
See: Pepine, chapter on "Intro. to Coronary Angioplasty."

43. You are attempting to directly stent a calcified tight circumflex lesion. When advancing the stent catheter it fails to pass the lesion and backs the guiding

catheter out of the ostium. What are the safest and most appropriate strategies to recommend to your new Dr? Select 3 answers below.
a. Increased backup with a larger diameter dilation catheter
b. Using a smaller diameter guiding catheter and deep throat it
c. Use an AL4 or EBU guiding catheter
d. Use a JL3 short tip or IMA guiding catheter
e. Predilate with a smaller profile dilation catheter

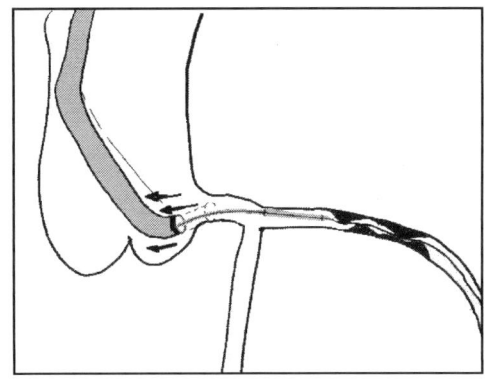

Guider backs out of ostium

ANSWERS: a, c, & e. Try to get increased backup support with a larger guider or extra-backup design. Predilation with a smaller dilation catheter will also help.

Grossman says: "Stenting of noncomplex lesions is typically performed through 6 French guiding catheters. Smaller-diameter guides, however, provide reduced backup support, a disadvantage that may necessitate active guide catheter manipulation (deep guide intubation), a technique that is usually safe when performed by experienced operators, although it may occasionally result in proximal coronary dissection requiring placement of additional stents."

"If significant guide catheter backup support is anticipated (e.g., fibrocalcific or tortuous vessels, distal lesions or total occlusions), or simultaneous delivery of multiple stents or use of atherectomy devices is planned, larger-dimension guiding catheters (typically 7F or 8F for greater passive support) or specialized shapes (e.g., Extra-back Up or Amplatz shapes for the right coronary artery and saphenous vein grafts) should be chosen. Larger guiding catheters may also be required for stenting of bifurcation lesions."

"Excessive force should never be applied in trying to pass a stent across a rigid, nondilated lesion; such efforts are likely to be unsuccessful and increase the risk of stripping the stent from the balloon. If guide support is adequate and the stent doesn't easily pass across the lesion, it should be carefully withdrawn back into the guide catheter under fluoroscopic visualization and the lesion predilated before an attempt to readvance the stent is made."
See: Grossman chapter on "Coronary Stenting"

44. Identify the guider catheter used for a Shepherd's Crook Right coronary #1 on the diagram.
a. JR4
b. Hockey stick / El Gamal
c. EBU / Right Voda
d. Amplatz

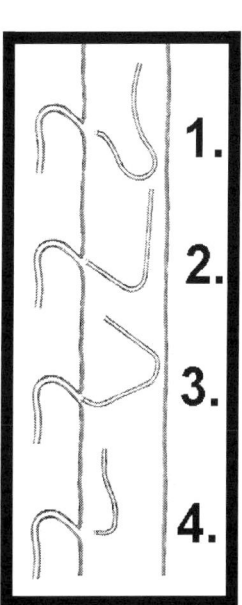

ANSWER d. AMPLATZ: Gentle "S" duckbill shape
BE ABLE TO CORRECTLY MATCH ALL ANSWERS BELOW:
2. HOCKEY STICK / EL GAMAL: Hockey stick shape. For Rt. superiorly angulated right coronary (Shepherd's Crook). Has a

75° or 90° horizontal angled tip off an S shaped body.
3. EBU / RIGHT VODA: Similar to Judkins Left for extra backup support. Also termed XB, LBR, LBU or LAD catheter.
4. JR4: Standard Judkins 4 cm. bend
See: Freed, Chapter on PTCA Equipment

45. When using a JL3.5 catheter via the femoral route on a left coronary PCI in a large man:
   a. It is difficult to engage
   b. The tip will be angled up superiorly
   c. There will be excellent backup support
   d. It will double back on itself in the sinus of Valsalva

Answer b. The tip will be angled up superiorly. Kern says, "A left 4-cm Judkins catheter fits in most adult patients. When the catheter [bend] size is adequate the catheter tip is aligned with the long axis of the left main coronary trunk. A smaller (3.5 cm catheter in the same patient will tip upward, and a larger (5. cm) catheter will tip downward (into the coronary cusp.)" Note in the diagram how the tip is pointing up and is not aligned with the left main coronary artery. But, this upward directed tip would give the best coaxial support in a superiorly directed Left Main coronary artery.

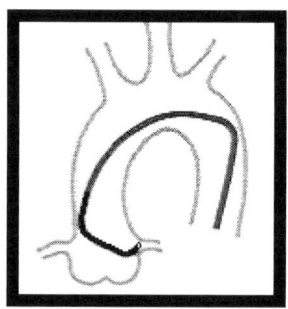
Figure 23 Too small JR3.5

Judkins left catheters are easy to engage, and it doesn't matter whether the LM takeoff is high or low on the aortic root. It will slide down the AO wall into place. Judkins said that his JL catheters "know where to go, unless thwarted by the operator." The reason the questions say "American" is that Asian stature is usually much smaller, and uses a JL3.5 as normal. Unless the JL is way too small, it will not double back on itself.
See: Kern, Interventional Cardiac Catheterization Handbook, chapter on "Arterial and Venous Access..."

46. Your patient with chronic hypertension has a dilated aortic root.. With the root aortogram shown which catheter would you recommend?
   a. EBU 2
   b. EBU4.5
   c. AL2
   d. AR4
   e. Pigtail

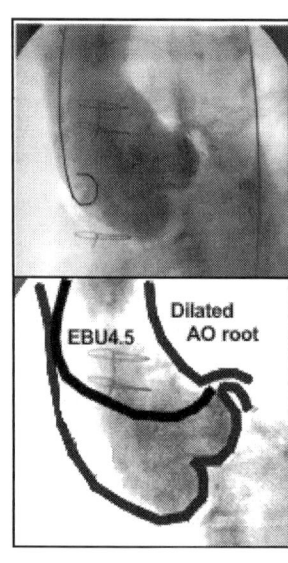

ANSWER b. EBU4.5 This is an enlarged aorta which needs a large left coronary bend such as the Extra Backup 4. Other catheters that might work are the AL4, JL5.

Grossman says: "In patients with a widened aortic root owing to aortic valve disease or long-standing hypertension, the 4-cm left Judkins [the average bend] may be too short to allow successful engagement. ... In this case, a left Judkins catheter with a larger (JL4.5, JL5, or even JL6) curve should be selected. A pigtail is a flood angiographic catheter, not a selective guiding catheter. See: Grossman chapter on Coronary Angiography"

47. Identify the coronary bypass catheter labeled #1 on the diagram.
   a. Left coronary bypass
   b. Internal mammary bypass
   c. Coronary Bypass II
   d. Right coronary bypass
   e. Multipurpose A-1

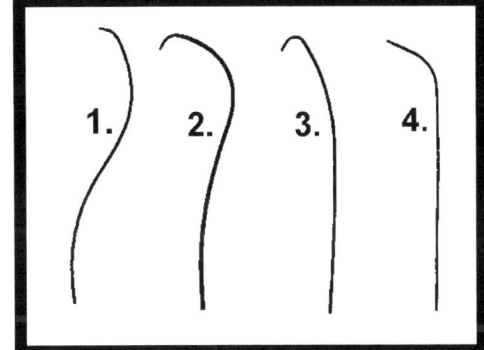
Coronary Bypass & IMA catheters

ANSWER: d. Right coronary bypass designed for right coronary venous bypass grafts attached to the right coronary artery. Tip and secondary bends approximate 120°. It is shaped much like a Judkins Rt. Coronary catheter with shallower tip bend.
-2. LEFT CORONARY bypass: Designed for left coronary venous bypass grafts attached to the LAD or circumflex artery. Tip has 90° bend with 70° secondary bend. It is shaped much like a cobra.
-3. INTERNAL MAMMARY bypass: Designed for both Rt. and left Internal Mammary arteries. Shaped much like a Judkins Rt. coronary catheter with a steeply angled tip (80 to 85°)
-4. MULTIPURPOSE A-1 is designed with a straight tip so it easily falls into right coronary bypass grafts.
See: Pepine, chapter on "Intro. to Coronary Angioplasty."

48. This diagram shows five poorly positioned Judkins coronary catheters. What positioning problem is shown at #3?
   a. Shepherd's hook tortuosity
   b. Too small a secondary bend size
   c. Too large a secondary bend size
   d. Selective conus injection
   e. Pressure damping

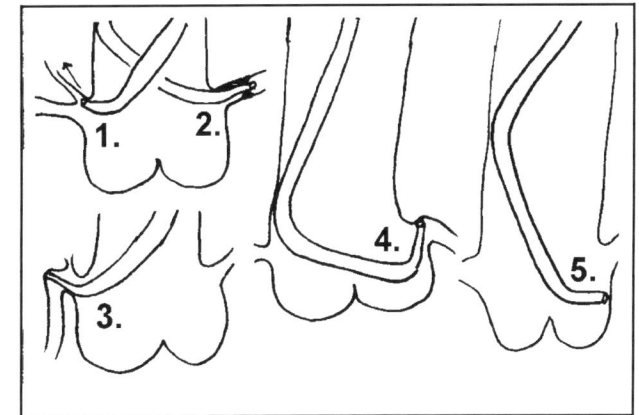

ANSWER a. Shepherd's hook tortuosity in RCA.
BE ABLE TO CORRECTLY MATCH ALL ANSWERS BELOW:
-1. SELECTIVE CONUS may appear to be RCA, leading to false diagnosis of occluded right coronary artery.

-2. PRESSURE DAMPING DUE TO WEDGING THE CATHETER into a tight ostium or stenosis.
-3. SHEPHERD'S HOOK TORTUOSITY of the RCA MAY CAUSE DAMPING or intimal dissection.
-4. TOO SMALL A SECONDARY BEND SIZE: This tip is directed too superiorly.
-5. TOO LARGE A SECONDARY BEND SIZE: The secondary bend is high in the arch. And the tip points inferiorly.
See: Pepine, chapter on "Catheters...equipment."

49. Judkins believed that coronary angiographic catheters should be single ended with NO side-holes because side-holes tend to:
a. Invalidate coronary angiography
b. Cause coronary ischemia
c. Increase likelihood of ostial dissection
d. Invalidate coronary pressure monitoring

ANSWERS d. Dr. Judkins insisted on careful hemodynamic pressure monitoring to warn the operator about "damping" because it cuts off flow to the coronary and can cause ischemia, injury and infarction. Judkins says, "Coronary catheters *should not have* side holes! Side holes in a coronary catheter predispose to increased clotting, obscure and do not prevent subintimal tip placement, and invalidate tip pressure monitoring." Freed says: "When dampening is due to the presence of a small coronary artery or an ostial obstruction, the guiding catheter should be replaced with a sidehole catheter; side-holes allow passive entry of aortic blood into the guiding catheter and coronary artery. If a sidehole catheter is not available, side-holes can be created with a sidehole cutter or the beveled end of the vascular access needle. Potential problems with sidehole catheters include suboptimal opacification (contrast escapes through the side-holes); decreased back up support due to weakness of the catheter shaft; and kinking at the side-holes, particularly in giant lumen guides. When sidehole guides are used for ostial lesions, the presence of side-holes will permit passive perfusion, but does not decrease the chance of guiding catheter injury to the vessel ostium. "
See: King, chapter by Judkins on, "Coronary Arteriography." and Freed, chapter on "PTCA Equipment"

50. Identify the PCI guider catheter shown on this diagram.
a. Amplatz
b. Voda Right
c. Judkins Right
d. Hockey Stick
e. Multipurpose

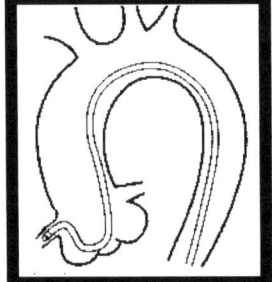

Answer: a. Amplatz. This is an inferiorly directed RCA ostium. Nguyen says, "Selection of [RCA] Guides for Inferiorly Oriented Takeoff Angle: In this orientation of the proximal segment of the RCA aggressive engagement of the tip from a regular JR tip can abut the lateral wall and cause dissection. The guides with inferiorly directed tips, such as the right venous bypass, Multipurpose, and Amplatz guides, may achieve more effective coaxial alignment with the proximal vessel segment." Nguyen, chapter on "Guides" Keywords: Amplatz = inferior takeoff RCA

51. What coronary catheter shape resembles a duck with bill as shown?
a. Judkins Left Coronary
b. Judkins Right Coronary
c. Amplatz Left Coronary
d. Amplatz Right Coronary

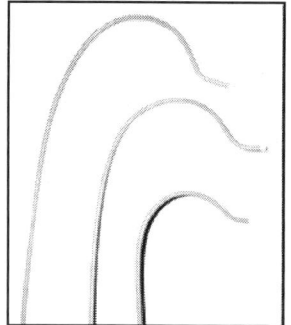

ANSWER: c. Amplatz Left Coronary must be reformed in the arch so it can be pulled back into the LCA. We always called these "duck-bill" catheters.

52. Identify the PCI guider catheter shown on this diagram.
a. Amplatz Right and Amplatz Left
b. Voda Right and Voda Supreme
c. El Gamal and El Gamal Short
d. Extra Backup and Extra Support
e. Judkins Left and Judkins Left Short

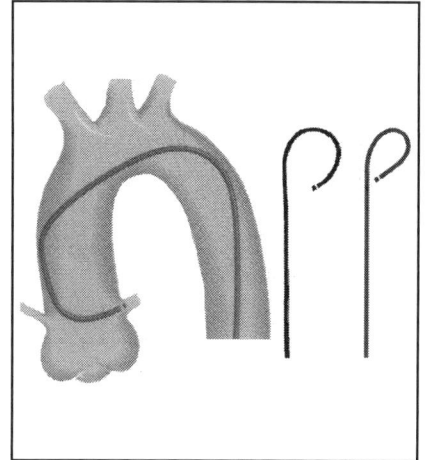

Answer: d. This shows an Extra Backup (XB-LAD or EBU) Left coronary catheter and an Extra Support(XB). These are variations on the Judkins Left design used when more backup support is needed. Note the diagrams of commonly used catheters at the end of this chapter. See: Cordis.com

Figure 29 Cordis catheters with permission

53. What nitinol device is designed to retrieve a coronary stent lost in the distal circulation?
a. King bioptome
b. Guide wire loop
c. Goose-neck snare
d. Amplatz grasping basket

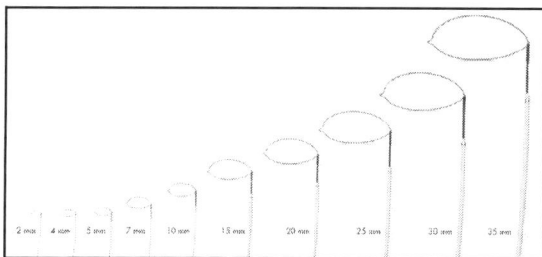

ANSWER: c. Goose-neck snare. This snare loop is at 90 degrees to the snare shaft, and the loop diameter is chosen to match or approximate the diameter of the vessel. Remember to upsize the sheath or guide catheter to be able to receive and withdraw the retrieved object.

PERIPHERAL CATHETERS

54. Match the type of diagnostic catheter to its bend (side-holes not shown):
a. Selective catheter with complex bend
b. Selective catheter with double curve bend
c. Selective catheter with simple bend
d. Flood/flush catheter

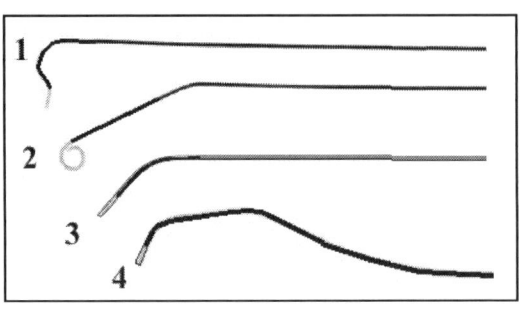

Caths shown are:
-1.a. Complex bend selective (Amplatz)
-2. d. Flood/flush catheter bend (Pigtail)
-3.b. Simple selective (Multipurpose/Berenstein)
-4.d. Double curve selective (H1 headhunter)

The pigtail is a flood catheters with multiple side-holes used to pressure flush large volumes of contrast into a large cardiac chamber or aorta. The other catheter bends are designed to selectively catheterize a vessel and hand inject small volumes of contrast. Schneider says: "Selective catheters have either a simple or complex curved head shape. A simple way to distinguish between the two is that a complex curve needs to be reshaped in the aorta before it can be used to selectively cannulate a side branch.

The bent-tip Berenstein or H1 catheters are a simple-curve selective catheter, but it can be used simultaneously for general applications. The bend at the tip of the catheter confers directionality to the guidewire tip. Hook-shaped catheter heads are useful for turning an acute angle at a tight corner. Complex-curve catheter heads have a curve in one direction, then back in the other direction. These are used primarily to select out aortic side branches for cannulation. Examples include the Simmons and the shepherds hook cerebral catheters." See: Schneider, chapter on "Guidewire - catheter skills"

55. Complex selective "S" shaped catheters are used mainly for cannulating:
a. Coronary arteries
b. Up and over aortic bifurcations
c. Femoral and other leg arteries
d. Aortic side branches

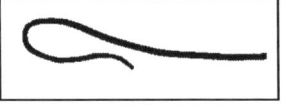

ANSWER d. Aortic side branches. Schneider says: "Complex-curve catheter heads have a curve in one direction, then back in the other direction. These are used primarily to select out aortic side branches for cannulation. Examples include the Simmons and the H3 Headhunter cerebral catheters." Note that when an engaged complex-curve catheter is pulled back, it dives deeper into the vessel and can damage it if forced. When removing one always advance first to get out of the selected vessel then torque it to straighten. See: Schneider, chapter on "Guidewire - catheter skills"

56. Match the selective renal and adrenal arteriography catheter bend on the diagram with its name below.
  a. Hook
  b. Cobra
  c. Double curve / RDC
  d. Simmons / Shepherd hook

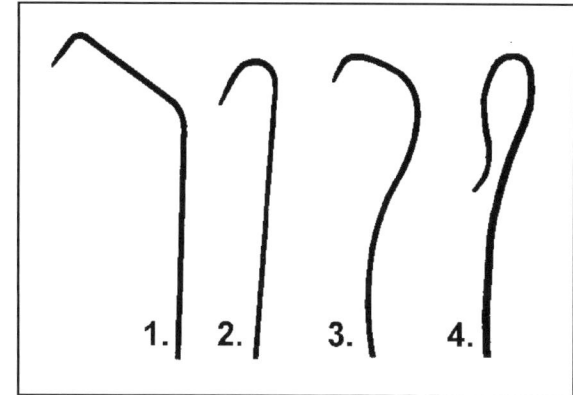
Renal arteriography catheters

ANSWER
  1.c. DOUBLE CURVE: Femoral renal end-hole only catheter, sometimes called the RDC (Renal Double Curve). Also, it is available in A-2 with 2 side-holes. It has a straight 90° tip and a sharp 120° secondary bend. The two bends are sharp and distinct.
  2. HOOK - Femoral visceral End-hole only. It is a rounded C or J, fishhook shape.
  3.a. COBRA: Femoral visceral End-hole only (also available A-2 with 2 side-holes). It looks like a cobra posed and ready to strike. It has a 90° tapered tip and a 90° gradual secondary curve which gives backup support from the opposite wall of the aorta.
  4. SIMMONS Sidewinder / SHEPHERD HOOK: End-hole only. It looks like a shepherd's staff or a duck's head. The secondary bend is around 180 degrees.
See: Johnsrude, chapter on "Equipment

57. From femoral access, match the three visceral selective angiography catheter bends that would best fit in the superior, horizontal and inferiorly directed vessels shown.
  a. Cobra
  b. Berenstein
  c. Simmons Sidewinder

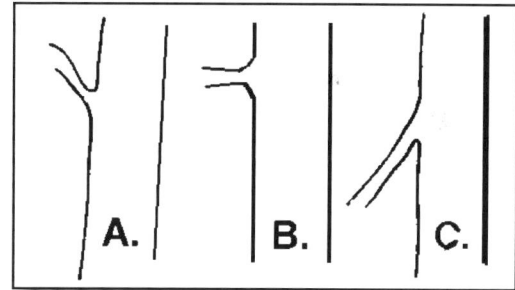

ANSWER For each of these three types of side branches (up, flat and down) Kessel & Robertson list three bends ththat best fit each arterial takeoff.
-A. (up) Berenstein, Headhunter H1, Mani
-B. (horizontal) Cobra, Multipurpose, or Renal Double Curve
-C. (down) Sidewinder, SOS Omni, RDC.

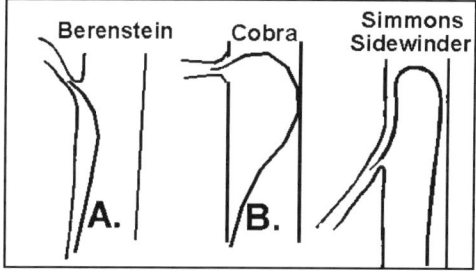

Kessel says: "The most important factor in catheter choice is the angle at which the target vessel arises from the parent vessel." He also lists his top 5 selective visceral and peripheral catheters as Cobra, Simmons Sidewinder, Sos-omni, Berenstein and Renal double curve (RDC) and headhunter H1. Simple superiorly directed vessels only require a small curve on the catheter tip like the Berenstein or H1, while inferiorly directed vessels require a hooking catheter, like the Simmons or Renal Double curve so the catheter tip points down. See: Kessel, chapter on "Equipment for Angiography"

58. Match each selective cerebral angiographic catheter in the diagram to its name below.
  a. JB1 / Berenstein
  b. Headhunter H1
  c. Simmons
  d. Vertek / Mani

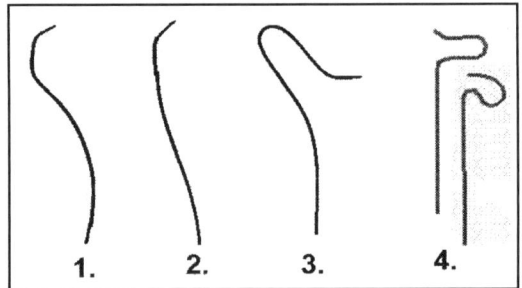

59. In a patient with normal carotid anatomy which cerebral catheter is most useful to selectively catheterize all arch vessels by "direct advancement" as shown?
  a. Headhunter (H1)
  b. Headhunter (H2)
  c. Simmons #2
  d. Newton #2

ANSWER a. The Headhunter H1 can be manipulated into every one of the 4 head vessels using direct advancement - that is, without using hooking maneuvers. This diagram shows the "direct advance" technique. These vessels show a normal "take-off." If the arch vessels are acutely angled, hooking may be necessary with a double bend catheter, such as the sidewinder.
See: Johnsrude, chapter on "Aortic Arch and Brachiocephalic Angiography."

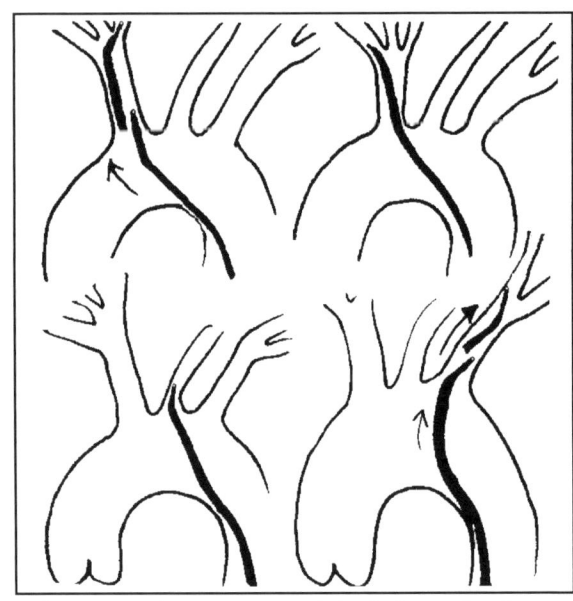

Selective catheterization of Arch & cerebral vessels

60. Complex selective peripheral aortic catheters use a "pulling" maneuver to hook the catheter tip in the target aortic side branch. What size of catheter bend is recommended?
  a. Bend to tip should normally be 4 cm
  b. Bend to tip should be 110% the width of AO
  c. Primary to secondary bend measurement should exceed the width of AO
  d. Primary to secondary bend should normally be 4 cm.

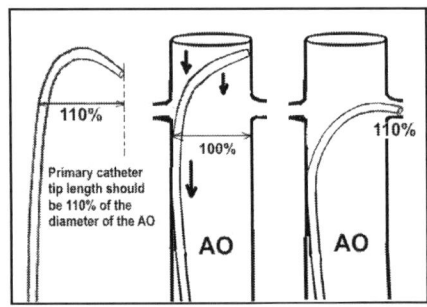

Answer b. Bend to tip should be 110% the width of AO.

After the hook is removed by being reformed in the AO and pulled back, "backup" forces will help push the catheter tip into the side branch. Braun says: "Rule of 110. Pull-type catheters are available in different tip lengths. The primary catheter tip length should be 110 percent of the diameter of the abdominal aorta. The catheter that matches this percentage is easiest to reform and reposition within the abdominal aorta. The catheter tip that is slightly greater than the width of the aorta will allow the catheter tip to engage the orifice of branched vessels."
See: Braun, Interventional Radiology Procedure Manual, chapter on Equipment

61. In a patient with tortuous carotid anatomy, which complex bend cerebral catheter is most useful to selectively catheterize all arch vessels by the hooking maneuver?
 a. Headhunter (H1)
 b. Headhunter (H2)
 c. Simmons #2
 d. Newton #2

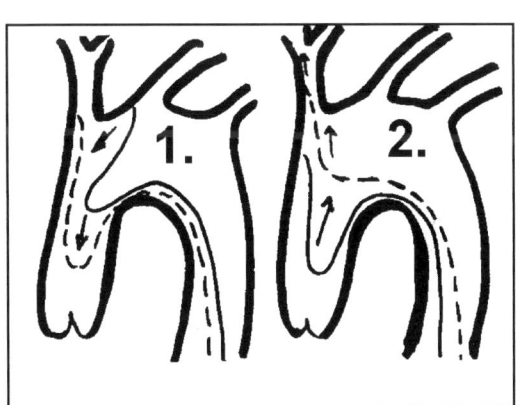

ANSWER c. Simmons #2. The primary curve (tip) is hooked in an arch vessel and advanced. This allows the catheter to double over at the secondary bend. The secondary curve now leads as it is advanced, doubled over, into the ascending aorta. The catheter tip is then positioned in the innominate artery (or other acute takeoff vessel) and drawn back.
Withdrawal forces the tip higher into the carotid artery. Removal of the tip then requires advancing the secondary curve down the aortic arch. This hooking maneuver also works with the #3 headhunter catheter.
See: Johnsrude, chapter on "Aortic Arch and Brachiocephalic Angiography."

TRANSSEPTAL CATHETERS

62. Identify the transseptal catheterization equipment labeled at #4 in the diagram.
 a. Mullins sheath
 b. Brockenbrough needle
 c. Brockenbrough catheter
 d. Bing stylet

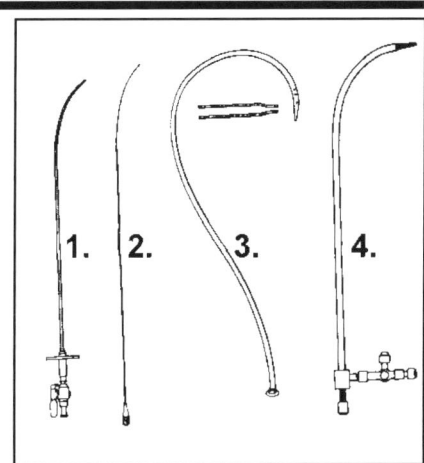

ANSWER a. Mullins sheath and dilator

1. BROCKENBROUGH NEEDLE: is a 70 cm long curved 18 gauge needle (21 gauge at tip). This is the instrument that punctures the atrial septum as it is advanced through the RA catheter. It has a needle flange (hilt) with a pointed end showing the direction of the curve. It has a built in one way stopcock.

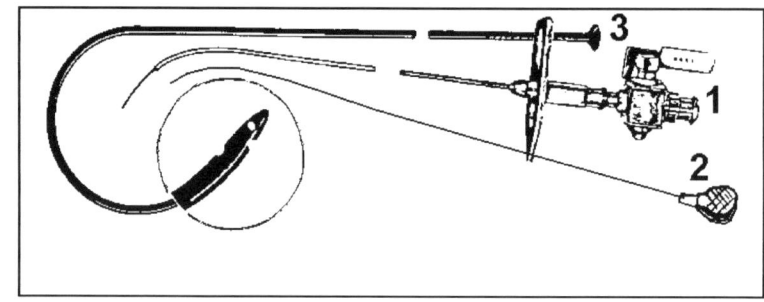

2. BING STYLET: is a curved blunt obturator slightly longer than the needle to safely pass the long Brockenbrough needle up the catheter without catching on the catheter wall. This blunt stylet is withdrawn just before the atrial puncture is made.

3. BROCKENBROUGH CATHETER: is a fairly rigid Teflon 70 cm. tapered tip catheter to allow percutaneous entry and smooth passage through the atrial septum. It has an end-hole and 6 side-holes for angiography. The bend shape is circular with radii of 2.0, 2.5 and 3.0 cm. The tapered hub must be attached to a flare adapter once the puncture is done.

4. MULLINS SHEATH: This is a long Teflon sheath that can be advanced with its introducer catheter over the needle across the fossa ovalis and into the LA. It is usually used to introduce other catheters into the LA such as a special pigtail or valvuloplasty catheter. These sheaths are also used in mitral valvuloplasty catheter introduction.

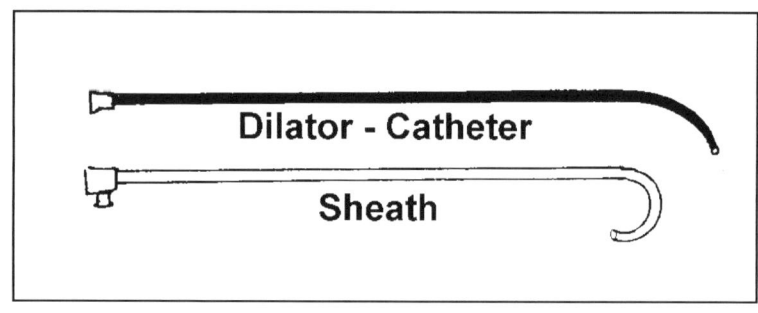

MULLINS DILATOR (CATHETER): Similar to the Brockenbrough catheter but with less curve. It is designed specifically to introduce and extend beyond the Mullins sheath.
See: Grossman, chapter on "Percutaneous Approach (& Transseptal Cath)"

63. This Brockenbrough catheter and stainless steel curved needle are used to puncture the:
   a. Ductus Arteriosus
   b. Ligamentum Arteriosum
   c. Fossa Ovalis
   d. Foramen Ovale

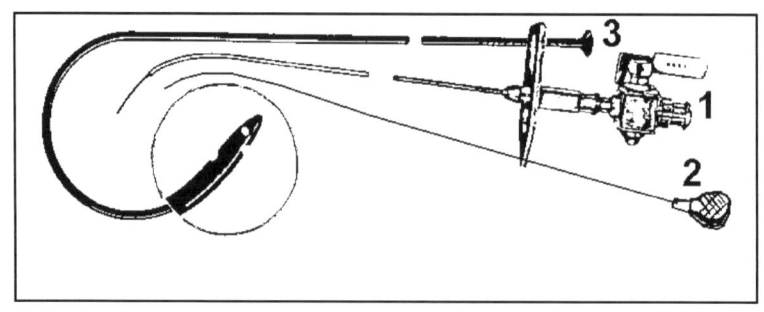

ANSWER c. The Brockenbrough transseptal set shown above is for atrial transseptal puncture. Puncture is made through the fossa ovalis the thinnest part of the atrial septum. This is where the foramen ovale was in the fetus.
See: Grossman, chapter on "Percutaneous Approach."

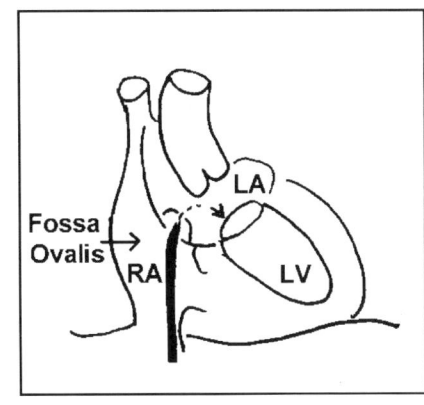

CATHETER CARE AND HANDLING

64. Care of indwelling right heart catheters is different from the care of arterial catheters in that right heart catheters:
  a. Require pressurized flush bags
  b. Require a continuous heparinized saline drip
  c. Safely allow injection of small air bubbles
  d. Are inserted by the Seldinger technique

ANSWER c. Air bubbles are not usually a problem on the right side of the heart. Small air bubbles will be effectively filtered out by the lungs that then slowly absorb the air. It may take a hundred cc's of air to cause a critical pulmonary embolism. This is NOT true on the left side where air emboli lodges in peripheral capillaries and obstructs critical flow, leading to tissue infarction or the "bends." Even so, technologists should get in the habit of keeping bubbles out of all catheter lines.
  Rt. heart (venous) lines can be dripped continuously with a gravity drip. But a continuous drip on Rt. Ht. catheter is not necessary. Many Rt. Ht. caths are done without heparin. However, frequent hand flushing of these catheters is necessary.
  Arterial pressure will "back up" an IV because arterial pressure is so great. Pressure bags are necessary. Pressure bags are often used in Swan-Ganz long term monitoring lines as well. This is because the catheter may be in place for a week. Heparin flush is essential to prevent clotting for this long term monitoring.
See: Grossman, chapter on "Cardiac Ventriculography."

65. On this femoral access patient you expect to use a 5F angiographic catheter, and then a 7F interventional guider if an intervention is needed. To prevent bleeding at the catheter site:
  a. Start with a small diameter sheath and exchange up in Fr. size
  b. Start with a 7F diameter sheath so you can insert either catheter as needed
  c. Place a 5F sheath in RFA and 7F sheath in LFA
  d. Do not anticoagulate the patient

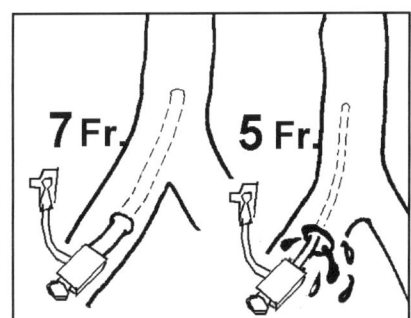

ANSWER a. Start with the smaller 5F sheath and exchange up in Fr. size only if you proceed with the intervention. You don't want to exchange down in French size as this would allow the puncture site to bleed around the smaller sheath (see diagram). Catheter exchanges between different sizes are usually no problem when done through a sheath. But, if they cancel the intervention you will not need the larger sheath. Make no larger hole than necessary. Neither do you need 2 sheaths. You will only need one catheter at a time - diagnostic then interventional.

Johnsrude recommends starting with the smaller catheters (usually selective) first, then exchanging UP in French size, to prevent bleeding and hematoma at the puncture site. **See:** Johnsrude, chapter on "Equipment."

66. **Catheters with PA balloons or closed ends SHOULD NOT BE INTRODUCED by the_____ method.**
   a. Femoral cutdown
   b. Brachial cutdown
   c. Seldinger over-the-wire
   d. Femoral sheath

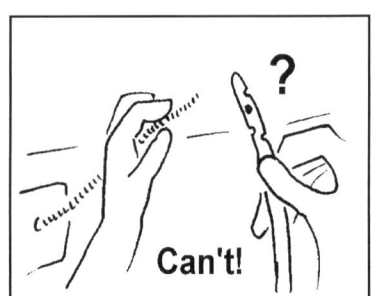

ANSWER c. Seldinger over-the-wire method. Clearly "No End-hole" catheters like the NIH and Berman cannot be introduced percutaneously over a guide wire - since they have no end hole. They must be introduced by the sheath or cutdown methods.

Introducing Swan-Ganz, angioplasty balloons or stents over the wire risks damage to the balloon passing through the tissue. Swan-Ganz catheters usually require a sheath one Fr. size larger than the catheter Outside Diameter (O.D.) Small diameter guide wires may be placed though the distal lumen after catheter insertion.
See: Tilkian and Daily, chapter on "Tools for Catheterization."

67. **Which catheter may be introduced over-the-wire?**
   a. Fogarty
   b. Berman
   c. Swan-Ganz
   d. Brockenbrough

ANSWER: d. Brockenbrough is a transseptal catheter introduced over-the-wire. Once in place the transseptal needle is placed within it to make the inter-atrial puncture. The Fogarty and Swan are balloon catheters. Fogarty and NIH have no end hole.
See: Grossman, chapter on "Percutaneous Approach" Keywords: Swan, Fogarty and NIH not over-wire

68. Identify catheter #3 in the diagram?
a. IMA
b. Judkins
c. Amplatz
d. Multipurpose
e. Coronary bypass

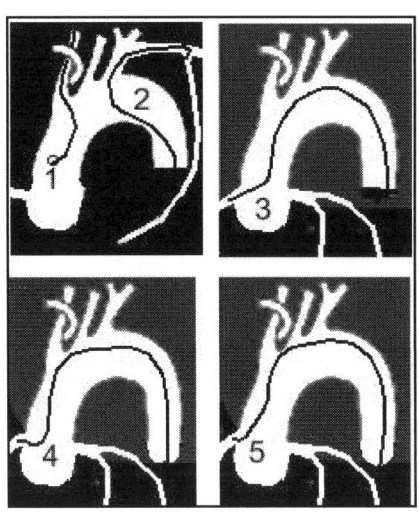

Answer: d. Multipurpose.
-1. Coronary bypass, by left brachial
-2. IMA, by femoral approach
-3. Multipurpose, by femoral approach
-4. Amplatz right coronary, by femoral approach
-5. Judkins right coronary, by femoral approach
See: Cordis "Catheters to know" on last page this chapter

Cordis catheters with permission

69. Which peripheral catheter inserted in the arm is used for long term administering of nutrient fluids, chemo- agents, or other central venous medications in the SVC?
a. Midline catheter
b. Port catheter
c. PICC
d. Tunneled Hickman catheter

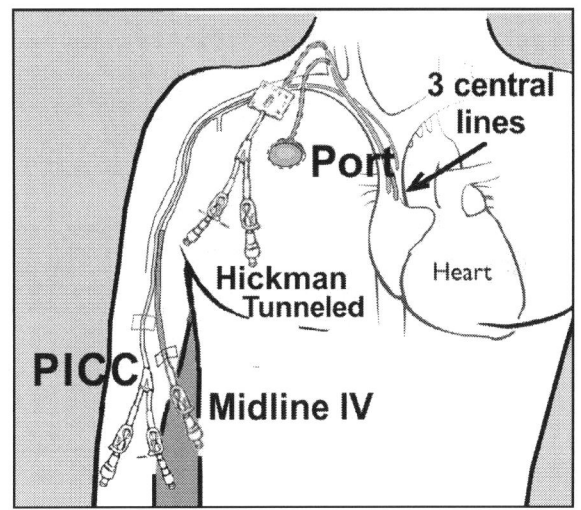

Answer c. PICC = "Peripherally Inserted Central Venous Catheter." A PICC is inserted in the upper arm to drip in various therapeutic IV nutrient fluids, chemo- agents or other strong drugs. The catheter is advanced to the SVC or RA because some caustic IV solutions may damage smaller veins, and in the RA they are immediately diluted. Since PICCs may be in the vein for weeks, they are made of silicone or other inert hypo-c allergenic plastics and may have several ports for 2 or more simultaneous IVs. PICC insertions have decreased complication risk and can remain for a much longer time than peripheral IVs or central lines from the neck.

Midline" catheters are also advanced from the arm like PICCs, but a midline catheter tip ends in the upper arm and is only suitable for non irritating IVs.

Tunneled" catheters have a cuff that stimulates tissue growth that will help hold it in place in the body for a long time. Examples of the tunneled catheter include HICKMAN® catheters, BROVIAC® catheters and GROSHONG® catheters. They are often used for renal dialysis access or when central venous access is needed for longer period of time and when the catheter line will be used many times each day - usually in RIJ.

The most invasive central line is the "port" catheter, or subcutaneous implantable port. It is a permanent catheter attached to a small reservoir placed under the skin, similar to a "tunnel" catheter except it has a reservoir with a silicone covering that can be punctured with a special bent Huber needle. Everything is under the skin and the port is punctured through the skin to fill the medication reservoir.

REFERENCES:

Baim, D. S. and Grossman W., *Cardiac Catheterization, Angiography, and Intervention*, 7th Ed., Lea and Febiger, 2006

Braun, Nemcek, and Vogelzang, Interventional Radiology Procedure Manual, Churchill Livingstone, 1997

Freed, Grines, and Safian, The New Manual of Interventional Cardiology 2nd printing, Physicians Press, 1996

Johnsrude, I. S., Jackson. D. C., Et. al., *A Practical Approach to Angiography,* 2nd Ed., Little Brown and Co., 1987

Kern, Morton, *The Cardiac Catheterization Handbook,* 6th Ed., Mosby, 2016

King, S.B. III and Yeung, Alan, *Interventional Cardiology*, McGraw-Hill Book Co., 2007

Lanzer, Peter, *Mastering Endovascular Techniques, a guide to excellence*, Lippincot, 2007

Nguyen, & Colombo, et all., Practical Handbook of Advanced Interventional Cardiology, 3rd Ed., Blackwell Futura, 2009

Pepine, J. C., and Hill, J. A., et. al., *Diagnostic and Therapeutic Cardiac Catheterization*, 2nd Ed., Williams and Wilkins, 1994

Schneider, Peter, Endovascular Skills, Guidewire and Catheter Skills for Endovascular Surgery, 2nd Edition, Marcel Dekker, Inc., 2003

Tilkian, A. G., and Daily, E, J, *Cardiovascular Procedures, Diagnostic Techniques and Therapeutic Procedures*, C. V. Mosby Company, 1986

OUTLINE: Catheters

1. CATHETER BASICS
   a. Components
      i. -Body
      ii. -Primary bend (1°)
      iii. -Secondary bend (2°)
      iv. -Tip (blunt, tapered, soft tip)
      v. -Heat shrink/sleeve
      vi. -Hub
   b. Side-holes
      (1) increase cor. blood flow
      (2) reduce cor. ischemia
      ii. -Disadvantages of side holes
      (1) less dye opacification
      (2) more contrast needed
      (3) less backup support
      (4) loss of cor. pressure monitoring (damping)
      (5) possible kinking
      (6) Judkins disliked sideholes
   c. CONSTRUCTION AND PLASTICS
      i. Manufacturing process
      (1) -Extrusion
      (2) -Multi-lumen Extrusions
      (3) -Braid
      (4) -Tip Welding
      (5) - Increasing softt tip
      ii. Catheter construction materials:
      (1) PVC - Swan Ganz
      (2) Polyurethane (PU)
      (3) Polyethylene (PE)
      (4) Teflon (PTFE) -sheaths & linings of guiders
      (5) Nylon - strong (may not need steel braiding)
      (6) Rubber - Swan balloons
      (7) Hydrophilic polymer -slime
      (8) Wire braid - st. steel
   d. QUALITIES OF CATHETERS
      i. Flexibility
      ii. Memory
      iii. End and side-holes
      iv. Torque control
      v. Bend sizes
      vi. Trackability
      vii. Backup support
      viii. Soft or blunt tip
      ix. Reusability (EP electrodes)
      TYPES of CATHETERS

- x. Flood/flush
- xi. Selective - simple bend
  - (1) angled
  - (2) hooked
  - (3) double bend
- xii. Selective - complex bend
  - (1) hooking maneuver
  - (2) 110% rule (bend 10% larger than AO diameter)
  - (3) reform cath (hook) in aorta
  - (4) disengage by pushing - pulling cath. may advance tip
  - (5) Used mainly in AO side branches & inferior takeoff
- xiii. Diagnostic catheters
  - (1) smaller
  - (2) flexible tips
- xiv. Guiding catheters
- e. SHEATHS
  - i. advantages of sheath
    - (1) Smaller arteriotomy
    - (2) Have hemostatic side valve
  - ii. advantages guiding catheters
    - (1) wire braid for torque control
    - (2) more bend sizes
    - (3) kink resistant
2. CATHETER SIZING
   - a. OD - french size
     - i. convert 3Fr/1mm
     - ii. ID - thousandths of inch
     - iii. Convert 25.4 mm/in
   - b. ID - Sheaths
     - i. 6F sheath ID really 7F OD
     - ii. 6F cath. in 6F sheath is difficult to flush sheath - too tight
   - c. Poiseuille's Law
     - (1) -effect of changing Inside diameter
   - d. lengths (80, 100, 110 cm...)
3. CATHETERS: TYPES
   - a. Balloon catheters.
     - (1) Berman
     - (2) Swan-Ganz
     - (3) Rashkind
     - (4) Fogarty
     - (5) PTA, PTCA, dilatation
     - (6) IABP, counterpulsation
     - (7) Valvuloplasty
   - ii. Swan-Ganz Catheters:
     - (1) use
     - (2) sizes
     - (3) advantages - disadvantages
     - (4) Catheter ports
       - (a) distal port (for PA pressure)
       - (b) balloon port (air filled rubber balloon)
       - (c) thermistor connector (to CO computer)
       - (d) Guide-wire port
       - (e) proximal port
   - b. RIGHT HEART CATHETERS
     - (1) Rt. Ht. monitoring catheters
       - (a) Multipurpose
       - (b) Swan-Ganz
       - (c) EP electrodes
         - (i) steerable
       - (d) RF Ablation catheters
         - (i) large metal tips
         - (ii) steerable
     - (2) Right heart temporary pacing electrodes or catheters.
       - (a) Pacing electrodes - standard and semi-floating
       - (b) Floating electrodes - balloons
       - (c) Thermodilution catheter
       - (d) Super Swan - Floating, thermo, sensing, pacing
       - (e) use in patients with LBBB
   - c. TRANSSEPTAL EQUIPMENT
     - i. Brockenbrough catheter
     - ii. Brockenbrough needle
     - iii. Bing Stylet
     - iv. Mullins sheath
     - v. Tip occluder
4. ANGIO-FLOOD CATHETERS
   - i. Angiographic flood catheters.
     - (1) Halo
     - (2) NIH
     - (3) Pigtail
     - (4) Berman
     - (5) Multipurpose
     - (6) Brockenbrough
   - ii. Pigtail catheters.
     - (1) Least recoil with flood injection
     - (2) Pigtail angiographic
       - (a) angled pigtail
       - (b) Grollman PA pigtail
       - (c) micro pigtail
     - (3) Flush vigorously - clots in tip
   - b. CORONARY CATHETERS
     - i. Diagnostic & Guiding catheters.
       - (1) Multipurpose
         - (a) B1, B2
         - (b) A1, A2
       - (2) JR4, 5, 6
       - (3) JL4, 5, 6
       - (4) Left Amplatz
       - (5) Rt. Amplatz
       - (6) Extra Backup (EBU)
         - (a) Voda
       - (7) Hockey Stick
       - (8) Internal Mammary
       - (9) El Gamal
       - (10) Arani (Double Loop)
       - (11) Use large bends for large aortas
       - (12) Coronary Bypass
         - (a) Rt. & Lt. bypass
         - (b) Multipurpose
         - (c) Internal mammary
         - (d) Coronary Bypass II
       - (13) Radial coronary
         - (a) Judkins Rt & LT
         - (b) Tiger & Jacky
5. SPECIAL VASCULAR CATHETERS
   - a. Selective VASCULAR catheters.
     - i. JB1

            ii. Manni & Newton
            iii. Headhunter H1
            iv. Simmons sidewinder
            v. Berenstein
            vi. Hook
            vii. Cobra
            viii. Renal double curve
        b. Central venous lines
            i. PICC
            ii. Midline
            iii. Port tunneled
            iv. Hickman tunneled
6. CATHETER CARE AND HANDLING
    a. Cleaning and Sterilization of Catheters
        i. Reusable - EP electrodes
        ii. Resterilize other plastics with ETO gas
        iii. Washing blood, flushing
        iv. Packaging, sterilization control
    b. Principles/precautions of catheter use
        i. Flush catheter before use
        ii. Inspect before use
        iii. Advance with leading guide
        iv. Advance exchange over a guide
        v. Gently advance/ don't force
        vi. Flush vigorously every 3 minutes
        vii. Aspirate before flushing
        viii. avoid knots and kinks
        ix. Observe pressures for damping
        x. Never reuse catheters
        xi. Direct advance maneuvers
        xii. Hooking maneuvers
        xiii. 110% rule
    c. Problems associated with use of pigtail and multiple sidehole catheters.
        i. Thrombosis at tip (flush vigorously)
        ii. Accidental selective injection by tip
        iii. Intimal staining
        iv. Knots
        v. Catheter removal (wire in)

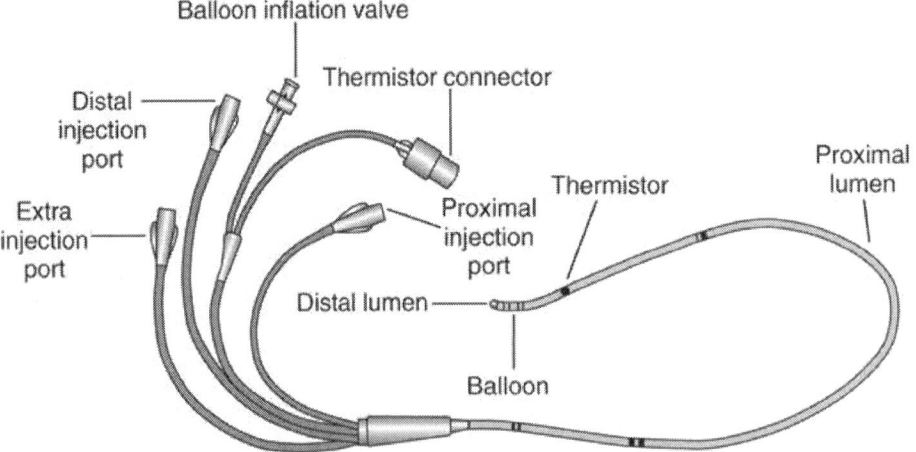

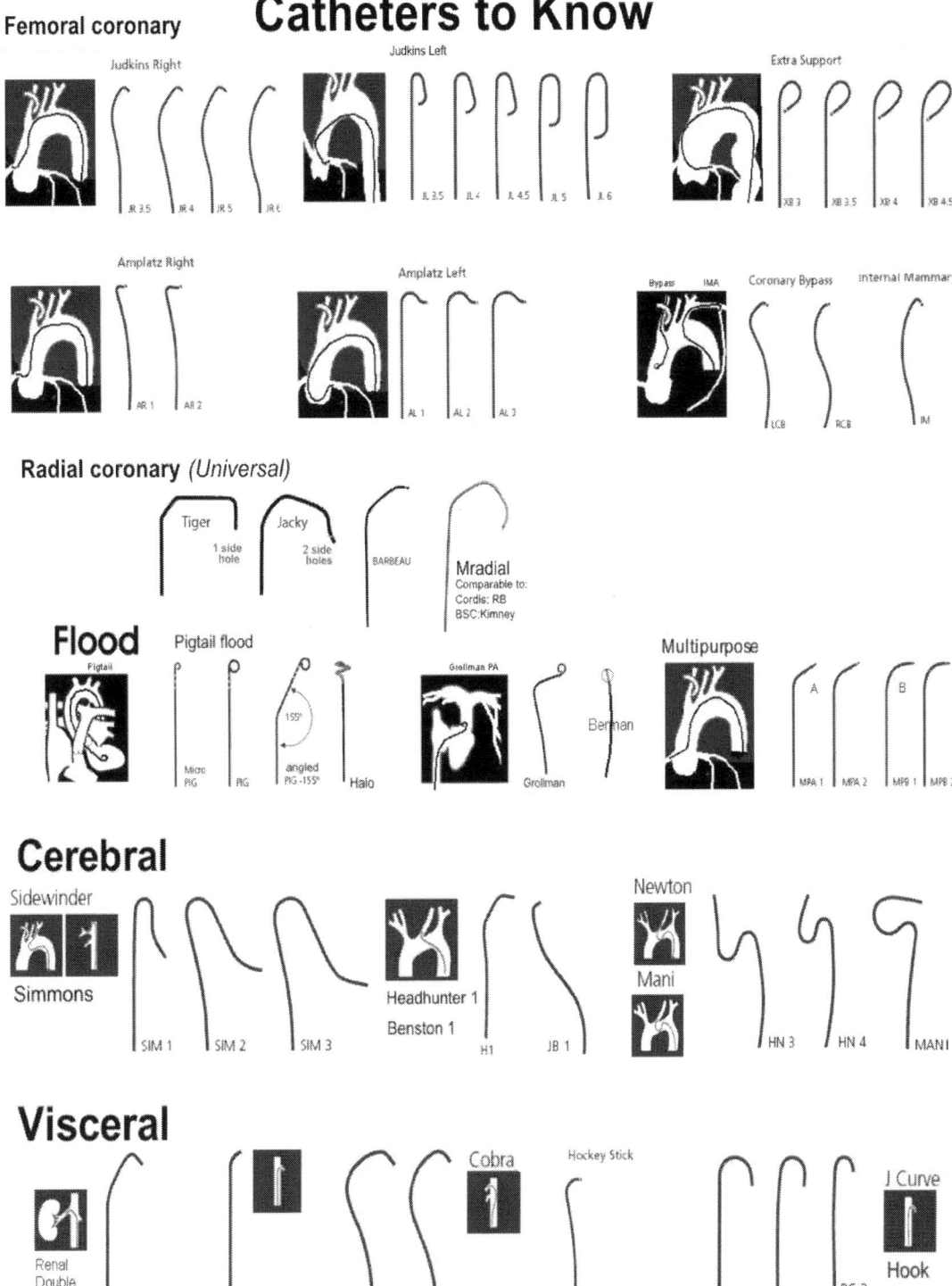

Catheterization Equipment: Other

INDEX: D2: Catheterization Equipment: Other
- 1. General . . . . . p. 41 Know
- 2. Needles . . . . . p. 43 Know
- 3. Sheaths . . . . . p. 46 Know
- 4. Stopcocks, Adapters . . . p. 48 Know
- 5. Guide Wires . . . . p. 55 Know
- 6. Handling Equipment . . . p. 68 Know
- 7. Chapter Outline: Other Equipment p. 73

General Catheterizing Equipment

70. Identify the part of an introducer sheath set labeled #3 on the diagram?
    a. Wire-guide, short
    b. Sheath
    c. Dilator
    d. Seldinger needle

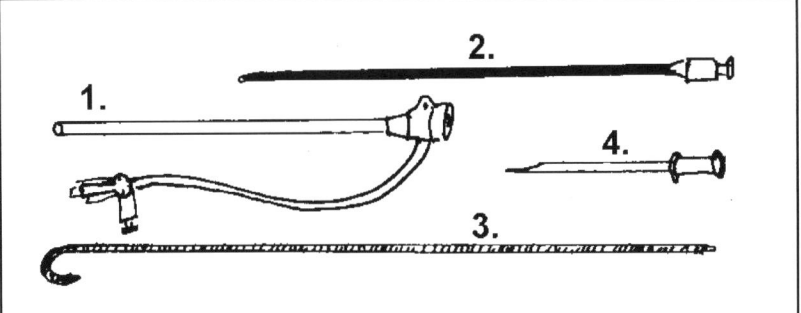

Parts of a sheath set

ANSWER a. Short wire-guide. **MATCHED ANSWERS ARE:**
1. **SHEATH:** The Teflon sleeve that admits the dilator and catheter. Most sheaths have a hemostasis valve proximal to the sidearm. They are made of slits in a rubber diaphragm or several layers of rubber. A good hemostasis valve prevents bleed-back through the proximal end of the sheath during catheter exchange. You can insert and remove catheters without bleed back through the sheath.
2. **DILATOR:** The short section of tapered catheter that expands the vessel puncture site. The taper makes the transitions between guide-wire OD size and sheath ID size. The dilator is the same French size as the largest catheter you can introduce through the sheath. A 6F sheath can introduce a 6F catheter.
3. **Wire-guide, SHORT:** These short .035 inch OD guides are used only for inserting the sheath. They extend through the dilator but are too short to be used with a catheter.
4. **SELDINGER NEEDLE:** The 18T needle used for wire insertion by the Seldinger method (may be a 1 part, 2 part, or 3 part needles.)

See: Grossman, chapter on "Percutaneous Approach." **Keywords:** sheath set components

71. The outside diameter of the catheterization equipment labeled #1 in the box is usually measured in:
a. Inches
b. mm.
c. French
d. Gauge

CATH EQUIPMENT
*1. Diagnostic catheter OD
2. Inflated Balloon cath. OD
3. Needle OD
4. Guide wire OD

ANSWER c. French size. One french size equals 1/3 (0.33) of a mm or .013 inches. The outside diameter (OD) of cath equipment is traditionally measured using four different scales.

    1. Catheter OD in French . . 1 Fr. = 0.33 mm = .013 in.
    2. Balloon diameter in mm . . 1 mm = .0394 inches
    3. Needle OD in "gauge." . . 18 gauge = .050 in. (nonlinear system)
    4. Guide-wire OD in thousandth of inches .035 inch = 0.89 mm

We mix the English, French, metric, and gauge measuring systems. This tradition of mixing systems makes it difficult to convert between the systems. It becomes especially confusing when attempting to pass one system through another, as in PCI.
See: Co. literature and Tilkian, chapter on "Tools for Catheterization." **Keywords:** measuring OD, French size

72. To enlarge the puncture site for a femoral artery catheter through the subcutaneous tissue most catheterizing physicians use a:
a. #10 scalpel blade
b. #11 scalpel blade
c. #12 scalpel blade
d. #15 scalpel blade

ANSWER b. #11 scalpel blade.
CORRECTLY MATCHED ANSWERS ARE:
    1. **#10 SCALPEL BLADE:** A large curved blade for major surgery.
    2. **#11 SCALPEL BLADE:** The pointed blade used for the stab wound.
    3. **#12 SCALPEL BLADE:** A hooked "eagle beak" shaped point for fine slicing
    4. **#15 SCALPEL BLADE:** A small curved blade used for making skin incisions as in cutdown procedures.
See: Grossman, Cardiac Cath, Angiography . . . chapter on "Percutaneous Approach." **Keywords:** enlarge puncture site → #11 scalpel blade

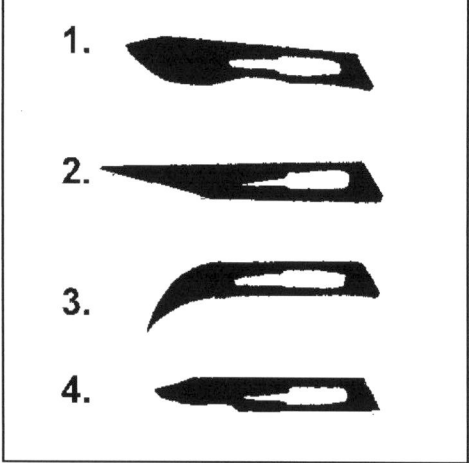

Common Scalpel blades

Needles

73. All vascular needles and catheters are fitted with _____ connectors as shown.
   a. Male slip luer
   b. Male luer lock
   c. Female luer lock
   d. Beveled tip

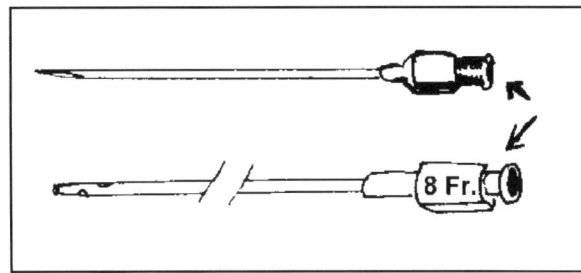
Needle and Cath luer fittings

ANSWER c. Female luer lock. Needles and catheters have FEMALE luer connectors. They mate with the male luer lock ends of syringes and stopcocks. Luer was a little-old German instrument maker. The Luer taper allows an air-tight seal between the syringe and needle, and easy connect/disconnect.
See: Co. literature and Tilkian, chapter on "Tools for Catheterization." **Keywords:** Needles have female LL connectors

74. The standard arterial Seldinger needle diameter that just admits a .038" guide-wire is:
   a. 20T gauge
   b. 18T gauge
   c. 5 French thin wall
   d. 7 French thin wall

ANSWER b. 18 gauge. Thin walled needles are the standard vascular needles. They will admit .032, .035, and .038 inch guide-wires. Micropuncture kits use a 21 gauge needle.
See: Tilkian, chapter on "Tools for Catheterization." **Keywords:** standard arterial needle = 18 T

75. What are the standard equipment sizes of micropuncture introducer sets?
   a. 18-gauge needle, .035 inch wire
   b. 18-gauge needle, .018 inch wire
   c. 21-gauge needle, .024 inch wire
   d. 21-gauge needle, .018 inch wire

ANSWER d. 21-gauge needle, .018 inch wire. Company literature says: "The micropuncture introducer set is used for placement of .035 or .038 inch diameter wire guide wires into the Vascular system when a small

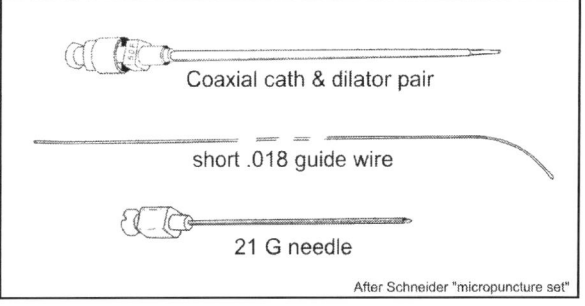
Micropuncture introducer set

21-gauge needle stick is desired. After initial access and placement of the .018 inch diameter Torq-Flex (40 cm long) wire guide, the coaxial catheter pair is introduced.

Removal of the inner dilator and wire guide facilitates placement of the .035 or .038 inch diameter wire guide through the outer catheter."

Once the micropuncture coaxial catheter is placed a larger guidewire and dilator/sheath maybe put in. Introducer sets are available for 4, 5, 6 & 7 F catheters. It is most commonly used in pediatric cases and known peripheral artery disease. There is purported to be a reduction in bleeding complications with the smaller needle puncture and smaller catheter. It is placed like any sheath, except the size of the instruments (needle, wire & sheath) are smaller.
See: www.cookmedical.com Co. literature and Schneider, chapter on "Percutaneous Vascular Access". **KEYWORDS:** Micropuncture

76. **Which needle size would be SMALLEST and least traumatic to inject local subcutaneous anesthetic beneath the skin (wheal) before deep infiltration with xylocaine and arterial puncture?**
    a. 16 gauge
    b. 25 gauge
    c. .025 inch
    d. .038 inch

ANSWER b. 25 gauge diameter needles are the smallest we usually use in the Cath lab (.020"). 16 gauge is about the largest we ever use (.065"). The larger the gauge the smaller the needle diameter. Note this is an INVERSE relation. Stubs developed the "Stubs" gauging system for electrical wire that is still used commercially for wire and metal tubing. **See:** Tilkian, chapter on "Tools for Catheterization." **Keywords:** needle size - smallest = 25

77. **What system uses a Doppler probe within the needle to guide vascular access?**
    a. 2 D Ultrasound
    b. DopplerView
    c. ArterioStick
    d. SmartNeedle
    e. NeedleView

ANSWER d. SmartNeedle
www.dicardiology.com says, "The SmartNeedle Vascular Access System, by Vascular Solutions, consists of a hand-held monitor and one-time use needles designed to provide auditory ultrasound-guided access during catheterization procedures. The reusable, hand-held monitor transmits a continuous wave Doppler signal, providing continuous auditory feedback to help locate and access the artery or vein quickly. If desired, the monitor can be covered with a disposable sterile bag for use in the sterile field.
Sterile, single-use needles range from 18G to 24G, with bare tip and sheathed IV options. Bare-tipped needles are available in 18G, 20G and 22G sizes, and consist of a detachable

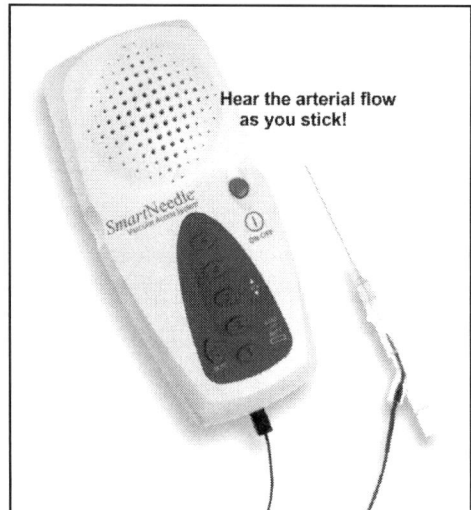
Doppler from tip of needle

Doppler probe that is housed within the lumen of a standard sized introducer needle. IV sheathed needles, used when attempting to access a vessel with the intent of leaving a small catheter in place, are available in 20G, 22G, 24G and 26G sizes." For more information: www.vascularsolutions.com

78. **Which type of IV cannulation system is labeled at #1 on the diagram. It is now rarely used because it may accidentally shear off the catheter which could then embolize into the vein?**
    a. Catheter over needle
    b. Catheter through needle
    c. Catheter over guide wire
    d. Sheath and dilator over wire

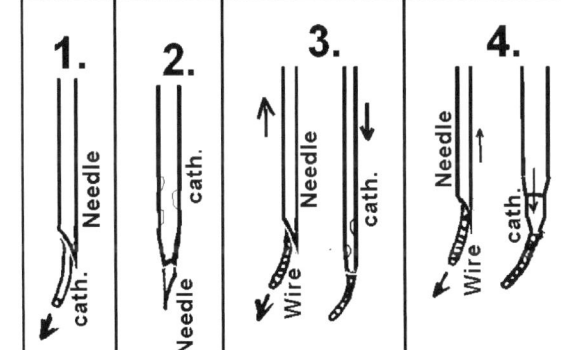

Catheter/needle combinations

ANSWER b. Catheter through needle.
Be able to match all answers below.
MATCH ALL CORRECT ANSWERS BELOW:
   1. **Catheter through needle**: The older Intra-cath was a method of IV access now rarely used because of the risk of cutting the catheter with the sharp needle tip. Many law suits resulted from catheters cut and lost in the patient's vascular system.
   2. **Catheter over needle**: This is the commonly used "Angiocath." It is used for most arterial line and IVs.
   3. **Catheter over guide wire**: This is the Seldinger technique commonly used in vascular catheterization labs. **No sheath is used.**
   4. **Sheath and dilator over wire**: This is the preferred method when frequent catheter exchanges are made with larger catheters. Now commonly used in cardiac catheterization.
   See: ACLS chapter of IV access

79. **The nurse inserted an IV in a hand vein with no blood return. She then reinserted the needle into the sheath. She then withdrew the needle and sheath. It looked like this. What went wrong?**
    a. She should have inserted a guidewire first
    b. Embolization of sheath fragment
    c. Defective sheath from manufacturer
    d. Reinsertion of needle punctured the sheath

ANSWER d. Reinsertion of needle punctured the sheath. The plastic catheter is punctured and almost sheared off. If this happens in the vein it may potentially embolize and travel proximally in the circulation. This sequence of events occurs when the needle is withdrawn from the catheter and then reinserted. Therefore, once the needle is removed it should never be reinserted. Catheter embolism carries a high complication rate, and fluoroscopic catheterization and retrieval of the foreign body is usually recommended.

SHEATHS

80. What is the minimum size of the sheath that will just allow passage of a 7 French catheter?
a. 7 F.
b. 8 F.
c. .038"
d. .045"

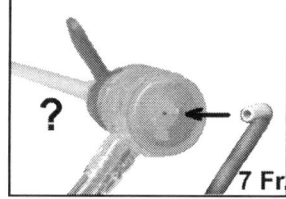
Sheath & 7F catheter

ANSWER a. 7 French. Sheaths are numbered by the size of a catheter they will admit. E.g., A 6 French sheath will admit a 6 Fr. cath of 2.0 mm. Outside Diameter (OD). A very small clearance (.05-.1 mm) is allowed between the sheath ID and the catheter OD. The sheath will have an Inside Diameter (ID) of approximately 2.1 (0.1 mm of play) but an OD of 2.33 mm (7.5 French). Note: OD= Outside Diameter; ID = Inside Diameter.
See: Co. catalog. **Keywords:** 7 Fr. pigtail → 7 Fr. sheath

81. Sheaths for doing interventions on the contralateral leg, by going "up-and-over" the aortic bifurcation, are the:
a. Raabe or Mullin's reinforced introducer sheaths
b. Radifocus or GlideSheath introducer sheaths
c. Balkin or Destination curved introducer sheaths
d. Input or ArrowFlex 90 degree introducer sheaths

ANSWER c. Balkin or Destination introducer sheath with a generous curve like a hockey stick or RDC bend. These sheaths are designed to go up-and-over the iliac bifurcation into the contralateral femoral artery. They are commonly used for lower extremity interventions.

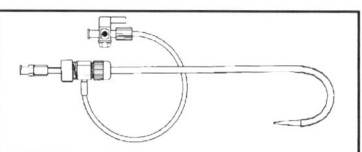
Curved "up-and-over" sheath

Once angiography is performed to assess a lesion a curved sheath is advanced retrograde to the bifurcation, where the curved sheath directs the wire and interventional catheter antegrade down the contralateral Femoral artery as shown. The Cook "Ansel" is another curved sheath. The Raabe reinforced sheath is a straight long sheath unsuitable for going up and over the iliac bifurcation. The Mullin's sheath is specific to the transseptal technique.
See: Co. literature **Keywords:** Balkin curved contralateral sheath

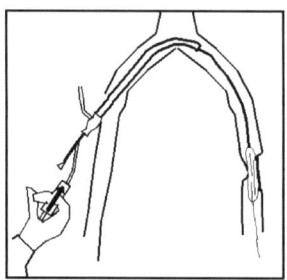
Femoral angioplasty contralateral sheath

82. You plan on doing a vascular intervention on a patient who has had multiple catheterizations and has a scarred groin. You have a .035 guidewire in the RFA, but you are having trouble advancing the 6F, 90 cm long sheath into the artery. What should you do?
   a. Predilate the site with an angioplasty balloon
   b. Use scalpel and hemostat to enlarge the puncture site
   c. Use a series of dilators to predilate the entry site to 7F
   d. Use a 6F sheath that is braid reinforced
   d. Force the 6F dilator and sheath through the scar tissue with a rotating motion

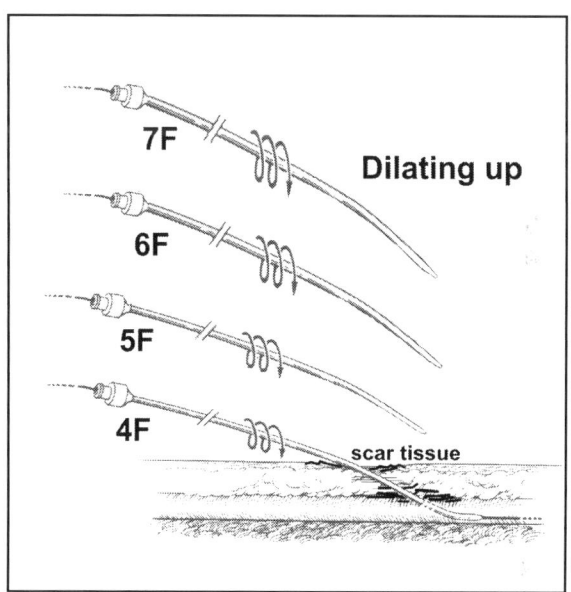

Progressive dilation of arterial access site

ANSWER c. Use 4, 5, 6 & 7 French dilators to enlarge the puncture site. Remember sheaths outside diameters are larger than the inside diameter. A 6F sheath which admits a 6F catheter, has an outside diameter of approximately 7F. Schneider says: "When planning sheath placement through a difficult entry site (e.g., a scarred groin or a previously placed bypass graft), a series of vascular dilators should be used to predilate the entry site to one French size larger than the label on the sheath. This eases placement and helps prevent a buckle at the tip of the sheath that can damage the arteriotomy site and unnecessarily enlarge it." Although rotating the sheath in helps, forcing the sheath through may damage the tip of the sheath and the arterial wall. Using a scalpel and hemostat helps enlarge the skin wound, but not the scarred artery.
See: Schneider, chapter on "Access for Endovascular Therapy" P 190

83. Arterial sheaths on heparinized patients should be meticulously aspirated and flushed immediately after insertion and _____ .
   a. Every 1-2 minutes thereafter
   b. Whenever the ACT falls below 120 sec.
   c. Aspirated and flushed after each catheter is removed.
   d. Flush continuously with continuous flow device infusing flush at 10-20 ml/min

Answer: c. Aspirated and flushed after each catheter is removed. Kern says, "The sheath should be aspirated and flushed after each catheter is removed." Whenever you remove a catheter the sheath can strip off thrombus adherent to the catheter wall. By aspirating you remove any thrombus remaining in the sheath. Discard this bloody fluid. Then flush with heparinized saline to clear blood from the sheath. It heparinizes and lubricates the sheath for the next catheter insertion.

A sheath can clot if blood is allowed to stagnate in it. Periodic flushing is recommended every 5 minutes or more frequently if clots are seen in the aspirant.

Grossman recommends a continuous flow device at 30 ml/hour [0.5 ml/min] on the arterial sheath. He recommends power flushing with this device after any new catheter is introduced or removed.

STOPCOCKS

84. Which port of the 3-way plastic stopcock shown is usually attached directly to the catheter or needle?
a. 1
b. 2
c. 3
d. Either 2 or 3

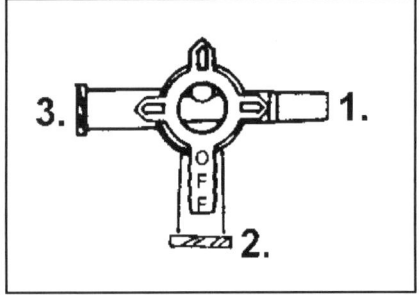
Stopcock connections

ANSWER a. #1 The male-end mates with the female needle or catheter hub. All the females are alike, and can mate with any male. But there are various types of males: Luer slip, Luer Lock, and Linden fittings. Thus is the sex-life of a stopcock!
See: Co. catalogs **Keywords:** needle connects to male stopcock port

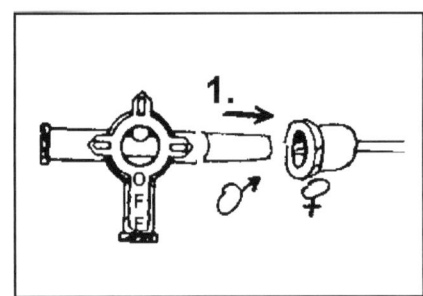
Stopcock connections

85. In this plastic "Handle-OFF" stopcock manifold, when saline is injected into the port #4 as shown on the diagram, where will the saline EXIT?
a. #1
b. #2
c. #3
d. No-where (turned off).

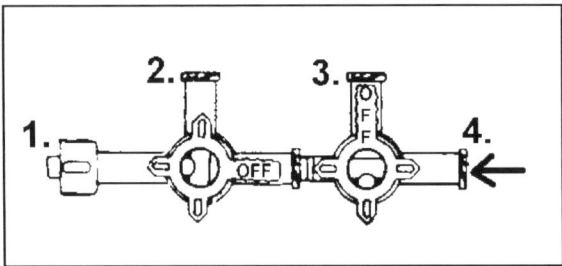
Handle-OFF stopcock manifold

ANSWER d. No-where (turned off). Saline is blocked by the distal stopcock. In "handle-OFF" stopcocks wherever the handle points no fluid can pass. These stopcocks usually have "OFF" written on the handle. They are more common than the "handle-ON" stopcocks that usually have an arrow drawn on the handle. Normally, stopcock keys are limited to 180 degrees of rotation. This makes it impossible to connect all 3 ports together, which would be in effect a Y adapter. In this manifold Ports #1 and #2 are also open together as indicated by the arrows drawn on the handle.

D2.: DIAGNOSTIC TECHNIQUES: Cath. Equipment: Other   49

See: Company literature **Keywords:** Handle-OFF stopcock positions
Keywords: "handle-off" stopcock positions

86. What type of 3-way stopcock is labeled #2 in the drawing? (Note LL = Luer Lock)
- a. Male slip,   Handle-off
- b. Male slip,   Handle-ON
- c. Male LL,   Handle-OFF
- d. Male LL,   Handle-on

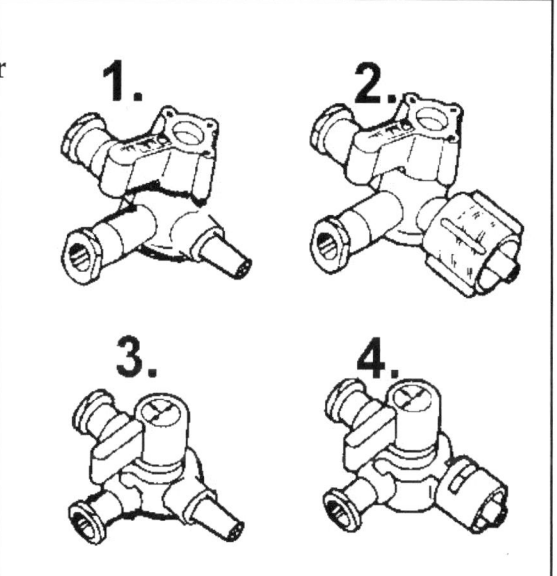

Types of 3 way stopcocks

ANSWER c. Male LL, Handle-OFF.
MATCHED ANSWERS ARE:
1. **MALE SLIP, Handle-OFF:** The male slip adapters slide into a female without rotation. They pull apart easily and are thus seldom used in catheter/manifold connections. Handle-OFF stopcocks are used most commonly because they are simple. The handle has an "OFF" printed on it. Wherever the handle is turned, that port is OFF. The other 2 ports are connected.
2. **MALE LL, Handle-OFF:** In Male LL, a locking mechanism surrounds the male element. These male adapters require ½ turn to make the connection secure. These are commonly used in vascular labs to prevent accidental disconnection and leaks. Handle-OFF stopcocks are used most commonly because they are simple. The handle has an "OFF" printed on it. Wherever the handle is turned, that port is OFF. The other 2 ports are joined.
3. **MALE SLIP, HANDLE-ON:** The male slip adapters slide into a female without rotation. Handle-ON stopcocks usually have an arrow marked on the handle to show that they drill a hole through the key parallel to the handle. These markings are the key to understanding where flow is directed.
4. **MALE LL, HANDLE-ON:** The luer LOCK requires ½ turn to make the connection secure. Handle-ON stopcocks usually have an arrow marked on the handle to show that they drill a hole through the key parallel to the handle. Most metal reusable stopcocks are of this variety.

See: Co. literature **Keywords:** types of 3-way stopcocks handle-ON/off, Slip/LL

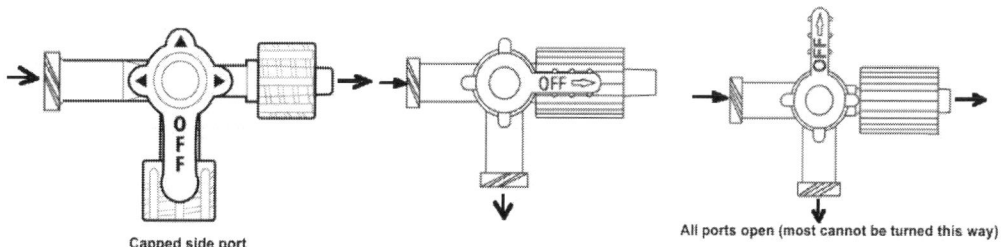

Capped side port   All ports open (most cannot be turned this way)

87. What type of male stopcock adapter is labeled at #5 on the diagram?
a. Luer slip
b. Luer lock
c. Linden fitting
d. Swivel collar luer lock
e. Rotating adapter

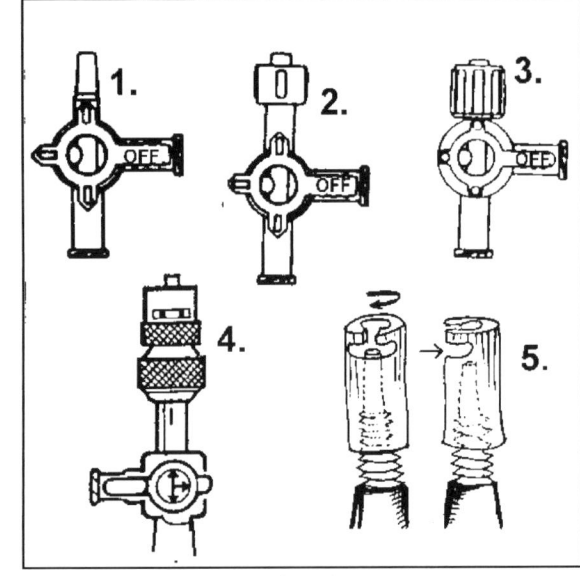

Types Male adapters

ANSWER c. Linden fitting. **CORRECTLY MATCHED ANSWERS ARE:**
1. **LUER SLIP**: a simple male luer fitting which can "mate" with any female
2. **LUER LOCK:** a male tapered fitting that must be screwed on ½ turn to lock it into the female.
3. **SWIVEL LUER LOCK:** This fitting over male luer ports allows you to tighten the luer lock down without turning the whole stopcock. The locking mechanism turns. This allows you to align other stopcocks and adapters in one plane for easier manipulation.
4. **ROTATING ADAPTER:** This is another male fitting usually found on catheter manifolds. It has a luer lock connector, but can swivel 360 degrees to allow catheter torquing.
5. **LINDEN FITTING:** This is the most secure fitting. Because the "Linden fitting" is so secure and tight it is usually used on pressure injector syringes. But, it is tricky to mate the female onto the male. It must be opened enough for the slot in the side to clear the male luer inside. Then the female is slipped into the slot sideways. Once in, screw the Linden fitting down 4-8 turns until the female is secured.
See: Grossman, chapter on "Percutaneous Approach." **Keywords:** Male fittings Linden fitting

88. On the plastic 2-stopcock coronary-catheter manifold-system shown, what stopcock port should be connected to the pressure transducer?
a. #1.-Distal, rotating adapter
b. #2.-Distal, side-arm.
c. #3.-Proximal side-arm
d. #4.-Proximal end female adapter

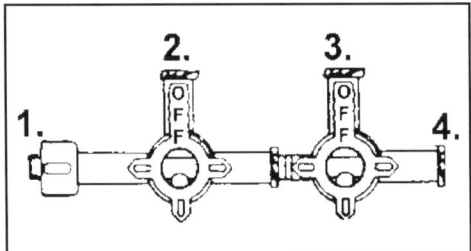

Coronary Manifold

ANSWER b. #2 Distal, side-arm.
CORRECTLY MATCHED ANSWERS ARE:
1. Distal, rotating adapter (catheter)
2. Distal, side-arm (Pressure)
3. Proximal side-arm (contrast)
4. Proximal end female adapter (syringe)

The pressure transducer should be closest to the catheter to monitor arterial pressure. Then the more proximal stopcocks can be used for filling the syringe and other manipulations without affecting pressure. When angiographic injections occur, of course, the pressure monitoring port must be turned off. At all other times aortic pressure should be monitored.
See: Grossman, Cardiac Cath, Angiography..., chapter on "Percutaneous Approach." **Keywords:** pressure monitoring stopcock → most distal side-arm

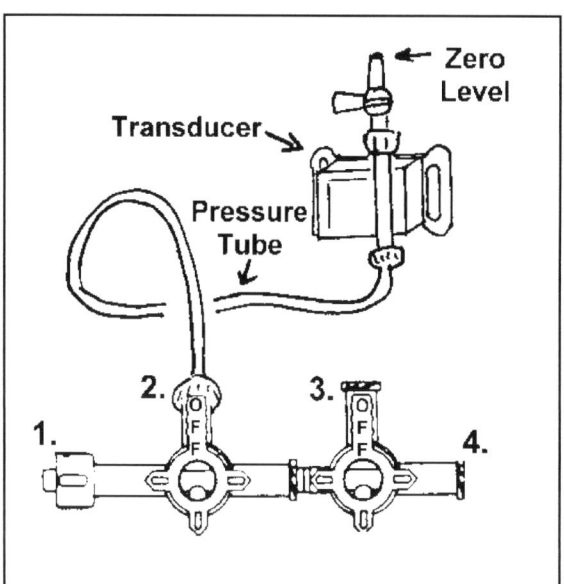

Manifold, Off-table Transducer

89. In the 3-way stopcock turned 45° as shown, which ports are open?
a. 1 & 2
b. 2 & 3
c. 1 & 3
d. None, all blocked off

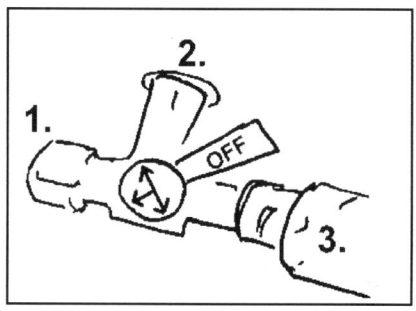

3 way stopcock opening

ANSWER d. None, all blocked off. Sometimes a new system is confusing. Sometimes, blood spurts all over, and the Dr. yells at you. PANIC! You need a minute to figure things out. When in doubt, turn the key 45° (panic position) and all 3 ports will be blocked off as shown.

The normal 3 positions of a 3-way stopcock will connect any 2 ports together. Normally, all 3 ports cannot be opened at once (creating a Y or T).
See: Co. catalogs **Keywords:** male LL, handle-OFF stopcock

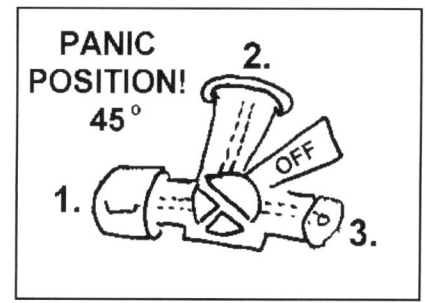

3 way stopcock opening

90. A PA catheter is connected to a "handle-ON" stopcock. What will happen when the stopcock handle is turned to position #1 as shown in the diagram?
a. Blood will drip out the side-arm
b. All ports are open
c. You can draw-back blood or flush the catheter with the attached syringe
d. The blood is blocked OFF and the syringe is connected to the side-arm

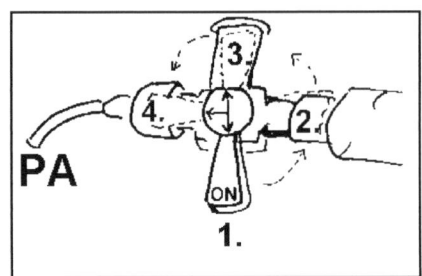
Stopcock positions

ANSWER a. Blood will drip out the side-arm.
In the "handle-ON" stopcocks they drill a hole through the key <u>parallel</u> to the handle. They drill one other hole half way through to form a "T" within the key.
CORRECTLY MATCHED ANSWERS ARE:
  1. **BLOOD WILL DRIP OUT THE SIDE-ARM:** As shown in diagram

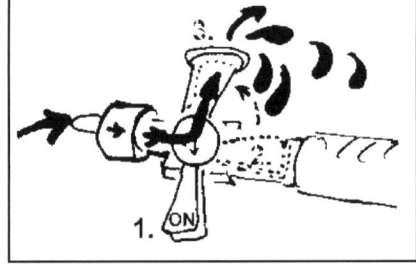
Stopcock positions

  2. **YOU CAN DRAW BACK BLOOD OR FLUSH THE CATHETER WITH THE ATTACHED SYRINGE:** When the handle is turned in the direction of the syringe - the catheter and syringe are connected.
  3. **THE BLOOD IS BLOCKED OFF AND THE SYRINGE IS CONNECTED TO THE SIDE-ARM:** With the handle up the syringe and side-port are connected.
  4. **ALL PORTS ARE OPEN:** If the handle is forcibly turned toward the catheter (not recommended), all ports would be open. This effectively turns the stopcock into a T or Y adapter.
See: company literature   Keywords: Handle-ON stopcock positions

91. The catheterizing radiologist has just placed a Cobra catheter in the aorta. He has his thumb over the catheter hub to prevent bleeding. He asks for a "handle-off" stopcock. In general, how should the handle be turned before handing it to him?
a. Position #1
b. Position #2
c. Position #3
d. Position #4

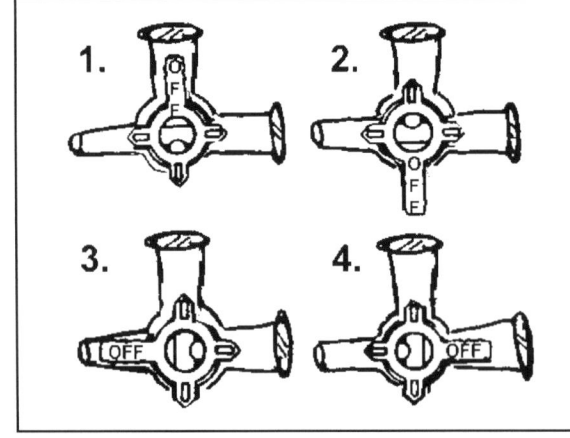
Key positions 3-way Stopcocks

ANSWER c. #3. Handle toward catheter.
   When the physician puts the stopcock on he will want it turned OFF to prevent more bleeding. Of course, he can do this, but his hand may be busy holding the catheter hub. Generally the assistant should hand all stopcocks and sheaths to the physician with the stopcock turned off. This will prevent blood from leaking back accidentally causing an

embarrassing "bleed on the Dr's. shoe. OH NO!"
- **#1.** - distal and proximal port open.
- **#2.** - All port open. Stops are normally built into stopcocks to make it impossible to turn it to position #2. However, plastic stopcocks can be easily stripped out and forced to turn 360 degrees. When forced into this position #2, the stopcock becomes a "T" or "Y" adapter - all ports are open.
- **#3.** -Two female ports open. Male closed off.
- **#4.** -Distal male port and side-arm open.

Note that on this stopcock the handle or key has small arrows showing the open ports. The handle is marked "OFF," so wherever the handle is turned that port is OFF.

See: Personal experience **Keywords:** Turn OFF stopcocks

92. **This rotating Y adapter used in angioplasty is termed a:**
    a. Hemostasis valve
    b. 3-way manifold
    c. Dotter "Y" adapter
    d. Tuohy-Borst adapter

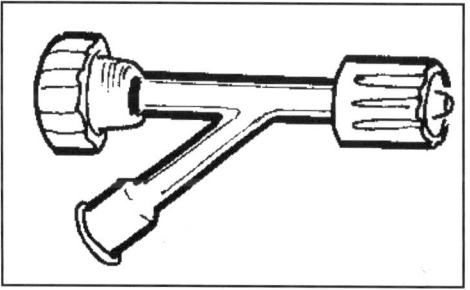

Rotating Y adapter

ANSWER d. Tuohy-Borst adapter. This Y adapter was developed by Tuohy and Borst to allow double access to a catheter. Screwing down the proximal "O-ring" gradually compresses the "O-ring" and closes off flow around the inserted catheter, as shown in this diagram. Note how when tightened, it compresses the O-ring washer around the balloon catheter or whatever is within the Tuohy's lumen. If you screw it down too tight you will constrict the balloon lumen and slow deflation time - dangerous!

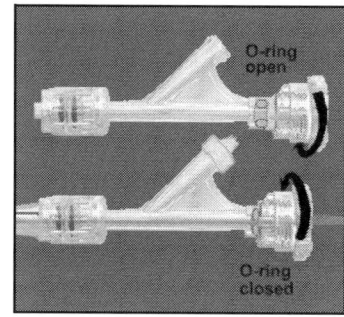

Tightening down a Tuohy-Borst "Y" adapter prevents bleedback

These are normally used in Angioplasty, where a balloon catheter is introduced straight into the "through" port of the Tuohy-Borst and into the guider catheter. The sidearm port is used to flush, inject dye, and measure orifice pressure through the guider catheter.

Some companies are making spring loaded Y-adapters which prevent bleed-back and hold constant tension without too tightly compressing the dilation catheter.

See: Co. Literature **Keywords:** Tuohy-Borst adapter

93. **Long-term Swan-Ganz and arterial lines should be connected to a continuous flush device which at 300 mmHg infusion pressure will deliver approximately:**
    a. 1-2 ml flush/min
    b. 5-10 ml flush/min
    c. 3-8 ml flush/hour
    d. 20-40 ml flush/hour

54 ◂◂ D2.: DIAGNOSTIC TECHNIQUES: Cath. Equipment: Other ▸▸

ANSWER c. 3-8 ml flush/hour. These continuous flush devices have made extended hemodynamic monitoring possible. At this low flow rate catheters can be kept open while simultaneously measuring pressure through the transducer. The pressure increase due to this slow infusion is negligible in most catheters.
See: Daily, Bedside Hemodynamic Monitoring, chapter on "Arterial Pressure Monitoring."

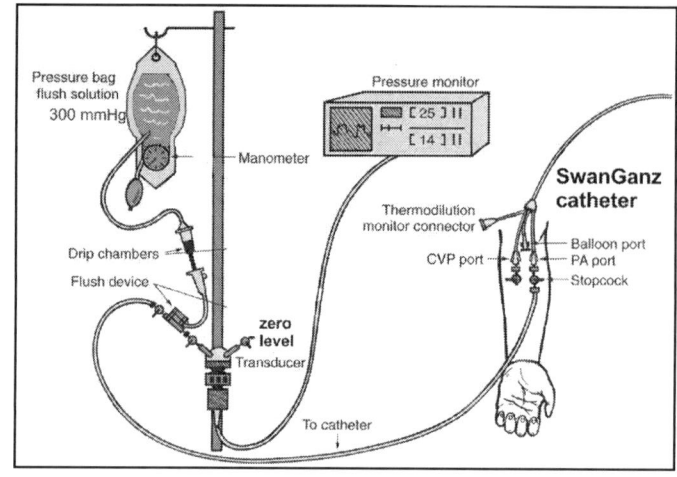

94. In this stopcock maze if saline is injected into port labeled #1 it will exit a port # ___.
a. 1
b. 2
c. 3
d. 4
e. 5
f. 6
g. 7
h. 8
i. 9
j. 10
k. 11

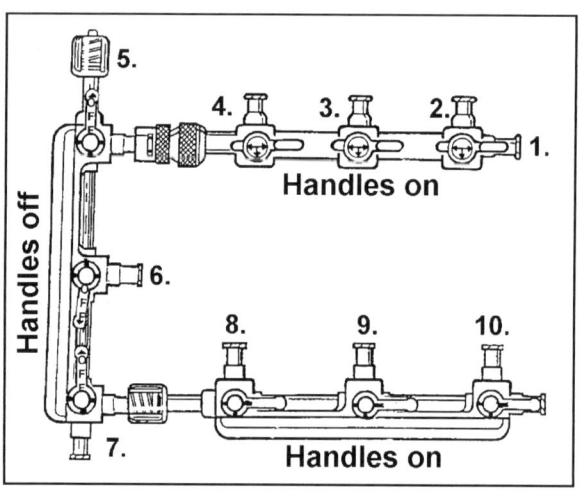

Three gang (handle-off & ON) Stopcock Maze

ANSWER f. #6 is the exit point. First the
flush enters and passes the open handle-on 3-manifold or 3-gang stopcocks.
then it makes the corner at the handle-off manifold and is directed out the side-arm of the center stopcock #6.

Besides ports 1-6 and 7-11 all other ports of this assembly are closed. Practice turning the various handles and figure out passages through this maze. It's fun to try this with a real manifold maze and friend who doesn't mind getting squirted. Note the mixture of handle-OFF and handle-ON stopcocks.
See: personal experience. SCC lab ICT 134. **Keywords:** Stopcock maze

95. This 3 way coronary stopcock manifold:
   a. Is set up for a waste bag
   b. Utilizes 4 one way stopcocks
   c. Measures pressure at the manifold
   d. Is connected to a continuous flow device

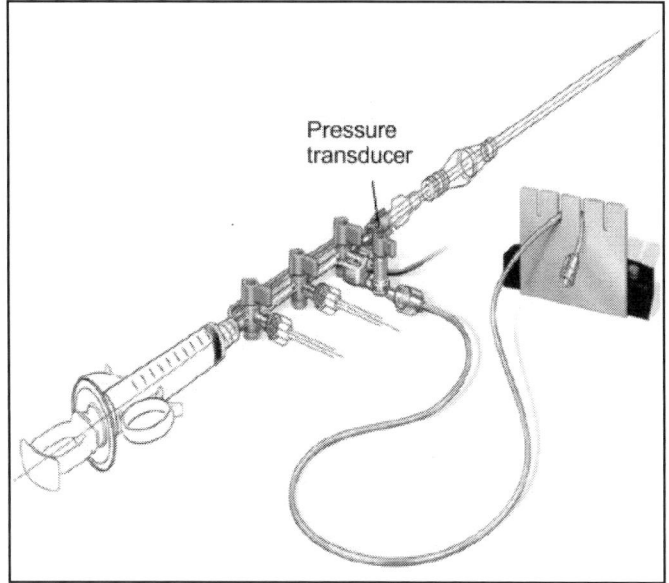

Stopcock manifold - after Namic with permission

ANSWER. c. Measures pressure at the manifold with a transducer built into the 1st stopcock position. This eliminates the problem of resonance in long pressure tubes and improves the fidelity of pressure measurement. The long tube attached to the transducer is not required but can be used for off-the-table zeroes, so the operator can connect to zero and flush out bubbles at any time. Zero level is at tip of the long tube, off the table, so manifold does not need to be at heart level. See: http://www.navilystmedical.com

GUIDE-WIRES

96. Identify the type of guide-wire labeled #1 in the diagram.
   a. Movable-core stainless steel guidewire
   b. Fixed-core stainless steel guidewire
   c. Nitinol hydrophilic guidewire
   d. Steerable stainless steel PTFE coated form-able tip mandrel guidewire

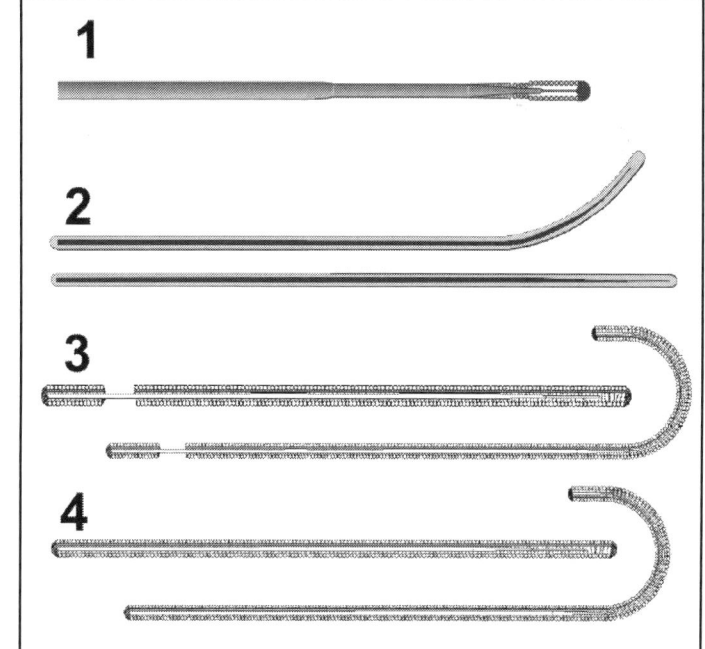

Types of Guide wires

ANSWER d. (diagram #1) Steerable stainless steel PTFE coated form-able conventional steerable stainless steel taper mandrel guidewire. Most common interventional tracking wire. Other wires shown are:
   2. Nitinol core hydrophilic coated guidewire. Curved and straight tip, parabolic tip which cannot be formed by the operator. Great torque control and slipperiness (Terumo GlideWire)

3. **Movable-core stainless steel guidewire.** Straight and J wire. Floppy tip area can be increased by pulling the movable core. Its increased floppiness is useful for crossing the valve in AS, but dangerous when the core is fully inserted. In many movable core wires the mandrel is coated with Teflon to facilitate easy sliding of the core within the spring.

4. **Fixed-core stainless steel guidewire.** Straight and J wire. Most commonly used diagnostic wire.

See: Lanzer, P., Mastering Endovascular Techniques, chapter on "Coronary Arteries"

97. Guide-wire diameters are usually measured in:
a. mm.
b. cm.
c. Hundredths of inches
d. Thousandths of inches
e. Gauge

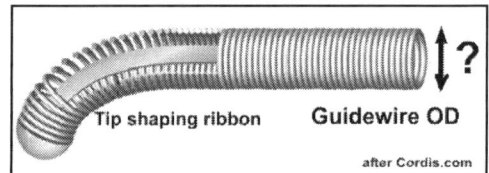
Guidewire Outside Diameter

ANSWER d. Thousandths of inches = .001". Most companies measure guide-wire diameter in thousand's of inches. A .038" guide-wire is approximately 1.0 mm in diameter. To convert from inches into mm. multiply by 25.4 mm/inch. The standard .038" guide will pass an 18T gauge needle with an inner diameter of .042".
See: Tilkian, chapter on "Tools for Catheterization." **Keywords:** Measure GW diameters in thousandths of inches

98. It is occasionally difficult to cross the aortic valve in patients with severe aortic stenosis. In general what is the LONGEST AMOUNT OF TIME a standard diagnostic guide wire should be used in the body before it is removed and carefully wiped with a heparinized gauze?
a. 3 min
b. 10 min
c. 20 min
d. No limit

ANSWER a. 3 min. Kern recommends that diagnostic guide wires be removed and wiped every 3 minutes to reduce the chance of clot formation on the wire. This is especially recommended in unheparinized patients, and in critical procedures, like crossing the aortic valve in AS. In AS the wire is in a critical area (Ascending AO) and is heavily manipulated for long periods. Some labs start a stopwatch to time the wire manipulation time for 3 minutes before removing and wiping it with a heparinized gauze. However, smaller diameter coated PTCA tracking wires are left in for much longer periods with few complications. **See:** Kern, chapter on "Hemodynamic Data." **Keywords:** reduced wire manipulation time < 3 min.

99. Which guide-wire becomes slippery (lubricous) when wet? It has a "nitinol" spring steel core in a polyurethane jacket with a special coating.
   a. Hydrophilic "Glidewire"
   b. Cook BH coated wires
   c. Hydrophobic (Silicone) coated wires
   d. Teflon (PTFE) coated wires

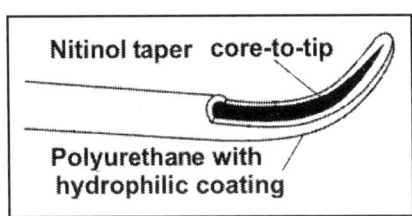

Terumo Glide-wire

ANSWER a. The Terumo hydrophilic glide-wire wire is covered with a tungsten impregnated Polyurethane plastic. Then it is coated with a hydrophilic polymer. (Hydrophilic means it attracts and absorbs water.) Instead of a wire coil this wire's body derives from one strand of a tapered elastic spring Nickel-steel alloy. It has excellent memory, torquability, and is less traumatic due to its smooth surface.

The "Glidewire" may be so "slimy" that the operator may be unable to manipulate it. A damp sponge, pin-vise or turning tool may provide a better grip. It needs to be stored moist in it's hoop. The "Glide-wire" is available in various lengths, diameters, bends, core tapers, core stiffness and with a gold tip. Many companies now use these materials. **See:** Co. product literature **Keywords:** "Glide-wire" → Glide (Terumo) wire

100. Which guide-wire is most kink-resistant?
   a. Braided stainless steel wires
   b. Coiled stainless steel wires
   c. Hypo-tube and safety ribbon wires
   d. Nitinol core-to-tip wires

ANSWER d. Nitinol core-to-tip wires use this very springy steel throughout, from proximal to distal tip. Freed says: "Guidewires with nitinol cores are virtually kink-resistant, while those with stainless steel cores are more susceptible to kinking." Once a guidewires becomes kinked it can hang-up on the catheter hub and lose it's 1 to 1 torque response. It should be replaced. Stainless steel coiled and hypo-tube wires kink easily.
See: Freed, Chapter on PTCA Equipment

101. Many small diameter PCI guide-wires incorporate PLATINUM or GOLD metal within the spring tip to increase their:
   a. Torquability
   b. Trackability
   c. Radiolucence
   d. Radiopacity

ANSWER d. Radiopacity. Many coronary PCI tracking wires are so fine that they are difficult to visualize under fluoroscopy. Although very expensive, platinum metal is more radiopaque than stainless steel. It absorbs more X-rays to cast a more visible fluoro shadow. Some labs recycle these platinum tips. Incorrect answer, "Radiolucence" means it is invisible

on X-ray - that X-rays pass through it, just like glass is "translucent" to light.
See: Johnsrude, chapter on "Equipment." **Keywords:** Platinum GW tip → more radiopaque

102. The ability of a guidewire to been seen under fluoroscopy is usually improved by:
  a. Increasing X-ray KV
  b. Using nitinol core construction
  c. Using core-to-tip construction
  d. Adding precious metal to the tip

Answer: d. Adding precious metal to the tip increases radio-opacity by absorbing more X radiation. Thin stainless steel mandrel wires are barely visible on fluoro. Heavy or precious metals are added to the tip of most guidewires to increase tip visibility. Metals like gold, platinum, or tungsten are incorporated into most guidewire tips.

103. Generally, stiff guidewires should be placed:
  a. After the catheter is positioned with a floppy tip wire
  b. As the 1st wire whenever increased backup support or trackability is anticipated
  c. When stent placement is anticipated
  d. To start a TAVR procedure

ANSWER a. After the catheter is positioned with a floppy wire. Davies says: "It is generally easier to track a catheter or device over a stiffer guidewire; however, a very stiff guidewire may be more difficult to manipulate into a vessel origin or through a diseased vessel. Exchanging wires is often necessary for different parts of a procedure, but a stiff wire should always be placed through a catheter that has been positioned using a more conventional wire to prevent damage to the vessel during advancement of the stiff wire." See: Davies & Brophy, Vascular Surgery, Chapter on "Endovascular Approaches and Techniques" Published by Springer, 2005

104. What type of guidewire is used to straighten tortuous coronary vessels and provide a platform for advancing stents in calcified arteries. They are stiff in the distal region 2-15 cm from the tip, but have a tapered flexible 1-2 cm tip?
  a. Stiff wire
  b. Floppy tip wire
  c. Backup wire
  d. Support wire
  e. TCO wire

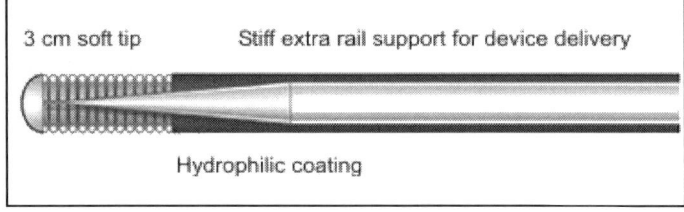

Boston Sci. Mailman guidewire

ANSWER d. Support wire.
   Holmes says: "The thickness of the core at the tip of the guidewire determines whether a wire is soft or stiff; the thicker the core, the stiffer the wire. Stiff wires transmit torque better than soft guidewires and provide excellent crossability in complex lesions and chronic total occlusions. ...The disadvantage of

stiff guidewires is an increased risk of wire perforations. A soft guidewire is often the first wire used because it provides good tip control with little risk of injury to the arterial wall. Support guidewires should not be confused with stiff guidewires. Guidewire support is determined by the thickness of the core in the working segment of the wire, from 2 to 15 cm. Support guidewires are often constructed with a soft, atraumatic tip so that significant tapering of the core occurs in the last 2 cm of the wire. However, unlike stiff guidewires, support wires have a significant core tapering at the tip, from 1 to 2 cm. This abrupt transition causes the guidewire to prolapse when attempts are made to cannulate severely angled bifurcations. Support wires are usually placed through an over-the-wire balloon or transfer catheter after first crossing the lesion with anther wire. Supportive guidewires are ideal for straightening tortuous vessels and for providing a platform for pushing stents in calcified arteries."

See: Homes & Verghese, chapter on "Equipment Selection and Techniques of Percutaneous Coronary Intervention"

105. The core of a wrapped guide wire is termed its:
 a. Co-axial trocar
 b. Movable handle
 c. Mandrel
 d. Stylus

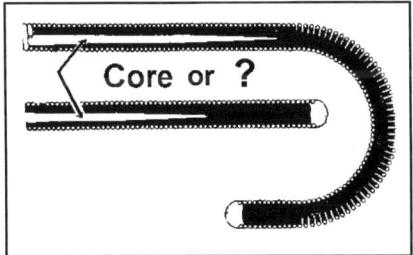
Guidewire Core

ANSWER c. Mandrel. The core or mandrel provides the body and stiffness of a guide wire. A "mandrel" is a spindle or support around which something is bent - in this case the coiled spring wire. Mandrel cores are usually tapered at the distal end to make a smooth transition between stiff and floppy. The tapers may be short (ST), or long (LT), or very long (LLT). The cores are usually fixed, but may be movable. If the mandrel ends before reaching the tip of the wire coil, it is a very floppy tip.
See: Co. Literature Keywords: guidewire mandrel

106. Angioplasty wires with a spring coil mounted on a flexible stainless steel shaft as shown are termed:
 a. Solid core wires
 b. Support wires
 c. HI-torque wires
 d. Mandrel wires
 e. Glide wires

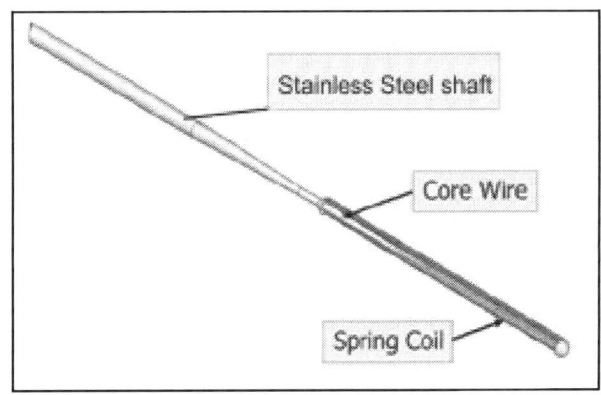

Answer: d. Mandrel wires are the 0.014" - 0.018" angioplasty wires with a long flexible stainless steel shaft with a spring coil on the end. They are available in many different shaft strengths and many different types of coils, bends, and coatings. They are the thin wires that are advanced through balloon catheters and through the lesion to be stented. Then the balloon/stent is advanced over this wire and into to the lesion. So the tip must usually be soft and maneuverable, and the wire body must be strong enough to support delivering the balloon and stent.

FDA says, "The Mandrel wire family is made of a coated (PTFE or Silicone) or uncoated Nitinol or Stainless Steel core wire that is tapered at the distal tip where a coil is secured to the distal end. The distal coil can be anywhere from 2 cm to 30 cm depending on specific design and can consist of Stainless Steel, Palladium, Platinum, or the proposed Tungsten materials. The guidewire may contain proximal core markers."
See: https://www.accessdata.fda.gov/cdrh_docs/pdf14/K140482.pdf and Endovascular today, 2017 Buyers Guide

107. Tapered tip 0.018" tapered tip mandrel wires as shown are designed to be used on:
a. Long thrombotic occlusions
b. Acutely angled bifurcation lesions
c. Retrograde recanalization of CTOs
d. Fibrous caps on CTOs

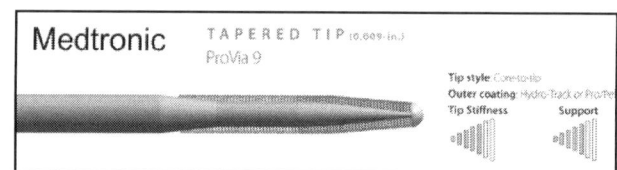

Answer d. Fibrous caps on CTOs
King says, "There are four groups, classified by purpose. The first group is the standard-use guidewire, which is used for usual PCI cases [workhorse wire]. The second group is stiff-tip wire, used especially for chronic total occlusion. **The third group is tapered-tip wire, used for chronic total occlusion. The tapered tip wire is intended to clear chronic total occlusion, especially for those cases which require penetration through a hard, fibrous cap**. The fourth group is the support wire, which is used as a support to cross devices over lesions with strong back-up force. Support wires are specific-use wires, such as a Rota-wire for Rotablator and marker wire."

108. Guidewire tip softness or flexibility is measured by:
a. Tip load in gm
b. IFR resistance in dynes
c. Ductility index
d. Aldrete Score

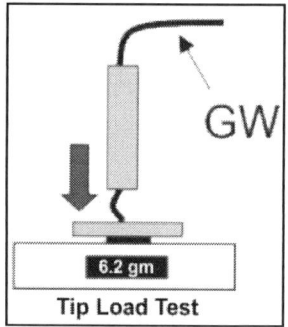

Answer a. Tip load in gm measures how flexible the tip is.
One way of quantifying some of the physical features of a coronary guidewire is by using a strain gauge to measure the force needed to bend a wire when exerted on a straight guidewire tip, at a point 1 cm from the tip. Using this method, the tip loads in ascending order are (from less stiff to more stiff) 3 gm, 4.5 gm, 6 gm, 9 gm and 12 gm (ultra stiff). As stiffness increases the wire becomes prone to perforating the vessel. Note that straight tip wires have a higher tip-load number than angled wires because the initial strain tends to compress the coil instead of bend it.

D2.: DIAGNOSTIC TECHNIQUES: Cath. Equipment: Other

109. The solid core guidewire tip construction shown with increased pushability and torquability is termed:
  a. Support wire construction
  b. Tapered tip construction
  c. Single core construction
  d. Core-to-tip construction

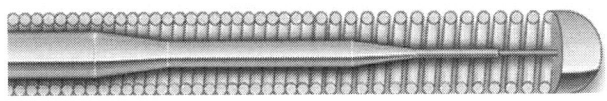

Answer: d. Core-to-tip construction has a core welded at both ends of the wire which transmits push and torque to the distal coil tip. Also termed solid-core construction. dicardiology.com says, "Core-to-tip Guidewires: When the core is extended to the tip, that increases pushability, precise steering, tip control, tactile feel and torquability. This can be a useful feature for example in probing chronic total occlusions. [Alternatively] If there is a two piece tip to the guidewire, then shaping is easy and the wire is likely to retain its shape, a property called "wire memory". See:
https://www.dicardiology.com/videos/video-basics-interventional-guidewire-design-and-function

110. To avoid damage to a plastic coated "Glidewire" be careful to NEVER:
  a. Use it with a single wall needle
  b. Use it with a metal pin-vice
  c. Pull it back through a needle
  d. Torque it excessively

ANSWER c. Pulling back these plastic wires through a needle can sever them or shave off pieces of plastic, as they are likely to catch in the needle's sharp beveled edge. They may be advanced though the needle, then the needle removed. Only then can the "Glide wire" can be manipulated back and forth. Never use a metal pin-vise - plastic or gauze is OK. Davies says: "However, a hydrophilic guidewire may not be appropriate for initial introduction because its coating may be sheared off by the end of the metallic needle if the wire is retracted (even partially). It is safer to initiate the intervention with a standard steerable, soft-tip metallic guidewire and then, following sheath introduction, exchange if for a GlideWire..."
See: Davies & Brophy, Vascular Surgery, Chapter on "Endovascular Approaches and Techniques" Published by Springer, 2005"

111. Why is the "Glidewire" resistant to kinking?
  a. Hydrophilic coating prevents excessive torquing
  b. Stiff and strong stainless steel core
  c. Nitinol core springs back to original shape
  d. No core joints or thin coiled wires

Answer c. Nitinol core springs back to original shape. The single piece core-to-tip design is made of nitinol (an elastic nickel-titanium alloy with memory). This gives it more torque control and makes the wire very steerable. The Terumo coating is slippery due to its hydrophilic coating (draws in water), not hydrophobic (repels water). Remember a

"phobia" is something you fear and push away. Terumo says, "Hydrophilic "M" polymer coating for frictionless endovascular steerability and trackability."
See: Davies & Brophy, VASCULAR Surgery, Chapter on "Endovascular Approaches and Techniques" Published by Springer, 2005

112. Which type of guide-wire is 260-300 cm long?
   a. PTCA balloon tracking guide-wire
   b. PTCA guider catheter wire
   c. Exchange guide wires
   d. Safety guide wires

ANSWER c. Exchange guide-wires are three times as long (260 - 300 cm) as a diagnostic catheter (100 cm). This length simplifies catheter exchange, but complicates handling. They are especially helpful in tortuous anatomy, where wire position may be difficult to achieve. The long wire (260 cm) is threaded down a positioned catheter. The catheter is removed, leaving the wire in place. A new catheter is threaded over the exchange wire which then tracks back to the original catheter tip position. It is like leaving a railroad "track" to slide different trains along. 145 cm diagnostic guide-wires are not long enough for this.
See: Pepine, chapter on "Equipment." **Keywords:** Exchange wire = 260 cm

113. You have had a difficult time passing a 190 cm, .014" guidewire through a tight coronary lesion, but finally are through. When you attempt to pass the monorail/RX dilation catheter (balloon) over the wire into the lesion, it is too tight to pass. Your Dr. wants to replace it with a lower profile balloon, but your lab only caries them in over-the-wire style (OTW). How can you exchange dilation catheters without removing the initial 190 cm wire from the target lesion you should: Select 2 correct answers below.
   a. Exchange the 190 cm wire for a 300 cm exchange wire
   b. Extend the 190 cm wire with an extension wire
   c. Use a fixation device to "fix" the wire to the guiding catheter.
   d. Have the assistant advance the wire completely into the hub of OTW dilation catheter (balloon), while the Dr. pulls the OTW dilation (balloon) catheter
   e. Push the guide wire out until it wedges in the distal coronary artery, then slowly pull the OTW dilation catheter (balloon) out while observing the wire on fluoro. to keep the same location

ANSWERS: b & c. An exchange wire length is needed, but it is too late to insert a 300 cm wire. A monorail system can only be inserted after the initial dilation catheter is removed. And here it cannot be removed because the wire is too short. Never pull a catheter over a wire and let the wire disappear into the hub of the catheter. You could lose it!
   b. Extend the 190 cm wire with an extension wire such as a 125-140 cm "doc" or "cinch" extension wire. This extra length added to the wire will allow you to remove the dilation catheter and leave the wire tip in place. Currently 190-135 = 55 cm wire "hanging out" - not enough to safely remove the 135 dilation catheter. Add an extension wire to add length to the short 190 cm wire available. Then you will have

enough wire to remove the OTW dilation catheter.
c. Another method is to fix the wire to the guiding catheter with a fixation device, such as the Boston "magnet" system, so it will not move during the exchange.

Kern says: "An exchange guidewire is similar to guidewires mentioned previously except that its length is 280 to 300 cm. This long wire replaces the initial wire when the exchange of an over-the-wire balloon catheter is necessary. Alternatively a 120 to 145 cm extension wire can be connected to the end of the initial guidewire to allow balloon catheter exchange.... Several guidewire fixation or exchange systems are available. One uses a special short balloon on a wire that is not long enough to leave the guide. When inflated, the balloon traps the wire inside the guide catheter, permitting the balloon catheter to be pulled off without moving the guidewire.... Another wire fixation device has a twisting wire that entraps the guidewire and fixes it while the balloon is removed....A third system has a magnet and a special guidewire, and can be used with any guide catheter and balloon system. The magnet fixes the guidewire in place while the balloon catheter is exchanged."

See: Kern, chapter on "Interventional Techniques"

114. Advancing a kinked guide-wire may cause a "dagger effect." The sharp core/mandril may poke through the spring coils making a sharp fork at the tip of the wire. The "dagger effect" is reduced by using: (*select 4 answers below*)
   a. **Safety wires or ribbons**
   b. **Small diameter "J" wire bends**
   c. **"Ball tipped" tapered core wires**
   d. **Nitinol movable core wires**
   e. **Fixed core wires**
   f. **Core-to-tip wires**

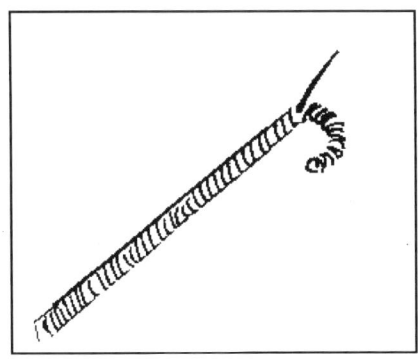
GW Dagger Effect

ANSWERS: a, c, e & f. Safety wires or ribbons and "Ball tipped" tapered core wires. The sharp core/mandril may poke through the spring coils making a dangerous sharp fork. When this happens the core should be retracted and the wire replaced. In general kinked guide-wires should not be used. They can "hang up" on the catheter, cause "dagger effect" and manipulate poorly.

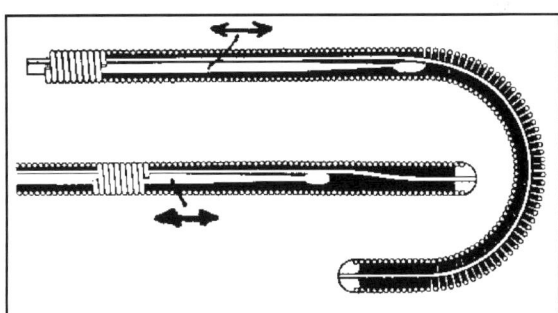
Ball-tip movable-core GW

1. YES: SAFETY WIRES OR RIBBONS: The safety wire runs the length of the coil and is welded at both ends to hold the spring together. Without it these coils would be as springy as "slinky." If a safety wire breaks the guide wire should be replaced. A kinked wire may still "dagger" and poke through the coil even with an intact safety wire.
2. NO: SMALL DIAMETER "J" WIRE BENDS: Small diameter bends are worse for the "dagger" effect because the advancing core has a tighter radius to straighten.
3. YES: "BALL TIPPED" TAPERED CORE WIRES: The ball on the tip of a tapered movable-core wire was designed to prevent a puncture of the coil. Still, this risk exits in any

movable-core wire as the movable-core is advanced into a kinked wire. Some companies use needle-point movable-core tapered wires that are dangerous!
4. NO: NITINOL MOVABLE CORE WIRES: There are no nitinol movable core wires. Nitinol cores can be sharp and pierce a coil like any other metal.
5. YES: FIXED CORE WIRES are safest because they cannot move within the coil.
6. YES: CORE-TO-TIP WIRES are also fixed within the coil, being welded to the coil at both ends. **See:** Grossman, chapter on "Percutaneous Approach" and Co. literature

115. If a spring-guide tip breaks, it may move through (embolize) into the vascular system and cause problems. Modern cardiovascular guide-wires reduce this complication by using: *(Select 2 answers below)*
a. Cores/mandrels welded to the spring every few cm.
b. Safety wires and ribbons welded at each end of spring
c. Nitinol cores
d. Nitinol coil springs
e. Core-to-tip mandrels

ANSWER b.& e. Safety wires and ribbons and e. Core-to-tip mandrels are welded at each end of spring. Without these fixes the spring coil would stretch and unravel when pulled. The safety wire holds the spring together during manipulation. These both reduce kinking and separation of the tip.

This diagram shows a fixed-core tapered safety-wires in both the "J" and straight design. Often a malleable shaping ribbon is welded from the core to tip of the spring. No "ball tip" is needed if the core does not move within the coil. Core-to-tip wires are also welded at each end of the wire and likewise hold the spring coil together.

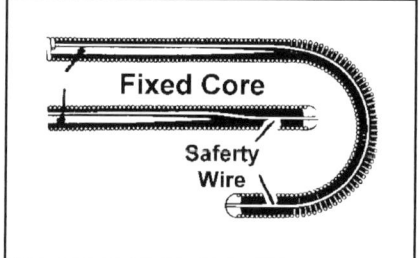

Guide-wire Safety Wire

See: Tilkian, chapter on "Tools for Catheterization." **Keywords:** Safety wire

116. What is the most common complication of guidewire handling during PCI?
a. Coronary dissection
b. Coronary perforation
c. Thrombus formation
d. Coronary spasm

ANSWER: a. Coronary dissection. King says, "Guidewire perforations are most frequent, especially when hydrophilic wires are used in complex cases. In the usual scenario, the guidewire migrates distally in a tiny branch and eventually perforates the distal tip of the branch. This complication may not be recognized until the guidewire is withdrawn. In one reported series, 20% of perforations causing pericardial tamponade were the result of guidewire perforation. Other guidewire complications include: vasospasm, pseudostenosis (wire caused kinks in vessel), and wire fracture & embolization. **See:** King, chapter on "Coronary Artery Perforation" **Keywords:** guidewire complication = dissection

D2.: DIAGNOSTIC TECHNIQUES: Cath. Equipment: Other

117. When inserting systems into a guiding catheter, how much clearance must be allowed between catheter ID and system OD?
   a. .01 - .05 mm.
   b. .08 - .10 mm.
   c. 0.10 - 0.13 mm.
   d. 0.15 - 0.20 mm.

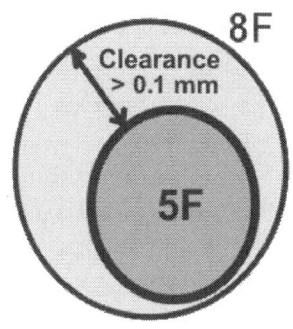

Adequate clearance

ANSWER c. 0.10 - 0.13 mm.
Johnsrude recommends that a clearance of at least .10-.13 mm (.004-.005 inches) is necessary between the ID (Inside Diameter) of any catheter and the OD of anything you wish to pass through it. Generally a difference of 3+ French sizes is required. E.G.: a 5 Fr. tube of 1.67 mm OD is a very tight fit within an 8 Fr. thin wall catheter (1.73 mm ID). This is because there is only 0.08 mm difference between ID and OD.
This becomes especially important in interventional procedures where several wires and/or angioplasty balloons may be passed through one catheter (E.g., Kissing balloon technique).
See: Johnsrude, A Practical Approach to Angiography, appendix, "Catheter dimensions and Coaxial systems." **KEYWORDS:** OD - ID system clearance

118. Standard diagnostic guide-wires used on routine adult femoral left heart caths and coronary arteriography are ___ long and ___ in diameter.
   a. 95-100 cm, .025" - .035"
   b. 95-100 cm, .035" - .038"
   c. 145-150 cm, .025" - .035"
   d. 145-150 cm, .035" - .038"

ANSWER d. 145-150 cm, .035" - .038". Since most coronary catheters are 100 cm long, and the wire must extend a foot or so beyond the catheter tip, diagnostic wires need to be at least 145 cm long. Diagnostic cardiac guide-wires are .035" in diameter, but .038" may be used if more stiffness is needed. Mini- and micro-puncture kits use 20 and 22 gauge needles. But these are not in common use. Remember wire lengths are in cm but wire diameters are in inches. To make it more confusing catheters are measured in French sizes.
See: Johnsrude, chapter on "Equipment."

119. Your patient has a dilated right heart. You are unable to float your 7F Swan-Ganz femoral catheter through his tricuspid valve. You suggest that your Dr. utilize a:
   a. .014" guidewire
   b. .025" guidewire
   c. 7F long sheath
   d. 8F guiding catheter

ANSWER b. 0.025" guidewire will pass into the distal lumen of most Swan Ganz catheters. Peterson says: If you use a sheath for a Swan-Ganz, you must have a sheath at least 1 size larger than the Swan catheter to prevent damage to the balloon. "In markedly dilated right

hearts even this maneuver may be unsuccessful and the floatation catheter must be stiffened by inserting a 0.25-inch flexible guide wire in its distal lumen."
See: Peterson, chapter on methods of Cardiac Catheterization

120. Which type of guide-wire has the longest atraumatic soft tip (5-15 cm of completely floppy tip), has a very gradually tapered mandrel (15 cm.) and has a stiff core. It is recommended as a starter wire for passing tortuous aortas.

a. Amplatz or Wholey
b. Bentson or Newton
c. Rosen or Coons
d. Lunderquist or ViperWire

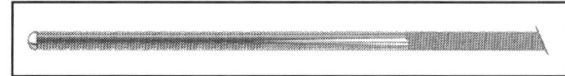

ANSWER b. Bentson and Newton wires are commonly used in many peripheral procedures and easy to pass up a very tortuous aorta. The extreme floppiness allows it to move almost anywhere. This classic design is still produced by many manufacturers. The operator can "tractor" this straight floppy tip guide-wire around lesions by advancing the body of the wire. It's shoulder will loop over the lesion, like treads on a tank and snake around an obstruction. Other floppy tip wires are available.

Kruse says, "The Bentson guide wire (Cook, Inc.), was originally designed for cerebral angiography, but we often find it extremely useful during difficult interventional procedures and selective angiographies when other standard guide wires fail; occasionally it is indispensable. We find the Bentson Starter wire especially useful because its straight floppy tip forms an atraumatic "functional J-tip" when advanced through a vessel, yet the wire is able to cross tight stenoses because the J is not fixed."

A similar cerebral guide-wire is the Newton. It also has a gradually tapered core. (LT=10 cm taper, LLLT=20 cm taper) But its tip is less flexible and its core less stiff. The Amplatz and Lunderquist wires are extremely stiff. Note: LT = Long Taper.
See: Cardiovascular and Interventional Radiology (1985) "Interventional and Angiographic Uses of the Bentson Guide Wire"
See: Kruse, "Thoracic Endovascular Aortic Repair (TEVAR) Guidewires", https://www.ctsnet.org/article/thoracic-endovascular-aortic-repair-tevar%C2%A0guidewires

121. What type of diagnostic guide-wires are recommended for torturous atherosclerotic vessels, plaques, and when passing a wire through a previously placed stent.

a. Straight stiff-tip guide-wire
b. "J" guide-wire
c. Support guide-wire
d. Glide wire

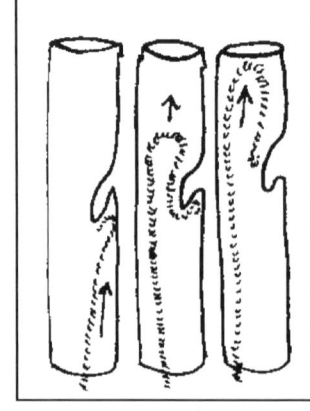

Passing plaques

ANSWERS: b. "J" guide-wire. Tortuous "twisty" arteries are often difficult to pass with a guide-wire. The tip of a straight wire may hang up in pockets of the tortuous aorta and on atherosclerotic lesions or flaps. "J" guides often pass easily. The "shoulder" of the guide seeks the center of the vessel. It is safer because the "J" deforms easily when pushed, and because the atraumatic shape it is less likely to knock off plaque or cause arrhythmia in the heart.

Schneider says: "J-tip guidewires are useful for passage through an occlusion or a previously stented arterial segment. The curved J tip is less likely to pass through the struts of a stent or create a false passage."

On young patients with normal vessels straight floppy guide-wires may work satisfactorily. The operator can "tractor" a straight floppy tip guide-wire like the Benston around lesions by advancing the body of the wire. Its shoulder will loop over the lesion, like treads on a tank move over an obstruction. Soft guide-wires may also be used successfully.
See: Schneider, chapter on "Guidewire - Catheter Skills"

122. What is a "knuckle wire" as used on CTO procedures?
  a. Tapered tip micro-wire with polymer coating
  b. Braided stainless steel wire that is spun by hand
  c. Micro-wire which is bent manually and forms a J shape when advanced
  d. Ball-tipped micro-wire that may be advanced with blunt atraumatic dissection

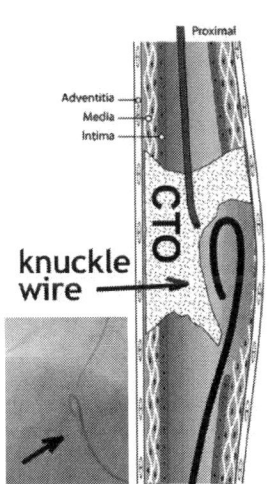

Answer: c. Micro-wire which is bent manually and forms a J shape when advanced. This resembles a bent knuckle on your finger. Initially the 3-4 mm tip is bent at about 45 degrees. This allows the wire to double over when pushed in the subintimal space making an atraumatic tip that passes in the subintimal plane and will not cause coronary artery perforation. Do not twist a knuckle wire or it may knot up.

123. Following PCI the most common cause of acute coronary closure, often attributed to coronary guidewire handling, is coronary artery:
  a. Spasm and plaque disruption
  b. Perforation and tamponade
  c. Dissection and thrombus formation
  d. Guide wire fracture and distal migration

ANSWER c. Dissection and thrombus formation. Freed says: "The most common causes of acute closure include coronary dissection, thrombus formation and/or spasm....While some degree of coronary spasm may contribute to abrupt closure from dissection and/or thrombus, isolated spasm is an infrequent cause of acute closure."
See: Freed, chapter on Dissection and Acute Closure

124. A fixed-core "J" wire may be difficult to thread into the hub of an arterial needle. The floppy tip may be inserted into the arterial needle more easily and safely using a:
  a. Plastic sleeve tip-straightener
  b. Funnel shaped needle threader
  c. Tapered core wire
  d. Non-tapered core wire

ANSWER a. Plastic sleeve tip-straightener. It is like trying to thread a needle with a wet noodle. These sleeves come with all "J" wires. When pulled over the "J" it straightens it for easier insertion. Of course, they must be removed before the catheter is threaded over the wire. Methods of straightening J-wires include:
  1. Straightener sleeves (describe above)
  2. Grasp the wire and stretch it between your thumb-forefinger and palm-little finger. This straightens most "J" wires so they easily advance into a needle or catheter hub.

See: Johnsrude, chapter on "Equipment."

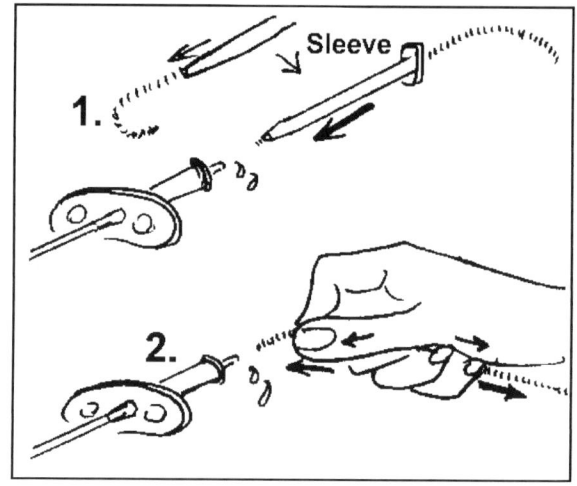
Methods of Inserting "J" wire

HANDLING CATH EQUIPMENT

125. It has been difficult crossing the aortic valve retrograde in a patient with aortic stenosis. This was finally accomplished with an Amplatz AR1 and a .035 straight tip guide-wire. LV pressure was recorded. To do LV angiography the next step is to:
a. Connect the AR1 to the pressure injector
b. Record pressures during an LV-AO pullback
c. Remove AR1 catheter over a .035 - 145 cm wire
d. Insert exchange wire and replace AR1 with a pigtail

ANSWER d. Insert a .035" - 260-cm exchange wire remove the AR1 and replace it with a pigtail. The AR1 is a single end hole catheter, unsuitable for flood angiography. A flood catheter is needed (E.g., pigtail). But, it may take hours to re-cross this tight aortic valve. A 260-300 cm exchange wire will maintain your position in the LV. Once the exchange wire is in the LV, then the AR1 can be removed, and replaced with a pigtail catheter. After doing LV angiography then the LV-AO pullback can be recorded.
See: Grossman, chapter on "Percutaneous Approach." **Keywords:** 260 cm. Maintain LV position AS use a 260 cm. Exchange guide-wire

126. When making a vascular puncture with a front/single wall needle how should it be inserted into the skin?
a. Bevel up
b. Bevel down
c. Holding onto the syringe
d. With the sharp stylus fully advanced

ANSWER a. Bevel up. With the beveled part of the

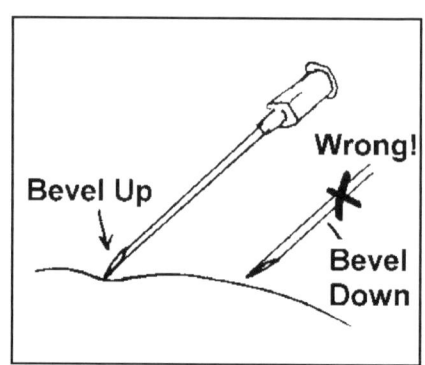
Needle puncture

needle up, you can see the lumen of the needle and the sharp point is down, touching the skin. This allows the needle to dive down into the tissue.
See: Grossman and Johnsrude, chapter on "Equipment." **Keywords:** when making needle puncture → Bevel up

127. Before catheters, needles, and sheaths are inserted into the patient they should be _____.
a. Flushed with pure heparin (1000 USP units/cc)
b. Flushed with heparinized saline
c. Flushed with sterile saline
d. Flushed with sterile contrast
e. Left dry

ANSWER b. Flushed with heparinized saline "flush." Flush within catheters helps prevent air embolization and thrombosis. It also checks the equipment for defects and leaks. It is also essential to wet hydrophilic coated wires and catheters before use.
See: Grossman, chapter on "Percutaneous Approach."

128. Air embolism into the vascular system is most likely when a stopcock is left open leading to a large bore:
a. Central venous line
b. PA line
c. Pigtail LV catheter
d. Arterial monitoring catheter

ANSWER a. Central venous line. An air embolism is a possibility into low pressure chambers like the RA. During deep inspiration the negative thoracic pressure may "suck" room air into the catheter and right heart. Consequently, during pacemaker insertion some physicians elevate the patient's legs to raise venous pressure. However, it takes a large amount of air to obstruct the lungs.

Pacemaker implantation requires a large bore central venous catheter. This is a time when air can be sucked into the right heart by the patient taking a deep breath. Elevating the patients legs usually increases the CVP enough to prevent air embolism. When air is sucked into the RA it tends to float in the RA or RV where on fluoro it resembles a puddle of "bouncing ghosts." Small amounts of air will slowly dissolve into the venous blood.
See: Grossman, Cardiac Cath, Angiography . . . chapter on "Percutaneous Approach."

129. The reason for enlarging a femoral artery puncture site with scalpel and forceps are to ease catheter passage and to:
a. Reduce trauma to the vessel at the puncture site
b. Reduce hematoma blood accumulation
c. Get closer to the artery for ease of arterial puncture
d. Prevent tissue damage to fragile catheters and guide-wires

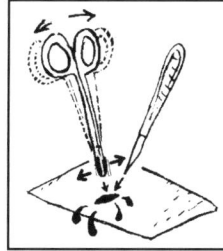

ANSWER b. Reduce hematoma blood accumulation. This tract from the subcutaneous tissue to the surface allows leaking blood to escape. This reduces hematoma that often accumulates during catheter exchanges and manipulations. At the end-of-the-case when holding pressure it simplifies hemostasis by allowing the compressor to see any developing hematoma.
See: Grossman, Cardiac Cath, Angiography . . . chapter on "Percutaneous Approach."

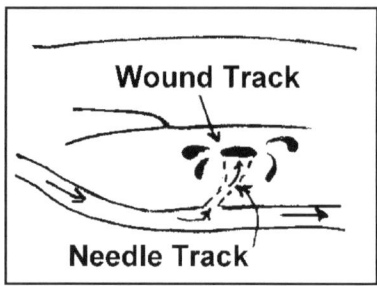

130. A cardiologist has just punctured a patient's RFA. He requests a movable-core guide-wire for Seldinger insertion. He asks you to fully advance the movable-core for easy insertion into the needle. To prevent "spearing" the back wall of the artery, when inserting a "stiff" guide-wire:
a. Soften the wire before insertion
b. "J" the wire in the needle
c. "J" the wire when it exits the needle
d. Soften the wire in the descending AO

ANSWER b. "J" the wire in the needle. I have seen many arteries dissected or punctured by the stiffened movable-core wire. When stiffened, these wires becomes "spears." When using a movable-core wire be sure your Dr. is aware of the risk. He may not pull back the core to soften it, resulting in a dangerously stiff non-floppy tip.

Once the stiffened movable-core is passed into the needle the Dr. must pause. Then the assistant must quickly soften or "J" the wire within the needle. You should then say "Soft" or "J-ed" to communicate to the Dr. that it is now safe to advance the wire into the artery. **DO NOT** let the operator spear or dissect your patient's artery by pushing a stiffened wire through the artery. If necessary tell the Dr. to WAIT until you have it "J-ed."
Dissection of puncture can easily occur if the physician accidentally inserts the stiff end of a guidewire.

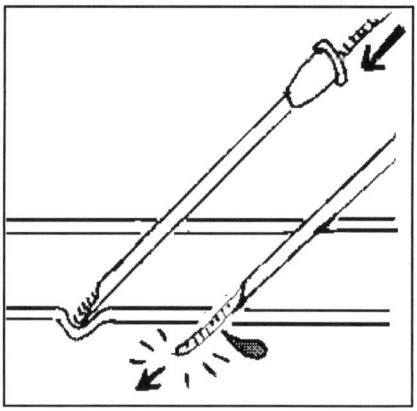

Wire Dissecting RFA

A safer alternative is to use a fixed-core "J" wire or to leave it "J-ed" before inserting it into the needle. This may require a plastic sleeve to straighten the "J."
See: Grossman, chapter on "Percutaneous Approach." **Keywords:** Movable-core = spear, "J" it before it leaves needle

131. When advancing a guide-wire through a needle into an artery, a patient experiences discomfort. When you meet resistance advancing a guide-wire your next step should be to:
a. Rotate and firmly advance the guide-wire
b. Remove the wire and check for good blood flow back though the needle
c. Depress the needle slightly and try again to gently advance the wire
d. Remove the needle and attempt to puncture the contralateral artery

ANSWER c. Depress the needle slightly and try again to gently advance the wire. Often the operator feels the back wall of the artery and has difficulty advancing into the vessel. When this happens, Grossman recommends depressing the needle hub. This may elevate the point of the needle in the artery so it is not touching the back wall of the vessel. The guide-wire may then be easily advanced.

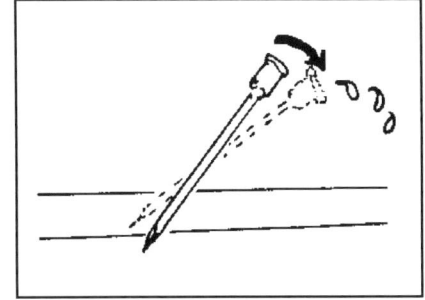
Depressing needle hub

If this is unsuccessful then check blood flow from the needle. It should spurt continuously. If that is unsuccessful then remove the needle and attempt to puncture the same vessel. Grossman recommends that after three unsuccessful punctures, the contralateral artery should be prepped, draped, and cannulated. NEVER advance the guide-wire against resistance. This may dissect the vessel and cause unwanted complications.
See: Grossman, chapter on "Percutaneous Approach." **Keywords:** resistance to advancing wire → depress needle hub

132. In interventional catheterization, after the target vessel is cannulated, the guidewire should be advanced as far as possible through the lesion into the vascular bed. This is termed:
a. "Distal protection"
b. "Backup support"
c. "Burying" the guidewire
d. "Pinning" the guidewire

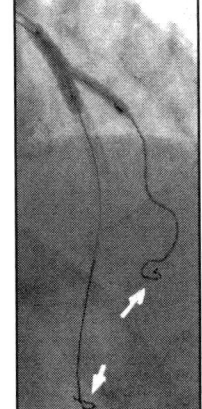
Buried wires

ANSWER c. "Burying" the guidewire. Schneider says: "After the vessel is cannulated, the guidewire should be advanced past that point as far as possible ("bury the guidewire") to prevent it from becoming dislodged during catheter advancement. This provides stable support for the advancing catheter." Sometimes the ends of these wires are "knuckled-over" as shown.
See: Schneider, chapter on "Selective Catheterization" p. 89

133. When a catheter is first placed in the aorta Dr. Grossman recommends that it be "double flushed." How do you use the FIRST syringe when giving a "double flush"?
a. Drawn back blood forcefully into the syringe, then discarded
b. Carefully drawn back blood until you see bubbles, then discard it
c. Carefully inject flush
d. Forcefully inject flush

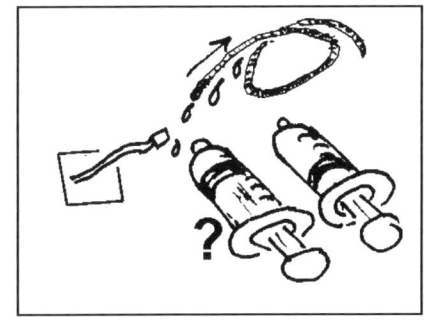
Double Flush

ANSWER a. Drawn back blood forcefully into the syringe and then discarded. The double flush technique is recommended whenever the catheter is in a critical area. Critical areas are the cerebral circulation and where catheter clotting is likely (E.g., after lengthy guide-wire manipulation). The purpose of it is to forcefully draw back any clots into the first syringe. A large syringe (20 cc) is attached to the catheter and at least 2-4 cc of blood drawn back forcibly. This aspirates any clots. The blood in that syringe along with the clot is then discarded or "wasted."

The second 20 cc syringe of clean heparinized flush is then connected, slightly drawn back to check for bubbles and then 2-5 cc are flushed into the patient. This leaves heparinized solution within the catheter to prevent clotting.

Flood catheters with many side-holes should be forcibly flushed - enough to clear all side-holes. E.g., Pigtail catheters. However, to avoid damaging a vessel NEVER forcibly flush wedged selective catheters. Be sure they are free in the lumen before flushing.
See: Dyer, ch. on "Catheters and Guide-wires." **Keywords:** Double flush 1st syringe=waste

134. Venous puncture is performed differently than arterial puncture. What equipment is UNIQUE to venipuncture?
  a. Smaller needles are used (22T)
  b. Single wall needles are used
  c. Saline filled syringe is fitted to the needle
  d. Contrast filled syringe is fitted to the needle

ANSWER c. Saline filled syringe is fitted to the needle. Because the femoral vein is much lower pressure than the artery, it is usually necessary to use a syringe to see the venous blood. Arterial puncture is noted immediately by the spurting blood. But venous blood just oozes. The saline filled syringe allows the Dr. to aspirate blood and see it "flash-back" immediately upon venous entry. Single wall needles are designed to only puncture the anterior wall. So, draw back on the syringe as you advance the needle.

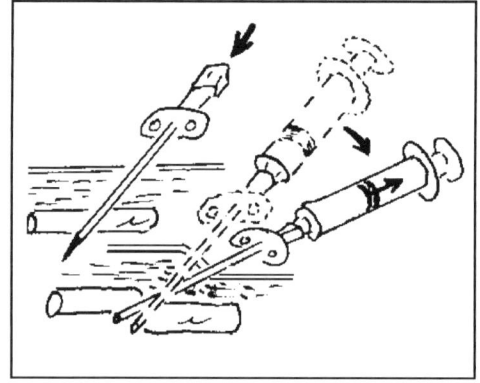

Venous puncture & aspiration

If the Seldinger needle punctures both walls of the vein, then the needle is attached, depressed, and aspirated during drawback as shown. **See:** Grossman, chapter on "Percutaneous Approach."

135. A deep right femoral arterial puncture has just been attempted with an arterial needle. No blood has exited the needle. The Dr. releases the needle in the skin to observe its pulsation. You observe the needle hub bounce sharply to your right (medially) with each systole. It is most likely that the needle is _____ the femoral artery.
  a. Through the anterior wall of
  b. Through both walls of
  c. Lateral to
  d. Medial to

ANSWER c. Lateral to the FA. As the artery pulses in systole it bounces the needle tip slightly. Here the needle hub pulses medially with each systole - as shown. The needle HUB PULSES TOWARD THE ARTERY as the needle tip pulses away. The next puncture should be made just medial to the first puncture. If the artery is transfixed through both walls, it will dance up and down with each heart beat. **See:** Johnsrude, chapter on "Equipment." **Keywords:** needle dancing to side➜ Medial bounce=next puncture more medial

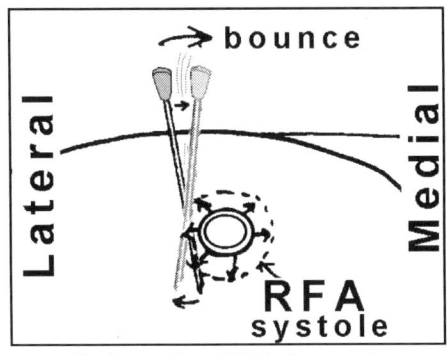

Needle lateral to RFA bouncing

REFERENCES:

Baim, D. S and Grossman W.., *Cardiac Catheterization, Angiography, and Intervention,* 7th Ed., Lea and Febiger Book Co., 2006

Dyer, R., ed., *Handbook of Basic Vascular and Interventional Radiology,* Churchill Livingstone Book Co., 1993

Homes D. & Verghese M., editors, *Atlas of Interventional Cardiology* 2nd Ed., Current Medicine, Inc., , 2002

Johnsrude, I. S., Jackson. D. C., Et. al., *A Practical Approach to Angiography,* 2nd Ed., Litt, Brown and Co., 1987

Kern, Morton, *The Cardiac Catheterization Handbook,* 6th Ed., Mosby, 2016

King, S.B. III and Yeung, Alan, *Interventional Cardiology,* McGraw-Hill Book Co., 2007

Lanzer, Peter, *Mastering Endovascular Techniques, a guide to excellence,* Lippincott, 2007

Nguyen, & Colombo, et all., Practical Handbook of Advanced Interventional Cardiology, 3rd Ed., Blackwell Futura, 2009

Pepine, J. C., and Hill, J. A., et. al., *Diagnostic and Therapeutic Cardiac Catheterization,* 2nd Ed., Williams and Wilkins Book Co., 1994

Peterson, & Nicod, Cardiac Catheterization, Methods, Diagnosis, and Therapy, W.B.Saunders Co., 1997

Schneider, Peter, Endovascular Skills, Guidewire and Catheter Skills for Endovascular Surgery, 2nd Edition, Marcel Dekker, Inc., 2003

Tilkian, A. G., and Daily, E, J, *Cardiovascular Procedures, Diagnostic Techniques and Therapeutic Procedures,* C. V. Mosby Company, 1986

OUTLINE: Catheterization Equipment: Other

7. NEEDLES
    a. Types
        i. Seldinger - 2 part
        ii. Single (front) wall
    b. Sizes
        i. Gauge size = OD (Stubs wire)
        ii. Larger Gauge= smaller diameter
        iii. 18T = standard for .038 wire
        iv. Needle lengths measured in inches
    c. Desired features
        i. sharp
        ii. smooth
        iii. beveled cannula
        iv. thin wall
        v. appropriate size
        vi. beveled inner hub
    d. Special needles
        i. Smart needle (ultrasound guidance)
        ii. Winged "Butterfly" needle
        iii. Biopsy needles
        iv. Spinal
8. SHEATHS
    a. Components - Introducer set
        i. Wire-guide, short
        ii. Sheath
        iii. Dilator
        iv. Single wall needle
    b. Desired features

i. Tapered tip & sleeve
ii. Smooth (PTFE, hydrophilic)
iii. Bendable & kink resistant
iv. Low leak, smooth hemostatic valve
v. Side port tube & stopcock
c. Types
i. Standard
ii. Balkin- contralateral
iii. Mullins - Transseptal
iv. Protective (accordion) sleeves
v. Pass long sheaths past tortuosity
vi. Micropuncture 21G, short .018" wire
d. Sheath sizing - Inner Diameter
i. Same French size as catheter
ii. For Swan balloon catheters use one Sheath size larger

9. STOPCOCKS, ADAPTERS
a. Types
i. Male - female
ii. 1 - 3 way
iii. Handle on - off
iv. Male Slip - Luer Lock
b. Male ends
i. Luer slip
ii. Luer lock
iii. Linden fitting
iv. Swivel collar luer lock
c. Manifolds
i. Standard connections
(1) Distal, rotating adapter (catheter)
(2) Distal, side-arm (Pressure)
(a) Air Zero
(3) Proximal side-arm (contrast)
(4) Proximal end female adapter (syringe)
(5) Waste bag
ii. Handle positions
(1) Manipulation
(2) "Panic" position
d. Adapters
i. Tuohy-Borst
ii. Male-female
iii. Dead-ender, plugs
iv. Rotating adapter

10. GUIDE WIRES
a. Configurations
i. Fixed or Movable-core
ii. Straight, J tip, or angled tip
iii. Core-to-tip (as GlideWire)
iv. Formable tip (malleable)
v. Safety guides
vi. Soft, stiff, support wires
b. Wire Uses
i. Interventional tracking wires .014" -.018"
ii. PTCA guiding catheter wire .063"
iii. Exchange wires 270 cm-400 cm
iv. Diagnostic wires .035"-.038"
c. Wire Coatings
i. Heparin (BH)
ii. Teflon (PTFE)
iii. Silicone (Propel)
iv. Hydrophilic polymer (E.g., Glide-wire)
d. Core construction
i. Stainless steel
ii. Nitinol = Nickel + Tin alloy
iii. Gold, platinum tip=radiopaque
iv. Taper: ST, LT, LLLT
e. Specific Named Guidewires
i. Bentson floppy
ii. Amplatz stiff
iii. Glide-wire, Terumo
f. Wire Qualities
i. Stiff for manipulating & tracking
ii. Flexible atraumatic (floppy tip)
iii. Memory of tip (Nitinol)
iv. Smooth, PTFE, hydrophilic
v. Kink resistant (Nitinol)
vi. Torque control
vii. Trackability
g. Wire Sizes
i. Lengths
(1) in cm.
(2) exchange guides
(3) extendable guides
(4) fixation devices (magnet)
ii. Diameters
(1) hundredths of inches
(2) diagnostic .035, .038"
(3) interventional .014, .018"
h. Wire - Other
i. Dagger effect
ii. Safety wire
iii. Malleable - formable tip
iv. J-guide
v. Straightening tip for insertion

11. HANDLING EQUIPMENT
a. Needles
i. Bevel up
ii. Safe disposal
iii. Flushing
iv. Air embolism
v. Venipuncture technique
(1) use of saline filled syringe
vi. Arterial puncture technique
(1) needle bounce
b. Scalpel blades
c. Scalpel shapes
i. #10
ii. #11
(1) stab wound vents blood
iii. #12
iv. #15
d. Guide Wires
i. Preventing dissection
ii. Handling, coiling, wiping
iii. Preventing kinking
iv. Danger of GlideWire pullback in needle
v. Longest use time = 3 min.
vi. Floppy wires used 1st, followed by stiffer wires thru cath, if needed
vii. Burying the guidewire
e. Introducer sheaths
i. Flushing
ii. Insertion
iii. Clotted or kinked sheath
f. Catheters
i. Flushing
(1) Double flush
ii. Preparing
(1) Flushing new catheters
(2) Inspecting, sizing
iii. Inside clearance ID-OD
(1) >0.10 mm00

Indications, Risks and Complications

INDEX: D3 - Indications, Risks and Complications
1. Indications & Contraindications   p. 75 - Know
2. Precautions . . . .   p. 79 - Know
3. Risks . . . . .   p. 85 - Know
4. Cardiac Complications . .   p. 88 - Know
5. Immune Response . .   p. 99 - Know
6. Vascular Complications . .   p. 101 - Know
7. Chapter Outline . . .   p. 113

1. Indications and Contraindications

136. Which 3 patients have a major indication for combined cardiac catheterization and coronary angiography? (Check 3 below.)
a. An older man being considered for valve surgery in 1 week
b. A young man with chest pain of uncertain origin for the last month
c. An older woman with Q-wave myocardial infarction 24 hrs old
d. A middle-aged woman being considered for PCI tomorrow
e. A cyanotic child with tetralogy of Fallot

ANSWERS: a, b, & d.
A. An older man being considered for valve surgery in 1 week - YES
B. A young man with chest pain of uncertain origin for the last month - YES
C. An older woman with Q-wave myocardial infarction 24 hrs old - NO
D. A middle age woman being considered for PCI tomorrow - YES

Q-waves indicate irreversible death of myocardium. After an infarction process begins, the window to salvage myocardium is usually considered to be 4-6 hrs. Prior to this brief time PCI, thrombolysis, or CABG may prevent the death of some myocardial cells and "salvage" myocardium. After that time infarcted tissue has died and recovery in CCU and medical therapy is usually all that can be done.

Indications for a heart cath include:
1. **Impending heart surgery** of any kind (especially in older patients to check for coronary disease.)
2. **Coronary arteriography** is the best diagnostic tool to see if chest pain is due to coronary obstruction.
3. **Acute MI** is an indication for diagnostic cath and intervention, but the window of time is only 4-6 hrs long. After that, recovery in a CCU is usually all that can be done.
4. **Diagnostic coronary arteriography** always precedes PCI to define coronary anatomy. The PCI may be done the next day to reduce the length and risk of the procedure.
5. Children seldom have coronary disease

See: Kern, The Cardiac Cath. Handbook, chapter on "Intro. to Cath Lab."

137. **A patient has aortic stenosis, mitral regurgitation and first degree heart block. He is scheduled for a heart catheterization prior to valve replacement surgery. Besides standard Judkins and pigtail catheters what additional catheter will the physician wish to use?**
  a. **Bioptome for ventricular biopsy**
  b. **Temporary pacemaker**
  c. **Thermodilution Swan-Ganz**
  d. **Valvuloplasty balloon**

ANSWER c. Thermodilution Swan-Ganz. Valvular heart disease cases require right and left heart caths. In mitral disease the wedge pressure is especially important, because it evaluates the severity of regurgitation (V-waves) and any LA-LV mitral gradient. Aortic valvuloplasty is seldom recommended due to its high re-stenosis rate.
OTHER TYPES OF CASES WHERE RIGHT HEART CATH IS HELPFUL ARE:
  • Valvular heart disease
  • Pulmonary disease (COPD, Pulm. hypertension...)
  • Congenital heart disease (pediatric or adult)
  • Electrophysiology study (sudden death, arrhythmia...)
  • Pericardial constriction or tamponade
  • Cardiomyopathy
  • Heart transplant follow up (including biopsy)
  • Acute care monitoring (Swan Ganz)

See: Kern, chapter on "Intro. to Cath Lab." **Keywords:** AS, MR patient ➜ needs right heart cath.

138. **Which type of patient below will probably need three combined procedures: right and left heart cath plus coronary arteriography?**
  a. **Unstable angina**
  b. **Aortic dissection**
  c. **Pediatric heart disease**
  d. **Pericardial disease**

ANSWER d. Pericardial disease patients need right and left heart cath. Pericardial disease can often be diagnosed by the pressure waveforms. The hemodynamics here are critical. Coronary arteriography outlines the epicardium and rules out coronary disease. Cardiac angiography may show right sided chamber collapse.

Pediatric heart disease requires right heart cath since most congenital shunts can be entered from the right side. However, coronary arteriography is seldom necessary.
See: Kern, chapter on "Intro. to Cath. Lab." **Keywords:** Right and left heart cath and coronaries needed in pericardial disease

139. Myocardial biopsy is commonly performed on what two types of heart cath patients?
   a. Infected prosthetic valve
   b. Cardiomyopathy
   c. Heart transplantation follow-up
   d. LA or LV myxoma

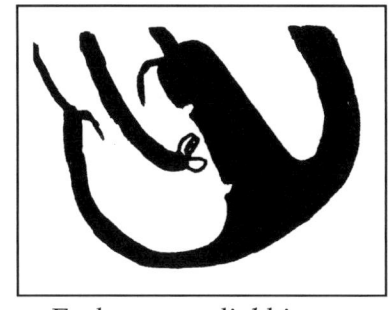
Endomyocardial biopsy

ANSWERS: b & c. Cardiomyopathy and heart transplant follow up both require biopsy.
a. NO: INFECTED PROSTHETIC VALVE: In prosthetic valve infections, blood cultures may diagnose the organism. Biopsy in the area of a prosthetic valve might cut the sutures.
b. YES: CARDIOMYOPATHY: Myocardial fiber disarray (myofibrillary disarray) seen in hypertrophic cardiomyopathy may be diagnosed by biopsy of the interventricular septum.
c. YES: HEART TRANSPLANTATION FOLLOW-UP: RV biopsy is routinely done following transplantation to evaluate the level of immune response in the sarcomere. When the myocardial cells begin to congest and swell it's time to add more immunosuppression medication.
d. NO: LA OR LV MYXOMA: Don't mess around a myxoma with a bioptome or catheter. They break loose and embolize too easily.
See: Kern, chapter on "Intro. to Cath. Lab." **Keywords:** Types of cases utilizing biopsy = cardiomyopathy and transplantation

140. A patient work-up indicates suspected silent ischemia with atypical Prinzmetal angina. What invasive procedures are indicated?
   a. LV + COR (Left heart cath)
   b. R + L, LV, COR (Right and left heart cath)
   c. LV and COR, Ergonovine
   d. R + L, LV, COR, BX (Right and left heart cath, with LV and coronaries, and ventricular biopsy)

ANSWER c. LV and COR, Ergonovine. The cause of atypical chest pain can be difficult to diagnose. The pain occurs at unusual times and often with no apparent cause. Holter/ambulatory monitors are now widely used to diagnose the ECG ST elevation characteristic of Prinzmetal angina. The invasive diagnosis of coronary spasm involves doing baseline coronary arteriography (which is often normal) and then to administer a vasospastic drug IV in increasing dosages. In susceptible individuals ergonovine like drugs provoke coronary spasm. When successful, the coronary vessel can be seen to constrict on angiogram and the characteristic ST segments can be recorded. Nitroglycerin is the antidote to reverse the provoked spasm.

Kern says, "Ergonovine malate is no longer manufactured in this country. Some investigators have used methylergonovine, but little is reported with this agent. Intracoronary acetylcholine produces coronary vasoconstriction in patients with propensity for spasm or in those with endothelial dysfunction. It should be reserved for laboratories with a particular interest in this problem and most often under a research protocol." **See:** Grossman, chapter on "Incidence..."

141. Relative contraindications to left heart cath and coronary angiogram procedures include uncontrolled:
1. PAT and PACs
2. Hypertension
3. Hypokalemia
4. Liver disease
5. Epilepsy
6. Fever
   a. 1, 4, 6
   b. 4, 6
   c. 2, 3, 4
   d. 2, 3, 6

ANSWER d. 2, 3, & 6 (Hypertension, hypokalemia, and fever are contraindications.)
   1. **NO: PAT AND PACs:** Atrial arrhythmias are usually no problem.
   2. **YES: HYPERTENSION:** This predisposes the patient to coronary ischemia or pulmonary edema and should be controlled prior to cath.
   3. **YES: HYPOKALEMIA (Low Potassium):** Predisposes the patient to ventricular arrhythmias.
   4. **NO: LIVER DISEASE:** Few cardiac related problems.
   5. **NO: EPILEPSY:** Few cardiac related problems
   6. **YES: FEVER:** Febrile illness predisposes the patient to infection at the access site and lowers his resistance.

See: Grossman, chapter on "Complications..." **Keywords:** Relative contraindications → hypertension, hypokalemia, fever

142. How should the relative contraindication to heart catheterization, labeled #5 (Hypokalemia) in the box, be corrected before the procedure?
a. Antibiotic therapy
b. Digitalis & diuretics
c. Lidocaine drip
d. Vasodilator therapy
e. KCl drip
f. Steroids and Benadryl

RELATIVE CONTRAINDICATIONS
1. Ventricular irritability
2. Hypertension
3. Fever
4. LV Failure
*5. Hypokalemia
6. Allergy to contrast

ANSWER e. KCl drip. HypoKalemia is a deficiency of potassium (chemical symbol K). KCL - IV infusion replaces the lost K and brings up serum K levels to avoid arrhythmia.
BE ABLE TO CORRECTLY MATCH ALL ANSWERS.
1. **VENTRICULAR IRRITABILITY:** Lidocaine drip
2. **HYPERTENSION:** Vasodilator therapy
3. **FEVER:** Antibiotic therapy
4. **LV FAILURE:** Digitalis & diuretics
5. **HYPOKALEMIA:** KCl drip

6. **ALLERGY TO CONTRAST:** Steroids (Prednisone) and anti-histamines like diphenhydramine (Benadryl)
See: Kern, chapter on "Intro. to Cath. Lab." **Keywords:** Correcting relative contraindications (KCl drip)

2. Precautions

143. Heart cath patients may be asked if they are allergic to seafood or fish because this indicates a possible allergy to:
   a. Coumadin or vitamin K
   b. Heparin or streptokinase
   c. Contrast or protamine
   d. Na sulfite or other preservative

ANSWER c. Contrast (iodine) or protamine. Seafood has a high concentration of iodine. Iodine is also the radio-opaque ingredient in contrast. There is a strong correlation between the two allergies. Seafood allergies may tip you off to use low osmolar contrast and/or limit the amount of contrast used, or premedicate the patient to avoid allergic reactions with steroids and antihistamines.
   Grossman says: "Release of histamine and other agents causes the clinical manifestations (sneezing, urticaria, angioedema of lips and eyelids, bronchospasm, or in extreme cases, shock with warm extremities due to profound systemic vasodilation). Risk of such reactions is increased in patients with other atopic disorders, allergy to penicillin, or allergy to seafood (which contains organic iodine) and may be as high as 15% to 35% in patients who have had a prior reaction to contrast." He recommends premedicating the patient with prednisone, H1 antihistamine (Benadryl), and H2 blockers (cimetidine) and using nonionic contrast agents (not ionic low-osmolar agent such as Hexabrix) Protamine is made from fish products (salmon eggs).
   Seafood and fish sensitive individuals may be allergic to protamine as well. Kern, recommends avoiding the use of protamine in fish sensitive individuals.
See: Grossman, chapter on "Complications..." **Keywords:** Seafood allergy → iodine allergy

144. A patient scheduled for angiography is NPH-insulin dependent. What specific precautions should be taken?
   a. Avoid the use of ionic, high osmolar contrast media
   b. Avoid reversing heparin with protamine
   c. Premedicate the patient with Benadryl and steroids
   d. Premedicate the patient with atropine and epinephrine

ANSWER b. Avoid reversing heparin with protamine. NPH-insulin is "Neutral Protamine Hagedorn Insulin." These individuals may have increased sensitivity to protamine. Up to 25% of these individuals may have a major anaphylactic type allergic response. Protamine should be avoided in these individuals. Protamine is made from fish products and fish sensitive individuals should also avoid protamine. Other reactions patients have to protamine are:
   • back and flank pain (minor reaction)

- flushing with peripheral vasodilation and hypotension (minor reaction)
- facial flushing and vasomotor collapse which may be fatal (major reaction)

In addition, insulin dependent individuals who are instructed to fast overnight (NPO after midnight) may experience hypoglycemia with normal insulin use. These individuals are recommended to use 50% of their normal insulin dosage in the AM.

See: Kern, chapter on "Intro. to Cath. Lab." **Keywords:** NPH-insulin ➜ use no protamine

145. Your cath patient is an NPH insulin dependent diabetic. On the morning of her cath she should be kept NPO and be administered:
   a. Quarter dose metformin instead
   b. Oral metformin instead
   c. Half dose NPH insulin
   d. No NPH insulin

ANSWER c. Half dose insulin. Kern says, "For patients taking subcutaneous insulin (NPH, regular), an overnight fast with their normal dose insulin would cause hypoglycemia. The dose of NPH insulin should be decreased by 50% for patients coming to the catheterization laboratory when they are NPO in the early morning." **See:** Kern, chapter on "Introduction to the Catheterization Laboratory"

146. Identify the advantages the non-ionic contrast agent (Omnipaque) has over standard high-osmolar contrast. (Select 4 from below.)
   a. Less thrombogenic
   b. Less vasodilation
   c. Less myocardial depression
   d. Less elevation of LV-EDP
   e. Less nausea and hot flash

ANSWERS: b, c, d, & e.
   a. Less thrombogenic - NO.
   b. Less vasodilation - YES
   c. Less myocardial depression - YES
   d. Less elevation of LV-EDP - YES
   e. Less nausea and hot flash - YES

The non-ionic agent (Omnipaque) seems to activate platelets and may allow blood mixed with the agent to clot more easily. Peterson says, "...observations would suggest that the nonionic agents, as compared with the ionic agents and irrespective of osmolarity, have a strong propensity to cause platelet activation, the earliest step in arterial thrombotic occlusion.... Patients...were more commonly found to develop new thrombus if a nonionic agent was used..." **See:** Peterson, chapter on "Radiographic Angiocardiography."

147. To reduce the incidence of transient neurologic deficit and pain during IMA angiography Baim and Grossman recommend:
   a. Use of full systemic heparinization
   b. Use of NO heparin
   c. Use of high-osmolar contrast

d. **Use of low-osmolar contrast**

ANSWER d. Use of low-osmolar contrast. In attempting to catheterize the IMA artery off the subclavian, the vertebral artery may carry contrast to the brain. The cerebral circulation is sensitive to high-osmolar contrast. Baim and Grossman say, "Transient neurologic deficits may also result from the injection of high osmolar contrast agents into the carotid or vertebral arteries... Use of low osmolar agents is thus required during internal mammary angiography, both to avoid cerebral contrast toxicity...."
See: Grossman, chapter on "Complications...", chapter #1 on "Contraindications".
Keywords: Use of low-osmolar contrast for IMA angiography

148. **Patients coming to heart cath who have had a previous allergic reaction to contrast media should:**
   a. Have their case deferred due to unacceptable risk
   b. Receive non-iodinated contrast only
   c. Receive reduced volume contrast injections and DSA procedures
   d. Be premedicated with atropine, Valium, and epinephrine
   e. Be premedicated with steroids and anti-histamines

ANSWER e. Be premedicated with steroids and anti-histamines. For patients with a history of contrast allergy, Dr. Kern recommends steroid and anti-histamine premedication along with the standard premed-cocktail. He recommends:
   • Prednisone (60 mg the night before and 60 mg pre-cath)
   • Diphenhydramine (Benadryl - 50 mg pre-cath)
These premedications greatly reduce the incidence of allergic reactions even among those extensive allergic histories.
   Patients may have just as severe a reaction with a small volume contrast injection as a large volume load. That is why contrast test doses have NEVER been a helpful screening method. All contrast contains iodine as the radiopaque metal. However, gadolinium is a contrast used in MRI that is non-iodinated.
See: Kern, chapter on "Intro. to Cath. Lab." Keywords: Patient with allergy to contrast ➜ steroid, Benadryl premed

149. **A patient with a St. Jude prosthetic mitral valve needs heart catheterization. He takes Coumadin daily, but has had no clotting problems. What are the ACC/SCA&I Consensus Standards recommendations regarding administration of oral anticoagulants pre-cath?**
   a. Maintain the patient's normal Coumadin therapy and administer vitamin K prior to angiography
   b. Maintain the patient's normal Coumadin therapy and administer fresh frozen plasma prior to angiography
   c. Discontinue Coumadin 48 hrs. prior to cath until INR < 1.8
   d. Wean patient from Coumadin 1 week prior to cath and replace with heparin drip

ANSWER c. Discontinue Coumadin 48 hrs. prior to cath until INR < 1.8. However, it

depends on how critical the oral anticoagulation is to the patient. If he is in great danger of clotting his valve, Dr. Grossman says it is OK to stop Coumadin and switch to heparin drip, two days prior to cath, because heparin is easier to reverse than Coumadin. He states that if the patient **MUST** be kept on Coumadin or if it is an emergency **DO NOT REVERSE COUMADIN WITH ITS ANTIDOTE VITAMIN K.** IV vitamin K occasionally induces a hyper-coagulable state, which is what you **don't** need. In emergencies Grossman recommends using fresh frozen plasma (FFP) which contains many clotting factors, including platelets, to counteract the Coumadin.
See: Grossman, chapter on "Complications...", chapter #1, Contraindications.

150. CVA and TIA can best be prevented during coronary angiography by:
  a. Administration of thrombolytic drugs
  b. Using full systemic heparinization
  c. Screening patients for carotid artery stenosis
  d. Removing aortic guidewires above the innominate artery

ANSWER b. Full heparinization prevents clot formation and stroke.
CVA = "Cerebral Vascular Accident" is a stroke or cerebral thrombosis. TIA = "Transient Ischemic Attack" is a small temporary stroke. Both involve thrombi to the brain. Heparin will prevent formation of new thrombi. But it does not affect existing clots. Plaques or thrombi can be broken off with a catheter from the LV (in MI or LV aneurysm), the aortic arch or the carotid vessels. Thrombolytic drugs do not prevent clots, they only dissolve them. They also recommend pulling wires below the arch (not in it) so thrombi adherent to wires will not enter the cerebral circulation.
See: Grossman, chapter on "Complications..."

151. Grossman and Peterson state that the most important factor in reducing complication rates during heart catheterization and angiography is the:
  a. Speed of doing the case (<½ hr.)
  b. Experience of the operating physician
  c. Systemic heparinization of the patient
  d. Meticulous attention to details of technique

ANSWER d. Meticulous attention to details. Grossman mentions this "meticulous attention to details" several times in his section on preventing complications. The other distractors (experience, heparin and speed) are all helpful, but are included in the correct answer. **See:** Grossman, chapter on "Complications..." and Peterson, chapter on "Basic Techniques and Complications." **Keywords**: To prevent cath complications → be meticulous

152. Identify the normal blood chemistry range for magnesium (#5 in the box).
  a. 0.8-1.0 mg/L
  b. 1.5-2.1 mEq/L
  c. 3.5-4.5 mEq/L
  d. 95-105 mEq/L

BLOOD CHEMISTRIES
1. Sodium
2. Potassium
3. Chloride
4. Total Calcium
*5. **Magnesium**

e. 135-145 mEq/L

ANSWER b. 1.5-2.1 mEq/L. "Because of the risk of cardiac arrhythmias when electrolyte deficits are present .... all patients .... should have a serum magnesium measurement on admission. We advocate read replacing magnesium deficits to maintain a serum magnesium level of 2.0 mEq /liter or more." **See:** Braunwald, chapter on "ST-elevation MI Management"

BE ABLE TO CORRECTLY MATCH ALL ANSWERS BELOW.

BLOOD CHEMISTRIES	Normal Value
1. Sodium	135-145 mEq/L
2. Potassium (K+)	3.5-4.5 mEq/L
3. Chloride	95-105 mEq/L
4. Total Calcium	0.8-1.0 mg/L
5. Magnesium	1.5-2.1 mEq/L

See: Underhill, chapter on "Laboratory Tests" also, Todd, Vol II, chapter on "Catheterization Protocol" **Keywords:** Blood chemistries pre-cath.

153. The incidence of renal failure after angiography (CIN) is most likely to occur in patients with:
  a. Elevated blood creatinine levels and/or elevated BUN levels
  b. Reduced blood creatinine levels and/or reduced BUN levels
  c. Elevated blood sodium levels and/or elevated potassium levels
  d. Reduced blood sodium levels and/or reduced potassium levels

ANSWER a. Elevated blood creatinine and/or elevated BUN (Blood Urea Nitrogen). These are waste products that are normally cleared by the kidneys. Since the kidney is the only organ that can eliminate contrast from the body, efficient kidney function is essential for angiography patients to be able to excrete the contrast.

Bhatt says of CIN, "The most important patient-related risk factor is preexisting renal insufficiency.... Age has also been shown to be an independent predictor of CIN. Possible explanations for this observation could be the gradual decline of renal function that naturally happens with aging.... Any condition associated with inadequate renal perfusion can be a major risk factor. Specifically, the presence of heart failure, hypovolemia, hemodynamic instability, and the use of an intraaortic balloon pump have been shown to increase the incidence of CIN. The presence of anemia is an additional well-described but underappreciated risk factor.... Procedure-related factors such as the type and volume of CM used can also influence the incidence of CIN. The use of HOCM is associated with a higher incidence of CIN when compared to LOCM. The importance of contrast volume was first shown by McCullough et al. in a cohort of 1,826 consecutive patients undergoing coronary intervention. In this study, increasing contrast volume was a major risk factor for CIN, and the risk of CIN was minimal in patients receiving less than 100 mL of CM. Subsequently, Freeman et al. developed a formula for calculating the maximum radiographic contrast dose (MRCD) allowed to avoid nephropathy requiring dialysis. According to this study, MRCD = 5 mL × body weight (kg)/serum creatinine (mg/dL)...." Using this formula a 100 Kg patient with a Cr of 2 would be allowed 500/2= 250 ml of contrast.

Normal creatinine levels are 0.8-1.5 mg/100 ml. So, many labs use 1.5 as the top end of normal, and begin preventive IVs with statins or sodium bicarbonate in high risk patients. **See:** Grossman, chapter on "Complications..." and Bhatt, chapter on "Contrast Selection"

154. **Patients with diabetes and/or renal insufficiency are at risk for contrast-induced renal failure or nephropathy (CIN). This risk is reduced by starting the patient on ___ the night before cardiac catheterization.**
 a. Low dose dopamine
 b. Ca-channel blockers
 c. D5W drip
 d. Normal saline drip

ANSWER d. Normal saline drip starting the night before cath will hydrate the patient and keep the kidneys flowing. But, the best prevention of NIC is to limit the amount of low osmolar contrast during the case. Grossman says, "The main defense against contrast induced nephropathy is limitation of total contrast a volume to 3 mL/kg. ... limit views and multiple contrast "puffs" during interventional wire and device placement.... Adequate prehydration is also critically important ...Hydration with half normal saline for 12 hours before and after the contrast procedure provided the best protection against creatinine rise...." Normal saline has proven more effective than half normal saline prehydration. **See:** Grossman, chapter on "Complications of Cardiac Catheterization" **Keywords:** NIC

155. **Which of the following are reported to reduce or improve contrast-induced nephropathy (CIN) following PCI? (Select 4.)**
 a. Limit contrast dose during cath
 b. Hydrating the patient pre- and post- cath
 c. Using low-osmolar contrast during angiography
 d. Administering a sodium bicarbonate IV pre- and post- cath
 e. Administering n-acetyl cystein (e.g. Mucomyst) pre- and post- cath
 f. Insure patient is NPO 24 hours pre cath

ANSWERS: a, b, d, & e.
 a. Limit contrast dose during cath - **YES**
 b. Hydrating the patient pre and post cath - **YES**
 c. Using low-osmolar contrast during angiography - NO
 d. Administering a sodium bicarbonate IV pre and post cath - **YES**
 e. Adminstering n-acetyl cystein (e.g. Mucomyst) pre and post cath - **YES**
 f. Patients are normally NPO (nothing by mouth) the day of cath has no effect on CIN. Grossman says "Prospective trials comparing high- and low-osmolar contrast agents have generally failed to show consistent benefit. Trials with the iso-osmolar agent iodixanol (Visipaque), however, have tended to show benefit.... The main defense against contrast induced nephropathy (CIN) is limitation of total contrast volume to 3 ml/kg (or 5 mg/Kg divided by the serum creatinine, in patients with elevated baseline creatinine)....Adequate hydration is also critically important in any patient with impaired baseline renal function." Administering N-acetyl cystein (a mucolytic agent) or sodium bicarbonate pre- and post- cath also appear to reduce CIN. **See:** Grossman, chapter on "Complications..." **Keywords:** Reducing CIN

156. In order to prevent excessive bleeding from the puncture site, angiography patients should come to the lab with a blood prothrombin time (PT): (Note > is greater than)
 a. < 5 sec
 b. < 18 sec
 c. > 18 sec
 d. > 50 sec

ANSWER b. < 18 sec. Grossman recommends a PT time < (less than) 18 seconds long. Normal PT time is 12-15 sec. This assures that heparinization can be optimized during the case and that it can be reversed adequately with protamine if necessary. It facilitates hemostasis at the end of the case. Pressure holding time will not be excessive and hematomas will be minimized. Normal ACT is 100 sec. **See:** Grossman, chapter on "Complications..." **Keywords:** PT time < 18 sec

3. Risks

157. What is the incidence of permanent major complications or sequelea (e.g. stroke, heart attack, death) due to diagnostic heart catheterization?
 a. 0.1 %
 b. 0.25%
 c. 1.0%
 d. 2.5%

ANSWER b. 0.25% major complication rate = 1/400. Remember the death rate is .1% (one in a thousand). By adding in stroke and MI the major complication rate almost doubles the severe complication rate. Grossman quotes this number to patients, because for many people having a stroke is just as bad as death. These "Major Adverse Cardiac Events" are often given the acronym MACE. **See:** Grossman, chapter on "Complications..."

158. The abbreviation/acronym that refers to the worst complications of a cardiac procedure such as death, emergency CABG surgery, abrupt closure and stroke is:
 a. ICHD
 b. SICP
 c. MACE
 d. NYHA

ANSWER c. MACE stands for "Major Adverse Cardiac (or Coronary) Events (death, emergency CABG, abrupt closure & stroke). It is an acronym commonly quoted in research papers and by companies boasting a low MACE rate for their interventional therapies.
See: ACC guidelines." **Keywords:** MACE

159. The in-hospital mortality rate for diagnostic cardiac catheterization with coronary angiography as of 1999 according to Kern was:
 a. 0.10%
 b. 0.72 %
 c. 2.5%
 d. 5.5%

ANSWER a. 0.10% death rate from diagnostic heart cath. This number has been constant at around 1 death for every 1000 patients.
See: Grossman, chapter on "Complications..." **Keywords:** Average cath mortality = 0.1%

160. What is the average rate of any adverse event in diagnostic catheterization and coronary angiography?
 a. 0.001 %
 b. 0.5 %
 c. 1.35 %
 d. 4.53 %

ANSWER c. 1.35 % averaging about one in a hundred for diagnostic cath. Kern reports MACE rate of 1.35% for diagnostic cath and 4.53% for PCI interventional cases. Thus, the risk of intervention is about 3 times as high as diagnostic heart cath.
See: Kern, chapter on "High Risk Catheterization"

161. The average mortality risk to standard PCI interventional cases is:
 a. 0.11 %
 b. 0.5 %
 c. 1.0 %
 d. 4.3 %

ANSWER a. 0.11%. Averaging one in a thousand. Thus, average risk of death from cath is about one tenth of the risk of an adverse event (adverse event = 1% versus mortality 0.1%). **See:** Kern, chapter on "High Risk Catheterization"

162. Which sub-set of coronary arteriography patients are at the greatest risk of dying?
 a. Patients with severe LV dysfunction: (LV EF < 50%)
 b. Elderly women patients (> 60 years old)
 c. Patients with both coronary disease and aortic stenosis
 d. Patients with significant left main coronary disease

ANSWER d. Left main stenosis (widow-maker) has a death rate 10-20 times that of patients with single vessel disease. Be extremely careful about entering the left main coronary artery in these patients. Some labs require "OR" standby when LM stenosis is suspected. Low osmolar contrast is recommended. Normal EF is >50% but severe LV dysfunction is <39%. **See:** Grossman, chapter on "Complications..."

Diagnostic Techniques: D3 - Indications, Risks and Complications

163. Which one of the following patients has the lowest mortality risk during cardiac catheterization?
   a. Infants (< 1 year of age) or elderly individuals > 60 years of age
   b. Valvular heart disease patients with coronary disease
   c. Hypertensive women
   d. Patients with severe coronary obstructions (widow-maker)
   e. Functional class IV patients
   f. LV dysfunction patients (EF < 30)
   g. Severe non-cardiac disease (diabetes, renal insufficiency, cerebrovascular or PV disease)

ANSWERS: c. Hypertensive women.
   a. NO: INFANTS (< 1 year of age) or ELDERLY INDIVIDUALS > 60 years of age have increased risk.
   b. NO: VALVULAR HEART DISEASE patients, especially those with combined coronary disease have increased risk.
   c. YES: HYPERTENSIVE WOMEN: Hypertension is only a relative contraindication that can usually be corrected pre-cath. However, women are more prone to cardiac and vessel rupture, hematoma, and false aneurysm.
   d. NO: SEVERE CORONARY OBSTRUCTED patients (widow-maker) have increased risk
   e. NO: FUNCTIONAL CLASS IV patients have increased risk.
   f. NO: LV DYSFUNCTION patients (EF < 30) have increased risk.
   g. NO: SEVERE NON-CARDIAC DISEASE (diabetes, renal insufficiency, cerebrovascular or PV disease) have increased risk.
See: Grossman, chapter on "Complications..."

164. A patient's elevated creatinine level on the patient's blood work alerts you to possible:
   a. Old MI
   b. Recent MI
   c. Poor liver function
   d. Poor kidney function

ANSWER: d. Poor kidney function. Since contrast is eliminated by the kidneys, good kidney function is vital to eliminate this toxic compound. Iso-osmolar contrast (not just low-osmolar) should be used in patients with poor kidney function. **See:** Grossman, chapter on "Complications..." **Keywords:** High creatinine = poor kidney function

165. Contrast Induced Nephropathy (CIN) is diagnosed after angiography by ___ and can usually be prevented and treated with ___.
   a. Rise in bilirubin and jaundice, diuretics and renal dialysis
   b. Rise in bilirubin and jaundice, steroids and antihistamines
   c. Rise in serum creatinine, hydration by normal saline IV
   d. Rise in serum creatinine, steroids and antihistamines

ANSWER: c. Rise in serum creatinine, hydration by normal saline IV. CIN is a kidney problem (nephropathy) prevented with saline hydration. It is usually reversible and only extreme cases require renal dialysis. Jaundice is a liver problem treated with dialysis.

Watson says, "Contrast Induced Nephropathy: Large amounts of iodinated contrast media are nephrotoxic and account for 12% of all hospital acquired renal failure cases. ... It is defined as an elevation of the serum creatinine 20-50% above baseline that is noted 48-72 hours after the administration of contrast media.... Prevention of contrast media nephrotoxicity requires the patient be adequately hydrated before and after the procedure. This can be done by using an IV infusion of 0.9% saline, which has been shown to be more efficient than 0.45% saline.... Extensive hydration of patients during long procedures requiring considerable amounts of contrast media is very important....In daily practice, dialysis is rarely required." **See:** Watson, chapter on "Radiography"

4. Cardiac Complications

166. The most common complication of percutaneous transluminal angioplasty (PTA and PCI) is:
  a. Stenosis of branch vessels (snowplow effect)
  b. Embolization of plaque constituents
  c. Coronary artery dissection at dilatation site
  d. Emergency CABG revascularization surgery

ANSWER c. Coronary artery dissection at dilatation site. Controlled dissection is an expected (even desired) complication of PCI. This is induced intentionally by the balloon dilatation catheter. When the plaque/intimal fractures are small and stable, they are usually good. They allow the vessel to expand. The injured intima usually heals within a few weeks to an enlarged smooth lumen. The "controlled dissection" may occasionally be seen on the angiogram as a **small** longitudinal tear within the lumen. But **large** dissections or **flaps** are considered a **complication** of angioplasty. See: Grossman, Cardiac Cath., Angiog..., chapter on "Complications..." **Keywords:** Most common PCI complication = dissection

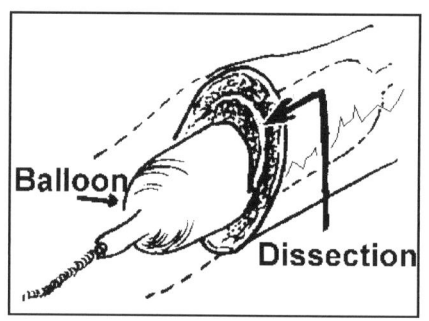
PCI dissection

167. Retroperitoneal hematoma is a possible complication to a HIGH femoral artery puncture. Its signs and symptoms are:
  a. The appearance of blood on the surgical dressing
  b. Complaints of chills, fever, and chest pain
  c. Slowing of the pulse and swelling at the puncture site
  d. Pallor, fall in blood pressure, tachycardia and abdominal pain

ANSWER d. Pallor, fall in blood pressure, tachycardia and abdominal or back pain. There may be left lower quadrant

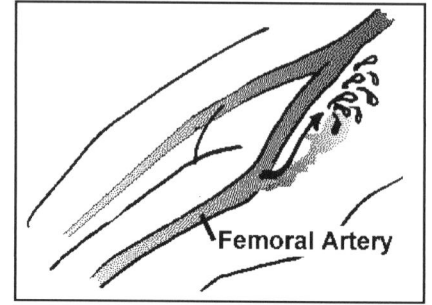
Retro-peritoneal - extravasation hematoma

swelling and tenderness. This rare complication is important because it can be lethal. If the puncture site is high and pressure is held too low, arterial blood may leak from the femoral artery and extravasate superiorly into the pelvis or the peritoneal cavity. This amounts to a loss of blood due to a hematoma that can't be seen. It is masked by the abdomen. Recent reports indicate that large retroperitoneal bleeds may be diagnosed with a KUB film. A "dent" in the bladder indicates an "abdominal mass" of blood.

The worst form of retroperitoneal bleed is a form of hypovolemic shock caused by insufficient circulating volume due to blood loss from the circulation. Signs and symptoms of hypovolemic shock include ↓BP, ↓RA, ↓LA filling pressures, ↓CO, vasoconstriction, ↑HR, lactic acidosis, pallor and cool skin all because of blood loss. Fluid administration can be lifesaving.
See: Braunwald, chapter on "Shock."

168. **The most common complication of cardiac ventriculography is:**
a. Hypotension (vasovagal)
b. Ventricular tachycardia runs
c. Endocardial staining
d. Myocarditis

ANSWER b. Ventricular tachycardia and/or runs of PVCs. These occur in 30 - 50 % of all ventricular catheterizations. They usually terminate with catheter withdrawal. Runs of PVCs become VT after 3 consecutive beats. If the run lasts over 30 beats it is termed ventricular tachycardia and should then be defibrillated before it degenerates into VF. Peterson reports an increased incidence of ventricular arrhythmias in critically ill patients with ischemic heart disease (52%) during Swan-Ganz balloon insertion. Runs of VT can be minimized by using less contrast, low-ionic contrast and balloon flotation catheters. But, VT can occur even in coronary angiography patients with no ischemic disease.
See: Grossman and Peterson, chapters on "Complications..." **Keywords:** VF/VT → RCA injection

169. **During a Judkins coronary arteriography procedure, most strokes and neuro-opthamalogic complications are caused by emboli from the:**
a. LV
b. Aorta
c. Coronary arteries
d. Carotid arteries

ANSWER b. Aorta. Plaques in the ascending aorta may be scraped off with a catheter tip or forceful catheter manipulation. These plaques then embolize to the head and result in stroke, TIA, or amaurosis fugax (partial blindness).

Baim and Grossman say, "most strokes or neuroopthamalogic complications (retinal artery embolization) appear to be caused by emboli released after disruption of unrecognized plaques on the walls of the aorta, liberating cholesterol crystals, calcified material, or platelet-fibrin thrombus." This is good reason to use a leading guidewire while crossing the aortic arch.
See: Baim and Grossman, chapter on "Complications..." and Grollman, editorial in Catheterization and CV Diagnosis: 1991 "Does Use of Vascular Introducer Sheath Obviate Need for Catheter Exchanges over a Guidewire?"
Keyword: Strokes result from aortic emboli

170. **Ventricular tachycardia and fibrillation most frequently occurs during excessive catheter manipulation and occlusive engagement during:**
   a. Left coronary arteriography
   b. Right coronary arteriography
   c. Renal stent placement
   d. Coronary sinus venography

ANSWER b. Right coronary arteriography. For an unknown reason when normal right coronary arteries are injected with contrast, VF or VT may ensue. RCA injection may also cause asystole and/or bradycardia due to SA and AV node ischemia. Grossman recommends only using as much contrast as is necessary.
   Kern says "occlusion of flow through the coronary artery (or vein graft) by the catheter is reflected by a damped pressure wave. Ostial occlusion in combination with contrast dye injection can lead to the development of ventricular fibrillation, particularly during the right coronary artery arteriography."
See: Grossman, chapter on "Complications..." **Keywords:** VF/VT → RCA injection

171. **This arrhythmia happens most often during excessive manipulation of a cardiac catheter in the:**
   a. RA
   b. RV
   c. LA
   d. LV

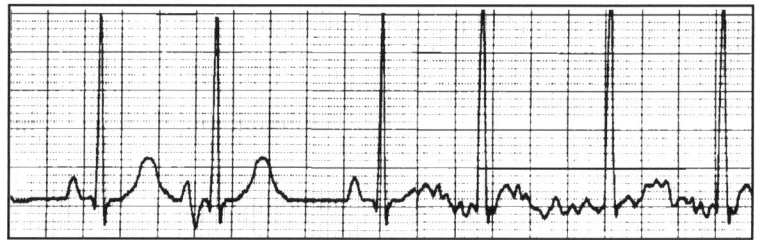

ANSWER a. RA. This arrhythmia shows one PAC followed by atrial fibrillation. PAC's are easily induced by irritating the atrial wall. Frequent PACs may lead to atrial tachycardia, atrial fibrillation or flutter. Since every right heart cath goes through the RA, (the LA is seldom entered), the RA is the most common source of mechanically-induced PAC's, atrial fib and flutter.
See: Grossman, chapter on "Complications..." **Keywords:** RA irritability → atrial fib/flutter

172. **What cath lab complication would cause you to call for a stat echocardiogram?**
   a. Cardiac tamponade
   b. Air embolism
   c. No Reflow
   d. Coronary artery spasm
   e. Abrupt closure

ANSWER a. Cardiac tamponade. Topol says, "The presence of coronary perforation should also trigger urgent echocardiography. If a large pericardial effusion is present associated with cardiac tamponade physiology, emergent pericardiocentesis is indicated. Should echocardiography not be available, the diagnosis of tamponade on clinical grounds, use of right heart catheterization, or fluoroscopy of the heart's borders may be helpful." See: Topol chapter on pericardiocentesis

173. Following several unsuccessful transseptal needle puncture attempts, a patient's BP is falling and his neck veins are distended. The most likely associated complication is:
   a. LV puncture with myocardial infarction
   b. Aortic puncture with pericardial tamponade
   c. HIS bundle transection
   d. Vasovagal bradycardia

ANSWER b. Aortic puncture with pericardial tamponade. The aortic root lies close to the fossa ovalis where the transseptal puncture is made. Any slight deviation in anatomy or needle location can puncture the aorta. This may seal, because the needle is small, or it may bleed into the pericardium, compressing the heart so much that it cannot fill properly. Cardiac tamponade can be a fatal complication if not recognized and treated promptly.

Pressure monitoring at the needle tip will tell you if the Dr. inadvertently punctured the aorta. If bleeding occurs around the needle, the Brockenbrough catheter can be used to plug the puncture site while the patient is taken to surgery. Pericardial centesis in the lab may be lifesaving.
See: Grossman, chapter on "Percutaneous Approach."

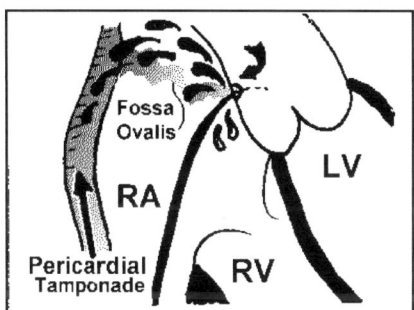
Unsuccessful transeptal puncture-induced pericardial tamponade

174. Perforation can be a complication of cardiac catheterization. The most common heart chamber to be perforated in a combined right and left heart cath is the:
   a. RA
   b. RV
   c. PA
   d. LA
   e. AO

ANSWER b. RV. 0.6% of bilateral heart cath patients experience cardiac perforation. The RV is the chamber most often accidentally punctured. It is a thin walled chamber in which the catheter is often severely torqued and manipulated. RV perforation happens most commonly in elderly female patients.

Most of these perforations in low pressure chambers seal themselves. However, some lead to dangerous pericardial tamponade. In high risk patients soft catheters should be used and carefully manipulated only by experienced physicians. Naturally, in transseptal catheterization the RA septum is intentionally perforated. **See:** Grossman, chapter on "Complications..."

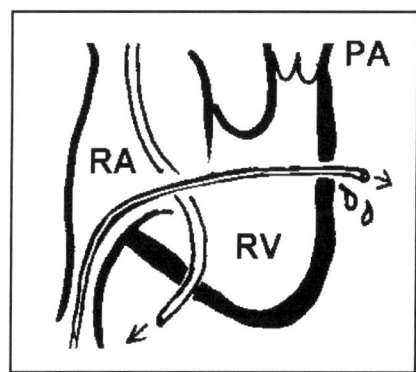
Cath perforation of RV

175. Following myocardial biopsy the patient develops hypotension, increasing venous pressures, tachycardia, and electrical alternans. The most likely complication is:
   a. Cardiac perforation
   b. Vasovagal discharge
   c. Pulmonary embolism
   d. Infection at the biopsy site

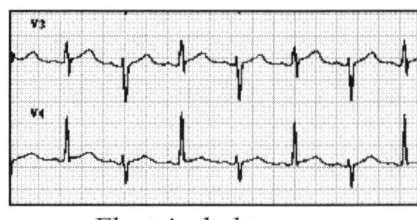
Electrical alternans

ANSWER a. Cardiac perforation of the RV is the most dreaded complication of **myocardial biopsy** since it can lead to fatal pericardial tamponade. The RV is only a few mm thick and with force any stiff catheter can perforate it. That is why only septal wall samples are taken and heparin is not given with RV biopsy. Simple pericardial centesis usually cures the tamponade problem. Electrical alternans shows on the ECG as alternating high and low QRS complexes. This may occur in a large pericardial tamponade where the heart swings back and forth periodically changing its electrical axis. Similar symptoms occur with a pacemaker lead that has eroded into the pericardium.

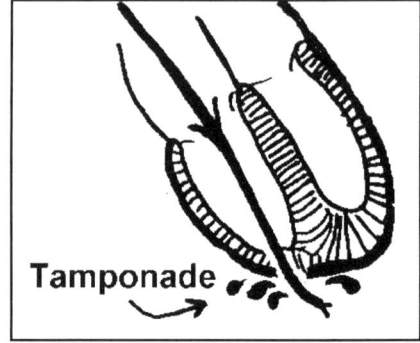
Bioptome RV perforation

See: Baim and Grossman, chapter on "Myocardial Biopsy."

176. Which of the following increases the risk of CARDIAC PERFORATION during cardiac catheterization? (Select 3 answers below.)
   a. Transseptal or endomyocardial biopsy procedure
   b. Elderly women over 65 years of age
   c. Temporary pacing wire placement
   d. Pulmonary or systemic hypertension
   e. Patients with severe diabetes

ANSWERS: a, b, & c.
   a. Transseptal or endomyocardial biopsy procedure - YES
   b. Elderly women over 65 years of age - YES
   c. Temporary pacing catheter placement, since it is commonly wedged between trabeculations, in order to keep it's positon. - YES
   d. Pulmonary or systemic hypertension - NO. (Results in ventricular hypertrophy, which strengthens the ventricle.)
   e. Patients with severe diabetes - NO.

Because the female RV is thinner, it is more susceptible to perforation, especially in the elderly female. Stiff catheters of any kind also increase the incidence of cardiac perforation and of tamponade. Hypertrophied hearts are more difficult to perforate, because of increased thickness.
See: Grossman and Peterson, chapters on "Complications..."

Diagnostic Techniques: D3 - Indications, Risks and Complications   93

177. An apprehensive elderly patient experiences pain during the femoral artery catheter insertion. After angiography the patient feels nauseous with pale cool skin. Her BP is 80/50 mmHg and falling. The HR remains at 65/min. What complication is developing?
   a. Cardiogenic shock
   b. Vasovagal reaction
   c. Anaphylaxis
   d. Allergic reaction

ANSWER: b. Vasovagal reactions are usually characterized by bradycardia. However, in older patients (as here) hypotension may be the only sign. Fear and anxiety are a setup for vaso-vagal reactions. Add a little pain and the vagus nerve goes wild. The overstimulated parasympathetic system depresses all cardiac function: HR, BP, contractility, EF... and the patient is in trouble.

Vasovagal reactions need to be identified and treated quickly. If allowed to persist, irreversible shock may develop. These vagal discharges can usually be quickly counteracted with 0.5-1 mg atropine IV, elevation of the legs, and fluid administration. Pressors may be used if hypotension persists. **See:** Grossman, chapter on "Complications..."

178. In which type of patient is a vasovagal reaction most dangerous?
   a. LV aneurysm with EF < 30%
   b. CHF patient with EF <30%
   c. Acute MI patients
   d. Critical aortic stenosis

ANSWER d. Critical aortic stenosis. Baim & Grossman say, "Patients with critical valvular heart disease may undergo severe and even irreversible decompensation if they are allowed to remain hypotensive for an indolently treated vasovagal reaction." He also warns that vasovagal bradycardia is one of the earliest signs in cardiac perforation and tamponade. Critical AS patients are prone to sudden death. **See:** Grossman, chapter on "Complications..."

179. Fever and cramps (rigor) following injection of foreign protein and endotoxin from previously used or unclean catheterization equipment is termed:
   a. Phlebitis
   b. Anaphylaxis
   c. Pyrogen reaction
   d. Vasovagal reaction

ANSWER c. Pyrogen reaction. A pyrogen is any substance that produces fever (pyro = fire). Foreign substances which are introduced into the patient's bloodstream (even though sterile) may trigger this. If fever and chills develop during the case Grossman recommends an immediate small dose of IV morphine and that the procedure should be immediately terminated. If this happens more than once, look for a source of contamination within your lab. Reused catheters has been implicated in many pyrogen reactions. With recent developments in disposable equipment this complication is now, fortunately, very rare.
See: Grossman, chapter on "Complications..." **Keywords:** Fever and chills = pyrogen reactions

180. An acute MI patient comes to your lab with bouts of ventricular tachycardia that are unresponsive to antiarrhythmic medications and must be defibrillated frequently. He is pale, severely SOB, HR = 110, with a BP of 90/70 mmHg on dopamine. The physician wants BOTH groins prepped and draped because he plans to use:
a. Kissing balloons
b. Right and left heart cath
c. Prophylactic balloon pump
d. Prophylactic temporary pacer

ANSWER c. Prophylactic balloon pump. Kerns says, "Prophylactic balloon pump (IABP) placement should be considered for patients with known severe left main coronary artery disease, recalcitrant pulmonary edema, or hemodynamic instability... arterial access in the contralateral femoral artery should be obtained with placement of a 4 F or 5 F sheath."
See: Grossman, chapter on "Complications..." Keywords: IABP

181. Which therapy below should be prepared for the heart cath complication labeled #4 in the box (pyrogen reaction)?
a. Heparin
b. Pericardial centesis
c. Fogarty embolectomy
d. Morphine
e. Antibiotic
f. Atropine

<u>CATH COMPLICATIONS</u>
1. CVA
2. Heart perforation
3. Pulseless artery following Sones procedure
*4. **Pyrogen reaction**
5. Phlebitis and fever 12 hrs. following temporary pacemaker implantation.
6. Vasovagal reaction

ANSWER d. Morphine. Grossman recommends administering IV morphine for pyrogen reactions. 2-4 mg IV may quiet and relax the patient. Pyrogen reactions may lead to anaphylaxis. Be able to match all answers below.
CORRECTLY MATCHED ANSWERS ARE:
1. **CVA:** Systemic heparinization 5000 units IV
2. **HEART PERFORATION:** Pericardio-centesis
3. **PULSELESS BRACHIAL ARTERY** following Sones coronary angio: Fogarty embolectomy
4. **PYROGEN REACTION:** Morphine 2-4 mg IV repeated as necessary
5. **PHLEBITIS AND FEVER** 12 hrs. following temporary pacemaker implantation: Antibiotic
6. **VASOVAGAL REACTION:** Atropine .5-1 mg. IV
See: Grossman, chapter on "Complications..." Keywords: Cath complications & therapy

182. In the cath lab, pericardiocentesis is usually done with what 2 kinds of guidance/imaging?
a. ECG & intracardiac echocardiogram
b. ECG & 2-dimensional echocardiogram
c. Fluoro & intracardiac echocardiogram
d. Fluoro & 2-dimensional echocardiogram

ANSWER d. Fluoro & 2-dimensional echocardiogram. Grossman says, "At most centers, pericardiocentesis is performed in the cardiac catheterization laboratory using a combination of echocardiographic and fluoroscopic guidance." ECG may be used but is not really guidance or imaging. The unipolar needle ECG lead is to tell if you accidentally touch or puncture myocardium with the needle. See: Grossman, chapter on "Pericardial Disease" **Keyword:** Centesis guidance

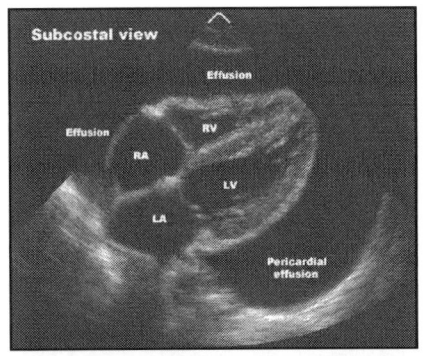

183. Echocardiography is brought to the cath lab to assist with pericardiocentesis. The echo tech says the effusion is "loculated." This means the effusion is:
    a. Clear fluid
    b. Bloody with clots
    c. In small compartments
    d. Filled with strands of tissue

ANSWER c. In small compartments. Loculation means "divided into small cavities or compartments." If the two pericardial walls adhere together with scar tissue, effusion fluid cannot fill that part of the pericardial sack. So, the effusion is not concentric, but localized in certain areas around the heart. Of course you direct the needle at the pericardial space holding the loculated effusion.

Grossman says, "It is helpful to obtain a two-dimensional echo just prior to the procedure to document the presence, location, and size of the effusion; to

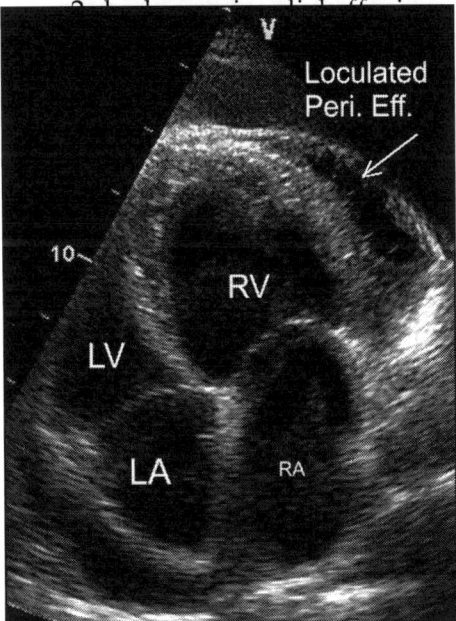

2-d echo, loculated peri. effusion

determine the presence of loculation or significant stranding; and to determine the location on the body surface where the effusion lies closest to the surface at which the fluid depth overlying the heart is maximal. Once an entry location is selected, the echo can indicate the optimal direction for needle passage and the approximate depth of needle insertion that will be required." Watch a dramatic animation of pericardial rupture with bloody pericardial tamponade resulting in cardiac constriction. See: Medical dictionary
http://www.youtube.com/watch?v=QwgfuDegC5Y&NR=1 **Keyword:** Loculated effusion = localized

184. How should the patient be positioned for a pericardiocentesis procedure?
    a. Propped up at 20-30 degrees
    b. Propped up to about 45 degrees
    c. Trendelenburg position
    d. Reverse Trendelenburg position

ANSWER b. Propped up to about 45 degrees with a wedge or bolster. This allows the pericardial fluid to drain into the inferior part of the pericardium to be "tapped" by the

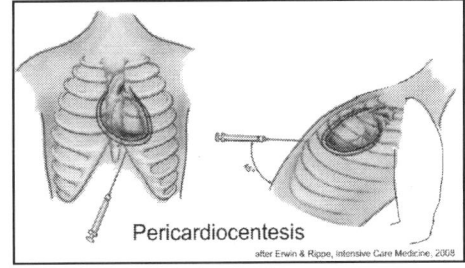

Positioning for pericardiocentesis

centesis needle. Grossman says, "The patient torso is propped to a level of about 45° using a bolster or other mechanism, and the transducers are zeroed to the level of the heart position. The subxiphoid approach is classic:...Removal of **as little as 50 mL is often sufficient to relieve frank tamponade** and improve hemodynamics. After removal of 100 to 200 mL of fluid, it is informative to remeasure the pericardial and right atrial pressure before resuming aspiration."
See: Grossman, chapter on "Pericardial Disease"

185. Which therapy below should be prepared for the allergic reaction presenting with signs listed in the box labeled at #2 (dyspnea, wheezing, syncope)?
  a. CPR as needed
  b. Valium
  c. Benadryl, Prednisone, Decadron
  d. Epinephrine, volume infusion (CPR as needed)
  e. Phenegran

ALLERGIC REACTIONS

1. Rash, urticaria
*2. Dyspnea, wheezing, syncope
3. Seizure, hypotension, bradycardia, dyspnea
4. Seizure, vital signs OK
5. Nausea, vomiting

ANSWER d. Epinephrine, volume infusion (CPR as needed). This is a major anaphylactic allergic reaction involving laryngeal and pulmonary edema. The laryngeal edema may lead to bronchospasm within minutes. Fatal respiratory arrest and cardiac arrest result if not treated promptly with epinephrine. Be able to treat all forms of allergic reaction.

These major reactions are often accompanied by some less severe minor reactions, such as rash. This is the same therapy given to people allergic to bee stings. Some minor reactions just need Benadryl, others have more severe anaphylactic reactions and may need Epi. and BLS (CPR). Be able to match all answers below.
CORRECTLY MATCHED ANSWERS ARE:
  1. **RASH, URTICARIA**: Benadryl, Prednisone, Decadron
  2. **DYSPNEA, WHEEZING, SYNCOPE**: Epinephrine, Volume infusion (CPR as needed)
  3. **SEIZURE, HYPOTENSION, BRADYCARDIA, DYSPNEA**: CPR as needed
  4. **SEIZURE, VITAL SIGNS OK**: Valium
  5. **NAUSEA, VOMITING**: Phenegran
See: Kern, chapter on "Introduction to Cath Lab.

186. In the invasive lab what 4 signs below indicate a patient in shock? (Select 4 below.)
  a. Cold and clammy skin
  b. Decreased heart rate
  c. Collapsed neck veins
  d. Decreased urine output
  e. Dilated, unresponsive pupils
  f. Hypotension

ANSWERS: a, c, d, & f

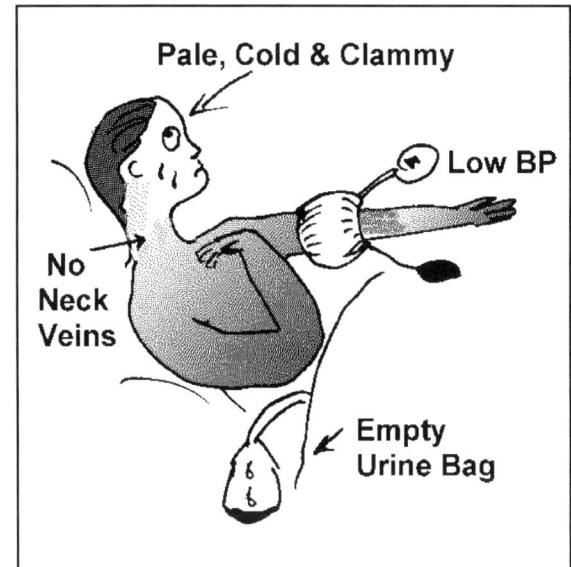

a. **YES: COLD AND CLAMMY SKIN.** It results from adrenergic vasoconstriction of periphery.
b. **NO: DECREASED HEART RATE.** Tachycardia is an important compensation mechanism for the decreased SV and CO.
c. **YES: COLLAPSED NECK VEINS.** Preload is reduced in most forms of shock. In cardiogenic shock CVP is usually normal. The exceptions are right heart infarction, pulmonary hypertension, and right heart failure. LV-EDP and wedge pressures are elevated due to the "backward failure" pattern of CHF.
d. **YES: DECREASED URINE OUTPUT.** This is a classic tool to evaluate the severity of shock. Urine output ceases in severe shock.

Signs and symptoms of shock

e. **NO: DILATED UNRESPONSIVE PUPILS** are a sign of brain death or narcotic overdose.
f. **YES: HYPOTENSION.** Blood pressure is commonly below 90 mmHg systolic.

Other clinical signs of shock are: prostration, pallor, mental confusion. **See:** Braunwald, chapter on "Acute Circulatory Failure (Shock)." **Keywords:** Shock, signs and symptoms

187. Within minutes after arteriography your patient develops wheezing, shortness of breath, pallor and diaphoresis. The BP falls to 90/50. RA pressure averages 2 mmHg. The pulse raises to 120/min with occasional PVCs. How should the patient be positioned?
  a. Supine, elevate the legs 6-12 inches
  b. Sit the patient up 30-45 degrees
  c. Turn in left lateral position - legs flexed
  d. Reverse Trendelenburg position

ANSWER a. Supine, elevate the legs 6-12 inches. These are classic signs and symptoms of anaphylactic shock. It is similar to hypovolemic shock. Both are treated by administration of IV fluid. Raising the patient's legs provides an immediate "transfusion" of lower limb blood into the thorax.

Positioning the patient is probably not enough for a severe anaphylactic reaction. Consider fluid infusion, IV epinephrine, Benadryl, and steroid therapy.
See: Braunwald, chapter on "Acute Circulatory Failure (Shock)." **See:** Study guide C4-Shock Pathology

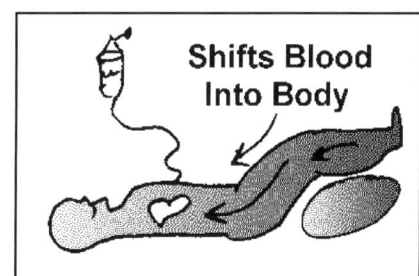

Raising legs in shock

188. In an acutely dyspneic patient going into anaphylactic shock what two medical therapies are indicated?
   a.   IV fluid administration (200-500 ml. IV)
   b.   IV lidocaine (100 mg. IV)
   c.   IV epinephrine (0.5 mg. IV)
   d.   Atropine (0.5 mg. IV)

ANSWERS: a & c. Fluid and Epi.
a. YES: IV fluid administration (200-500 ml. IV). This will replace the fluid lost due to the altered capillary permeability.
b. NO: IV lidocaine (100 mg. IV). Although the patient may have PVCs, this is not the life threatening problem. Anaphylactic shock is.
c. YES: IV epinephrine (0.5 mg. IV)
d. NO: Atropine (0.5 mg. IV). This would further speed the heart rate. The increased HR is a necessary compensation for the low CO.

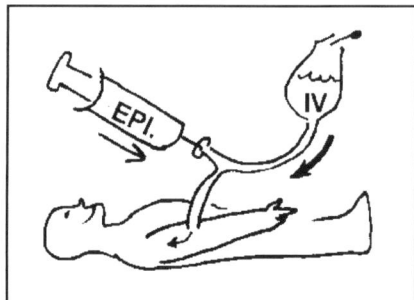

IV infusion & epi.

In the early stages "anaphylactic shock" is reversible with administration of large volumes of fluid and/or immediate administration of epinephrine 0.5 mg. IV (or 1.0 mg intratracheal).
See: Braunwald, chapter on "Acute Circulatory Failure (Shock)." See: Todd, chapter C4 "Heart Failure and Shock - General Types and Pathology of Shock" and previous question

189. During permanent pacemaker lead insertion through a central venous catheter, a bouncing shadow is seen in the cardiac silhouette as shown. What is this?
   a.   Air in RA
   b.   X-ray quantum mottle
   c.   Thrombus on electrode
   d.   Epicardial defibrillator patch

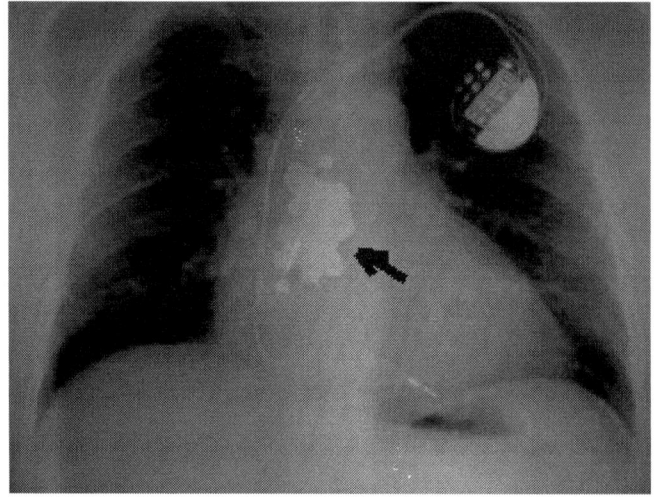

ANSWER. a. Air in RA. "Air embolism is more commonly seen with central venous catheters, however it may also occur with peripheral catheters. If air is introduced into the vascular system, it may accumulate and cause complications such as blockage of the right side of the vascular system (i.e. venous) leading to outflow obstruction of the right ventricle and pulmonary arteries. Possible symptoms include impaired gas exchange, hypotension, and circulatory collapse. Obstruction of the coronary or cerebral arteries by air can lead to myocardial infarction and acute stroke, respectively."

"While it is classically taught that 5 ml / kg of air is needed to produce an "air lock" of the right ventricle and pulmonary artery, circulatory collapse has been reported with as little as 20cc of air. Should significant air embolization occur, the patient should be placed in a left lateral recumbent position to trap the air in the right atrium. Available interventions include aspiration via a central venous catheter, hyperbaric treatment, and in severe cases, thoractomy."

Air embolism in the coronary artery is potentially fatal, depending on how much air was injected. To prevent air embolism, all tubing should be flushed prior to utilization, all connections must be tight, fluid bags should not be allowed to completely empty before replacement, and the patient's legs elevated to increase RA pressure. **See:** Topol, chapter on "Air Embolism"

5. Immune Response

190. What chemical mediator initiates the inflammation response?
a. Agglutinins
b. Antigens
c. Granuloma
d. Histamine

ANSWER d. Histamine release causes vasodilation of arterioles to bring increased blood flow and white cells to an area of injury. Injured basophils and platelets release histamine as a chemical mediator. Besides increasing blood flow to the injured area, it also increases permeability of the vessels in the area and makes the tissues swell and inflame. The intent is to induce healing. However, it often leads to a deleterious over reaction. Histamine blockers such as Benadryl can reduce this effect. **See**: Spense, chapter on "Defense Mechanisms." \

191. In the immune response the foreign protein that stimulates antibody production is:
a. Agglutinin
b. Antigen
c. Erythrocyte
d. Eosinophil

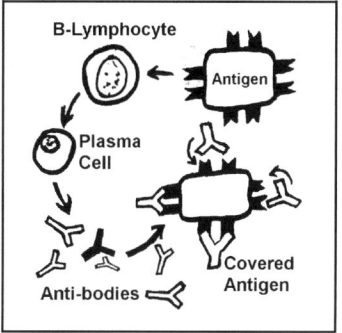

Antigen and antibodies

ANSWER b. An antigen is any invading substance which the body senses as foreign. An example of an "antigen" is a foreign bacteria, toxin or enzyme. When antigens enter the body they can trigger a cell mediated immune response after the body's lymphocytes become sensitized to this antigen. Antibodies are chemicals released by B-lymphocytes and their helper plasma cells into the blood. Antibodies have a configuration that can cover and inactivate these invading antigens. Note in the diagram how the small antibodies fit into, cover, and inactivate specific sites on the large invading antigen. See: Guyton, chapter on "Immunity and Allergy."

192. T-cells are:
a. Erythrocytes (RBCs) which produce antigens
b. Lymphocytes which destroy foreign antigens
c. Foreign antigens which are cytotoxic
d. Helper cells in antibody synthesis

ANSWER b. T-cell lymphocytes are essential to the immune system. "Killer T-cells" are activated by antigens. They react to antigens by destroying them directly or by recruiting other lymphocytes. They are important in graft rejection where they facilitate the immune reaction. They also help fight various infectious organisms.

   T cells are reduced in HIV infected patients. And their suppression makes the AIDS patient susceptible to opportunistic infections. **See:** Guyton, chapter on "Immunity and Allergy."

193. The adrenal cortex produces glucocorticoids (steroids) which may be given in large doses to treat:
   a. Infection and fever
   b. Hypertension and heart failure
   c. Inflammation and allergic reactions
   d. Peptic ulcers and esophageal varices

ANSWER c. Inflamation and allergic reactions. Glucocorticoids are the steroids like cortisol and hydrocortisone produced in the adrenal cortex. They normally regulate metabolism of carbohydrate, protein, fat and electrolyte balance. They are helpful in the treatment of many inflammatory conditions such as: allergic states, arthritis and shock. They are generally contraindicated in infection because they may mask fever. Loebl says to use steroids with caution in ulcers, heart failure, hypertension and renal insufficiency. **See:** Loebl, chapter on "Adrenocorticosteroids" **Keywords**: Glucocorticoids = steroids fight inflamation

194. The plasma protein that plays an important role in antibodies & immunity is:
   a. Albumin
   b. Gamma-globulin
   c. Fibrinogen
   d. Thrombin

ANSWER b. Most gamma-globulins are immunoglobulin, the antibodies that play an important role in immunity. Injections of gamma-globulin often give a short term boost to our immune system. These are solutions of globulins from nonhuman blood consisting of antibodies that react with specific pathogens, such as measles, hepatitis, tetanus, etc. They are prepared by injecting specific virus into animals, removing blood from the animals after antibodies accumulate, isolating these antibodies, and finally injecting them into a human for short term immunity. **See:** Guyton, chapter on "Immunity and Allergy."

6. Vascular Complications

195. Identify 5 clinical signs and symptoms of acute femoral arterial occlusion following catheterization.
a. Leg pain
b. Leg paralysis
c. Warm, sweaty leg
d. Pulseless leg
e. Leg numbness
f. Pale or mottled leg color
g. Progressive dyspnea

ANSWERS: a, b, d, e, & f.
The signs & symptoms of acute arterial occlusion are: (Note they all have words starting with P.)
 1. PAIN
 2. PARALYSIS
 3. PARAESTHESIA (numbness)
 4. PALLOR
 5. POLAR (coldness)
 6. PULSELESS

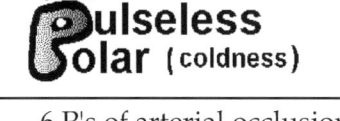

6 P's of arterial occlusion

A warm, sweaty leg and progressive dyspnea are NOT clinical signs or symptoms. Below the occlusion the leg is cool to the touch due to poor capillary flow. This is sometimes termed "polar coldness" - like the "North Pole." Dyspnea is difficult or labored breathing.
See: Underhill, chapter on "Abnormalities of coagulation, bleeding and clotting."

RADIAL Complications

196. At the end of a radial artery coronary arteriogram the catheter is stuck. It is painful and cannot be easily removed through the sheath. For the pain the physician orders more Versed and Fentanyl. For the spasm he gives 200 µg nitroglycerin and verapamil 2.5 mg through the catheter. If these fail to relax the artery what one additional therapy might you suggest?
a. Oral nifedipine 100 mg
b. Warm compress on arm
c. Removing the sheath first
d. Steady forceful traction on catheter

ANSWER: b. Warm compress on arm.
   Kern says, "Some spasm during sheath withdrawal is common. Despite all precautions, if radial artery spasm occurs or persists, consider the next suggestions. Do not allow the patient to experience significant pain; analgesics and sedation should be administered. If spasm is severe and the sheath (or catheter) is stuck, the following actions can be undertaken:
1. Administer nifedipine 10 mg orally.

2. Give more analgesia and sedation.
3. Place warm compresses over the forearm to relax the spastic artery.
4. Administer nitroglycerin 200 µg IA; repeat if necessary.
5. Give verapamil 2.5 mg IA (diltiazem can also be used). This should be mixed with blood prior to injection via the sidearm of the sheath because direct injection will cause significant discomfort.

If these do not work, wait for an hour and try again. During this time, maintain proper anticoagulation (heparin), sedation, and analgesia. If nothing helps, an axillary block, propofol, or general anesthesia might be required to relax the radial artery. One should never apply excessive force. This might result in rupture or avulsion of the radial artery. **See:** Kern, chapter on "Arterial and Venous Access"

Steinberg says, "The management of radial artery spasm centers on preventive antispasmodic administration of a cocktail consisting of nitrates and/or calcium channel blockers. The exact formula or ratio of individual agents is largely a matter of style. When patients develop spasm, management options include a tincture of time, increased sedation, additional or alternative antispasmodic medications, catheter downsizing, or abandoning the access site altogether. In rare cases, a patient may require deep conscious sedation or even intubation (in order to achieve profound sedation) to manage spasm." **See:** Steinberg, "Managing-complications-of-transradial-catheterization," Cardiac Interventions Today, 2015

197. **If the radial artery catheter remains stuck after all above attempts to relieve the spasm have failed, Kern recommends:**
a. **Inject 100 ug adenosine IA**
b. **Rapidly vibrating the catheter**
c. **Call a vascular surgeon for possible cutdown**
d. **Insert a small dilation balloon and dilate segments of distal spasm**
e. **Return to ward, wait for an hour and repeat antispasmodic measures**

ANSWER: e. Return to ward, wait for an hour and repeat antispasmodic measures again. Adenosine is only used on coronary arteries with 40-50 ug bolus.

Kern says after all therapy listed in previous question, "If these do not work, wait for an hour and try again. During this time, maintain proper anticoagulation (heparin), sedation, and analgesia. If nothing helps, an axillary block, propofol, or general anesthesia might be required to relax the radial artery. One should never apply excessive force. This might result in rupture or avulsion of the radial artery." **See:** Kern, chapter on "Arterial and Venous Access"

198. **Your heart cath patient has hypertension. Following radial artery catheterization, you remove the compression bracelet and notice a growing 3 cm swelling at the access site but no spreading to adjacent muscles or forearm. After applying manual pressure for 5 minutes you then reapply the compression bracelet. What 2 additional actions are indicated? (Select 2 below.)**
a. **Notify physician immediately**
b. **Apply local ice pack over the site**
c. **Apply additional compression bracelet**
d. **Apply tight ACE bandage around forearm**
e. **Administer protamine to reduce ACT below 250**

f. Inflate a BP cuff to the arm with pressure 20 mm below systolic

ANSWERS: b & c. Apply local ice pack over the site & apply additional compression bracelet. Ice is recommended for all hematomas along with an additional compression bracelet and mild compression bandages.

Kerns "Easy Hematoma Classification after Transradial/Ulnar PCI" table shows these mildest local superficial radial hematomas (up to 5 cm above puncture site) occur less than 5% of the time. He recommends mild compression measures and careful observation, but only informing the physician if it becomes worse. Hematomas >5 cm above the puncture site SHOULD be reported to the physician. For more extensive radial hematomas extending up to >10 cm he adds inflating a BP cuff (inflated to 20 mm below systolic and deflate every 20 minutes) to reduce radial pressure, protamine, wrapping an ACE bandage around the bracelets and arm and increasing tightness if necessary, or Velpeau pressure bandage for a few hours.

Kern says, "Radial Bleeding and Vascular Complications: Although vascular complications are rare, early recognition of a problem is vital... These can be more subtle than those seen from the femoral approach, and no overt bleeding occurs. Patients complaining of pain or parasthesia (numbness) warrant a close evaluation. Developing hematomas can be averted with gentle manual pressure followed by a careful arm-wrapping technique. While maintaining the wristband in place, wrap the arm loosely with gauze and secondarily with elastic tape or an ACE bandage, providing compression to the forearm. After several minutes, remove the tape and recheck the forearm; it should be softer. If not, rewrap with slightly higher tension. An unnoticed and untreated hematoma can produce a forearm compartment syndrome, threatening the viability of the forearm and hand." **See:** Kern, chapter on "Arterial and Venous Access"

Grade	I	II	III	IV	V
Definition	Local hematoma, superficial	Hematoma with moderate muscular infiltration	Forearm hematoma and muscular infiltration below the elbow	Hematoma and muscular infiltration extending above the elbow	Ischemic threat (compartment syndrome)
Treatment	Analgesia Additional bracelet Local ice	Analgesia Additional bracelet Local ice Inform physician	Analgesia Additional bracelet Local ice Inflated BP cuff inform	Analgesia Additional bracelet Local ice Inflated BP cuff inform	Consider surgery STAT call to physician

199. An untreated radial hematoma can produce a forearm compartment syndrome, threatening the viability of the forearm and hand. What is "compartment syndrome"?
   a. Buildup of fluid pressure cuts off blood perfusion
   b. Over tight pressure bandages can cause tissue ischemia
   c. A collection of hematoma can lead to thrombosis and septicemia
   d. Radial artery catheter manipulation can cause embolization leading to small artery occlusion

ANSWER: a. Buildup of fluid pressure cuts off blood perfusion. Medical dictionary says: "Acute compartment syndrome results from high tissue fluid pressure in a closed osseofascial compartment like the forearm that leads to reduced capillary perfusion below the level necessary for tissue viability." Radial hematoma can cause increased blood accumulation in enclosed tissue areas that compresses the capillaries leading to adjoining tissue ischemia and death. This is analogous to over packing your suitcase so tightly that your water bottle collapses.

200. After inserting the right radial sheath and catheter, angiography shows a perforation with small extravasation from the brachial artery. You recommend that the physician should:
   a. Continue with radial catheterization it will most likely resolve naturally
   b. Continue with radial catheterization after switching to a larger sheath and catheter size
   c. Inflate an angioplasty balloon to reduce bleeding and switch to the femoral approach
   d. Inflate a cloth covered stent at the site of the perforation and switch to the femoral approach

ANSWER: a. Continue with radial catheterization it will most likely resolve naturally.

Kern says, "Dissection or perforation of the radial or brachial artery can occur from wires or catheters. In this situation, the initial reaction is often to abort the procedure, but in fact, if the procedure can be continued safely, it is best to do so. The catheter will serve to tamponade the vessel, and the dissection/perforation will typically resolve by the end of the procedure. This can be confirmed by arteriography at the end of the case."

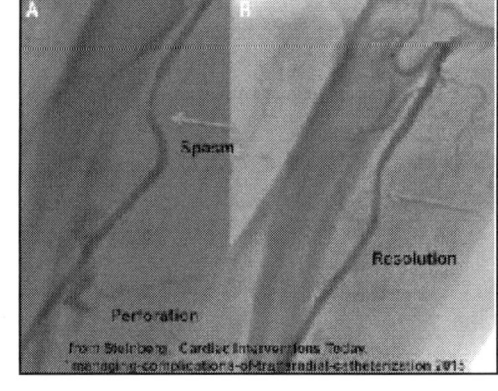

Steinberg says, "Perforation is usually discovered by contrast extravasation and staining beyond the normal architecture of the vessel. Once perforation has been established, management depends upon whether wire access is maintained. With wire access, the case can generally continue through the radial access site. Some operators recommend transitioning to a long sheath in order to tamponade the perforation and maintain access beyond the perforation site. In the case of lost wire access, the sheath should be removed with patent hemostasis maintained, and the patient should be monitored for hematoma formation." **See:** Steinberg, "Managing complications of transradial catheterization," Cardiac Interventions Today, 2015

201. To reduce the incidence of radial artery occlusion following a radial PCI case you should apply the compression bracelet tight enough to stop site bleeding and hematoma and:
   a. Totally occlude the radial artery
   b. Not totally occlude the radial artery
   c. Prevent retrograde flow up the ulnar artery
   d. Prevent radial artery compression syndrome

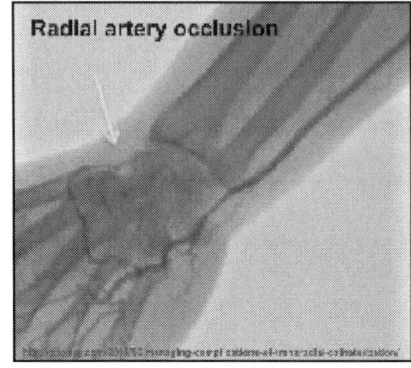

ANSWER: b. Not totally occlude the radial artery. This is termed patent hemostasis.

Steinberg says,"Another important practice for reducing radial artery occlusion is that of 'patent hemostasis.' Compared to traditional compressive hemostasis, patent hemostasis uses various compressive devices to provide sufficient hemostatic pressure over the arterial puncture site, but not enough to prevent antegrade flow through the radial artery into the distal arterial bed. In a randomized study of 436 patients undergoing transradial catheterization, Pancholy and colleagues compared compressive hemostasis to patent hemostasis and demonstrated a significant 59% reduction in early occlusion." **See:** Steinberg, "Managing complications of transradial catheterization," Cardiac Interventions Today, 2015

FEMORAL

202. Which of the following are therapy options for retroperitoneal bleed? (Select 4)
- a. **Blood transfusion**
- b. **Thoracentesis**
- c. **Protamine administration**
- d. **Continued pressure over puncture site**
- e. **Surgical arterioplasty**
- f. **Fogarty thrombectomy**

ANSWERS: a, c, d, & e.
- a. Blood transfusion - YES
- b. Thoracentesis - NO. Thoracentesis is not indicated since the bleeding is in the abdomen, not the thorax.
- c. Protamine administration - YES
- d. Continued pressure over puncture site - YES
- e. Surgical arterioplasty - YES
- f. Fogarty thrombectomy - NO. There is no clot in the artery.

Freed says: "After confirmation of retroperitoneal hematoma, cessation of heparin and removal of arterial catheters with prolonged compression of the involved vessel is mandatory. The majority of retroperitoneal bleeds will stop spontaneously. Although many patients may require a blood transfusion, most are hemodynamically stable. However, continued decline in hematocrit, signs of volume depletion, or hemodynamic instability despite reversal of anticoagulants indicate that hematoma expansion is likely and surgical exploration may be warranted."
See: Freed, chapter on "Medical and Peripheral Complications"

203. Twelve hours following angiography a patient develops a painful pulsatile mass just below the skin at the femoral artery puncture site. A femoral artery bruit can be heard with a stethoscope. What is the most likely complication?
- a. True aneurysm (TA)
- b. False aneurysm (FA)
- c. AV fistula (FA-FV)
- d. Hematoma (FA)

ANSWER b. False aneurysms (or pseudoaneurysms) are a

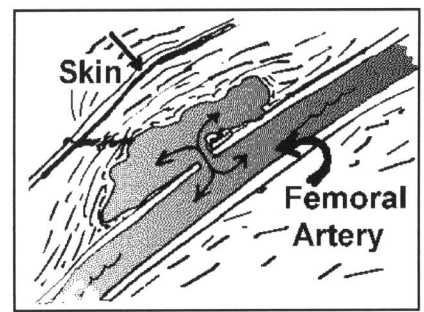

False aneurysm (FA)

pulsating encapsulated hematoma in communication with a ruptured artery. Blood swishes back and forth between the femoral artery (FA) and the false aneurysmal chamber, through a narrow neck.

These aneurysms frequently enlarge and rupture, although the rupture may not occur for several days post-cath. The causes include: enlarged puncture site and inadequate groin compression when the sheath is pulled. Surgical intervention may be necessary. Some practitioners attempt to close the false lumen with additional groin compression while observing Doppler flow through the aneurysm's "neck." A compressor clamp may be used to close the neck and allow it to clot off.

Grossman says, "Blood flowing in and out of the arterial puncture expands the hematoma cavity during systole and allows it to decompress back into the arterial lumen in diastole. Since the hematoma cavity contains no normal arterial wall structures (i.e., media or adventia), this condition is referred to as false or pseudoaneurysm." See Grossman chapter on Complications

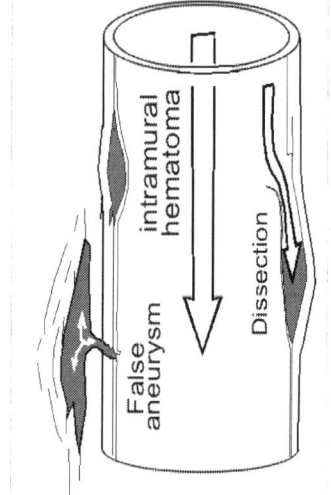

204. Bleeding between the walls of an artery that causes separation within the arterial layers and splits them apart is termed a/an:
a. AV fistula
b. Dissection
c. Aneurysm
d. Pseudoaneurysm

ANSWER b. Dissection within an arterial wall can be catastrophic. As it splits the intima from the media it makes a tear down the arterial wall like wet wallpaper being ripped off. Layers of intima may tear around a branch vessel and cut it off, leading to ischemia of the tissue it supplied. This is caused by a tear causing an entrance into the vessel wall. The area within the wall is called the false lumen. Sometimes a flap of the intima bows into the true lumen restricting it. Dissection may happen when a patient has "cystic medial necrosis" due to Marfan syndrome, where the media dissolves.

Coronary angioplasty often causes tears in calcified intima creating a false lumen. These may produce flaps of tissue that can cut off blood flow to areas of the heart. Like aortic dissections these may split the wall and extend down the vessel. When using a stiff guidewire an aggressive operator can penetrate the vessel wall and dissect down the coronary wall splitting it. In this common complication, balloon compression or stents may used to tack the intima back to the arterial wall.

False aneurysm or pseudoaneurysm occurs when the needle or guidewire track all the way through the wall of the RFA does not seal up. Then blood can leak out into the tissues in systole, and back during diastole. These are a pulsating loud type of back-and-forth bleeding hematoma. They need to be sealed with manual pressure using ultrasound guidance. See diagram.

There is another rare type of dissection not caused by a tear in the intima. This is called intramural hematoma or intramural hemorrhage. Trauma may cause rupture of the vaso vasorum blood supply within the media. Here, there is no entrance or exit point, since the hemorrhage comes from within the vessel wall itself. See diagram.
See: Grossman, chapter on "Complications" **Keywords:** dissection

205. Your patient develops a pseudoaneurysm 2 days after transfemoral catheterization. How can it be most easily repaired?
a. Use a Perclose vascular closure device
b. Manual compression with a Syvek® patch topical dressing
c. Inject procoagulant (thrombin) into the false aneurysm
d. Ultrasound localization with application of a Femo-stop
e. Ultrasound localization with application of Compressar clamp

ANSWER e. Ultrasound localization with application of Compressar clamp. Kern says, "With ultrasound imaging techniques these false channels can be easily identified and nonsurgical closure selected. Manual compression of the expansile growing mass guided by Doppler ultrasound with or without thrombin or collagen injection is an acceptable therapy for femoral pseudoaneurysm" Don't inject thrombin into a pulsating aneurysm. To use the perclose you would have to first stick the neck of the aneurysm which would be nearly impossible. See: http://heart.bmj.com/content/85/4/e5 Ferguson, "Ultrasound guided percutaneous thrombin injection of iatrogenic femoral artery pseudoaneurysms after coronary angiography and intervention" Heart 2001

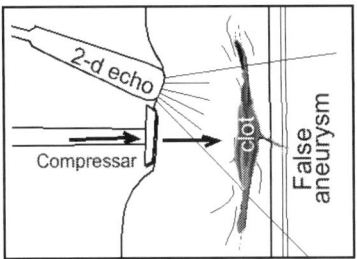

Noninvasive closure false aneurysm

206. Your overweight patient has undergone double stent placement in the LAD. The physician had a hard time gaining vascular access. He ended up puncturing the left femoral artery superior to the head of the femur. You are suturing in the femoral sheath when the patient complains of severe back pain with tenderness in the right inguinal area. ACT is 310, Hgb is 10, O2 sat is 94%. Suspect:
a. Aortic dissection
b. Pseudoaneurym of LFA
c. Retroperitoneal hemorrhage
d. Coronary artery perforation with pericardial tamponade

ANSWER c. Retroperitoneal hemorrhage or bleeding into the belly. This complication may occur with high femoral artery punctures. Freed says: "Effective compression may be impossible since the arterial structures area retroperitoneal and hemorrhage from the puncture site may accumulate posteriorly rather than in the inguinal region. . . ."

"Abdominal pain occurs in approximately 60% of patients with retroperitoneal hematomas, with back and flank pain in approximately 25%. . . . Often the diagnosis is suspected from an asymptomatic drop in hemoglobin." See: Freed, chapter on "Medical and Peripheral Complications" **Keywords:** Retroperitoneal bleed

207. **Which of the following are used to treat acute femoral arterial occlusion following catheterization? (Select 4.)**
   a. Arterial stent
   b. Rheolytic thrombectomy
   c. Bypass graft
   d. Endarterectomy
   e. Thrombolytic medication
   f. Icing the limb

   ANSWERS: b, c, d, & e.
   a. Arterial stent - NO. Stents are excellent to keep a vessel open. But it will not prevent a clot from lodging in the patent vessel.
   b. Rheolytic thrombectomy (AngioJet) - YES
   c. Bypass graft - YES
   d. Endarterectomy - YES
   e. Thrombolytic medication - YES
   f. Icing the limb - NO. Only if there is no hope for limb survival.
   Other emergency therapy includes: Pain control with narcotics. Keep the patient very warm to relieve arterial spasm. A room warmed to 80-85 degrees helps. Wrap the involved extremity loosely in cotton to preserve body heat and protect it from trauma. Icing the limb is contraindicated if there is hope for survival of the limb. But once gangrene has set in and amputation is inevitable, packing the limb in ice may reduce pain and delay emergency surgery. Elevation and application of heat are contraindicated here as they may hasten gangrene.
   See: Hurst and Logue, chapter on "Vascular Disease." and Braunwald, chapter on "Diseases of the Aorta."

208. **Following femoral arteriography a patient's leg becomes cool, pale, mottled, and painful from acute femoral artery occlusion. Initial therapy should include:**
   a. Heparin infusion
   b. Vasodilator infusion
   c. Cooling or icing the extremity
   d. Elevating the extremity

   ANSWER a. Heparin infusion. Initial therapy is to anticoagulate the patient to prevent further embolization and clot extension. The definitive treatment is surgical removal of the clot. Other therapies are: bypass graft surgery, endarterectomy, and thrombolytic medications. **See:** Hurst and Logue, chapter on "Vascular Disease." and Underhill, chapter on "Vascular Diseases."

209. **Your patient is a small elderly lady whose mid LAD has just been stented. After RFA sheath removal, her leg becomes pulseless, cold and painful. The cardiologist tells you to call a surgeon and prep the other groin (LFA). He probably intends to:**
   a. Insert a balloon pump
   b. Use a Fogarty catheter to remove an RFA clot
   c. Evaluate flow in the RFA with angiography
   d. Look for thrombus in the RFA with IVUS

ANSWER: c. Evaluate flow in the RFA with angiography. Grossman says, "Femoral artery thrombosis can occur in patients with a small common femoral artery lumen (peripheral vascular disease, diabetes, female gender), in whom a large-diameter catheter or sheath (e.g., intra-aortic balloon pump) has been placed, particularly when the catheter dwell time is long or when prolonged post procedure compression is applied. Such patients have a white painful leg with impaired distal sensory and motor function, as well as absent distal pulses. If this occurs during the catheterization procedure and is not corrected promptly by sheath removal, a flow-obstructing dissection or thrombus at the femoral artery puncture site or a distal arterial embolus should be suspected. This requires urgent attention via vascular surgery consultation (for exploration and correction of any local dissection or plaque avulsion and Fogarty embolectomy of the distal vessel as needed to restore distal pulses). Alternatively, operators skilled in peripheral intervention may be able to puncture the contralateral femoral artery, cross over the aortic [iliac] bifurcation and address a common femoral occlusion percutaneously." Ivus is poor at evaluating thrombus since it has the same density as blood. **See:** Grossman, chapter on, "Complications ..."

210. A pulmonary hypertensive patient is referred for pulmonary angiography. Immediately following PA angiography his HR drops and the systolic PA pressure rapidly increases, as shown. This severe complication is termed a/an:
a. Acute RV infarction
b. Acute cor pulmonale
c. Primary pulmonary hypertension
d. Anaphylactic allergic reaction

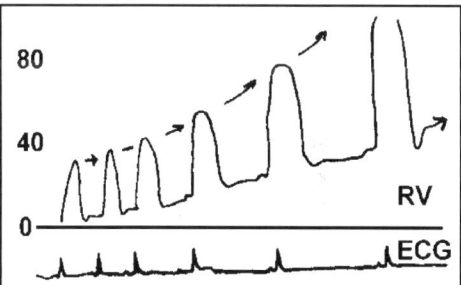
Rapidly rising RV & PA pressure

ANSWER b. Acute cor pulmonale is a critical and often irreversible complication of pulmonary arteriography in PA hypertensive patients (RV-edp >20 or 25). With PA angiography the PA pressure normally goes up slightly but the HR does not normally drop. When it does, begin immediate resuscitation maneuvers. **See:** Johnsrude, chapter on "Cath and Pulm. Angio."

211. Pulmonary angiography is a HIGH RISK procedure in pulmonary hypertensive patients with:
a. RA mean > 15 mmHg
b. RV-edp > 25 mmHg
c. PA diastolic > 20 mmHg
d. PA systolic > 30 mmHg

ANSWER b. RV-edp > 25 mmHg. Normally the RA mean pressure = RV-edp which are both below 7 mmHg. And the PA pressure is below 30/10 mmHg. High RV-edp and RA pressure indicate some right heart failure. When the RV-edp exceeds 20-25 mmHg the patient **MAY CRASH** with only slight amounts of contrast injected into the PA. These individuals are barely compensated. They are very unstable. Even small amounts of contrast may cause acute irreversible cor pulmonale with increasing RV pressure and bradycardia - leading to

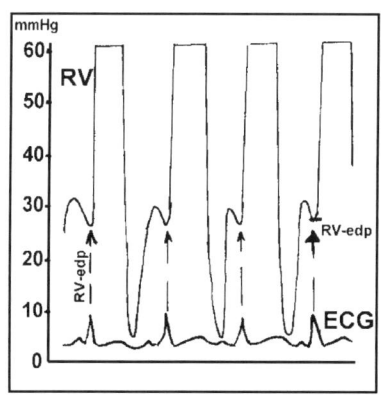
Pulm. hypertension - RVedp

cardiovascular collapse.

Johnsrude recommends using non-ionic contrast, using super-selective small volume injections, and administration of O2. An older treatment is to inflate tourniquets to 80 mm Hg on both legs. This traps venous blood and reduces the right heart load during pulmonary angiography. **See:** Johnsrude, chapter on "Cath and Pulm. Angio."

212. What type of pulmonary angiography patient has the greatest risk for in-procedure mortality?
a. Primary pulmonary hypertension patients
b. Secondary pulmonary hypertension patients
c. Acute RV infarction patients
d. Pulmonary valve stenosis patients

ANSWER a. Primary pulmonary hypertension patients are very intolerant of pulmonary arteriography, anesthesia, surgery, or lung scan. Small cardiovascular stresses may lead to sudden cardiovascular collapse. Any stress on the already over-constricted PA vessels may lead to further vasoconstriction, RV pressure overloaded, right heart failure, and lethal arrhythmias. Beware of primary pulmonary hypertensive patients.

"Primary" = essential = idiopathic meaning the cause is unknown and probably hereditary. Cardiac cath is the only test to rule out more treatable diagnosis. About all you can do for primary pulmonary hypertension (PPH) is a heart-lung transplant.

Grossman states than these procedures can be done safely in experienced hands. But, he recommends use of non-ionic contrast and super-selective hand injections of selected lung areas through balloon-flotation catheters. Others recommend vasodilators to reduce the pulmonary hypertension prior to cath. **See:** Braunwald, chapter on "Pulmonary Hypertension." **Keywords:** primary pulmonary hypertension = high risk PA angio

213. What complication can occur from frequent and prolonged wedging of Swan Ganz catheters?
a. Balloon rupture
b. Catheter thrombosis
c. Pulmonary infarction
d. Ruptured chordae tendineae

ANSWER c. Pulmonary infarction. During long-term Swan-Ganz monitoring the catheter may migrate with repeated RV contractions deeper into the lungs and become permanently wedged. This cuts off the blood supply and the downstream lung tissue may become infarcted and die. This damaged tissue may be seen as a "white-out" area on the chest film.

Prevention of this complication is to monitor the balloon position with X-rays or fluoroscopy. It may also be suspected when the pressure waveform is constantly wedged. To reduce the chance of catheter migration be sure it issutured tightly at the skin. **See:** Daily, chapter on "CVP and PA Pressure Monitoring." **Keywords:** Prolonged Swan wedging → pulmonary infarction

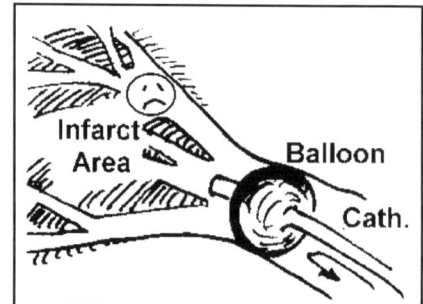

Pulmonary infarction

214. Which of the following are included in therapy for acute PA rupture? (Select 4)
a. Position patient on the side of the good lung
b. Intubate both lungs
c. Reverse anticoagulation with protamine
d. Inflate the Swan-Ganz balloon to decrease bleeding
e. Initiate intra aortic balloon pumping
f. Emergency surgery

ANSWERS: b, c, d, & f.
a. **NO: POSITION PATIENT** on the side of the effected lung to avoid bleeding into the good lung.
b. **YES: INTUBATE BOTH** lungs (with a bilateral tracheostomy catheter. Suction the bleeding lung, ventilate the good lung with O2).
c. **YES: REVERSE ANTICOAGULATION** with protamine to seal the wound with clot and slow the bleeding.
d. **YES: INFLATE THE** Swan-Ganz balloon to decrease bleeding: If the balloon catheter has not been removed it may be a lifesaving plug at the bleeding site. Simply inflating it again may cut off the PA pressure and blood from the bleeding site.
e. **NO: IABP may** increase bleeding.
f. **YES: EMERGENCY SURGERY** may be necessary.
See: Daily, chapter on "CVP and PA Pressure Monitoring."

215. A 75-year-old lady with pulmonary hypertension has a Swan-Ganz monitoring catheter. She suddenly develops coughing, massive hemoptysis, and dyspnea. What complication is likely?
a. Pulmonary infarction
b. RV infarction
c. PA rupture
d. PA dissection

ANSWER c. PA rupture is a rare, dramatic and often fatal complication of PA catheter use. The key here is "hemoptysis" which is spitting up blood. When the PA is ruptured venous blood enters the bronchi and lung bed. This causes coughing and can obstruct breathing. PA rupture by a Swan-Ganz may be caused by:
- **OVER-INFLATION OF THE BALLOON** (never use more air than the balloon is rated for and stop inflating when the wedge pressure appears on the monitor)
- **FREQUENT INFLATIONS OF THE BALLOON** (use PA edp to approximate wedge pressure)
- **DISTAL MIGRATION OF THE CATHETER TIP** (check pressures and X-ray position

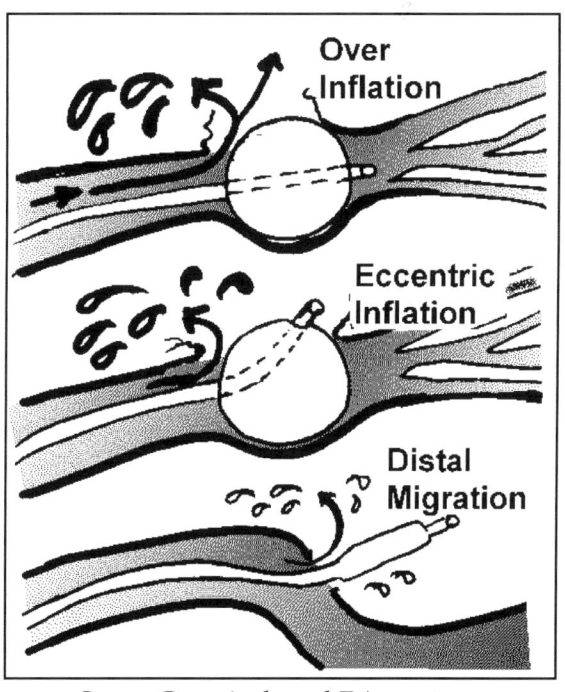

Swan-Ganz induced PA rupture

frequently)
- **FORCEFUL MANUAL FLUSHING OF A WEDGED CATHETER** (may blow out the vessel wall)
- **ECCENTRIC BALLOON INFLATION** (lumen in contact with wall causes "over-wedging" may erode out vessel wall or trap the tip in the PA)

Patients at high risk include those with:
- Elderly patients (weak vessel walls)
- Pulmonary hypertension (high PA pressure drives the catheter tip and balloon deeper into the lung)
- Anticoagulation and cardiopulmonary bypass (heart manipulation and hypothermia may drive the stiffened catheter deeper into the lung)

See: Daily, chapter on "CVP and PA Pressure Monitoring." **Keywords:** hemoptysis → causes of

216. Your pacemaker implant patient is snoring loudly. During subclavian puncture and sheath insertion what is an immediate sign of air embolism?
a. A hissing sound
b. Lung stridor sound
c. Cyanosis and/or drop in BP
d. Chest pain or coughing up bloody sputum

ANSWER: a. A hissing sound
 Ellenbogen says, "Air embolism can occur when a central vein is accessed by a sheath, regardless of the technique used to introduce it. This complication may be signaled by a hiss of air sucked into the sheath by negative intrathoracic pressure and may occur suddenly when a heavily sedated, snoring patient deeply inspires at a time when control over the sheath's orifice is not adequate." **See:** Ellenbogen, chapter on "Techniques of Pacemaker Implantation and Removal"

217. To help prevent air embolism during pacemaker implant, why is it important to be sure your patient is well hydrated?
a. Higher CVP makes it easier to feel venous pulse
b. Increased blood volume increases preload and BP
c. Increased blood volume minimizes effect of blood loss
d. Higher CVP less is likely to go negative on inspiration

ANSWER: d. Higher CVP less is likely to go negative on inspiration and suck in air.
Higher venous pressure makes less of a pressure gradient between intrathoracic pressure and atmospheric air pressure, so air is less likely to be sucked in during deep inspiration when the thoracic pressure drops. Intrathoracic pressure is always negative and goes more negative during deep inspiration. This negative pressure is transmitted to the intrathoracic vessels. The Trendelenburg position (elevated legs) also raises CVP and helps prevent air embolism during subclavian stick. "Three obligatory conditions need to coexist for pulmonary air embolism to occur: (1) there must be a source of gas/air; (2) an open access to the venous system; and (3) a pressure gradient between the source of gas/air and the venous system. It can be prevented through operator care and using introducers with hemostatic valves. The diagnosis is obvious because it is heralded by a hissing sound as the air is sucked in and with the fluoroscopic confirmation that follows."

http://cdn.intechopen.com/pdfs/13786/InTech-Common_pacemaker_problems_lead_and_pocket_complications.pdf

REFERENCES

Baim, D. S. and Grossman W., *Cardiac Catheterization, Angiography, and Intervention*, 7th Ed., Lea and Febiger Book Co., 2006
Braunwald, Eugene, Ed., *HEART DISEASE A Textbook of Cardiovascular Medicine*, 9th Ed., W. B. Saunders Co., 2012
CDC, Guideline for Prevention of Intravascular Device-Related Infections, 1996, www.cdc.gov/ncidod/hip/IV/Iv.htm
Daily, E. K., and Schroeder, J. S., *Techniques in Bedside Hemodynamic Monitoring*, 4th Ed., C. V. Mosby Company, 1989
Ellenbogen, Clinical Cardiac Pacing, Defibrillation, and Resynchronization Therapy, Elsevier, 2011
Freed, Grines, and Safian, The New Manual of Interventional Cardiology 2nd printing, Physicians Press, 1996
Hurst, J. W., and Logue, R. B., et. al., *THE HEART Arteries and Veins*, 3rd Ed., McGraw-Hill Book Co., 1974
Johnsrude, I. S., Jackson. D. C., Et. al., *A Practical Approach to Angiography*, 2nd Ed. Little, Brown and Co., 1987
Kern, Morton, *The Cardiac Catheterization Handbook,* 6th Ed., Mosby, 2016
King, S.B. III and Yeung, Alan, *Interventional Cardiology*, McGraw-Hill Book Co., 2007
Lanzer, Peter, *Mastering Endovascular Techniques, a guide to excellence*, Lippincot, 2007
Nguyen, & Colombo, et all., Practical Handbook of Advanced Interventional Cardiology, 3rd Ed., Blackwell Futura, 2009
Peterson & Nicod, *Cardiac Catheterization: Methods, Diagnosis, and Therapy*, 1st Ed, Saunders, 1997
Underhill, S. L., Ed., *CARDIAC NURSING*, 2nd Ed., J. B. Lippincott Co., 1989

OUTLINE: Indications, Risks, & Complications

1. INDICATIONS/CONTRAINDICATIONS
   a. Indications
      i. Pre- surgery (CABG)
      ii. Chest pain of uncertain origin
      iii. Recent Acute MI
      iv. Pharmacologic Therapy (hypertension)
      v. Interventional Therapy
      vi. PCI
      vii. Valvuloplasty
      viii. RT. heart Cath.
         (1) Valvular heart disease
         (2) Pulmonary disease (COPD, Pulm. hypertension...)
         (3) Congenital heart disease (pediatric or adult)
         (4) Electrophysiology study / ablation
            (a) sudden death, arrhythmia...
         (5) Pericardial constriction or tamponade
         (6) Cardiomyopathy
         (7) Heart transplant follow up
         (8) (including biopsy)
         (9) Acute care monitoring
      ix. Relative Contraindications to cath.
         (1) Uncontrolled Vent. Arrhythmias
         (2) Uncontrolled hypokalemia
         (3) Uncontrolled hypertension
         (4) Febrile illness
         (5) Uncontrolled CHF
         (6) Anticoagulation
         (7) Severe allergy to contrast
         (8) Renal insufficiency Cre> 1.5
         (9) pregnancy
   b. Absolute Contraindications
      i. Patient refusal (No Op. Permit)
      ii. Unsafe Lab conditions
         (1) untrained / incompetent staff
         (2) inadequate / unsafe equipment
2. PRECAUTIONS
   a. Anticoagulated patient
      i. if on Coumadin, switch to heparin
      ii. Adjust PT time < 18 sec
   b. Renal insufficiency (Cre. > 1.5)
      i. Use low Osmolar Contrast
      ii. CIN
      iii. Hydrate patient
   c. Previous stroke
      i. full dose heparin anticoagulation
   d. Sones -
      i. prevention of brachial thrombosis
         (1) Fogarty Brachial artery
      ii. prevention of infection
         (1) flush wound with Iodine-Povidone
   e. Allergic reaction
      i. Seafood allergy (Iodine)
      ii. NPH Insulin (no protamine)
      iii. Previous allergic reaction
   f. Previous Allergy to Contrast
      i. Premedication
      ii. Steroids (Prednisone) and Antihistamines like Diphenhydramine (Benadryl)
      iii. Prednisone (60 mg the night before and 60 mg pre-cath)
      iv. Diphenhydramine (Benadryl - 50 mg
3. RISKS
   a. Patients at increased risk during cath:
      i. infants (< 1 year of age) or elderly individuals > 60 years of age
      ii. Valvular heart disease patients with coronary disease
      iii. Patients with severe coronary obstructions (Widow-maker)
      iv. Functional class IV patients
      v. LV dysfunction patients (EF < 30)
      vi. Non-cardiac disease
         (1) diabetes
         (2) renal insufficiency
         (3) Cerebrovascular
         (4) Peripheral Vascular disease
   b. Mortality rate of coronary arteriography
      i. 0.1-0.3%
      ii. Greatest risk with Widowmaker lesion
   c. Mortality PCI
      i. 0.3%
   d. High risk PA angiography
      i. RVedp > 25 mmHg
      ii. Rt. heart Failure
      iii. Primary Pulmonary Hypertension
      iv.
4. CARDIAC COMPLICATIONS
   a. Mortality (Death) 0.1%
   b.
   c. CVA (Stroke) 0.07%
      i. Heparinization 5000 units IV
   d. Thrombosis
   e. Hematoma / bleeding
   f. Radial
   g. Patent hemostasis
   h. TR Band
   i. Ice
   j. ACE bandage
   k. BP cuff
   l. Radial Spasm
   m. Nifedipine
   n. Analgesia & sedation
      i. Warm compress
      ii. Nitro 200 ug
      iii. Verapamil 2.5 mg IA
      iv. Wait and try later
   o. Compartment syndrome
      i. retroperitoneal bleed
      ii. Intramural thrombosis
      iii. false aneurysm (pseudoaneurysm
      iv. A-V fistula
      v. Perforation
         (1) RV perforation most common

p. Pericardial tamponade therapy
   i. Pericardio-centesis
   ii. RV perforation
   iii. RV biopsy
   iv. Uses fluoro & 2-d echo
   v. Loculation=localized
   vi. Prop up torso 45 degrees
q. Dissection
   i. Balloon compression
   ii. Stent compression
r. Vasovagal
   i. Atropine, Fluid infusion, raise legs
s. Arrhythmia / blocks
   i. Catheter irritation
      (1) manipulation in ventricle, PVCs, VT
      (2) manipulation in atrium, PACs, AT
t. ALLERGIC COMPLICATIONS
   i. Rash, Nausea, Urticaria:
      (1) Benadryl, Prednisone, Decadron
   ii. Dyspnea, Wheezing, Syncope:
      (1) Epinephrine, Volume Infusion (BLS as Needed)
   iii. Seizure, Hypotension, Bradycardia, Dyspnea: (BLS as needed)
   iv. Seizure, Vital Signs Ok:
      (1) Valium
u. Infection
v. Hypotension
   i. Vasoconstrictors
w. PA Rupture by a Swan-Ganz Caused By:
   i. Over-inflation of the Balloon
   ii. Frequent Inflations of the Balloon
   iii. Distal Migration of the Catheter Tip
   iv. Forceful Manual Flushing of a Wedged Catheter
   v. Eccentric Balloon Inflation
x. Patients at high risk of PA rupture include
   i. Elderly patients (weak vessel walls)
   ii. Pulmonary Hypertension
   iii. Anticoagulation and cardiopulmonary bypass
y. Rx for PA Rupture
   i. Intubate Both Lungs
   ii. Reverse Anticoagulation with Protamine
   iii. Inflate the Swan-Ganz Balloon to Decrease Bleeding
z. Rx for Cor Pulmonale
   i. elevate the patient to sitting position
   ii. Administer 15 mg Morphine IV
   iii. Hang a Dopamine drip, administer 5-50 μg/kg/min
   iv. Advanced and Basic life support as needed
aa. SHOCK (Signs & Symptoms)
   i. Cold and Clammy Skin. It Results from Adrenergic Vasoconstriction of Periphery.
   ii. Collapsed Neck Veins. Preload Is Reduced in Most Forms of Shock.
   iii. In Cardiogenic Shock CVP Is Usually Normal.
   iv. Decreased Urine Output.
   v. Hypotension. (Syst. <90)
   vi. Prostration
   vii. Pallor
   viii. Mental Confusion.
bb. Pulseless Brachial Artery following Sones Coronary angio:
   i. Fogarty embolectomy
cc. Pyrogen Reaction:
   i. Morphine 2-4 mg IV repeated as necessary
dd. Phlebitis and Fever 12 hrs. following pacemaker implantation:
   i. Antibiotic
ee. Vasovagal Reaction:
   i. Atropine .5-1 mg. IV
   ii. Elevate legs, give IV fluid

5. VASCULAR COMPLICATIONS
   a. Arterial Occlusion
      i. Pain,
      ii. Paralysis
      iii. Paraesthesia (Numbness),
      iv. Pallor
      v. Polar (Coldness)
      vi. Pulseless
   b. Initial Therapy for arterial occlusion
      i. Pain control with narcotics.
      ii. Keep patient warm to relieve arterial spasm
      iii. Heparin
      iv. Surgery, Fogarty embolectomy procedure
      v. Heparin administration

Anaphylaxis: diagnosis and treatment

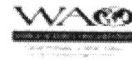

Initial treatment

1		Have a written emergency protocol for recognition and treatment of anaphylaxis and rehearse it regularly.
2		Remove exposure to the trigger if possible, e.g. discontinue an intravenous diagnostic or therapeutic agent that seems to be triggering symptoms.
3		Assess the patient's circulation, airway, breathing, mental status, skin and body weight (mass).
		Promptly and simultaneously, perform steps 4, 5 and 6.
4		Call for help: resuscitation team (hospital) or emergency medical services (community) if available.
5		Inject epinephrine (adrenaline) intramuscularly in the mid-anterolateral aspect of the thigh, 0.01 mg/kg of a 1:1,000 (1 mg/mL) solution, maximum of 0.5 mg (adult) or 0.3 mg (child); record the time of the dose and repeat it in 5–15 minutes, if needed. Most patients respond to 1 or 2 doses.
6		Place patient on the back or in a position of comfort if there is respiratory distress and/or vomiting; elevate the lower extremities; fatality can occur within seconds if patient stands or sits suddenly.
7		When indicated, give high-flow supplemental oxygen (6-8 L/minute), by face mask or oropharyngeal airway.
8		Establish intravenous access using needles or catheters with wide-bore cannulae (14 - 16 gauge); When indicated, give 1–2 litres of 0.9% (isotonic) saline rapidly (e.g. 5–10 mL/kg in the first 5–10 minutes to an adult; 10 mL/kg to a child).
9		When indicated, at any time, perform cardiopulmonary resuscitation with continuous chest compressions and rescue breathing.
		In addition,
10		At frequent, regular interval, monitor patient's blood pressure, cardiac rate and function, respiratory status, and oxygenation (monitor continuously, if possible).

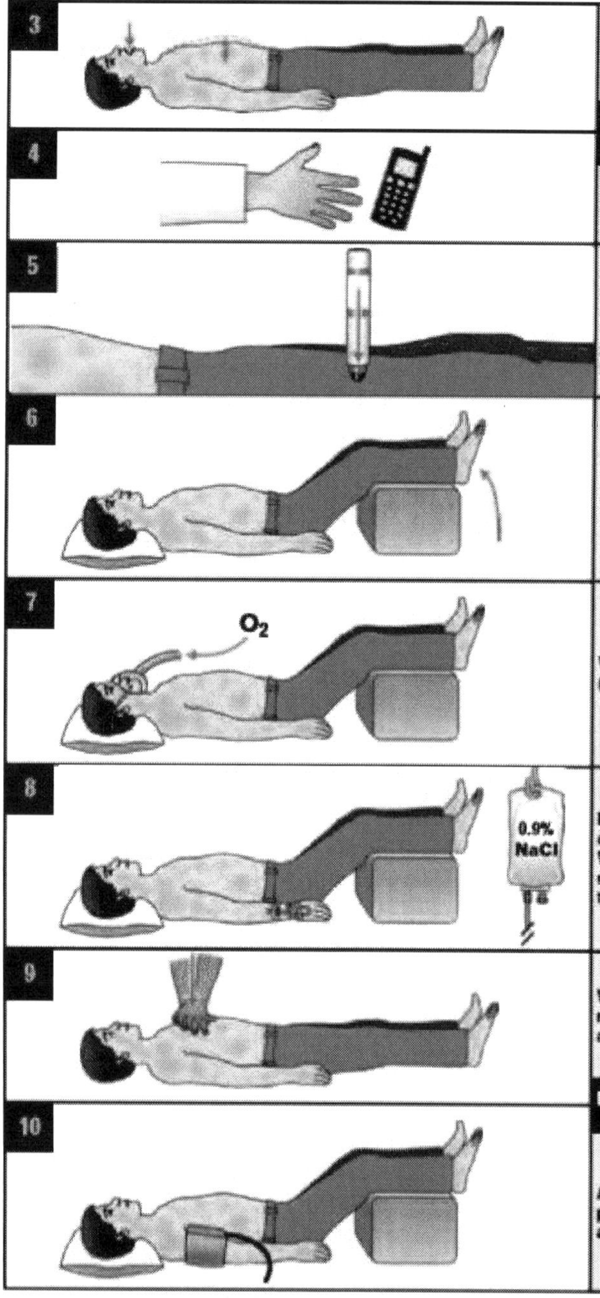

References: Simons FER et al, for the WAO. J Allergy Clin Immunol 2011;127:587-93.e22 and WAO Journal 2011;4:13-36. Illustrator: J Schaffer

Cath: Protocol and Preparations

INDEX: D4 - Cath: Protocol and Preparations
- 1. History . . . . . p. 117 - Review
- 2. Standards . . . . p. 117 - Know
- 3. Ethical & Legal . . . p. 121 - Know
- 4. Pre-cath . . . . p. 125 - Know
- 5. Premedications . . . p. 130 - Know
- 6. Chapter Outline . . . p. 138

1. History of Catheterization

218. Identify the chief accomplishment of the historic figure in cardiovascular catheterization - labeled #2 in the box (M. Sones).
- a. First heart cath (on horse) 1844
- b. First cath on human (himself) 1929
- c. Developed percutaneous technique 1953
- d. First coronary arteriogram 1959
- e. First coronary angioplasty 1977

> **HISTORIC FIGURES IN CARDIAC CATHETERIZATION**
> 1. Andreas Gruntzig
> *2. Mason Sones
> 3. Werner Forssman
> 4. Claude Bernard
> 5. S.I. Seldinger

ANSWER d. Mason Sones performed the first coronary arteriogram in 1959.
Be able to match all answers below. **CORRECTLY MATCHED ANSWERS ARE:**

HISTORIC FIGURE	ACCOMPLISHMENT - DATE
1. Andreas Gruntzig	First coronary angioplasty 1977
2. Mason Sones	**First coronary arteriogram 1959**
3. Werner Forssman	First cath on human (himself) 1929
4. Claude Bernard	First heart cath (on horse) 1844
5. Seldinger	Developed percutaneous technique 1953

See: Pepine, chapter on "Cath Techniques..." **Keywords:** Historic figures Sones = first coronary arteriogram

2. Standards

219. Which of the following are included in Grossman's general principles of designing a catheterization protocol? (Select 4.)
- a. Monitor arterial pressure in all patients
- b. Take hemodynamic measurements before angiography
- c. Measure O_2 saturations and pullback pressures on the way out
- d. Measure pressures and cardiac outputs simultaneously

e.   **Get most important angiograms first**

ANSWERS: a, b, d, & e.

Grossman recommends that the physician make everyone aware of what he's going to do on a case. "This carefully reasoned sequential plan designed specifically for the individual patient being studied" is the "protocol."

   a.   **YES: MONITOR ARTERIAL PRESSURE IN ALL PATIENTS:** He recommends that the sheath sidearm be connected to a pressure transducer to continuously monitor femoral artery pressure.
   b.   **YES: TAKE HEMODYNAMIC MEASUREMENTS BEFORE ANGIOGRAPHY:** He believes that angiographic contrast distorts all hemodynamic readings. Consequently he believes in doing the LV gram (and angiographic CO) before coronary arteriography, unless other reasons make the coronary angiography more important.
   c.   **NO: It should read - MEASURE O_2 SATURATIONS AND PRESSURES ON WAY IN**: He believes that you should get what information you can while you are there. You may have problems later and have to pull out of more distal chambers. (E.g., sample RA first, then RV...)
   d.   **YES: MEASURE PRESSURES AND CARDIAC OUTPUTS SIMULTANEOUSLY**: Hemodynamic states change constantly. By the time you get around to doing the CO the pressures may all have increased, or the patient may be put on O2 changing all hemodynamic parameters. "Get it while you can."
   e.   **YES: SHOOT THE MOST IMPORTANT ANGIOGRAMS FIRST:** This is obvious. If a person has isolated suspected LAD disease - shoot that first.

See: Grossman, chapter on "Percutaneous Approach." **Keywords:** 5 principles of protocol

220. **According to the ACC / SCAI Cath Lab Standards what is the minimum PCI case load necessary for a cath lab team to maintain competency?**
   a.   > 100 cases/year
   b.   > 200 cases/year
   c.   > 400 cases/year
   d.   > 800 cases/year

ANSWER b. > 200 cases/year in a hospital maintains staff competency. The ACC/SCAI guidelines say: "In general, the Committee thought that the minimum interventional caseload of 75 procedures/year for operators and a minimum performance **of 200 cases/year by institutions**, with the ideal being 400 cases/year per laboratory, both reasonable and supportable, based on current data. . . . The ACC/AHA guidelines for PCI have reviewed this issue in depth, noting multiple studies that support a relationship between complications and procedural volume." 2007 guidelines state" It is recommended that all institutions have a regular (at least monthly) catheterization laboratory conference." **See**: 2001 & 2007 ACC / SCAI Expert Consensus Document on Cath Lab Standards **Keywords:** Cath lab optimal case load >200 cases/year

221. The ACC/SCAI recommends that catheterizing physicians doing PCI need to maintain their skill level by performing more than _____ heart caths per year.
   a. >75
   b. >150
   c. >250
   d. >400

ANSWER a. > 75 /yr. Physicians performing catheterization also need to maintain their skills by doing more than 75 cases/year. This amounts to one PCI approximately every 5 days. (This does not apply to physicians who have accumulated a vast experience by performing more than 1000 cases in their career.)

The ACC/SCAI guidelines say: "A minimum interventional caseload is 75 cases/year per operator and ideally 400 cases/year for the laboratory. Because of the direct correlation between both laboratory and physician volume and outcomes, a low-volume operator (<75 cases/year) should only work in a high volume laboratory (600 cases/year), and even then with mentoring. Low-volume operators in any other setting should not perform **interventions." 2007 standards state, "It is recommended that the operator volume threshold [for PCI] continue to be 75 procedures per year."**
See: 2001& 2007 ACC / SCAI Expert Consensus Document on Cath Lab Standards
Keywords: Cath physician optimal case load >150 cases/year but < 1000 /yr

222. To what degree do the ACC / SCAI Cath Lab Standards endorse the performance of elective PCI in freestanding cardiac cath labs which lack adjacent cardiac surgical facilities? Such hospitals may be endorsed for PCI if:
   a. They perform >200 PCIs/year and are located where no other PCI is available
   b. Transport can provide <2 hr D2B time to approved hospital
   c. **Approved by the Joint Committee**
   d. Only STEMI cases are done

ANSWER a. Must perform >200 PCIs/year and be located where other PCI is unavailable standards say, "The 2013 PCI Competency Document identified a signal suggesting that an institutional volume threshold of <200 PCIs/year was associated with worse outcomes. Therefore, the 2013 Competency Document recommended that the continued operation of laboratories performing <200 procedures annually that are not serving isolated or underserved populations be questioned and that any laboratory that cannot maintain satisfactory outcomes should be closed." "the performance of PCI without on-site surgery in the US has gained greater acceptance, and questions about its safety in the presence of a proven, well defined, and protocol driven approach have diminished. PCI programs should be evaluated based on their ability to: (a) sustain adequate quality metrics, (b) provide access to elective and emergency PCI procedures that would otherwise be unavailable in their service area, and (c) maintain the operator and institutional volumes recommended in the 2013 PCI Competency Document." See" SCAI/ACC/AHA Expert Consensus Document: 2014
Update on Percutaneous Coronary Intervention Without On-Site Surgical Backup

223.
According to national guidelines cath labs should have regular team drills to establish protocol in emergency situations. Which 5 drills below are recommended for vascular complications? (Select 5 below.)
   a. Anticoagulation reversal protocol
   b. Paging protocol for immediate assistance from surgery or IR
   c. Protocol for emergency for suspected retroperitoneal hemorrhage
   d. Protocol for emergency CT angiography to identify bleeding site
   e. Protocol to balloon tamponade or stent a bleeding vessel
   f. Protocol for emergency pericardiocentesis

ANSWER f. Protocol for emergency pericardiocentesis, is not considered a vascular complication, although it could be. It is important enough to have its own classification. SCAI recommends 21 different drills and protocols that should be regularly practiced by the cath lab team. Consider the essential practice drills firemen go through. Cath lab team drills are just as essential. The first set of these drills is just for vascular complications. Your medical director should require and lead these.
   SCAI guidelines say, "CCL Emergency Preparedness Protocols: Though rare, serious complications do occur in the CCL and these can have devastating consequences if not handled in a timely manner. Select complications for which specific protocols should be developed are listed in Table V. Drills should be performed at routine intervals in the CCL to practice response to these complications.
Table V: Vascular Complications:
   -Anticoagulation reversal protocol
   -Paging protocol for immediate assistance from interventional cardiology, surgery or interventional radiology
   -Protocol for emergency non-contrast computed tomography when retroperitoneal hemorrhage is suspected and not responsive to supportive measures
   -Protocol for emergency computed tomographic angiography to identify bleeding site when appropriate
   -Protocol for immediate invasive angiography to balloon tamponade or stent bleeding vessel when available
See: SCAI Expert Consensus Statement: 2016 Best Practices in the Cardiac Catheterization Laboratory

224.
An "ambulatory or outpatient cath lab" is defined as one in which:
   a. The cath lab is mobile, and is parked by a hospital or clinic
   b. The cath lab is freestanding, not adjacent to any hospital
   c. The patients get up and walk within 4-6 hours
   d. The patients do not stay overnight in the hospital

ANSWER d. The patients do not stay overnight in the hospital. These same-day quick turnaround labs that take only elective diagnostic cases are few in number because of reduced reimbursement.
   The ACC/SCAI guidelines say: "Candidates for Same-Day or Ambulatory Cardiac Catheterization: Improvements in the safety and ease of performing invasive cardiac procedures plus the constant pressure to minimize costs have made it quite uncommon to hospitalize patients for only an invasive cardiac procedure. Indeed, for the vast majority of

adult patients, a diagnostic procedure can be safely completed in an ambulatory setting.....Patients are also being studied in freestanding laboratories (i.e., those that are not physically attached to the hospital). By definition a freestanding laboratory is one where quick transportation of a patient to a hospital by gurney is not possible. . . . It is vitally important to have mechanisms for backup and bailout in place to provide assistance should patients become unstable this setting. . . . Interventional procedures of any kind should not be performed in a freestanding facility." **See:** 2001 ACC / SCAI Expert Consensus Document on Cath Lab Standards **Keywords:** Ambulatory cath lab

225. According to ACC/AHA guidelines, which type of invasive procedure should NOT be performed in freestanding ambulatory cardiac cath labs?
  a. Permanent pacemaker insertion
  b. Endomyocardial biopsy
  c. Coronary interventions (PCI)
  d. Congenital heart disease

ANSWER c. Coronary interventions (PCI). The ACC/SCAI guidelines say: "Interventional procedures of any kind should not be performed in a freestanding facility.... a strategy of emergency transfer to an established center with a well-developed primary PCI program is preferred to the development of new freestanding primary PCI programs." This is because of the lack of cardiac surgical backup, and inability to monitor overnight. However, many invasive procedures do not require overnight monitoring, e.g. radial/branchial access cases have such a small hematoma rate, that they may be sent home the same day. **See:** 2005 ACC / SCAI Expert Consensus Document on Cath Lab Standards **Keywords:** freestanding cath lab, no PCI procedures

3. Ethical & Legal

226. In the CV lab, an example of privileged information that you must hold confidential or face a "breach of confidentiality" law suit is:
  a. A cardiologist tells you he is having an "affair"
  b. Your supervisor confides in you that your co-worker may have to be fired for poor performance
  c. The patient tells you that he has abused a child
  d. The patient's angiogram shows severe coronary disease

ANSWER d. The patient's angiogram shows severe coronary disease. The patient has the legal right to expect that all communications and records pertaining to his care should be treated as confidential. All case information is confidential and may not be discussed outside the lab. The patient's permission is required to transmit his or her private diagnostic information - either verbally or written. All these communications should be conducted discretely. Imagine that you are discussing this case in the elevator "Boy, Mr. Jones has a sick heart!" and his family overhears this.
  Ethically, you should not "tattle" on any confidential communication. But, you can't be sued for spreading co-worker gossip. And in some states you are legally responsible to

report suspected child abuse.
See: Torres, chapter on "Professionalism." Keywords: Confidential information

227. During diagnostic coronary arteriography you find that a stable angina patient has a discrete 90% LAD stenosis. The Dr. tells the patient "You need angioplasty NOW! You could have a lethal MI anytime!" The patient is undecided whether he wants to continue, especially since this is the first time he has even heard the term "angioplasty." He says "NO! I need more time to think about this." The Dr. stresses that this is "just routine" and it needs to be done NOW! What is the best course of action?
 a. The PCI should be deferred until informed consent is given
 b. Proceed with PCI on the basis that it is an emergency
 c. Reassure the patient then proceed with PCI
 d. Call the referring physician or surgeon into the lab to discuss PCI with the patient

ANSWER a. The PCI should be deferred until informed consent is given. Stable angina is not an emergency. Interventional procedures should always be discussed with the patient prior to cath at the time of obtaining informed consent. PCI and surgery are always possibilities when critical lesions are discovered during a diagnostic case. The patient should be prepared for the possibility of these interventions.

Pepine states "It is not appropriate to first approach the patient for additional procedures while diagnostic catheterization is in progress." However, it is not always possible to prepare every patient for every possible intervention. A true emergency procedure should be done unless the patient objects.
See: Pepine, chapter on "Cath Techniques..." Keywords: Informed consent - emergent PCI

228. Mr. Birch comes to the lab from the CCU with a recent MI. He signed the consent form last evening for a PCI. But, now he protests that HE DOES NOT WANT THE PROCEDURE! The cardiologist insists that he needs it to prevent further damage to his heart muscle. His family all agrees that this needs to be done. The cardiologist turns to you and asks: "What do you think?" You should respond:
 a. "We have to cancel this procedure now."
 b. "Scare him into it! Tell him he'll die without it."
 c. "Give him some Demerol! He'll forget all about it."
 d. "I'll help you hold him down. Go ahead!"

ANSWER a. "We have to cancel this procedure now." I've seen patients like this. When a patient refuses a procedure you have to cancel the case - even if you think it's in his best interest. You have to let him go! The more aggressive alternatives are unethical or illegal.

The Patient Bill of Rights says: "The patient has the right to refuse treatment to the extent permitted by law, and to be informed of the medical consequences of his action."
See: Torres, chapter on "Professionalism." Keywords: Patient refuses procedure

229. During a right heart cath a patient's heart is punctured with a stiff pacing catheter. The patient becomes hypotensive and groggy. The Dr. attempts to explain the seriousness of the situation to the patient, and that emergency pericardio-centesis or surgery is needed, but the patient is unresponsive. The standard informed consent form was signed and is on the chart. Without verbal informed consent of the patient to puncture his chest with a centesis needle you should:
 a. Proceed with lifesaving pericardio-centesis anyway
 b. Proceed with non-interventional life support maneuvers e.g. transcutaneous pacemaker, CPR...
 c. Defer the procedure until informed consent can be obtained
 d. Call a consulting physician and/or surgeon into the lab to get a second opinion

ANSWER a. Proceed with lifesaving pericardio-centesis anyway. Even if the consent form does not mention the possibility of these emergency maneuvers (most do), you should proceed with pericardio-centesis on the basis that this is a lifesaving emergency procedure. In this groggy state the patient is not competent to decide. This is "implied consent."
 It is analogous to the decision to do CPR on an unconscious patient. YOU DO IT unless you know of specific "Do Not Resuscitate" (DNR) orders. As a professional, it would be negligent to do otherwise.
See: Pepine, chapter on "Cath Techniques..." **Keywords:** No informed consent for emergency pericardio-centesis → do it anyway.

230. A patient arrives for a heart cath looking worried. You check his chart and the consent form has been signed and witnessed by a nurse. The patient asks you "What is this test for, and what is he really going to do?" As an experienced professional in the CV lab you should:
 a. Reassure the patient, make small talk, and proceed with lab preparations
 b. Answer his questions honestly and explain the procedure in laymen's terms
 c. Call in the hospital radiologist to explain the procedure and risks to the patient
 d. Call the patient's cardiologist and inform him of the patient's concerns

ANSWER b. Answer his questions honestly and explain the procedure in laymen's terms. If you try to sidestep the patient's questions, he will feel that you're holding back information. Many patients have questions which you can answer. The patient may prefer your answers to the physicians as "someone he can relate to, who really knows what's going on." As an experienced professional your duty is to prepare the patient in every way possible for the angiogram - including emotionally. Be informative, supportive, and meet the patient's needs.
See: Torres, chapter on "Professionalism." **Keywords:** Preparing the patient emotionally

231. **A patient arrives in the CV invasive lab for PCI. He has had several recent PCIs and bypass surgeries and is now back again. He looks depressed. You greet him and he does not respond. Your best response would be to:**
   a. Silently proceed with lab preparations
   b. Say "Aren't you feeling well today?"
   c. Say "Cheer up! We'll fix you up today."
   d. Postpone the preparations, until you have talked with the nurse and/or Dr.

ANSWER b. Say "Aren't you feeling well today?" The best course of action here is to listen to him. Ask an open-ended question that will help you understand where he is coming from. Perhaps it's just too early in the morning, he has chest pain, he didn't hear you, or he just normally looks like this in the morning. Don't try to cheer him up, or tell him that "we're going to make him **ALL BETTER** this time." It may not be true.
See: Torres, chapter on "Professionalism." **Keywords:** Preparing the patient emotionally

232. **In the cath lab, you note that the patient's "Operative Permit/Consent Form" is signed by the patient and a witness. Which condition might invalidate the legality of the signature? The patient:**
   a. Did NOT want the complications explained to her
   b. Refuses blood transfusions (Jehovah's Witness)
   c. Received preoperative Demerol prior to signing
   d. Does not speak or read English

ANSWER c. Patient received preoperative Demerol prior to signing.
   a. **NO, DID NOT WANT THE COMPLICATIONS EXPLAINED TO HER:** Most op-permits have a box to check if the patient does NOT want to be fully informed. Some people are scared by all the complications and don't want to know. Ignorance is bliss!
   b. **NO, REFUSES BLOOD TRANSFUSIONS (JEHOVAH'S WITNESS):** Most op-permits have a place for Jehovah's Witnesses or other religious patients to refuse blood transfusions. This can complicate cardiac surgery.
   c. **YES, RECEIVED PREOPERATIVE DEMEROL PRIOR TO SIGNING:** Legal informed consent is possible only from a lucid well informed patient, family, parents, and significant other. Narcotic drugs and sedatives even if given 6-8 hours earlier can interfere with the patient's ability to make informed decisions.

   Signatures made after the premeds take effect can be questioned, on the basis that the patient was in an altered state of mind. If the patient is brought to the lab with no signed consent form after the premedication has been given (depending on the type of premed), the signature may not be fully informed and therefore not valid.
   d. **NO, DOES NOT SPEAK OR READ ENGLISH:** This is OK if the patient had an interpreter that explained the form and what the Dr. or nurse told the patient about the procedure and risks involved. These patients should have an interpreter in the lab during the case.

See: Pepine, chapter on "Cath Techniques..." **Keywords:** Informed consent = no sedative premeds

233. You are circulating on a long interventional case. You fail to notice that the contrast bottle has become empty. The fellow injects air down the right coronary artery and the patient fibrillates. The patient is successfully defibrillated. Your response should be:
a. Sorry, I didn't notice it was almost empty.
b. I thought you were going to switch to Hexabrix.
c. We have been trying to save money on excess use of contrast.
d. Doctor, before injecting, you should always check to make sure they have enough contrast!

ANSWER a. Sorry, I didn't notice it was almost empty. It's best to fess up when you make a mistake. The cath team will respect you more and we learn best from our mistakes. This is a question of ethics.

4. Pre-Cath

234. During an invasive procedure a confused staff member should request a "reverse time out" by loudly saying:
a. "I'm confused."
b. "I need 2 minutes."
c. "Wait, something is wrong."
d. "I'm calling another TIME OUT."

ANSWER: b. "I need 2 minutes."
Kern says, "The Reverse Time Out or 'I Need 2 Minutes:' The time out before the procedure is a routine safety requirement. However, another kind of time out is sometimes needed when the case goes too fast...especially... physicians who sometimes want to work so fast that they outstrip the ability of the catheterization laboratory team to keep up with their demands or become confused ... Whenever this happens, anyone working in the laboratory can call a time out, which is stated out loud as 'I need 2 minutes.' The operators should stop and take a breath. This gives the person (and the team) who called time out a couple of minutes of uninterrupted time for him or her to get everything caught up and correct....The called 2-minute time out is the request back to the operators to give the nurse, technician, or team 2 minutes to get all the steps, equipment, or setup going and correctly brought together. During complex procedures, the nurse can say, "I need 2 minutes to do xyz." Everyone will hear and should understand. The operators will relax and wait for the team to catch up. Of course the called time out would not be appropriate if there was a critical situation occurring in which the patient could not wait for an emergency drug or other life-sustaining intervention (e.g., left ventricular [LV] support device or an intraaortic balloon pump [IABP] insertion)." **See:** Kern, chapter on "The Catheterization Laboratory"

235. According to the Joint Commission a pre-procedure "time-out" is required. When would a patient <u>not</u> be expected to participate in the "time out" discussion?
   a. CTO procedures in cath lab
   b. TAVR procedures in hybrid lab
   c. Mapping procedures in EP Lab
   d. Patient is never expected to participate in the time out discussion

ANSWER: b. TAVR procedures are often done in a hybrid lab and require general anesthesia where the patient is usually asleep prior to entry of the surgeon.

Kern says, "The time out, the immediate preprocedure pause, must occur in the location where the procedure is to be done (catheterization laboratory suite). The time out may precede anesthesia, or in the operating room it may occur after the patient is anesthetized (participation by the patient is not expected in surgical procedures, but is recommended for catheterization laboratory procedures) but just before starting the procedure." **See:** Kern, chapter on "The Catheterization Lab"

Kern says, "Standard for TAVR is a hybrid operating room/catheterization laboratory for simultaneous fluoroscopy guided catheter manipulation and conversion to open surgery, if needed. The room should be large enough to accommodate a team consisting of cardiac anesthesiologists, echocardiographers, cardiac surgeons, and interventional cardiologists." **See:** Kern, chapter on "Interventional Cardiology Procedures"

236. Prior to a PCI, the operating physician is out of the lab scrubbing his hands. He says that he is in a hurry and wants to skip the pre-procedure "time out." As the circulating nurse you should:
   a. Cancel the time out
   b. Do it anyway and start as he enters the room
   c. Do it without him in the lab to inform the rest of the team
   d. Inform him personally of the essential details while he is scrubbing

ANSWER: b. Do it anyway and start as he enters the room. It is required and he needs to be informed along with the staff.

Kern says, "The time out, the immediate preprocedure pause, must occur in the location where the procedure is to be done (catheterization laboratory suite).... Every laboratory is required to perform a preprocedure safety review, called the time out... At this time, the team agrees to proceed and then specifies what analgesia and sedation dose will be given. Time out is a Joint Commission requirement."

"Who should participate in the time-out process? The time out must involve the entire operative team. At a minimum, this includes the catheterization laboratory operator, his or her assistant, any anesthesia provider, and the circulating nurse. Participation with active (out-loud) verbal communication by all members of the team is required. ("I concur" is the proper acknowledgment.) In particular, if there is concern about a possible error, no one should be afraid to speak up and protect the patient. Even when there is only one person doing the procedure, a brief pause to confirm the correct patient, procedure, and site is appropriate. It is not necessary to engage others in this verification process if they would not otherwise be involved in the procedure." **See:** Kern, chapter on "The Catheterization Lab"

237. According to the Joint Commission two unique patient identifiers should be checked before you proceed with a case. *(Check 2 acceptable patient identifiers below).*
   a. **Birthday**
   b. **Home zip code**
   c. **Name on name band**
   d. **Hospital room number**
   e. **Procedure he/she expects**
   f. **What insurance he/she has**

ANSWERS: a. Birthday & c. Name on name band are both unique. Incorrect answers like zip code can include thousands of other addresses or are not specific enough.

    Joint Commission says: "Acceptable identifiers may be the individual's name, an assigned identification number, telephone number, or other person-specific identifier. Electronic identification technology coding, such as bar coding or RFID, that includes two or more person-specific identifiers (not room number) will comply with this requirement....The two identifiers may be in the same location, such as a wristband.... the two patient/client/resident-specific identifiers must be directly associated with the individual and the same two identifiers must be directly associated with the medications, blood products, specimen containers (such as on an attached label), other treatments or procedures." **See:**
https://www.utmb.edu/health-resource-center/partner-in-your-care-patient-safety/two-patient-identifiers-for-every-test-and-procedure

238. Efficient communication relies on 2 way communication. For the cath lab staff this usually means:
   a. **Anticipating what is needed next in the procedure**
   b. **Orders from the physician should be repeated back**
   c. **All orders should be documented in the medical record**
   d. **Speaking up whenever the patient's safety is threatened**

ANSWER: b. Orders from the physician should be repeated back.
Two-way communication occurs when the receiver sends response or feedback to the sender's message. All the above incorrect answers are good, but not 2 way communication.

    Kern says, "Communication among team members is critical. Clear and open two-way communication, especially under critical portions of procedures,... leads to improved safety through error reduction and timely performance of the catheterization."

    "Orders from the "table" should be acknowledged clearly by those designated to carry out the order. Just as military efficiency is built on this dictum, so should that of the well-run laboratory. It is disturbing to request medications and supplies and not know if someone has heard the request and is attending to it."

    "By letting the team know where the operator is in the procedure, the next steps can be anticipated. The recording technologists appreciate these announcements for documentation.... When at the "table," announce what the "table" is doing. For example, 'Left Jud going up' ... ," which the recording person then acknowledges." **See:** Kern, chapter on "The Catheterization Lab"

128   ◀◀ Diagnostic Techniques: D4 - Cath: Protocol & Preparations ▶▶

239. **To reduce the incidence of patient vomiting after receiving a contrast injection, patients should come to the cath lab _____ for 6 hrs. prior to cath.**
   a. TKO
   b. NPO
   c. PRN
   d. q.i.d.

ANSWER b. NPO = Nothing per Os (mouth)
a.   TKO = "To keep open" an IV (i.e., keep drip going)
b.   NPO = "Nothing Per Os" (mouth)
c.   PRN = "Per Request Needed" or "As Necessary."
d.   q.i.d. = "Four times a day" (q. for quarter)
See: Grossman, chapter on "Percutaneous Approach." **Keywords:** pre-cath fast is 6 hrs. NPO = "Nothing per Os"

240. **What blood chemistry result suggests that a non-ionic or low osmolar contrast be used for coronary angiography?**
   a. Calcium = 6.1 mEq/dL
   b. Calcium = 10 mEq/dL
   c. Creatinine = 1.4 mg/100 ml
   d. Creatinine = 4.3 mg/100 ml

ANSWER d. Elevated creatinine = 4.3 mg/100 ml. Normal creatinine is below 1.5 mg/100 ml. blood. So the higher creatinine of 4.5 is **markedly elevated** indicating **poor kidney function**. Contrast may be toxic to this patient's kidneys and cause renal failure and contrast induced nephropathy (CIN). Less toxic and minimal amounts of contrast are essential in this situation. If other risk factors for CIN are present you should prehydrate the patient. **See:** Grossman, chapter on "Angiography: Principles."

241. **Blood chemistries should be checked prior to cardiac catheterization. Identify the normal blood chemistry ranges for potassium. (#2 in the box)**
   a. 0.8-1.0 mg/L (8.8-10.3 mg/dl)
   b. 1.5-2.1 mEq/L
   c. 3.5-4.5 mEq/L
   d. 95-105 mEq/L
   e. 135-145 mEq/L

> **BLOOD CHEMISTRIES**
> 1. Sodium
> **#2. Potassium**
> 3. Chloride
> 4. Total Calcium
> 5. Magnesium

ANSWER c. 3.5-4.5 mEq/L. Decreased K^+ levels (<3.5 mEq/L) should be treated pre-cath with KCl drip. If left untreated the patient is at risk of developing lethal arrhythmias. Be able to match all answers below. **CORRECTLY MATCHED ANSWERS ARE:**
BLOOD CHEMISTRIES   Normal Value
1. SODIUM   135-145 mEq/L
2. POTASSIUM (K^+)   3.5-4.5 mEq/L

3. CHLORIDE   95-105 mEq/L
4. TOTAL CALCIUM   0.8-1.0 mg/L (8.8-10.3 mg/dl)
5. MAGNESIUM   1.5-2.1 mEq/L

See: Underhill, chapter on "Laboratory Tests." **Keywords:** Blood chemistries pre-cath.

242. A patient comes to the CV Invasive lab for a diagnostic heart cath with a prothrombin-time (PT) time of 12 sec. and an ACT (Activated Clotting Time) of 100 sec. To prevent excessive bleeding during and after the case, what should be done?
   a. Nothing - proceed with case, this is normal
   b. Call physician and suggest the case be deferred until clotting time returns to normal
   c. Administer 1 unit fresh frozen plasma to shorten clotting time
   d. Administer 10 mg protamine to reverse residual heparin and lengthen clotting time

ANSWER a. Nothing - proceed with case, this is normal. Trick question! Grossman recommends that patients arrive with a Pro-Time (PT) time < (less than) 18 seconds. (Normal PT time is 12-15 sec.) This assures a normal clotting baseline to return to at the end of the case. It facilitates hemostasis at the end of the case. Pressure holding time will not be excessive and hematomas will be minimized. Heparin may be reversed with protamine. Many cardiologists are not using heparin on short routine diagnostic cath procedures. **See:** Grossman, chapter on "Coronary Angioplasty. **Keywords:** ACT during PCI → 250-300+ sec.

243. During PCI 10,000 units of unfractionated heparin was administered to a PCI patient. You take a blood sample and analyze it on the ACT machine. Before proceeding with dilation the patient's whole blood clotting time (ACT) should be:
   a. 20-50 sec
   b. 60-100 sec
   c. 100-200 sec
   d. 250-300 sec

ANSWER d. 250-300 sec. Heparin (or other antithrombotic) is given prior to all interventional patients to prevent acute closure. According to Grossman enough heparin should be administered to keep the ACT between 250 - 300 sec. Topal recommends the ACT be over 300 sec. for PCI. This is 3 to 4 times the normal ACT of 75-120 sec. However, there seems considerable variability between the various measurement systems.

To achieve this desired level of anticoagulation it may take 10,000-20,000 units of heparin. Various factors affect the adequacy of heparinization in a patient: body size, prior heparin therapy, nitroglycerin levels, and heparin potency. The ACT should be measured periodically in PCI patients through the procedure to prevent acute closure. Many physicians keep their PCI patients on heparin 12-24 hours after the procedure to reduce the risk of acute closure. Others reserve post-procedure heparin for patients with suboptimal high-risk PCI results.

Most centers also start patients on aspirin (ASA) or Plavix 24 hours prior to PCI to reduce platelet aggregation and clotting. Aspirin and Plavix are usually continued after the procedure as well. In addition, many physicians premedicate patients with calcium channel blockers to reduce the incidence of coronary spasm during the case. **See:** Grossman, chapter on "Coronary PCI" and Topal, Textbook of Interventional Cardiology, chapter on "Abrupt Vessel Closure." **Keywords:** ACT for PCI should be 250-300 sec.

5. Premedications

244. Which drug below is an example of the class of premedication listed in the box at #2 (narcotic)?
   a. Demerol
   b. Valium or Versed
   c. Atropine
   d. Morphine
   e. Benadryl

CLASS OF PREMEDICATION
1. Antihistamine
*2. Narcotic
3. Short acting - pain duller (Narcotic like)
4. Benzodiazapine (Anti-anxiety agent)
5. Anti-cholinergic

ANSWER d. Narcotic = Morphine. Be able to match all answers below.
CORRECTLY MATCHED ANSWERS ARE:

CLASS OF PREMEDICATION	COMMON NAME
1. ANTIHISTAMINE	Benadryl
2. NARCOTIC	Morphine
3. SHORT ACTING (NARCOTIC LIKE) - PAIN DULLER	Demerol
4. BENZODIAZAPINE (ANTI-ANXIETY)	Valium
5. ANTI-CHOLINERGIC	Atropine

See: Pepine, chapter on "Cath Techniques..." **Keywords:** Classes of premedications - morphine=narcotic

245. What is the generic name below for the commonly used premedication listed in the box at #2 (Valium)?
   a. Diphenhydramine
   b. Atropine
   c. Meperidine
   d. Diazepam
   e. Midazolam

PREMED. - COMMON NAME
1. Demerol
*2. Valium
3. Versed
4. Benadryl
5. Belladonna

ANSWER d. Diazepam = Valium. Be able to match all answers below.
CORRECTLY MATCHED ANSWERS ARE:
COMMON NAME   GENERIC NAME
1. DEMEROL.......... Meperidine
2. VALIUM .... Diazepam
3. VERSED .... Midazolam
4. BENADRYL .... Diphenhydramine
5. BELLADONNA .... Atropine

246. Which sedative usually wears off within 30 minutes following IV infusion?
a. Valium
b. Versed
c. Benadryl
d. Demerol

ANSWER b. Versed (midazolam) is a short-acting bezodiazepine CNS depressant. The onset of its action is rapid (1-2 min) and its duration of action is only 30 minutes following a normal 5 mg IV dose. This short duration of action makes it an ideal sedative for angiographic procedures. It is easy to titrate the dose to the length and pain level of the case. And it wears off soon after the procedure terminates. It is eliminated 10 times faster than Valium. It is contraindicated in patients with narrow-angle glaucoma.
See: Kandarpa, chapter on "Commonly Used Medications." **Keywords**: Versed, short acting

247. Why might aspirin be given to a patient pre-PCI?
a. To reduce platelet-induced clotting factors
b. To reduce extrinsic thrombin clotting factors
c. As an anti-allergen
d. As an analgesic

ANSWER a. To reduce platelet-induced clotting factors. Aspirin selectively inhibits thromboxane (TXA2) and cyclo-oxygenase formation. This reduces platelet adherence and clot formation at the site of intimal injury, such as a PCI site. Some labs require that PCI patients be on an ASA regimen for several days prior to the procedure and remain on it indefinitely. However, aspirin blocks only one of the pathways by which platelets adhere to injured endothelium. Abciximab (Reo-Pro) is an IV platelet drug that is even more potent at reducing platelet adhesion by blocking the GP IIb/IIIa receptors on platelets. It reduces the incidence of thrombus-mediated ischemic complications. **See**: Grossman, chapter on "Coronary Angioplasty" **Keywords**: Aspirin = reduces platelet adhesion

248. What platelet receptor site does abciximab (ReoPro) block?
a. Plasminogen (t-PA)
b. Alpha 2-Antiplasmin
c. Glycoprotein IIb/IIIa
d. Thromboxane TXA2

ANSWER c. Glycoprotein IIb/IIIa. These important receptors are on the surface of all platelets. When activated they bind to subendothelial connective tissue exposed by injury. Platelets that adhere to an injured vessel lose their discoid shape, form pseudopods, and spread out over the injury. They then express other platelet receptors and release mediators that attract fibrinogen and other adhesive proteins that link platelets together into an aggregate. The IV drug abciximab (ReoPro) is a monoclonal antibody 7EE3Fab. ReoPro is a much more potent antiplatelet drug than aspirin. In adequate doses it completely blocks the GP IIb/IIIa receptors, inhibits platelet aggregation, prevents thrombosis and augments the activity of thrombolytic agents. Its chief complication is associated bleeding problems. **See**: Braunwald, chapter on "Hemostasis, Thrombosis, Fibrinolysis, and CV Disease."

249. Which premedication relaxes smooth muscles and helps avoid arterial and coronary spasm during PCI?
a. Persantine (Dipyridamole)
b. Angiotensin-converting enzyme inhibitors (Captopril)
c. Ca channel blocker (Nifedipine, Verapamil)
d. Beta blocker (Inderol, Metoprolol)

ANSWER c. Ca channel blockers (Nifedipine, Verapamil) help prevent spasm and are common ingredients in the radial artery cocktail. Baim and Grossman recommend a Ca channel blocker on the evening prior to the procedure to prevent vessel spasm due to irritation of the treated artery. Calcium channel blockers also have a negative inotropic effect and relax all vascular smooth muscle. For this reason they are commonly used to treat hypertension. Common Ca blockers include nifedipine, verapamil and diltiazem.

Grossman says, "The patient should have been prepared by proscription of oral intake after midnight on the evening before the procedure, and pretreatment with a calcium channel blocker (to prevent vessel spasm at the treatment site) and aspirin 325 mg/day to diminish platelet deposition on the disrupted endothelium. Other antiplatelet agents, including low-molecular-weight dextran and dipyridamole 200 mg/day, were one administered in conjunction with angioplasty but have now been abandoned due to lack of demonstrated efficacy, potential allergic or volume-overload side effects with dextran, and the availability of more potent antiplatelet agents. . . . Because aspirin reduces late cardiac mortality in patients with coronary disease, it is generally continued indefinitely after the procedure. . . ." **See**: Grossman, chapter on "Coronary Angioplasty." **Keywords**: Ca blocker for spasm

250. What is the average adult cath premedication dosage for the drug listed in the box at #3 (Benadryl)?
a. 0.5-1.0 mg IV or PO
b. 5-10 mg IV or PO
c. (10-50 mg IV) 25-50 mg PO
d. (50-300 mg IV) 300 mg PO

PREMED. - COMMON NAME
1. Valium
2. Cimetidine (Tagamet)
*3. Benadryl
4. Belladonna

ANSWER c. Benadryl = Diphenhydramine → (10-50 mg IV) 25-50 mg PO. Antihistamine is given to prevent and reduce allergic reactions. BE ABLE TO MATCH ALL ANSWERS BELOW. **CORRECTLY MATCHED ANSWERS ARE:**
    1. **VALIUM (Diazepam):** . . . . 5-10 mg IM, IV, or PO

Diagnostic Techniques: D4 - Cath: Protocol & Preparations

   Benzodiazapine, anti-anxiety drug
2. **CIMETIDINE (Tagamet):** .. .. (50-300 mg IV) 300 mg PO
   Given along with prednisone for dye allergic patients
3. **BENADRYL (Diphenhydramine):**... (10-50 mg IV) 25-50 mg PO
   Antihistamine, given to prevent allergic reactions
4. **BELLADONNA (Atropine):** .... 0.5-1.0 mg IV
   Cholinergic blocker, prevents vasovagal reaction

See: Pepine, chapter on "Cath Techniques..." and Yaniga, chapter on "Premedications"
Keywords: Premeds - dosage Benadry l 25-50 mg. PO

251. Prior to left heart cath and diagnostic coronary arteriography, how many cc's of heparin (1000 units/ml) should be administered IA for complete systemic anticoagulation on an average sized adult?
a. 1 cc
b. 2 cc
c. 5 cc
d. 10 cc

ANSWER c. 5 cc. Grossman recommends 5000 units (5 cc of 1000 u/cc) of heparin IA as soon as the catheter is in the aorta. He says this should provide complete anticoagulation for an hour. (60-90 minutes is considered the half life of heparin). Additional heparin may be given for longer cases and PCI.
   This 5 cc can be calculated by the formula:
- DOSE = Concentration X Amount.
- Dose (5000 units) = Amt. (?) X conc. (1000 units/cc)
- Solving for the unknown Amt. = dose/conc. = 5000u/1000u/cc = 5 cc.

Note how the units all cancel out to give cc or ml. Unit cancellation is always a safe way to calculate a medication dosage.
   Many physicians are now practicing diagnostic heart catheterization with reduced amounts or even NO heparin for short cases (<20 min.) Kern says: "In most centers, heparin can be omitted from routine left-sided heart catheterization when the procedure is performed in a timely and accurate manner." Heparin is recommended for cases longer than 20 min. PCI cases usually require 10,000 units of heparin. **See:** Kern, chapter on "Arterial & Venous Access."

252. To give heparin at the time of radial sheath insertion:
a. Give 5000 units mixed with 15 ml saline
b. **Give 50 U/kg mixed with the antispasm cocktail and mixed with blood**
c. Wait to give heparin after the catheter is in the aorta
d. Never give heparin in the cocktail. Only give it IV.

ANSWER b. Give 50 U/kg mixed with the antispasm cocktail and mixed with blood.
   Kern says, "Heparin is always given to prevent radial artery occlusion and is generally dosed at 5000 U or 50 U/kg IV. Heparin may be given intra-arterially (IA) within the cocktail, but if doing so, it should be mixed with plenty of blood to reduce burning. Alternatively, heparin can be given via IV to reduce local irritation and pain" **See:** Kern, chapter on "Arterial and Venous Access."

253. **Your 55 Kg patient comes to the cath lab premedicated with 300 mg clopidogrel (Plavix) for a PCI. The physician orders 2000 units of unfractionated heparin IV. To check for the proper level of anticoagulation draw the first ACT:**
   a. Immediately after the heparin is given
   b. 5 min after the heparin is given
   c. 1 hour after the heparin is given
   d. At end of case, prior to pulling the sheath

   ANSWER b. 5 min after the heparin is given to evaluate the anticoagulation level. Most authors recommend waiting 3-5 min after giving a heparin bolus, to draw and measure the ACT. For a PCI full anticoagulation is required with an ACT around 300 sec. (If GP IIb/IIIa inhibitors are given with heparin, the ACT level need not be that high, around 200-250 sec.) More heparin will probably be given if the resulting ACT is under 250 sec. Since the half life of heparin is 1 to 1 ½ hours, after readjusting your patient's coagulation status the ACT should be rechecked in ½ to 1 hour intervals. Of course, to avoid bleeding ACT is always checked before pulling the sheath.

   Schneider says, "When heparin administration is required, this should occur at least 3 minutes prior to balloon inflation... The half-life of heparin is 1 to 1 ½ hours and is prolonged in patients with renal or hepatic dysfunction."

   ACC, AHA & SCAI Guidelines say, "Heparin Dosing Guidelines In those patients who do not receive GP IIb/IIIa inhibitors, sufficient unfractionated heparin should be given during coronary angioplasty to achieve an ACT of 250 to 300 s with the HemoTec device and 300 to 350 s (200,201) with the Hemochron device. A weight-adjusted bolus heparin (70 to 100 IU per kg) can be used to avoid excess anticoagulation. If the target values for ACT are not achieved after a bolus of heparin, additional heparin boluses (2000 to 5000 IU) can be given. Early sheath removal should be performed when the ACT falls to less than 150 to 180 s." **See: ACC, AHA & SCAI Guidelines**

254. **At the beginning of a short coronary arteriogram procedure a patient was given 2500 units of IV heparin. What amount of protamine (10 mg/cc) should be given to reverse 2500 units of unfractionated heparin?**
   a. 1.25 cc
   b. 2.5 cc
   c. 5 cc
   d. 10 cc

   ANSWER b. 2.5 cc. Grossman recommends 10 mg (1.0 cc) of protamine to counteract every 1000 units of heparin. It's easy to remember because they react 1:1 by volume, or 1000µ:10 mg by dosage. If the concentrations are standard (1000 units heparin = 1 cc and 10 mg protamine = 1 cc), then each 1 cc of protamine counteracts each 1 cc of heparin.

   Grossman says: "If systemic heparinization is used, its effects must be reversed at the termination of the left heart catheterization and associated angiography. This is usually accomplished by administration of protamine (1 ml = 10 mg of protamine for every 1,000 units of heparin). The operator should be watchful for potential adverse reactions to protamine, characterized by hypotension and vascular collapse... Protamine reactions appear to be more common on insulin-dependent diabetics . . ."

   Because of this, many physicians are reducing the amount of protamine because of these several potentially lethal side effects. Since the half life of heparin is 40 minutes, only a fraction of the total reversal dose of protamine may be administered e.g. some give 25 mg protamine for 5000 units heparin at the end of a 40 minutes case. Grossman recommends withholding protamine on insulin-dependent patients, and just letting the heparin effect wear off. **See:** Grossman, chapter on "Percutaneous Approach."

255. Match the rating system to its use.
   a. Eligibility for conscious sedation
   b. Predicts ease of intubation
   c. Monitor depth of conscious sedation

RATING SYSTEMS
1. Mallampati class
2. American Society of Anesthesiologists Class
3. Aldrete Score

Correctly matched answers are:
1. Mallampati class = b. Predicts ease of airway intubation 1-4
2. American Society Anesthesiologists Class (ASA) = a. Eligibility for conscious sedation 1-4
3. Aldrete Score = c. Monitor depth of conscious sedation (1-10). Patient should return to baseline before discharge usually at least score of 9 out of 10.

Kern says, "An airway assessment should be part of the preprocedural routine. Most preprocedural check lists include the Mallampati classification, which is used to predict the ease of intubation. Mallampati scoring is as follows:
Class 1: Full visibility of tonsils, uvula, and soft palate
Class 2: Visibility of hard and soft palate, upper portion of tonsils, and uvula
Class 3: Soft and hard palate and base of the uvula are visible
Class 4: Only hard palate is visible..."

"The American Society of Anesthesiologists Physical Status Classification ... is helpful in determining the patient's eligibility for conscious sedation. It uses a 1 to 5 classification range, with 1 being a healthy patient and 5 being a moribund patient. Procedural sedation is appropriate for patients in classes 1, 2, and 3. Patients in classes 4 and higher are better suited for general anesthesia...."

"The Aldrete Scoring System ... can be used to assess the effects of sedation on the patient's major systems (neurologic, respiratory, and circulatory). A score of 0, 1, or 2 is given for level of activity, level of consciousness, respiratory ability, blood pressure, and color." **See:** Kern, chapter on "The Catheterization Laboratory"

256. **A patient comes to your lab with a American Society of Anesthesiologists Physical Status Class 5. You should:**
   a. Call Respiratory Therapy to intubate
   b. Request transesophageal echo placement
   c. Administer extra-heavy conscious sedation
   d. Recommend general anesthesia

ANSWER d. Recommend general anesthesia because conscious sedation will have problems on such a frail patient. Kern says of ASA Physical Status assessment, " Patients in classes 4 and higher are better suited for general anesthesia...."
See: Kern, chapter on "The Catheterization Laboratory"

Understand why each question on this model preprocedure checklist is important and what to do if the response to the question poses a problem?
a. Yes
b. No

ANSWER a. Yes. Check those you need to research below.

Model Preprocedure Check List for Cardiac Catheterization (*understand all below*)

Patient name: _____ RN: _____ Procedure Date: _____

Procedure Planned:
    Diagnostic cardiac catheterization
    Diagnostic cardiac catheterization with possible PCI
    Percutaneous coronary intervention

History and physical examination:
    Elective outpatient procedures: H&P documented within 30 days?
    Inpatient procedures: H&P documented within 24 hr of admission?
        If yes, were History of prior PCI or CABG: reports obtained?

Candidacy for DES:
    1. Is there significant anemia (Hct <30)?
    2. Any major surgery in the past month or next year?
    3. Is there any clinically overt bleeding?
    4. Is patient on chronic anticoagulation (e.g., warfarin, dabigatran)?
    5. Is there history of medication nonadherence?

Allergies:
    1. Contrast: If yes, was the patient pretreated?
    2. Aspirin: If yes, does the patient need desensitization?
    3. Heparin (HIT): if yes, consider antithrombotic agents?
    4. Latex: If yes, remove all latex products from procedural use?
    5. Multiple allergies: If yes, consider prednisone pretreatment ?

Medications:
    1. Did patient take aspirin within the past 24 hr?
    2. Did patient take clopidogrel within the past 24 hr?
    3. Did patient take metformin within the past 24 hr?
    4. Did patient take sildenafil (or equivalent) within the past 24 hr?
    5. Did patient receive LMWH within the past 24 hr? If yes for LMWH, time of last dose

Informed consent:
    Was informed consent obtained within 30 days?
    Is there a healthcare proxy?
    Is the patient DNR or DNI? Yes, but revoked for procedure?

Sedation, anesthesia, and analgesia:
    Are ASA and Mallampati class documented?
    Is there any contraindication to sedation?

Laboratories and studies:
    CBC and basic electrolytes within 30 days (outpatient) or 24 hr (inpatient)?
    Was EKG; performed within 24 hr?
    PT/INR performed within 24 hr (for patients on warfarin)?
    Does the patient require preprocedure hydration?

Clinical Expert Consensus Statement on Best Practices in the Cardiac Catheterization Laboratory: Society for Cardiovascular Angiography and Interventions, 2012

Other Cardiac Cath checklists available:

http://www.bcs.com/documents/396_Standalone_checklist.pdf
Cahill & Stables, The British Cardiovascular Society (BCS) Cardiac Catheterisation Lab Safety Checklist, Cath Lab Digest, Aug 2018

http://extcontent.covenanthealth.ca/Policy/EAC_PC_VIII-10.pdf

https://www.intersocietal.org/cath/forms/CathAccreditationChecklist.pdf

http://www.scai.org/qit/Default.aspx

http://www.umanitoba.ca/faculties/health_sciences/medicine/units/cardiac_sciences/pdf/preangiochecklist.pdf

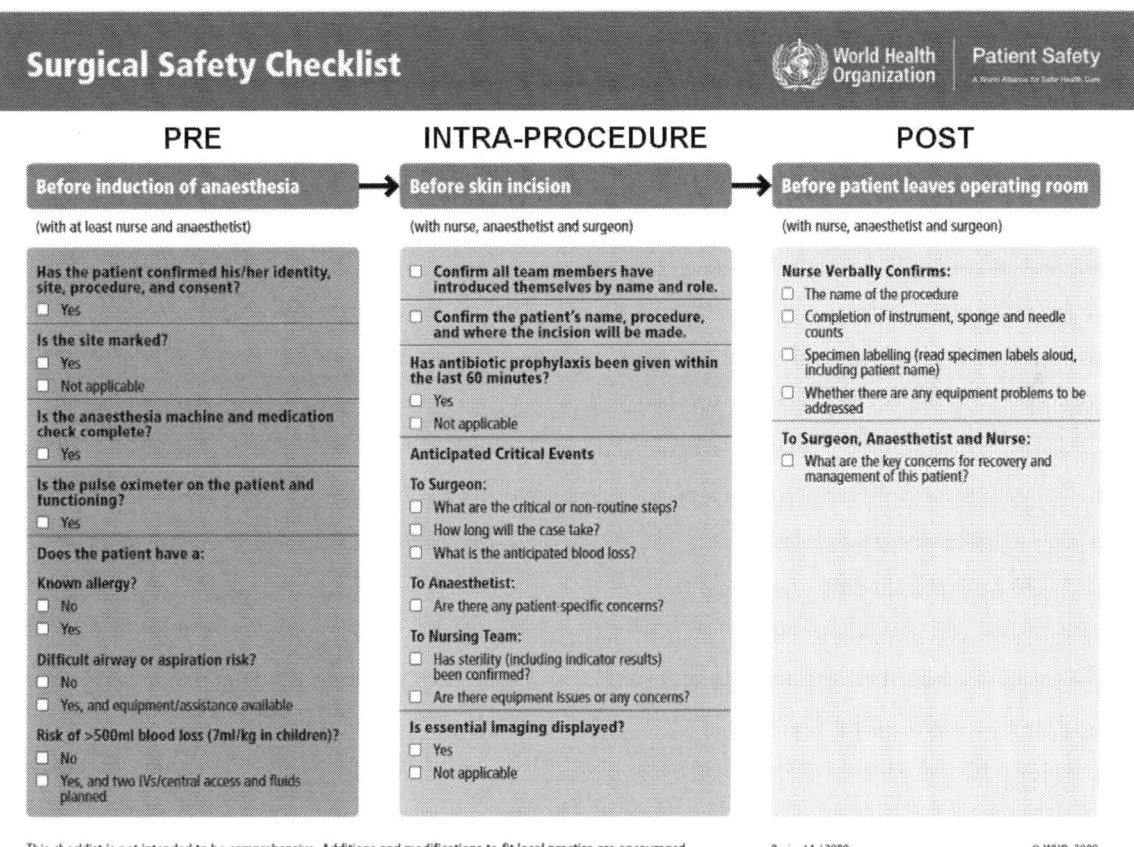

References:

Baim, D. S. and Grossman W., *Cardiac Catheterization, Angiography, and Intervention*, 6th Ed., Lea and Febiger, 2006
Bashore, Thomas, et al., ACC/SCAI Expert Consensus Document, in Am. Journal of Cardiology, Vol 37 #8, 2001, Pub. by Elsevier Science Inc.
Braunwald, et al, Ed., *Heart Disease, a Textbook of CV Medicine*, 9th Ed., Saunders, 2012
Daily, E. K., and Schroeder, J. S., *Techniques in Bedside Hemodynamic Monitoring*, 4th Ed., C. V. Mosby Company, 1989
Kern, M. J., Ed., *The Cardiac Catheterization Handbook*, 6th Ed., Mosby-Year Book, Inc., 2016
Pepine, CJ, et al, *ACC/AHA Guidelines for Cardiac Catheterization Laboratories*. ACC/AHA Ad Hoc Task Force on Cardiac Cath..., Circulation 84: 2213, 1991
Pepine, J. C., and Hill, J. A., et al, *Diagnostic and Therapeutic Cardiac Catheterization*, 2nd Ed., Williams and Wilkins, 1994
Torres, L. S., *Basic Medical Techniques and Patient Care for Radiologic Technologists*, 3rd Ed., J. B. Lippincott Co., 1989
Topal, E. J., Ed., *Textbook of Interventional Cardiology*, 2nd Ed., W. B. Saunders Co., 1994
Underhill, S. L., Ed., *CARDIAC NURSING*, 2nd Ed., J. B. Lippincott Co., 1989
Yaniga, Leslie, Cardiac Catheterization Medications Guide Workbook, Smith Notes Co., 1998

OUTLINE: Cath. Protocol and Preparations

1. HISTORY:
   a. 1600 AD William Harvey 1844 AD Claude Bernard
   b. 1895 AD   William Roentgen
   c. 1929 AD   Werner Forssman
   d. 1945 AD   Andre Cournand
   e. 1950 AD Helen Taussig
   f. 1953 AD Seldinger
   g. 1956 AD Forssman, Cournand, Richards won Nobel prize.
   h. 1959 AD Mason Sones and Braunwald
   i. 1964 AD Charles Dotter
   j. 1966 AD Rashkind
   k. 1967 AD Melvin Judkins Kurt Amplatz
   l. 1970 AD Swan and Ganz
   m. 1971 AD Andreas Gruntzig

2. STANDARDS
   a. Grossman's "general principles" of protocol.
      i. Everyone gets an IV or Arterial Line first
      ii. Hemodynamic measurements precede angiography
      iii. Measure pressures and Sats. immediately upon entry into a chamber.
      iv. Measure pressures and CO simultaneously
      v. Perform most important angiography/tests first.
      vi. Pull / Exchange catheters/guidewires in descending AO
         (1) avoids CVA
      vii. Always exchange catheters over a guidewire
   b. CATH LAB GUIDELINES
      i. reference - ICHD Special Report
      ii. Where cath labs should be set up.
      iii. recommended staffing patterns
      iv. medical director of cath lab
      v. Cathing Drs.
      vi. training requirements
         (1) Nursing personnel
         (2) X-ray techs
         (3) CV techs.
         (4) Monitoring techs.
         (5) Dark room tech.
         (6) Cross training
      vii. Recommended certification of personnel in cath labs
         (1) BLS
         (2) ACLS
         (3) RN
         (4) RT®)
         (5) RCVT
      viii. Recommended utilization levels in cath labs:
         (1) High case loads

- (2) Cathing Drs: Minimum case loads
  - (a) ->75 adult cases/year
  - (b) ->30 ped's. cases/ year
  - (c) Lab: minimum case loads
  - (d) ->200 general caths/yr.
- ix. LAB SAFETY
  - (1) -# normal studies / yr.
  - (2) -Major complication rate
  - (3) -repeat heart caths
  - (4) List and describe conditions prone to higher complications
  - (5) MD. inexperience
  - (6) Patient stability
  - (7) Extent of coronary disease
  - (8) Adequacy of LV function
  - (9) Patient. age
  - (10) hypoxemia
  - (11) Pulm. congestion
  - (12) Renal insufficiency
  - (13) incident reports
  - (14) "average" complication rate
- x. Describe when Pulmonary angiography is risky:
  - (1) Severely ill patient's.
  - (2) cyanotic/polycythemic patient's.
  - (3) High PVR (Pulm hypertensive
- xi. cath terms:
  - (1) "diagnostic" cath
  - (2) "interventional" cath
  - (3) "Acute MI" cath
  - (4) "provocative" testing
- xii. ETIQUETTE IN CATH LAB
  - (1) Introduce self to Dr., techs, Patient.
  - (2) Stay out of way
  - (3) Minimize talking (talk quietly)
  - (4) Avoid inappropriate discussion of case
  - (5) Evaluate tension level
  - (6) Be aware of family in wait room
  - (7) Appropriate dress, lead...
  - (8) Not assisting if you are ill
  - (9) Sensitivity to needs of Patient
  - (10) Don't overstep your knowledge & ability
- xiii. When should a RHC be done?
  - (1) valvular disease
  - (2) Pulmonary disease
  - (3) shunts/ped's.,
  - (4) Pericardio-centesis
  - (5) Myocardial biopsy
  - (6) Transseptal
  - (7) Electrophysiology
- xiv. MONITORING PATIENT SAFETY
  - (1) Use of 12 lead ECG amplifier problems
  - (2) errors from poor frequency response
  - (3) grounding problems
  - (4) ST changes
  - (5) T wave changes
  - (6) Arterial pressure monitoring
  - (7) low BP
  - (8) increase in PAW pressure (LVEDP)
  - (9) pH, PO2 changes
  - (10) use of single end hole catheters for coronaries.
  - (11) Dye causes changes in hemodynamics
  - (12) blood volume
  - (13) wedge (LVEDP)Recommended amount of dye
  - (14) max of 3 ml/kg
  - (15) Monitoring Transseptal puncture
- xv. EMERGENCY PACING
  - (1) standby pacing
  - (2) LBBB - use prophylactic pacer
- xvi. PHYSIOLOGIC EVALUATION
  - (1) Number of ECG amps (2 minimum)Number of pressure amps.
- xvii. EQUIPMENT RECOMMENDATIONS
  - (1) ECG transducer (strain gauge) accuracy
  - (2) O2 consumption measurement
  - (3) Blood gas analyzer (oximeter)
  - (4) Physiologic recorder
  - (5) Emergency cart/defib
- xviii. Video monitors/remote
- xix. Physiologic Recorder with Computer

3. ETHICAL / LEGAL
   a. TIME OUT
      i. All included
      ii. Patient may not be in if sedated
      iii. Reverse Time OUT
         (1) "Wait 2 minutes please"
   b. Medical "negligence" suites:
      i. Assumption of duty of care
      ii. failure to perform the assumed duty
      iii. Legal cause of harm to the patient
      iv. Proof of damages
      v. "Informed consent" for cath
         (1) Parents/guardians
         (2) Ability to make informed decisions
            (a) mind altering premeds
      vi. Legal/medical records found in cath labs.
         (1) breach of confidentiality
         (2) Privileged information
      vii. Product liability
      viii. Hospital Liability
      ix. Preparation of the patient
         (1) emotional preparation
   c. Medicare & Legislation impacts
      i. PRO
      ii. DRG
      iii. PCI
      iv. CABG

4. PRE-CATH PREPARATIONS
   a. Abbreviations
      i. TKO = "To keep open" an IV (i.e., keep drip going)
      ii. NPO = "Nothing Per OS" (mouth)
      iii. PRN = "Per Request Needed" or "As

Necessary."
  iv. q.i.d. = "four times a day" (q. for quarter)
 b. PREPARATIONS FOR CATH
  i. Fasting (NPO)
  ii. Vital signs
  iii. Glasses/dentures/rings/etc.
  iv. Lab tests precath.
   (1) P.T. (Pro time)
   (2) PPT
   (3) Hgb, Hct
   (4) CBC, RBC, WBC
   (5) CK, CK/MB
   (6) Creatinine, BUN
   (7) SODIUM 135-145 mEq/L
   (8) POTASSIUM (K^+) 3.5-4.5 mEq/L
   (9) CHLORIDE 95-105 mEq/L
   (10) TOTAL CALCIUM 0.8-1.0 mg/L (8.8-10.3 mg/dl)
   (11) MAGNESIUM 1.5-2.1 mEq/L
  v. Patient Work up
   (1) chart available
   (2) Informed Consent
  vi. Pre-room Check
  vii. X-ray Setup
  viii. Transfer Patient to Table
  ix. Evaluate and Inform Patient
  x. Set up ECG
  xi. Table Setup
  xii. Prep and Drape
  xiii. Monitoring Patient Condition
  xiv. Pulling Catheter and Sheath post cath
  xv. Returning Patient To Room
  xvi. Clean up
  xvii. Post Op. Monitoring and Care
  xviii. Outpatient Procedures
5. PREMEDICATION
 a. Premedication Drug Classes
  i. Sedative
  ii. Analgesic
  iii. Hallucinogenic
  iv. Anti-allergenic
  v. Anti-Vagal
 b. Action, side effects, contraindications, dose, and route of administration of:
  i. Antihistamine Benadryl
  ii. Narcotic Morphine
  iii. Short ACTING (NARCOTIC LIKE) Demerol
  iv. Benzodiazapine (Anti-anxiety) Valium
  v. Cholinergic Atropine
  vi. Demerol Meperidine
  vii. Valium Diazepam
  viii. Versed Midazolam
  ix. Benadryl Diphenhydramine
  x. Belladonna Atropine
  xi. Demerol (Meperidine) 25-100 mg IM (depending on size) Short acting narcotic analgesic
  xii. Valium (Diazepam) 5-10 mg im, I.V., or PO
   (1) Benzodiazapine, anti-anxiety drug
  xiii. Cimetadine (Tagamet) 300 mg PO
   (1) given along with prednisone for dye allergic patients.
  xiv. Benadryl (Diphenhydramine) 25-50 mg I.V. or PO
  xv. Antihistamine, given to prevent/neutralize allergic reactions
  xvi. Belladonna (Atropine) 0.4 mg Subq. or IV
   (1) Cholinergic blocker, prevents vasovagal reaction
  xvii. Prophylactic antibiotics
  xviii. Beta blockers
  xix. Ca blockers
  xx. Antiarrhythmic
  xxi Vasopressors
  xxii. Diuretics
  xxiii. Ergonovine
  xxiv. Digoxin
 c. Heparin
  i. Diagnostic case -2,000-5000 u
  ii. Sones - 5,000 u
  iii. PCI - 10,000 u
 d. Protamine
  i. Neutralizes Heparin
  ii. dose = 10 mg/1000 u. heparin
 e. Lidocaine
  i. Allergies
  ii. Other "-caines"
 f. Contrast
  i. Nonionic, Low Osmolar
  ii. Dye reactions
 g. Nitrates
  i. Nitroglycerine (SL)
  ii. Tridel (IV Nitro)
 h. Rating systems
  1. Mallampati class
  2. American Society of Anesthesiologists Class
  3. Aldrete Score

Vascular Access, Scrub Assist & Hemostasis

INDEX: D5 - Vascular Access, Scrub Assist & Hemostasis
1. Vascular Access
    a. General . . . . . p. 141 - Know
    b. Femoral/Seldinger . . . p. 146 - Know
    c. Radial . . . . . p. 150 - Know
    d. Cutdown . . . . . p. 152 - Know
    e. Venous Sites . . . . p. 156 - Know
2. Scrub Assist at Table
    a. Vascular Access and Sheath Handling p. 158 - Know
    b. Catheter Handling Techniques . p. 160 - Know
    c. Guide-wire Handling Techniques . p. 161 - Know
    d. Catheter Exchange . . . p. 163 - Know
3. Hemostasis
    a. Hematoma . . . . p. 167 - Know
    b. Pulling Sheaths . . . . p. 170 - Know
    c. Femoral Artery . . . . p. 175 - Know
    d. Radial Artery . . . . p. 181 - Know
    e. Vascular Closure Devices . . p. 186 - Know
    f. Bandaging and Patient Teaching . p. 189 - Know
    g. Post Cath Patient Care . p. 191 - Know
4. Chapter Outline . . . . p. 193
5. Manual Pressure Graphic

1A. Vascular Access - General

257. According to Kern, what are the two major "lifelines" which the staff should connect to the patient prior to beginning a cardiac cath procedure? (Select 2 below.)
    a. Pulse oximeter
    b. ECG monitor
    c. IV access
    d. Arterial line
    e. Defibrillator

ANSWERS: b. hookup to ECG monitor and c. IV access. The ECG is essential to monitor arrhythmias, bradycardia, ST changes, etc. And, the IV is necessary to administer medications during the case. IV drug administration reaches the heart before IA (arterial) administration and is safer than IA. **See:** Kern, chapter on "Arterial & Venous Access."

258. Which of the following catheterization procedures is done solely ANTEGRADE?
   a. Four-vessel head study
   b. Brockenbrough transseptal
   c. Coronary atherectomy
   d. Arterial femoral runoff

ANSWER b. Brockenbrough transseptal. Antegrade means "with the flow." All venous catheterizations are antegrade. Most use a "flow directed" or "floatation" catheter, because they float downstream with the flow. The antegrade Transseptal technique starts in the RA, then punctures across the atrial septum. The catheter continues into the LA and crosses the mitral valve into the LV, as shown.
See: Kern, chapter on "Arterial & Venous Access." **Keywords:** Antregrade = transseptal cath.

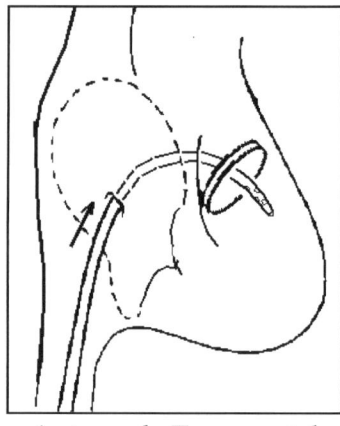
Antegrade Transseptal

259. Which of the following types of heart catheterization is done retrograde?
   a. Swan Ganz (RHC)
   b. Coronary arteriogram
   c. Brockenbrough (transseptal LV cath)
   d. Temporary pacemaker insertion

ANSWER b. Coronary arteriogram. Retrograde means "against the flow." So all arterial catheterizations of the heart and coronary arteries are retrograde. Retrograde catheters must be stiffer than antegrade (venous) catheters because they must go AGAINST the current. **See:** Kern, chapter on "Arterial & Venous Access." **Keywords:** Retrograde = arterial/coronary cath

260. When performing an arterial puncture you can best tell when you are within the artery by the:
   a. Color of the blood (red)
   b. Presence of pulsatile blood
   c. Depth of puncture
   d. Up and down dancing of the needle

ANSWER b. Presence of pulsatile blood. You can't always tell by the color of the blood. Lung disease, shunts, and low CO are associated with dark arterial blood. High pulsatile pressure is the best clue that it is arterial blood. With normal arterial blood pressure, blood will squirt out an 18 g. needle. Venous blood will drip out. Wear your mask and goggles to protect your mucus membranes from accidental blood exposure.
See: Kern, chapter on "Arterial & Venous Access." **Keywords:** Arterial blood squirts

Diagnostic Techniques: D5 - Vascular Access, Scrub & Hemostasis   143

261. What are the 2 main arterial access vessels used in adult coronary angiography? (Select 2 below.)
   a. Radial
   b. Axillary
   c. Brachial
   d. Femoral
   e. Subclavian

ANSWER: a & d. Radial and femoral, usually either the right arm or groin. Arterial access is normally either from the femoral or radial artery. However, other arterial access sites are available like the axillary or brachial arteries. **See:** Kern, chapter on "Arterial and Venous Access"

262. Which arterial access site is the easiest and quickest but has the most complications during PCI?
   a. Radial
   b. Axillary
   c. Brachial
   d. Femoral
   e. Subclavian

ANSWER: d. Femoral. Kern says, "The essence of the radial versus femoral vascular access debate can be summarized as follows: (1) Femoral access is quicker, easier, but has more complications, and (2) radial access is more difficult, takes more skill and time, but has nearly no complications." **See:** Kern, chapter on "Arterial and Venous Access"

263. Which type of arterial catheter would be used in the vascular access site labeled #2 in the box? (Right Femoral Artery - Percutaneous Antegrade)
   a. Judkins Coronary
   b. Sones Coronary
   c. Selective Celiac/Mesenteric
   d. Peripheral Angioplasty Balloon
   e. Jacky Universal Coronary

ARTERIAL ENTRY SITE
1. RFA (Percutaneous -Retrograde)
*2. RFA (Percutaneous - Antegrade)
3. RBA (Cutdown)
4. RBA (Percutaneous)
5. Right Radial (Percutaneous)

ANSWER: d. Peripheral Angioplasty Balloon. Puncture is made above the inguinal ligament with the needle pointing down toward the leg. **MATCH ALL CORRECT ANSWERS BELOW.**
   SITE = CATHETER
   1. RFA = Right Femoral Artery (Percutaneous -Retrograde): Judkins style coronary catheters are designed for the femoral retrograde approach.
   2. RFA = Right Femoral Artery (Percutaneous - Antegrade): Peripheral Angioplasty balloon must be directed down the leg - antegrade (or a Balkin up-and-over

contralateral curved sheath may be used. **See:** Todd, chapter on "Other Equipment")

3. **RBA = Right Brachial Artery (Cutdown):** Sones catheters are designed for cutdown insertion into the right brachial artery.
4. **RBA = Right Brachial Artery (Percutaneous):** Castillo percutaneous coronary catheters arteriography inserted from a sheath inserted in the left arm (brachial artery.)
5. **Right Radial:** Jacky or Tiger (TIG) are universal coronary catheters for RCA & LCA via the radial route. These universal radial coronary catheters avoid catheter exchange. Pigtail is still necessary for LV gram.

See: Kern, chapter on "Arterial & Venous Access." **Keywords:** Arterial sites → catheters used through RB cutdown = Sones

264. When palpating distal pulses during hemostasis, the posterior tibial artery is located _____ malleolus ankle bone.
 a. Behind the lateral
 b. In front of the lateral
 c. Behind the medial
 d. In front of the medial

ANSWER c. Behind or posterior to the medial malleolus ankle bone. In fact it is sometimes called the medial malleolar branch of the posterior tibial artery. This artery arises from the popliteal artery behind the knee, which arises from the femoral artery. If the femoral becomes partially occluded, these pedal pulses will be diminished. There are 4 locations commonly palpated in the lower extremity:
 • **Femoral artery** (above the femoral head in each groin)
 • **Popliteal artery** (posterior aspect of leg behind each knee)
 • **Dorsalis pedis artery** (on the anterior aspect of the foot between the first and second metatarsal.)
 • **Posterior tibial artery** (behind or posterior to the medial malleolus ankle bone.)

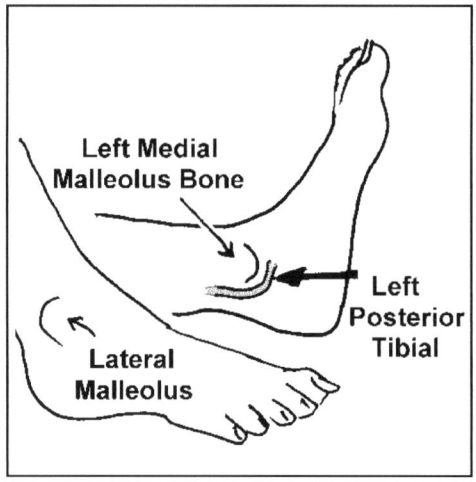

Posterior Tibial Artery

See: Snopek, chapter on "Femoral Angiography." **Keywords:** post. tibial location

265. Arterial pulse amplitude is graded on a scale from zero (absent pulse) to ___ (normal pulse).
 a. 2
 b. 4
 c. 10
 d. 100

ANSWER b. +4 out of 4, (4/4) is a normal pulse amplitude. When feeling these pulses use your index and middle fingers to palpate directly over the location where the artery is closest to the surface. They are evaluated manually according to intensity or amplitude of the pulse, with +4 being a normal strong pulse. Sometimes marked as ++++.
    0 = completely absent pulse
    +1 = markedly impaired pulse
    +2 = moderately impaired pulse
    +3 = slightly impaired pulse
    +4 = normal strong pulse
Grading allows follow up nurses to evaluate changes in the pulse over time e.g. if you find a +3 pedal pulse after establishing hemostasis, and later the floor nurse measures it to be +1, the artery may be occluding with thrombus or by hematoma. This grading scale is analogous to grading the intensity of murmurs, with the loudest murmur being 6/6. The 4+ grading scale is most common. However, other grading scales exist, some that rate 2+ as normal, and 4+ as a bounding pulse. Be sure everyone in your institution agrees on the same pulse grading scale.
See: Underhill, chapter on "History and Physical Examination" **Keywords:** Grading pulses +1 to +4

266. In patients with prosthetic mitral or aortic valves, it may be impossible to enter the LV by the retrograde or antegrade approaches. An alternative, but rarely used approach to the LV, is the:
a. Left atrial appendage
b. Translumbar approach
c. Direct LV apical puncture at PMI
d. Brockenbrough transseptal technique

ANSWER c. Direct LV apical puncture at PMI. This is done with echo guidance. The entry point is at the PMI apex. "PMI" is the Point of Maximal Intensity of the apical impulse on the chest marked by echo. After the initial transthoracic stick, a short wire and pigtail catheter are passed into the LV. LV angiography and pressure recording can then proceed. After removal of the large sheath a amplatzer type closure device may be placed between LV endocardium and epicardium. This direct puncture methods is an alternative in TAVR procedures in tortuous aortas.
See: Grossman, chapter on "Percutaneous Approach."

267. Some PCI sheaths are available with a flexible blunt tip obturator that is inserted into the sheath at the end of an interventional case and left in place overnight. Its main function is to:
a. Prevent sheath kinking
b. Allow clots to be removed easily
c. Prevent back-bleeding through sheath
d. Prevent accidentally pulling the sheath out of the artery

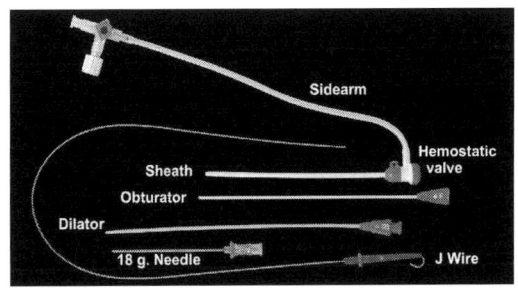

ANSWER, a. Prevent sheath kinking. If a patient's sheath does not have an obturator placed, and he bends his leg, the sheath may kink where it enters the artery, leading to hematoma formation.

Watson says: "Most of the PTCA sheaths are available with blunt tipped obturators that can be inserted at the end of the procedure to prevent the sheath from kinking if it is left in place overnight. The obturator is designed to allow fluids to flow around it and it does not hamper pressure monitoring through the introducer's side port." **See:** Watson, Invasive Cardiology, chapter on "PTCA"

Merit Medical says, "The Prelude® Obturators provide support as well as optimal flow for monitoring patient's blood pressure when sheath is left in place. Blood can be drawn from sheath side arm with obturator in place, avoiding additional venipunctures." **See:** https://www.merit.com/cardiac-intervention/access/obturators-guide-wires/prelude-obturators/

1B. Vascular Access - Femoral / Seldinger

268. The Judkins method of coronary arteriography typically uses the _____ technique through the _____ artery
a. Seldinger, Brachial
b. Seldinger, Femoral
c. Cutdown, Brachial
d. Cutdown, Femoral

ANSWER b. Seldinger insertion through femoral artery. Judkins designed his catheters for use from the femoral artery. They were designed to be put in by the percutaneous Seldinger technique of: needle, guide-wire, catheter. Although, now most are put in by sheath, the sheath is always put in by the Seldinger technique.
See: Grossman, chapter on "Percutaneous Approach."

269. Percutaneous femoral artery catheter insertion through a sheath is known as the: (Select 2 answers below.)
a. Arterial technique
b. Judkins technique
c. Modified Seldinger technique
d. Catheter through needle technique
e. Double wall puncture technique

ANSWERS: b & c. Judkins technique & Modified Seldinger technique. It may also be called the "single wall technique." Seldinger was a European radiologist who developed the original insertion method

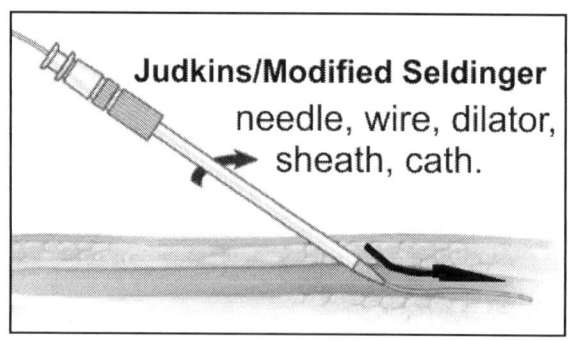

using a double wall stick which is more traumatic than the preferred single wall stick. Judkins modified it to use a single wall stick and a sheath. It has made possible all the

catheter/wire combinations we use today, including PCI. The sequence of a modified Judkins or Seldinger insertion is:
1. Needle insertion into a vessel
2. Insertion of a wire through the needle
3. Removal of the needle over the wire
4. Insertion of the dilator and sheath
5. Removal of wire and dilator
6. Insertion of catheter through sheath

The original Seldinger technique did not use a sheath, but inserted the catheter directly over the wire. This method is still used in some instances because it leaves a smaller wound.

Kern says, "Because of its relative ease, speed, reliability, and low complication rate, the Judkins technique has become the most widely used method of left-heart catheterization and coronary arteriography.... A transverse skin incision is made over the femoral artery with a scalpel. With a modified Seldinger technique an 18-gauge thin-walled needle is inserted at a 30- to 45-degree angle into the femoral artery, and a 0.035- or 0.038-inch J-tip polytetrafluoroethylene (Teflon)–coated guidewire is advanced through the needle into the artery. The wire should pass freely up the aorta without tactile resistance and feel like a hot knife passing through butter.. After arterial access is obtained, a sheath at least equal in size to the coronary catheter is usually inserted into the femoral artery." The catheter is then inserted through the sheath.
See: Kern, chapter on "Arterial and Venous Access"

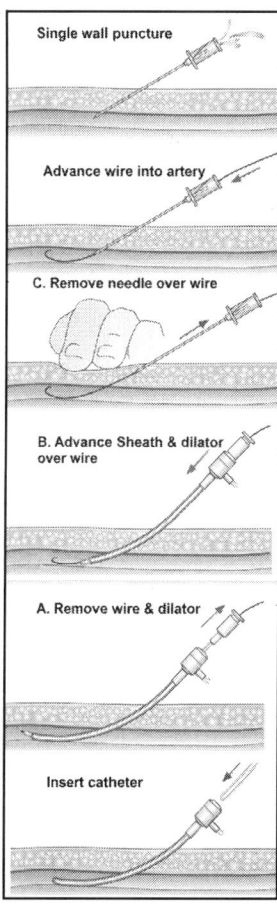

270. Rearrange the letters A, B and C below to get the correct order for Modified Seldinger or Judkins sheath insertion technique:
• Stick artery
• Advance wire through needle
• ____   A. Remove wire and dilator
• ____   B. Advance sheath/dilator over wire
• ____   C. Remove needle while wiping wire
• Insert preloaded catheter into sheath
    a. A, B, C
    b. B, C, A
    c. C, A, B
    d. C, B, A

ANSWER d. C, B, A
• Stick artery
• Advance wire through needle
• **C. REMOVE NEEDLE OVER WIRE**
• **B. ADVANCE SHEATH/DILATOR TOGETHER OVER WIRE**
• **A. REMOVE WIRE & DILATOR**
• Insert preloaded catheter into sheath

See: Grossman, chapter on "Percutaneous Approach." **Keywords:** Seldinger technique

148 ◄◄ Diagnostic Techniques: D5 - Vascular Access, Scrub & Hemostasis ►►

271. In an attempt to establish arterial access, the Dr's. first stick caused the patient to feel a shock down his right leg. In order to enter the RFA, his next stick should be directed just _____ to the first stick.
a. Medial
c. Lateral
c. Superior
d. Inferior

ANSWER a. Medial. Remember the right groin anatomic sequence is NAV or NAVL: Nerve, Artery, Vein, Ligament. So, the right femoral artery is just to your right of the nerve. Puncture 1-2 cm below the inguinal ligament, not the crease. If you go too far medial (rightward), you'll hit the vein, and finally the inguinal ligament itself. Remember NAVL for RFA.
See: Kern, chapter on "Arterial & Venous Access."
Keywords: Hit right femoral nerve → stick just medial for RFA

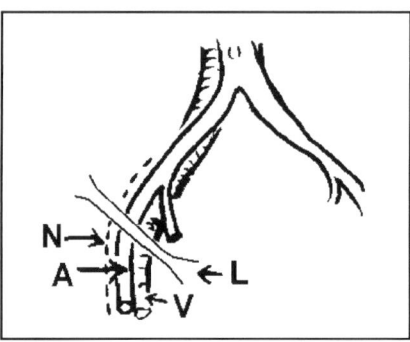
N-A-V-L

272. A patient has a hematoma on her right groin. The Dr. chooses the left femoral approach for coronary arteriography. In his first puncture attempt he accidentally punctures the <u>left femoral vein</u> as shown. He withdraws the needle and holds pressure for three minutes. His next LFA puncture attempt should be ____ to the last puncture site.
a. 1 cm medial
b. 2 cm medial
c. 1 cm lateral
d. 2 cm lateral

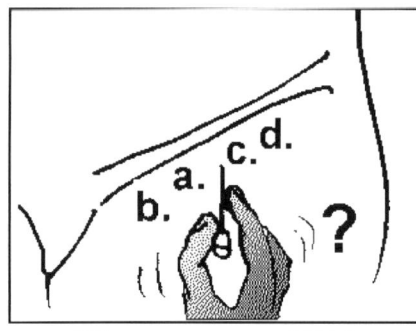
Where puncture LFA?

ANSWER c. 1 cm lateral to vein. Remember NAV (or NAVL) is for the right groin. For the left groin it would be reversed to - VAN. So he should stick 1 cm to the right of (lateral to) the original venepuncture site. NAVL stands for: NERVE - ARTERY - VEIN - (LIGAMENT). The femoral vein is about 1 cm medial to the femoral artery.
See: Kern, chapter on "Arterial & Venous Access."

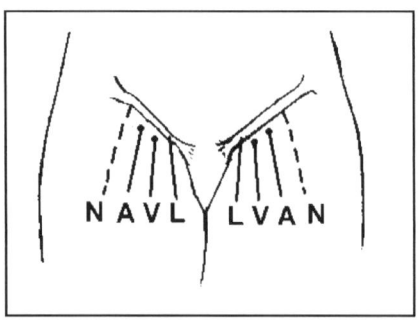
"NAV" - "VAN"

273. From the diagram, where should you stick the femoral artery for a heart cath?
   a. #2 - just below inguinal ligament
   b. #3 - 3 cm below inguinal ligament
   c. #6 - just below inguinal ligament
   d. #7 - 3 cm below inguinal ligament
   e. #8 - 6 cm below inguinal ligament

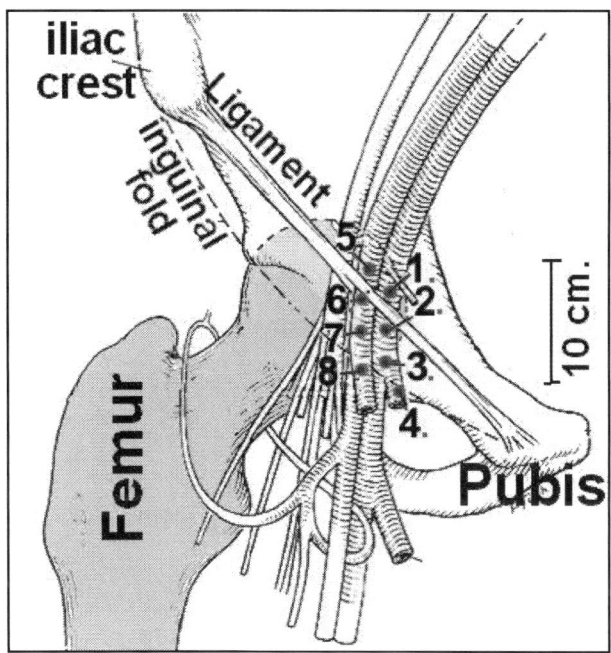

Femur and femoral triangle

ANSWER: d. #7 - 3 cm below inguinal ligament. Correct needle position for single wall common FA puncture is:
- Over the arterial pulsation
- Over the pubic bone and femoral head bones.
- FA is between the nerve and femoral vein as shown (NAVL)
- 3-5 cm below inguinal ligament

You do not want to puncture the superficial femoral artery at #8. It is too small to accept cardiac catheters without damage. Neither do you want to be above the inguinal ligament, the femoral head (#5), or the external inguinal artery because it is difficult to hold pressure there. The external inguinal artery is seen underneath the #1. High puncture increases the incidence of retroperitoneal bleed into the belly. The bone beneath the CFA provides a platform to push against when holding pressure. Many physicians observe the femoral head on fluoro before the stick, and mark it with a hemostat as the correct level to puncture the CFA. Note that the location of the inguinal fold is not a reproducible marker, as its location varies depending on patient weight and age. Obviously you do not want to puncture the vein medial to the artery (#1, #2, #3, and #4 in the diagram).

See: Kern, chapter on "Arterial and Venous Access and Hemostasis" **Keywords:** Femoral arteriography approaches

274. Femoral artery puncture above the inguinal ligament is associated with increased incidence of:
   a. A-V fistula
   b. Iliac artery thrombosis
   c. Femoral nerve laceration
   d. Retroperitoneal hematoma

ANSWER: d. Retroperitoneal hematoma or bleeding is associated with high femoral artery puncture. If the needle punctures the peritoneum, the artery may bleed into the abdominal cavity unnoticed. Watch for these signs in high femoral puncture post cath: hypotension, hypovolemic shock, low abdominal or flank pain, tachycardia, abdominal tenderness and low hematocrit.

Farouque says, "Several factors may predispose to RPH in the current era of PCI, including female gender, low BSA, and higher femoral artery puncture . . . Retroperitoneal hematoma (RPH) is one of the most serious complications after PCI. Unlike other bleeding sites, the retroperitoneum can harbor a large volume of blood with few external manifestations until hypovolemia occurs, leading to delayed recognition, added morbidity, and a potentially fatal result....Treatment includes transfusion of blood to correct anemia and surgical correction." **See:** Farouque, "Risk factors for the development of retroperitoneal hematoma after PCI", J Am Coll Cardiol, 2005

275. This sheath aortogram shows _____ and is associated with_____.
   a. Profunda femoral artery puncture, leg ischemia
   b. Common femoral artery puncture, routine arterial access
   c. Superfical femoral artery puncture, hematoma & pseudoanurysm
   d. High iliac puncture (above inguinal crease), retroperitoneal bleeding risk

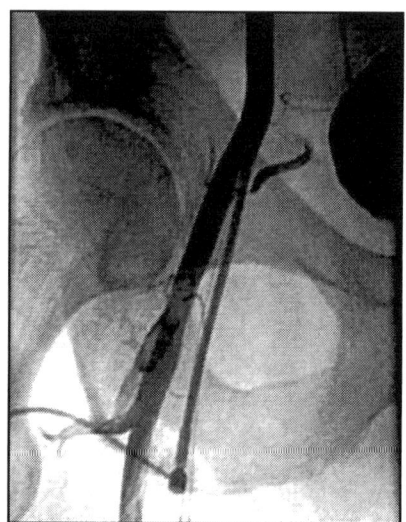

Arterial Access - After Ragosta

ANSWER: d. High iliac puncture, above inguinal crease, retroperitoneal bleeding risk. Note how the sheath entry is well above the femoral head, and above the inferior epigastric artery (on the right near the sheath entry into the iliac). High punctures like this are more prone to dangerous retroperitoneal bleeding complication. The femoral bifurcation shows the profunda on the left and superficial femoral on the right. If one of these smaller arteries were accessed, there is increased risk of hematoma or leg ischemia. An ideal puncture is on the save level as the femoral head (round ball joint). This gives you a large artery to access and a good base to hold pressure against when you pull the sheath.
See: Ragosta, Cardiac Catheterization, and Atlas, chapter on "Vascular Access" **Keywords:** Femoral access over femoral head

1C. Vascular Access - Radial

276. Before attempting a radial artery puncture, the pulses should be strong. The patency of the ulnar artery and palmar arch can be checked by doing the:
   a. Allen's maneuver
   b. Valsalva maneuver
   c. Brockenbrough maneuver
   d. Arm flexion maneuver

ANSWER a. Allen's maneuver checks the color of the hand after release of the ulnar artery. Here is how the Allen's test is done:
1. Patient raises his arm and clenches his fist as you compress both radial and ulnar wrist arteries.
2. Lower the patient's hand while still holding both arteries of the wrist.
3. Patient opens his hand. The hand will be white - no blood.
4. Then release the little finger side (ulnar artery). Color in the hand should return within

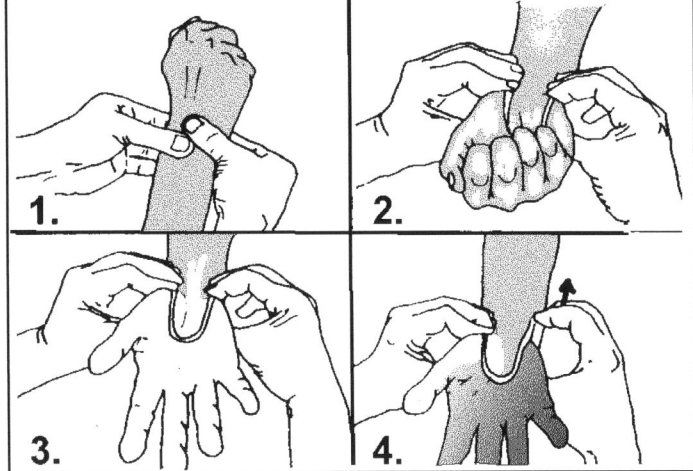
Modified Allen's test (after AHA, Textbook of ACLS)

6 seconds. If it takes too long, radial or brachial artery cannulation is risky because there is inadequate collateral circulation in the hand. Some use Doppler or pulse oximeter readings in the hand.

If radial artery thrombosis develops and there are no collaterals, the arm will become ischemic. Doppler examination of the palmar arch while compressing radial and ulnar arteries may be more reliable and can be used in lieu of the Allen's test. Pulse oximeters may also be used to evaluate palm flow. **See:** ACLS textbook, chapter on "Invasive Monitoring" also see Kern, chapter on "Arterial & Venous Access." **Keywords:** Allen's maneuver

277. The <u>Allen test</u> should be administered to a patient prior to coronary arteriography when using:
a. Radial artery access
b. Brachial artery access
c. Axillary artery access
d. Right femoral artery access
e. Contralateral femoral artery access

ANSWER: a. Radial artery access. King says, "It is critical that the Allen test be performed before electing the radial approach to assure that there is adequate collateral circulation to the hand, because occlusion of the radial artery is not uncommon." **See:** King, chapter on "Diagnostic Procedures: Special Considerations" **Keywords:** Allen test for radial cases

278. What are the 2 needle & sheath methods commonly used for radial artery access. (Select 2 below.)
a. Micropuncture needle with 1 wall stick, wire & short hydrophilic sheath
b. Micropuncture needle with 2 wall stick, wire & standard arterial sheath
c. Angiocath with 1 wall stick, remove needle, wire & standard arterial sheath
d. Angiocath with 1 wall stick, remove needle, wire & long hydrophilic sheath
e. Angiocath with 2 wall stick, remove needle, wire & short hydrophilic sheath

ANSWER: a & e. Micropuncture needle with 1 wall stick, wire & short hydrophilic sheath and Angiocath with 2 wall stick, remove needle, wire & short hydrophilic sheath

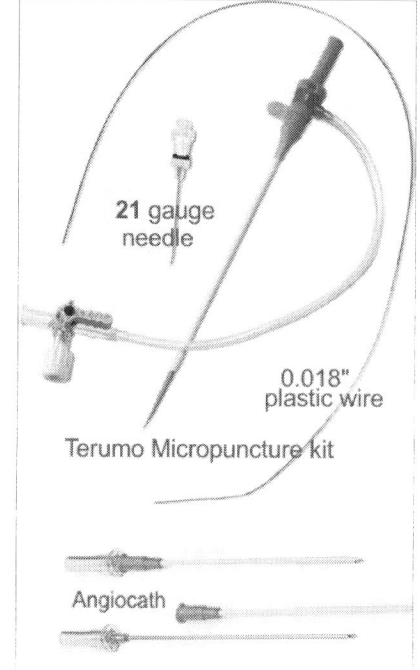

Kern says: "There are two techniques for arterial puncture: the use of a micropuncture needle or the use of an angiocath needle. The choice is really based on personal preference, although some data suggest that the angiocath needle technique is easier to learn and decreases the time and number of attempts used to gain access. Using the micropuncture technique, the operator punctures the front wall of the radial artery only, whereas with the angiocath technique, a through-and-through puncture must be used – whereby the needle is sent through the posterior wall of the radial artery. This is done to ensure access to the lumen and does not increase vascular complications as it might if the same approach were used for the femoral artery."

"Several radial sheath systems (10 to 30 cm) with graduated dilator system are available, although there is no data demonstrating an advantage to using a longer sheath.... A final important aspect of any sheath used is that it must be hydrophilic. This minimizes spasm, patient discomfort, and trauma to the vessel wall." **See:** Kern, chapter on "Arterial and Venous Access"

1D. Vascular Access - Cutdown

279. Which older arterial access method inserts an arteriography catheter through a brachial artery cutdown?
a. Sones
b. Judkins
c. Seldinger
d. Arteriectomy

ANSWER a. Dr. Mason Sones developed this approach for his method of coronary arteriography. Here the doctor surgically exposes the brachial artery and makes a small incision in it for direct insertion of the Sones catheter. This direct method gives unequaled control of a catheter in the aortic root. The brachial approach is still preferred if the femoral vessels are too tortuous, bypassed, or blocked. However, it has been largely replaced by the easier femoral Seldinger approach. Another advantage of the Sones method, is that once the arm cutdown is made, both the artery and vein are readily available for a bilateral heart catheterization. The larger impella catheters usually require brachial artery cutdown. **See:** Grossman, chapter on "Percutaneous Approach."

280. During a cutdown procedure for Impella 5.0 a patient's brachial artery has been isolated, tagged, and incised. The cardiologist is about to insert the Impella into the arteriotomy. When he says "NOW!" the scrub assistant should:
   a. Tighten the upstream tie
   b. Tighten the downstream tie
   c. Loosen the upstream tie
   d. Loosen the downstream tie

ANSWER c. Loosen or release the upstream ties (rubber bands or umbilical tape) to allow the catheter to pass up the artery. This is done by releasing the tension held on the medial ties and tighten the lateral ties. If you release too early, everyone gets squirted - too late the cath may tear the brachial artery. Peterson says, "It is important for the assistant to concomitantly relax the proximal elastomer tape, otherwise injury to the intima can be produced by the catheter tip pressing against the occluded lumen." Cutdowns may still need to be done in some cases.
See: Grossman, chapter on "Percutaneous Approach."

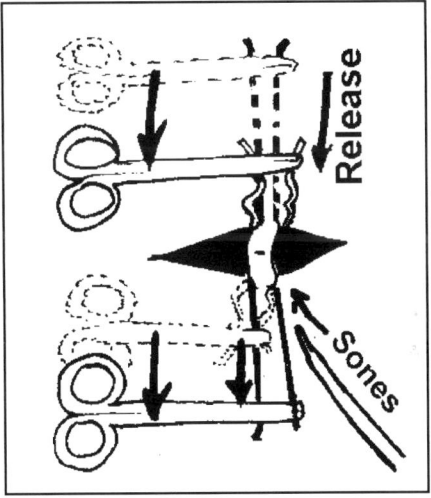

Sones catheter insertion

281. The suture used to repair a brachial arteriotomy is ___ and the skin suture is ___.
   a. 4-0 Dexon Plus absorbable, 6-0 (Prolene or Tevdec) non-absorbable
   b. 4-0 (Prolene or Tevdec) non-absorbable, 6-0 Dexon Plus absorbable
   c. 6-0 Dexon Plus absorbable, 4-0 (Prolene or Tevdec) non-absorbable
   d. 6-0 (Prolene or Tevdec) non-absorbable, 4-0 Dexon Plus absorbable

ANSWER d. 6-0 (Prolene or Tevdec) suture is used for the small arteriotomy. It is very fine, non-wettable, non-absorbable, polyester suture. You wouldn't want it to be absorbed in a few days and have the artery break open.

A 4-0 Dexon Plus is the larger standard thread size used for the skin. Grossman recommends that the skin suture be absorbable so the patient does not have to return to get them removed. They will be absorbed into the tissues within a week or two.
See: Kern, chapter on "Arterial & Venous Access."

282. When performing a brachial artery cutdown you make a _____ incision in the arm. Then after blunt dissection to bring up the artery, make a _____ incision in the artery.
  a. Lateral, Lateral (perpendicular to artery)
  b. Lateral, Longitudinal
  c. Longitudinal, Longitudinal (parallel to artery)
  d. Longitudinal, Lateral

ANSWER a. **Lateral** in skin, **Lateral** in the artery. The skin incision is **lateral** (perpendicular to the artery). Then use blunt dissection by opening hemostats longitudinally to move the vessel away from the tissue. Finally a #11 blade is used to make a small **lateral** incision in the artery. This cuts the artery parallel to the media smooth muscle fibers. Impella recommends a purse-string suture surround the arteriotomy.

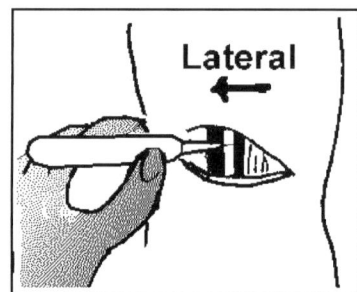

Sones arm cutdown

Peterson says, "A longitudinal arteriotomy is *not* advisable because it will often result in stenosis of the vessel when repaired." Some practitioners pinch the vessel to avoid cutting the back wall. Others enlarge the heparin needle puncture site in the artery with small scissors or forceps

Abiomed recommends a cutdown for the larger Impella catheters using a purse-string suture technique. **See:** Kern, chapter on "Arterial & Venous Access."

283. After performing a right heart cath via antecubital venous cutdown on a small vein the physician usually _____ the access vein.
  a. Ties off the upstream end of
  b. Ties off both ends of
  c. Sutures with nonabsorbable suture
  d. Sutures with absorbable suture

ANSWER b. Tie off **both ends** of the access vein. Most physicians waste the arm vein by tying it off with the tag suture. Both ends are tied to prevent bleeding. There are so many veins in the arm that to sacrifice several veins makes little difference in the venous return. The venous channels all anastomose. This is not the case in a brachial artery cutdown, where this artery is the only source of blood supply to the arm. Kern says, "small veins simply are tied distally and proximally using 4-0 silk. Large veins are closed using the pursestring technique as described for arteriotomy. Thrombotic occlusion develops in most repaired veins." **See:** Kern, chapter on "Arterial & Venous Access." **Keywords:** Tie off veins

284. To make the skin incision for a brachial cutdown, most catheterizing physicians use a:
  a. #10 scalpel blade
  b. #11 scalpel blade
  c. #12 scalpel blade
  d. #15 scalpel blade

ANSWER d. #15 curved - small blade. **Be able to match all answers below.**
1. **#10 SCALPEL BLADE:** A large curved blade for major surgery.
2. **#11 SCALPEL BLADE:** The pointed blade used for the stab wound.
3. **#12 SCALPEL BLADE:** A hooked "eagle beak" shaped point for fine slicing
4. **#15 SCALPEL BLADE:** A small curved blade used for making small skin incisions as in cutdown procedures.

See: Grossman, chapter on "Percutaneous Approach." **Keywords:** Cutdown use #15 curved scalpel blade

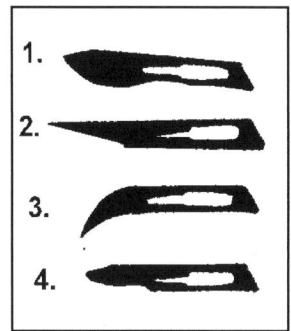
Common scalpel blades

285. **When performing right heart catheterization by the cutdown technique, when would the venous tourniquet MOST likely be applied?**
   a. After making the skin incision
   b. At the start of prepping the arm
   c. During the making of the incision
   d. Immediately prior to the arteriotomy
   e. Not needed, since it should be lateral to the exposed artery

ANSWER: b. At the start of prepping the arm or even sooner to identify a good vein. This will bring them up. "A visible vein should also be easily compressible in order to qualify for use. The vein should be palpated by the operator's index finger to determine the relative size of the vessel and the direction in which it runs. A firm to hard non-compressible vein is indicative of thrombosis and not suitable for further efforts at venous access. If the peripheral veins are not prominent and need to be made more prominent, gentle slapping of the skin overlying the vein may make it more prominent....Milking the vein from proximal to distal may also increase venous prominence. Venous prominence is further augmented by the use of a proximal venous tourniquet. ....The tourniquet should be applied 5-10 cm proximal to the selected site. This compression must be sufficient to permit arterial inflow whilst restricting venous outflow. Prolonged application of a venous tourniquet, for more than 5 minutes, increases venous tortuosity and fragility and should thus be avoided. If venous prominence is not improved by these measures, asking the patient to grip and relax their hands repeatedly, and application of a warm compress (pads soaked in lukewarm water) for at least 2-3 minutes will improve venous visibility. This is achieved by increased local blood flow which increases venous return...." **See:** http://www.ncbi.nlm.nih.gov/pmc/articles/PMC1741330/pdf/v075p00459.pdf

Grossman says, "If a right heart cath is contemplated, the incision is wide and made over the palpable brachial artery; if a right heart study alone is planned, the incision is narrow and made directly over a previously identified medial vein. [not one of the lateral arm veins which have more tortuosities]" **See:** Grossman, chapter on "Brachial Cutdown"

286. Where is the antecubital fossa?
a. In the arm pit
b. In the crease of the elbow
c. In the inter-atrial septum
d. In the inter-ventricular septum

ANSWER: In the crease on the front of the elbow. This is a common location for making a cutdown on a vein or establishing percutaneous brachial artery access. **See:** Medical dictionary

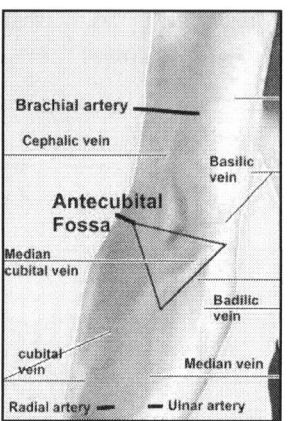

1E. Vascular Access - Venous Sites

287. Identify the neck venous access site labeled #3 in the diagram.
a. Subclavian vein
b. Innominate vein
c. Internal jugular
d. External jugular

ANSWER #3 = a. Subclavian Vein.
MATCH ALL CORRECT ANSWERS BELOW.
 1. Internal Jugular
 2. External Jugular
 3. Subclavian Vein
 4. Innominate Vein
See: ACLS, chapter on "Vascular Access."
Keywords: Venous access, neck

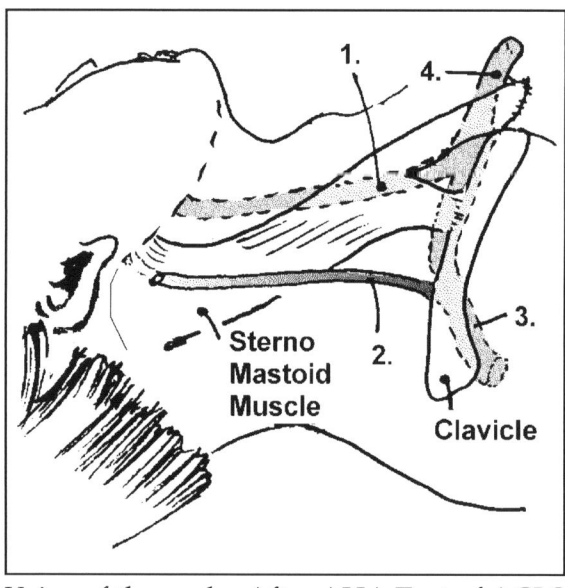

Veins of the neck - After AHA Text of ACLS

288. Identify the location for venepuncture to reach the vein labeled #3 (subclavian) in the box.
a. In the triangle at insertion of sterno-mastoid muscle into clavicle
b. Inferior to and beneath clavicle
c. On the surface of sterno-mastoid muscle

NECK VENOUS ACCESS SITES

1. Internal Jugular
2. External Jugular
*3. Subclavian

ANSWER b. The subclavian is reached by the subclavicular approach. Be able to match all answers below.

VENOUS ACCESS and PUNCTURE SITE
1. **Internal Jugular:** in the triangle of sterno-mastoid muscle
2. **External Jugular:** on surface of sterno-mastoid muscle
3. **Subclavian:** inferior and beneath clavicle

See: ACLS, chapter on "Vascular Access."
Keywords: Internal jugular access

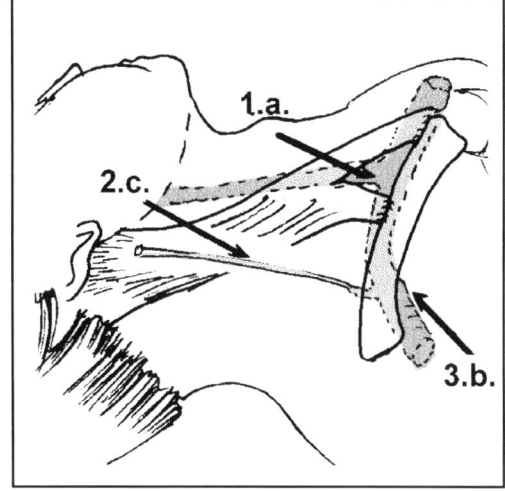
Internal jugular venipuncture

289. Which venous access site is shown? Percutaneous entry made through a triangle formed by the two sternocleido-mastoid muscle insertions and the sternum.
a. Subclavian vein
b. Azygous vein
c. Internal jugular vein
d. External jugular vein

ANSWER c. Internal jugular vein. This diagram shows the I.J. venepuncture. Understand all routine catheter entry routes and methods. **See:** ACLS, chapter on "Vascular Access." **Keywords**: Internal jugular access

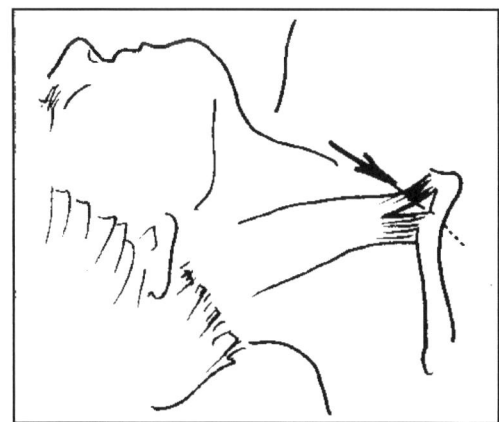
Venous access site

290. During internal jugular vein puncture on a patient with low venous pressure who occasionally gasps for air, how should the patient be positioned?
a. Trendelenburg
b. Reverse Trendelenburg
c. Flat with rolled towel behind neck
d. Flat with a pillow under shoulders

ANSWER a. Trendelenburg = head down, feet up. ACLS positioning for puncture of the central internal jugular vein is in a Trendelenburg position (15 degree - head down). This reduces the chance of air embolism and engorges the veins for easier puncture. Turn the patient's head away

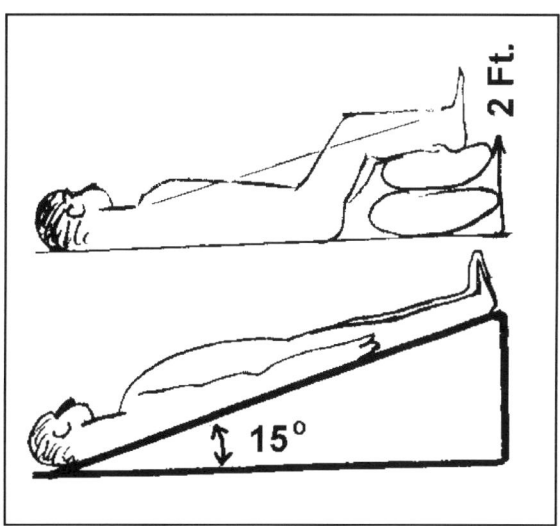
Position for internal jugular and subclavian venipuncture (Trendelenburg position)

from you about 30 degrees. Although some physicians prefer placing a towel between the shoulder blades, the ACLS manual recommends that you NOT do this, because it decreases the space between the clavicle and the first rib, making the subclavian vein less accessible.

If a patient has low venous pressure and takes deep breaths during central venous access, he may suck air through the venous catheter into the right heart. Large volumes of air in the venous can be lethal. Patients cannot suck air into the arterial circulation, but small injected volumes can block arterial flow and cause tissue ischemia.
See: ACLS manual, chapter on "IV Techniques." **Keywords:** Position for internal jugular puncture

291. How should the patient's head be positioned for right internal jugular vein access?
a. Looking straight ahead (up)
b. Turned 5-10 degrees to left
c. Turned 30 degrees to left
d. Turned 45-60 degrees to left

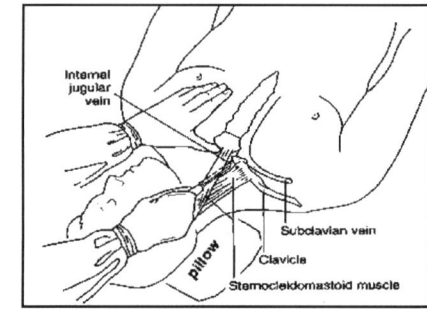

ANSWER c. Turned 30 degrees to left. Kerns says, "To identify landmarks, the operator instructs the patient to lie supine without a pillow under the head and, in the case of the right internal jugular, with the head turned 30 degrees to the left. Patients with low venous pressures may be placed in the Trendelenburg (head down) position." **See:** Kern, chapter on "Arterial and Venous Access" **Keywords:** IJ, turn head 30 degrees

2A. Scrub Assist - Vascular Access & Sheath Handling Techniques

292. The cardiologist is advancing a catheter into a sheath. You are his assistant. As you advance the guide-wire through the catheter into the artery, the patient jumps in pain and the wire becomes hard to push. When the wire meets resistance like this, your next step should be to:
a. Rotate and firmly advance the guide-wire
b. Remove the wire and check for good blood flow back though the catheter
c. Stop advancing. Tell the doctor that you feel "resistance"
d. Release the wire. Let the doctor feel the resistance as he advances the catheter

ANSWER c. Stop advancing. Tell the doctor that you feel "resistance." Often the operator feels the back wall of the artery and has difficulty advancing into the vessel. NEVER advance the guide-wire against this resistance. It can dissect the vessel and cause unwanted complications. Stop advancing, and tell the doctor immediately! Go slow, and be gentle. By tilting the needle or sheath up or drawing back slightly it will pop

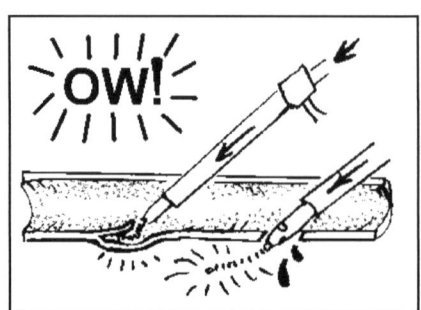

Wire dissecting RFA

safely in the main lumen. **See:** Baim & Grossman, chapter on "Percutaneous Approach."
Keywords: Resistance to advancing wire → stop and tell Dr. immediately

293. You are assisting a cardiologist to place a right femoral artery sheath. He has just inserted the sheath and dilator in a rotary motion over the wire. Now he removes and hands you the bloody guide-wire with the dilator still on it. The most efficient way to clean the bloody wire is to:
  a. Grab the dilator hub with a wet gauze. Pull it off the floppy end of the wire, while wiping the wire.
  b. Grab the dilator tip with a wet gauze. Pull it off the stiff end of the wire, while wiping the wire.
  c. Remove the dilator with your right hand and soak the wire in a basin of flush.
  d. Remove the dilator with your right hand and advance the wire into the wire storage-coil filled with flush.

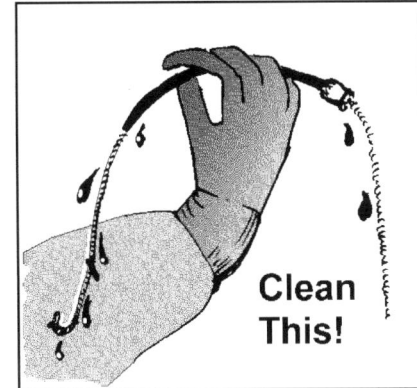
Cleaning bloody wire/dilator

ANSWER a. Grab the dilator hub with a wet gauze. Pull it off the floppy end of the wire, while wiping the wire. This will wipe the wire as you remove the dilator.
  This same method is used to remove bloody wires from used catheters during catheter exchanges.
See: Personal experience **Keywords:** Removing bloody dilator and wiping wire.

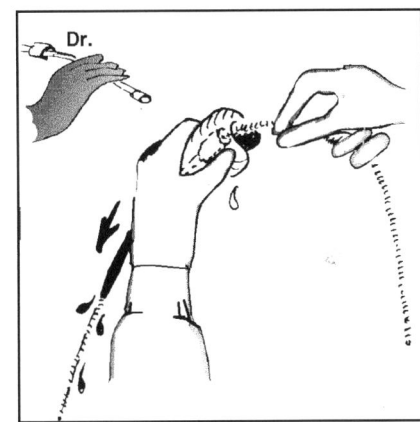
Cleaning bloody wire/dilator

294. A cardiologist is inserting a preloaded pigtail catheter into an RFA sheath. He requests a movable-core guide-wire. He asks you to fully advance the movable core for easy insertion into the sheath. To prevent "spearing" the back wall of the artery, when inserting a "stiff" guide-wire:
  a. "J" the wire before insertion
  b. "J" the wire in the sheath
  c. "J" the wire when it exits the sheath
  d. "J" the wire in the descending AO

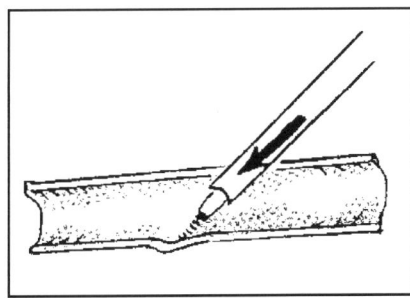
Spearing with stiff wire

ANSWER b. "J" the wire in the sheath. Many arteries have been dissected or punctured by the stiffened movable-core wire. When stiff these wires may become "spears."

Once the stiffened movable core is passed into the sheath the doctor must pause. Then the assistant must quickly soften or "J" the wire within the sheath. You should then say "soft" or "J-ed" to communicate to the doctor that it is now safe to advance the wire into the artery. **DO NOT** let the operator spear or dissect your patient's artery by pushing a stiffened wire through the artery. If necessary tell the doctor to WAIT until you have it "J-ed."

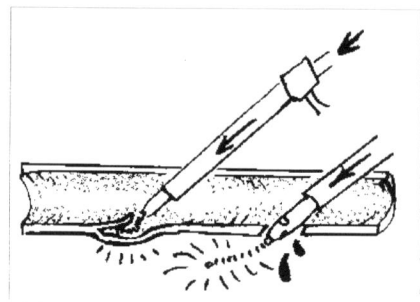
Wire dissecting / laceration

A safer alternative is to use a fixed core J-wire or to leave it "J-ed" before inserting it into the sheath. This may require a plastic sleeve to straighten the "J."
See: Grossman, chapter on "Percutaneous Approach." **Keywords:** Movable core = spear, "J" it before it leaves sheath

2B. Scrub Assist - Catheter Handling Techniques

295. When flushing an angiographic catheter you should always hold the syringe _____ and _____.
a. Horizontal, Draw back first
b. Horizontal, Flush vigorously
c. Vertical (tip down), Draw back first
d. Vertical (tip down), Flush vigorously

ANSWER c. Vertical (tip down), Draw back first.
1. The tip must be down so you can see any bubbles float up to the plunger of the syringe.
2. When you pull back and see the flash of blood, most of it will go to the top of the syringe because of its momentum. Watch and feel for any clots, which of course, must be removed.
3. When injecting flush, the syringe must be tip-down again, to prevent injecting bubbles. Finally when injecting saline never inject all of it. Leave a few cc's in the syringe to prevent injecting any residual air bubbles. Remove any bubbles from the syringe before proceeding. This is the single flush technique. The double flush requires 2 syringes and discards the bloody contents before injecting saline.

Flush catheters frequently to prevent clotting.
See: Johnsrude, "A Practical Approach to Angiography" chapter on "Catheterization Techniques." **Keywords:** Flushing syringes - tip down

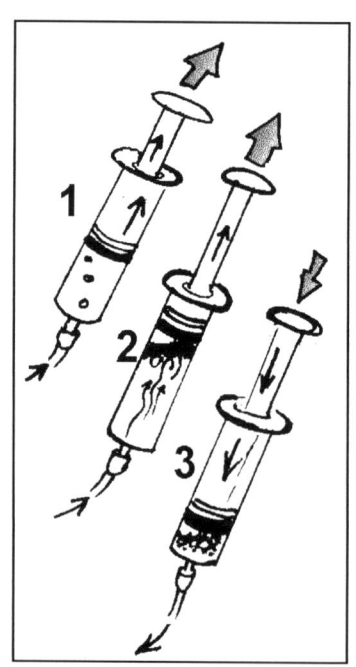
Flushing syringe

296. How should you clear a damped indwelling arterial catheter that is suspected of being clotted? Pull the catheter back below the renal arteries, then attempt to:
a. Flush gently with heparinized saline
b. Flush gently with thrombolytic agent
c. Push guide wire through catheter, then flush
d. Aspirate the clot then flush with heparinized saline

ANSWER d. Aspirate clot then flush with heparinized saline. Clots should NEVER be flushed into the body! They embolize, lead to arterial occlusion and tissue infarction. At least you have pulled the catheter back below the vital organs of brain, heart, kidney, liver, etc. If the clot cannot be aspirated, remove the catheter through a sheath. **See:** Grossman, chapter on "Percutaneous Approach" **Keywords:** Removing clotted catheter → aspirate clot

2C. Scrub Assist - Guide-wire Handling Techniques

297. You are next to a cardiologist, assisting him to advance a JR4 catheter into an RFA sheath. The JR4 is preloaded with a fixed core wire. He asks you to remove the wire. The preferred method to remove a wire is to:
a. Insert the stiff end of the wire into the plastic tube coil in which it came. Flush the coil to remove blood.
b. Pull the wire straight out with your right hand, while you wipe it with a wet gauze in your left hand.
c. Pull and coil the wire in you right hand as you wipe it with a wet gauze in you left hand.
d. Pull and coil the wire in your left hand as you wipe it with a wet gauze in your right hand.

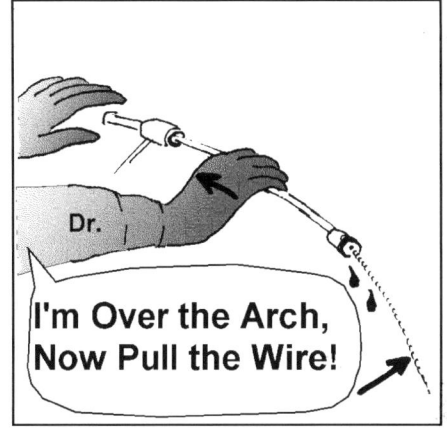
Pulling and coiling a wire

ANSWER c. Pull and coil the wire in you right hand as you wipe it with a wet gauze in you left hand. This allows you to do three things: pull and coil the wire and wipe it at the same time. This takes practice.

With movable core wires it is often just as easy to pull and wipe the entire wire without coiling it. This is because you have to straighten the movable core in order to wipe the tip free of blood. These cores can only be inserted while the wire is straight, because of the high resistance.

Once the wire is wiped-clean of blood, it can be coiled and stored. **See:** personal experience
Keywords: Pulling, wiping, and coiling wire.

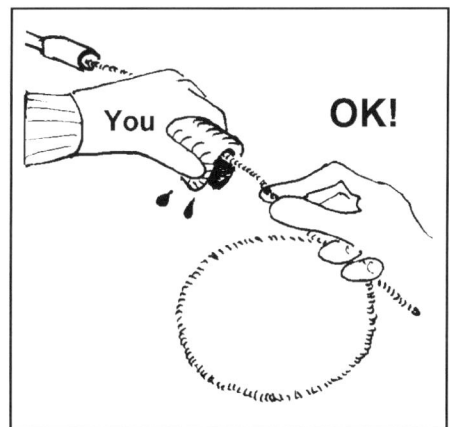
Pulling and coiling a wire

298. You are next to a cardiologist, assisting him to insert a right femoral arterial sheath. He has punctured the artery with the needle and advanced the wire into the vessel. He holds pressure at the puncture site with his left hand while just pulling the needle out of the skin with his right hand. Prior to removing the needle over the wire use your left hand to:
a. Place a wet gauze at the needle tip
b. Place a wet gauze at the needle hub
c. Hold the wire at the puncture site
d. Hold the stiff end of the wire

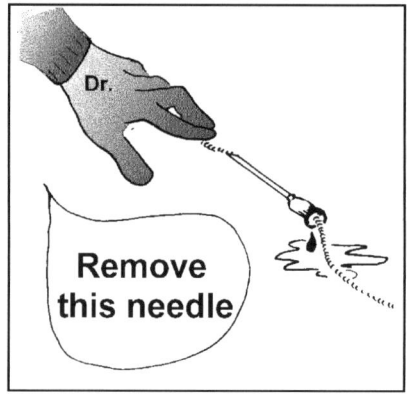
Prior to removing needle

ANSWER c. Hold the wire at the puncture site. It is necessary to "pin" the wire at the puncture site before removing anything over the wire. If you don't, you may pull out the wire. Then you lose your "track" up the aorta - your string back into the cave, so to speak.

If a sheath was not used and you pull the wire entirely out of the body - you're in big trouble! Then the doctor has to re-stick the patient to recannulate the vessel. Blush! See next questions. **See:** Personal experience. **Keywords:** Pinning wire at sheath/groin.

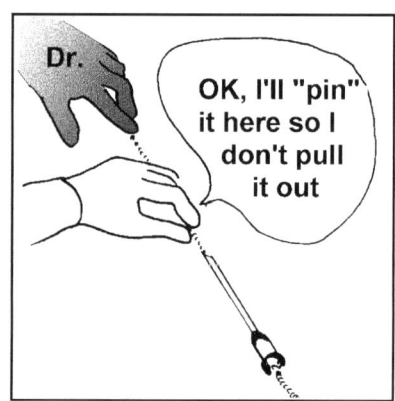
Prior to removing needle

299. You are first scrub assistant on an arteriogram. After arterial puncture, while removing the single wall needle over the wire, use your right hand to:
a. Grab and remove the needle, let the doctor wipe the wire with a wet gauze
b. Grab and hold up the stiff end of the wire for the doctor
c. Place a wet gauze over the needle tip, pull the needle and wipe the gauze in one motion
d. Place a wet gauze over the needle hub, pull the needle and wipe the wire in one motion

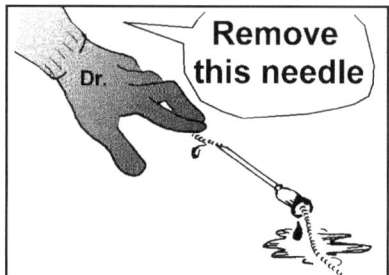
Remove this needle "over wire" for the Dr.

ANSWER c. Place a wet gauze over the needle tip, pull the needle and wipe the gauze in one motion. The wet gauze is used to both pull the needle and wipe the wire at the same time. Remember to pin the wire at the sheath or groin with your left hand to avoid pulling out the guide wire.

Beware of the sharp needle tip! Protect your gloves and skin from puncture by carefully covering the needle tip. Avoid the hazard of blood transmitted diseases. **See:**

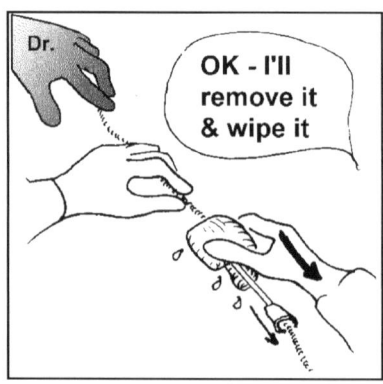
Removing needle "over wire"

◀◀ Diagnostic Techniques: D5 - Vascular Access, Scrub & Hemostasis ▶▶

Personal experience **Keywords:** Pulling needle over wire

300. While advancing a coronary arteriography catheter over the arch, the end hole appears to catch on the surface of the aorta. To avoid stroke and retinal artery embolization the catheter should be advanced with a leading:
a. High-torque floppy guide wire
b. Floppy straight tipped wire
c. Exchange wire
d. "J" tipped wire

ANSWER d. "J" tipped wire. Johnsrude says, "A general rule is that the catheter should not be advanced in the arteries without a guidewire; however this is not true in the venous system, in the right side of the heart, and in the smooth vessels of children." Even then, if any roughness or catching is noted as the catheter is advanced Grossman says, "The catheter should be pulled back into the descending aorta, double-flushed, and then readvanced around the arch over a leading J-tip guide wire."
See: Baim and Grossman, chapter on "Complications of Cardiac Catheterization."
Keyword: Safest catheter advance is with leading J wire

2D. Scrub Assist - Catheter Exchange Techniques

301. A physician wishes to exchange a pigtail catheter for a multipurpose (MP). He has inserted the wire and removed the pigtail catheter over the wire, leaving the wire in the vessel. After wiping the wire with a wet gauze, you thread the MP over the stiff end of the wire, slide the catheter tip down to the insertion site, and the Dr. starts inserting the MP over the wire into the artery as shown. You should:

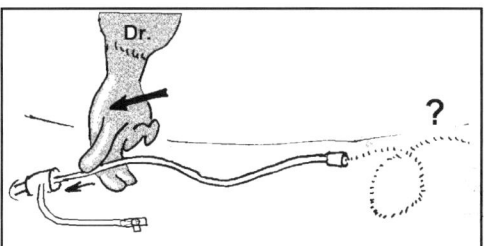
Dr. begins inserting wire and catheter

a. Let the wire advance to the level of the aortic valve and hold it there
b. Advance the wire all the way into the MP
c. Hold the tip of the wire in the descending AO by fixing it at the patient's legs/feet
d. Remove and wipe the wire with a dampened gauze

ANSWER c. Hold the wire firmly and fix it at a constant position in relation to the patient's legs/feet. The physician will advance the catheter over the guide-wire using it as a track up the aorta. As the catheter advances it may pull the guide-wire with it. You need to hold the guide

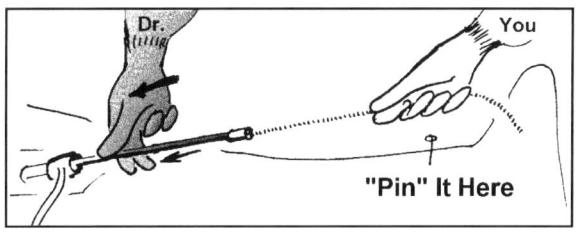
Pinning wire as Dr. inserts catheter

wire tightly and not let it move. This is called "pinning" the wire to the patient's leg. In an alternate method the physician may ask you to lead the catheter with the guide-wire as he advances it over the arch. This prevents catheter damage to the aortic intima and scraping off plaques. Even then, the wire must be "pinned" to prevent it from inadvertently entering the LV where it may cause arrhythmia.
See: Grossman, chapter on "Percutaneous Approach." **Keywords:** Pin/fix the wire

302. You are assisting the physician to exchange a JL4 for a pigtail catheter. He removes the JL4 without using a guidewire and drops it on the table. You should hand the doctor:
a. The pigtail catheter tip freshly flushed with saline
b. The preloaded pigtail with the soft tip of the guidewire just protruding
c. The soft tip of guidewire to insert into the sheath
d. The stiff tip of the guidewire for back-loading into the pigtail

ANSWER b. Hand him the preloaded pigtail with the soft tip of the guidewire just protruding. This will straighten the pigtail and allow for easy sheath insertion. Then the wire is inserted to lead the catheter up the aorta. This makes a safe, non-traumatic insertion.

Pulling a JL4 like this doctor did, without a wire can rake plaque or intima off the arterial wall. It may also catch on and damage the tip of the sheath. Your physician may be in a hurry. However, it is everyone's responsibility to assure the patients safety. Grollman says, "Always exchange catheters over a guidewire..."

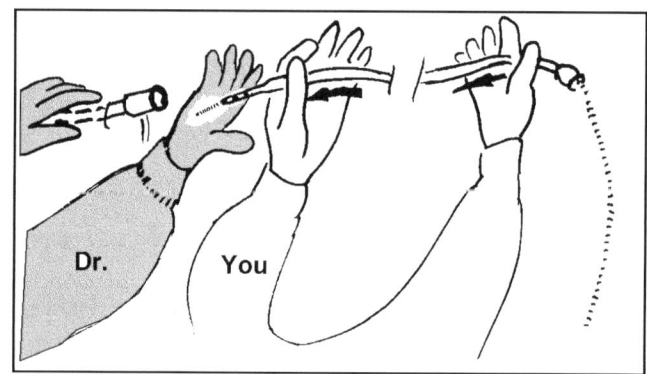
Handing the "preloaded" pigtail catheter

See: Grollman, editorial, "Does Use of Vascular Introducer Sheath Obviate need for Catheter Exchanges over a Guidewire?" **Keywords:** After cath removal hand the "preloaded catheter"

303. A doctor wants to exchange a pigtail catheter for a JL4. He removes the pigtail "over the wire" through the sheath. He leaves the wire in the sheath. You thread the JL4 over the stiff end of the wire and advance it. There is not enough wire, as shown. Before advancing the JL4 into the sheath, one of you needs to:
a. Advance the JL4 into the sheath
b. Pull the JL4 back more
c. Advance the wire into the sheath
d. Pull more wire out of the sheath

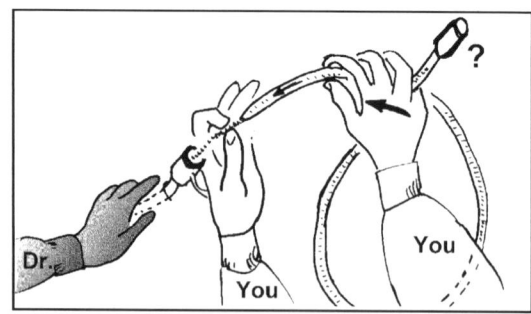
"Over the wire" exchange

ANSWER d. Pull more wire out of the sheath.

Tell the Dr. "I don't have enough wire." Then one of you must pull more wire out of the sheath and into the JL4. Only then can you secure the stiff end of the wire. As in the above question, you could lose the wire in the body by pushing the "loaded" catheter into the sheath.

Note how the hub of the catheter is held between the little finger and the ring finger of the right hand. This allows you to control both ends of the catheter with one hand.

See: Personal experience **Keywords:** Need more wire - pull some out sheath

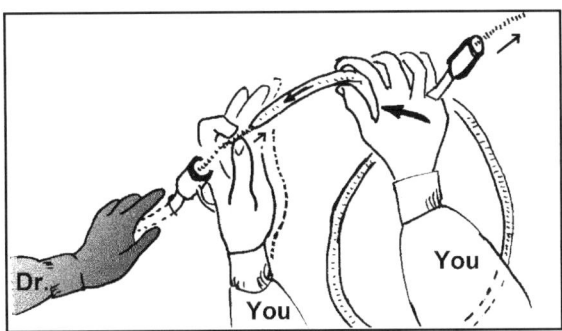

Pulling more wire from sheath to get it out the hub so you can hold it.

304. You are assisting a cardiologist to exchange a used pigtail catheter over-the-wire. He pulls the used pigtail back to the descending aorta and begins removing it. As he pulls out this used catheter over the wire you should:
 a. Tell the Dr. that you need to preload the next catheter with this wire first
 b. Tell the Dr. you need more wire
 c. Insert all the wire into the catheter hub as quickly as possible
 d. **Insert most of the wire into the pigtail but keep hold of the stiff end to prevent loss of the wire**

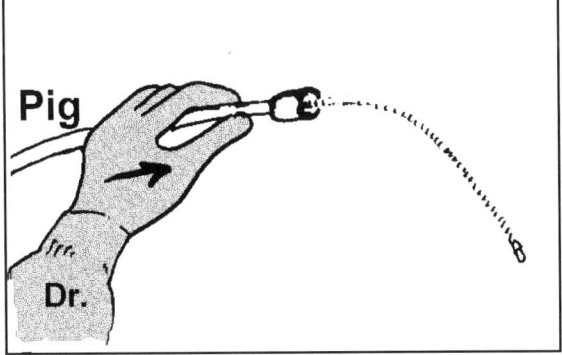

Inserting wire for "Over the wire" catheter exchange

ANSWER d. Insert most of wire into the pigtail but keep hold of the stiff end to prevent loss of the wire. Smoothly insert the wire at a rate equal to the removal of the catheter. This will leave the maximum amount of wire in the vessel for leading the JR4 up the aorta.

Then as the catheter exits the sheath insert the last few cm of wire into the pigtail.

See: Personal experience **Keywords:** Over the wire exchange

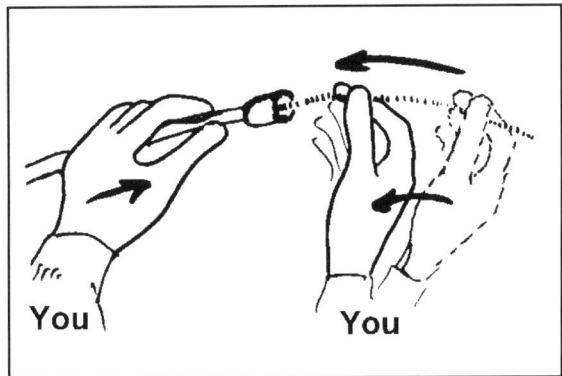

Inserting wire for "Over the wire" catheter exchange

305. You are assisting the physician to exchange a catheter over a fixed core guidewire. The flexible wire tip is in the patient. He inserts the catheter AND the wire into the vessel over the wire and through the sheath, as shown. You should:
  a. Say "I don't have a hold of the stiff end of the wire."
  b. Say "I have not softened the wire."
  c. Hold the catheter hub firmly
  d. Hold the floppy tip of the wire as he advances
  e. Pin the wire to the catheter hub as he advances

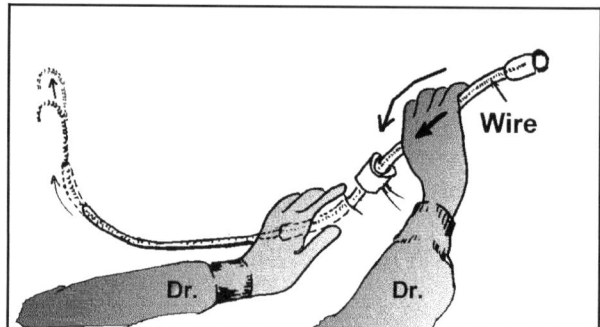
Dr. inserts catheter and wire into sheath

ANSWER a. Say "I don't have a hold on the stiff end of the wire" or "I need more wire." Without a hold on the wire, you may not be able to get it back. Beware, you don't lose the wire in the body.
See: Personal experience **Keywords:** "I don't have hold of the wire"

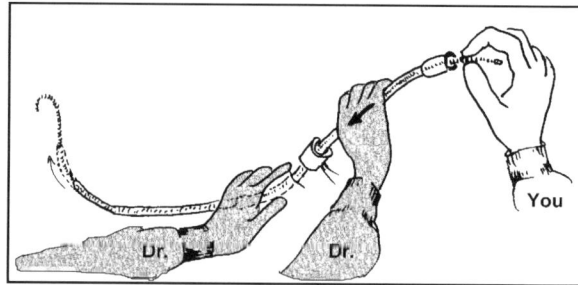
Dr. inserts catheter and wire into sheath

306. Identify the method of removing and exchanging a catheter shown at #4 in the diagram.
  a. "Without the wire" (no wire used)
  b. "Over the wire" (leaving the wire in the vessel)
  c. "With the wire" (remove both wire and catheter together)
  d. "Monorail" (alongside the wire)

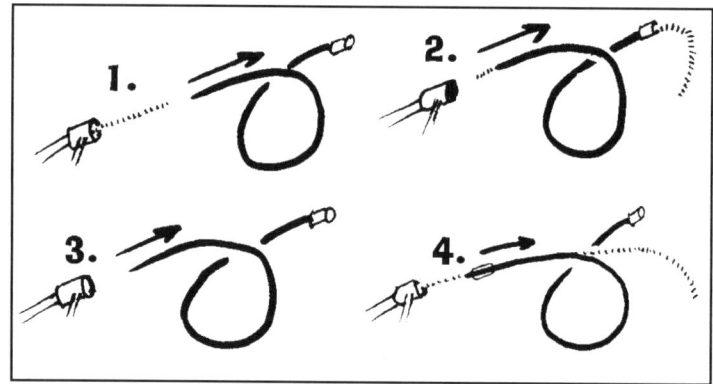
Methods of exchanging caths

ANSWER d. "Monorail" (alongside the wire). Be able to match all answers below.
  1. "OVER THE WIRE" (LEAVING THE WIRE IN THE VESSEL): This leaves the wire in the descending AO as a track for the catheter. It is like leaving a string trail in a cave so you can find you way back. Also, since the catheter always follows the wire, it cannot plow up plaque or clot.
  2. "WITH THE WIRE" (REMOVE BOTH WIRE AND CATHETER TOGETHER). This is a safe way to remove the catheter. And on reinsertion the wire always leads the catheter. It still must find a new path, and may still get trapped in tortuous vessels.

◀◀ Diagnostic Techniques: D5 - Vascular Access, Scrub & Hemostasis ▶▶ 167

    3. **"WITHOUT THE WIRE"** (NO WIRE USED): This is the most traumatic, because the wire does not lead the catheter. The cath tip may plow up plaque on the way up, and scrape it off on the way out. It is however, safe to pull relatively straight catheters with this method (e.g., Judkins Rt. and Multipurpose). But, Grollman says it **UNSAFE** to pull sharply curved catheters like, pigtails and Judkins Left coronaries. A wire should be inserted to straighten it before it is pulled..

    4. **"MONORAIL"** (ALONGSIDE THE WIRE): This is an angioplasty exchange technique. It is an "over the wire" exchange through the balloon end of an angioplasty catheter. Monorail catheters have a hole for the wire half way up the balloon catheter shaft. The distal half of the catheter has 2 lumens, one for the wire and another for the balloon inflation. The proximal (hub) end of the balloon catheter has only one lumen for the balloon. The catheter remains "beside the wire" during exchange, just as a monorail train is "alongside" its track.

        The monorail system gives the operator more control of wire and balloon catheter. However, this method only works inside a guider catheter. If too much catheter is outside the guider, you lose "pushability", because, in a vessel the proximal wire and catheter may separate and buckle.

See: Personal experience **Keywords:** Identify monorail exchange

307. Several methods have been developed for exchanging diagnostic arterial catheters through a femoral sheath. The SAFEST method in a patient with a tortuous aorta begins by removing (pulling) the catheter:
  a. "Over the wire" (leaving the wire in the vessel)
  b. "With the wire" (remove both wire and catheter together)
  c. "Without the wire" (no wire used)
  d. "Monorail" (alongside the wire)

ANSWER a. "Over the wire exchange" (leaving the wire in the vessel). This leaves the wire in the descending AO as a track for the catheter. It is like leaving a string trail in a cave so you can find you way back. Also, since the catheter always follows the wire, it cannot plow up plaque or clot. Grollman states: "Meticulously performing every exchange over a guidewire will prevent any iliac complications by carefully maintaining the wire tip well above the aortic bifurcation or above any segment where difficulty in passing the initial wire was encountered. This simple precaution adds a great deal of safety and at most a few seconds to each exchange or catheter removal."

See: Grollman, editorial, "Does Use of Vascular Introducer Sheath Obviate need for Catheter Exchanges over a Guidewire?" **Keywords:** "Over the wire" exchange safest

3A. Hemostasis - Hematoma

308. Bleeding under the skin from a vascular catheterization site is termed a/an:
  a. Hemopoiesis
  b. Hematoma
  c. Phlebotomy
  d. Extravasation

ANSWER b. Hematoma. Know all the terms described below.
  a. **HEMOPOIESIS:** Production and development of blood cells (in the bone marrow) Suffix: -poiesis = formation.
  b. **HEMATOMA:** A swelling or mass of blood confined to a tissue space and caused by a break (needle hole) in a blood vessel.
  c. **PHLEBOTOMY:** Opening a vein to withdraw blood.
  d. **EXTRAVASATION:** The escape of fluid into a surrounding space (like an IV needle that comes out of the vein, flooding the tissues).

See: Taber's Medical Dictionary. **Keywords:** Define hematoma

309. **After holding pressure on a femoral artery for 15 minutes, the groin is swollen with a 4+ pulse. Pedal pulses are +1 and the leg is cool. What vascular complication is likely?**
  a. Hematoma
  b. Retroperitoneal bleed
  c. False aneurysm
  d. AV fistula
  e. Femoral thrombus

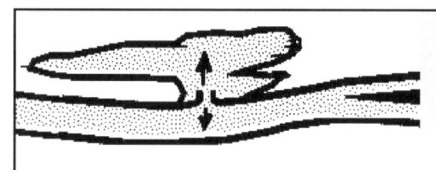

ANSWER c. False aneurysm or pseudo-aneurysm
are pulsatile. Hematomas are usually NON-pulsatile (they are hard.) When one is throbbing, it indicates blood is swishing back and forth into and out of an aneurysm. The effect of these aneurysms acts similar to a hematoma because the swelling around the vessel may collapse it and cut off femoral flow to the leg.

The aneurysmal chamber and its neck may be visualized with 2D ultrasound and Doppler. Once visualized it may be compressed, preferably with a compressor clamp, to close the tract and allow it to clot off.
See: Kern, chapter on "Arterial and Venous Access." **Keywords**: False aneurysm

310. **Certain patients are prone to developing hematomas. On which type of patient should extra care be taken to establish full hemostasis?**
  a. Diabetic males
  b. Tight aortic stenosis
  c. Patients with aortic regurgitation
  d. Patients with low cardiac output

ANSWER c. Patients with aortic regurgitation have a bounding "water-hammer pulse" that makes establishing hemostasis difficult. You should hold longer pressure (30 min.) on these patients before letting up to see if the bleeding has stopped. Other patients which require longer pressure application are:
  • Obese patients or those with large thighs
  • Hypertensive patients or those with bounding aortic regurgitation
  • Elderly patients - especially women
  • Patients who have undergone prior or recent puncture
  • Patients who suffer from coagulopathy or are on anticoagulants
  • Patients with peripheral atherosclerosis (diabetic calcified arteries may be so hard as

to be incompressible) **See:** Kern, chapter on "Vascular Access." **Keywords:** Hold pressure longer in patients with → AR

311. You have held pressure on a heart cath patient's RFA for 15 minutes. You slowly remove your fingers and see that the bleeding at the skin has stopped. But, you note a soft and stable 1/4 inch high swelling, about 1 inch in diameter. You should_____ and then watch the puncture site for 2-3 minutes more for further swelling.
   a. Circle the swollen area with a pen
   b. Continue compression for 5 more minutes
   c. Continue compression for 15 more minutes
   d. Continue compression for 25 more minutes.
   e. Set up and apply a FemoStop pressure device

ANSWER a. Circle the swollen area with a pen. This is a good reference to measure further swelling. Check and measure the pedal pulses. Note the observed hematoma size in the chart. It is common and normal to have a small swelling at the puncture site. Continue to observe it for several minutes to see if it enlarges. It is probably not a hematoma because it is soft and small. **See:** Grossman, chapter on "Percutaneous Approach." **Keywords:** Hematoma as big as quarter = normal

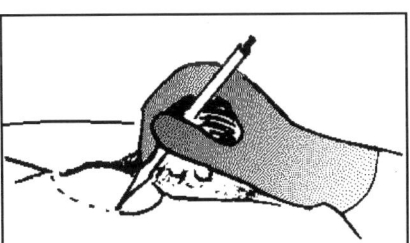
Circle hematoma

312. You have held pressure on a heart cath patient's RFA for 15 minutes. You slowly remove your fingers and see that the bleeding has stopped. You feel a new hard 2 inch wide swelling beneath the puncture site. You should_____ . Circle the swollen area with a pen. Then observe the puncture site for more 2-3 minutes.
   a. Remove your hands
   b. Continue compression for 5 more minutes
   c. Continue compression for 20 more minutes
   d. Administer protamine IV, apply pressure bandage

ANSWER c. Continue compression for 20 more minutes.
   A hematoma "extravasates" into the tissues forming a tense lump of pressurized blood. It may be localized under the puncture site or spread in a circle around where you were applying pressure. Kandarpa recommends 20 more minutes of pressure if a hematoma is discovered following the regular 15-20 minutes of pressure application. As with any suspected hematoma - circle it with a pen to observe its progress.
See: Kandarpa, chapter on "Angiography." **Keywords:** Hematoma

313. On which IV access site is hemostasis most difficult to achieve?
a. Femoral vein
b. Subclavian vein
c. Internal jugular vein
d. External jugular vein

ANSWER b. Subclavian veins must be entered blindly beneath the clavicle. Holding pressure beneath the clavicular bone is almost impossible. Johnsrude says, "On removal of the catheter, secure hemostasis by firm infraclavicular pressure at the site where the catheter enters the vein." Venous extravasation hematoma into the thorax is a possible complication.
See: Johnsrude, chapter on "Catheterization Techniques." **Keywords:** Hardest to control hemostasis → subclavian vein

3B. Hemostasis - Pulling Sheaths

314. At the end of a left heart cath before removing a pigtail catheter and sheath:
a. Double flush the sheath through the side-arm, then pull the pigtail.
b. Insert a guide wire to straighten the pig-tail, then pull it.
c. Administer protamine into the catheter. After flushing it with 10 ml of saline pull the pigtail.
d. Remove the sheath first, observe for hematoma, then remove the pigtail catheter.

ANSWER b. Insert a guide wire to straighten the pig-tail, then pull-it with the wire. Pigtail and Judkins left coronary catheters have such a severe bend that they may rake off plaque when they are pulled. Pigtails can also double over, kink, or knot when pulled back. The wire safely prevents this.

The soft end of the wire needs to be inserted far enough so that it's stiff core straightens the catheter bend. Observe this under fluoro. You can feel the wire meet resistance as the core hits the angled part of the catheter and straightens it. After the pigtail is removed then the sheath may be removed and hemostasis established. Grollman says, "Catheters with sharp curves such as the pigtail and left Judkins coronary catheters should not be withdrawn without first inserting a guidewire even if it is at the conclusion of the study."
See: Grollman, editorial, "Does Use of Vascular Introducer Sheath Obviate need for Catheter Exchanges over a Guidewire?" **Keywords:** Straighten pigtail before pulling

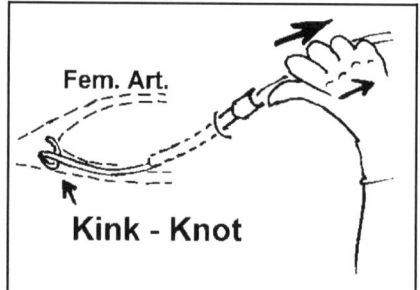

Pulling coiled pigtail cath.

315. Prior to pulling a femoral artery sheath on a patient an aspirated blood sample contained a thrombus. How should the sheath be "pulled" in this patient with a suspected femoral thrombus?
  a. Apply only light pressure to the puncture site when pulling the sheath. Do not cut off the pulse.
  b. Allow a spurt of blood to follow the sheath as it is removed.
  c. Inject 1000-3000 units of heparin into the sheath prior to removing it.
  d. Remove the sheath while someone else slowly draws back blood into a 20 cc syringe through the sheath's sidearm.

ANSWER b. Allow a spurt of blood. Most authors recommend that you "let it bleed" for just a second (2-3 ml) to purge out any clots in the artery. This is especially needed for large catheters which are in for long periods (e.g. IABP catheters). In these large catheters they recommend holding pressure distal below the puncture site as the catheter/sheath is pulled. This prevents the clot from embolizing downstream. Instead it is squirted out the puncture site by the blood pressure.

Johnsrude even recommends "milking" a known femoral clot out by applying digital pressure to the artery distal and proximal. Then work your fingers towards the puncture site hoping to press or milk out the clot.

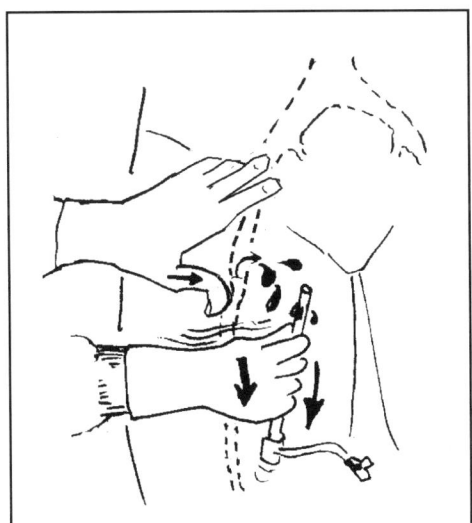
Purging clot

See: Kern, chapter on "Vascular Access" and Johnsrude, chapter on "Catheterization Techniques." **Keywords:** Spurt of blood to purge the site of remaining thrombi

316. In an arterial radial case how long should the wristband be left on to achieve hemostasis?
  a. 15 - 20 minutes of occlusive pressure, released slowly
  b. 10 minutes per sheath size of nonocclusive pressure, released slowly
  c. 30 minutes for diagnostic cases, 60 minutes for interventional procedures
  d. 90 minutes for diagnostic cases, 180 minutes for interventional procedures

ANSWER: d. 90 minutes for diagnostic cases, 180 minutes for interventional procedures. Grossman says, "Radial sheaths are removed immediately after diagnostic arteriography or coronary intervention in the cardiac catheterization laboratory. Since the radial artery is superficial and easily compressible and since transradial procedures are associated with only rare bleeding complications, ACT is not used to guide sheath removal in radial procedures. The compression strap or device is placed directly over the radial artery puncture site and occlusive pressure is applied for approximately 90 minutes for diagnostic procedures and approximately 180 minutes for interventional procedures." **See:** Grossman, chapter on "Percutaneous Approach" **Keywords:** Radial wristband = 90 min

317. After a radial PCI case when should you pull the sheath?
a. At conclusion of the case
b. When ACT falls below 160 sec
c. When ACT falls below 120 sec
d. After protamine administration

ANSWER: a. At conclusion of the case. Grossman says, "Since the radial artery is superficial and easily compressible and since transradial procedures are associated with only rare bleeding complications, ACT is not used to guide sheath removal in radial procedures."
 Kern says about using a band while pulling the sheath, "Position the device snuggly around the wrist before sheath removal; the compression portion of the device should be positioned to cover both the skin nick and arteriotomy site. Gauze can be placed under the device as a wick to collect any blood leakage and then pulled once hemostasis is achieved. The sheath should be removed slowly and smoothly while slowly tightening the device. One common mistake is tightening the device too aggressively before the sheath is removed, leading to patient discomfort. For both patient comfort and adequate hemostasis, the removal of the sheath and the tightening of the device should be done simultaneously. The device should be tight enough to ensure hemostasis but not too tight as to occlude the flow through either the radial or ulnar arteries. This is called patent hemostasis, and it is an essential technique for reducing radial artery occlusion. Once the device is in place and hemostasis is achieved, perform a reverse Barbeau to ensure patent hemostasis. Patent hemostasis of the radial artery will be confirmed by a Barbeau type A, B, or C while the ulnar artery is being compressed. If there is a Barbeau type D, try loosening the device. If the device cannot be loosened any further without blood leakage, send the patient to recovery and try again in 15 minutes. Generally, further loosening can be performed after a short period of time to obtain patent hemostasis. Recovery room nurses should be adept at performing the Barbeau test and maintaining patent hemostasis." **See:** Kern, chapter on "Arterial and Venous Access" **Keywords:** Pulling radial sheath = no ACT needed

318. At the end of a radial PCI case the compression band is placed over the access site and tightened or inflated with 13 ml of air (TR band). The sheath is then pulled while you observe the site for bleeding. The compression band pressure is then adjusted using the reverse Barbeau technique and left in place for 3- 4 hours. After pulling the sheath you should adjust the tightness of the band by slowly releasing band pressure:
a. Until Doppler flow begins in the palmar arch
b. Until the pulse disappears on a thumb plythemograph
c. Until a pulse is seen on an index finger plythemograph
d. Until the hand color pinks up and O2 sat rises above 95%

ANSWER: c. Until a pulse is seen on an index finger plythemograph. You leave the wrist band at that pressure for 3-4 hours which allows patent hemostasis.
 SCAI standards say, "Hemostasis by manual compression for the radial access site is usually obtained with wristband compression devices. Sheaths are removed immediately after the procedure, regardless of anticoagulation status. The "patent hemostasis" [reverse

Barbeau] technique should be used, performed by placing a pulse oximeter on the corresponding index finger [or thumb] and compressing the ulnar artery while lowering the hemostatic wristband compression pressure to the point where the plethysmographic waveform returns without pulsatile bleeding at the radial access site." **See:** SCAI expert consensus statement: "2016 best practices in the cardiac catheterization laboratory"

319. Following radial artery sheath removal with the wrist band fully inflated/compressed "patent hemostasis" or the reverse Barbeau technique requires you to follow 4 steps. Arrange these 4 steps in the correct order for the reverse Barbeau method of patent hemostasis.
  a. Occlude the ulnar artery
  b. Fully inflate/compress the wrist band
  c. Slowly release pressure in the wrist band
  d. Stop deflating when you see a pulse wave on the plethysmograph

ANSWER: b, a, c, d. After full inflation and compressing the ulnar artery, slowly release pressure on the band until plethysmographic arterial waveform returns with no pulsatile bleeding at the radial access site

This is called the reverse Barbeau test, because instead of testing for collateral flow from the ulnar artery, you are testing for flow through the radial artery. Remember, in the initial Allen's or Barbeau test, both arteries are compressed and the ulnar released. In the "reverse Barbeau," both arteries are compressed, and the radial is slowly released. A Doppler probe may also be used to test radial flow in the radial, and the oximetry level should remain over 90% if flow is adequate.

Current guidelines say "The "patent hemostasis" technique should be used, performed by placing a pulse oximeter on the corresponding index finger [or thumb] and compressing the ulnar artery while lowering the hemostatic wristband compression pressure to the point where the plethysmographic waveform returns without pulsatile bleeding at the radial access site."
See: SCAI expert consensus statement: "2016 best practices in the cardiac catheterization laboratory"

320. Following radial access cardiac catheterization, patients who are released to go home on the same-day should:
  a. No same-day discharge, all should remain in the hospital and be monitored overnight
  b. Be taught about the bleeding risks of coughing, Valsalva, and walking
  c. Refrain from load bearing exercises on the accessed limb for 2-4 days
  d. Receive a follow up phone call within 24-48 hours

ANSWER: d. Receive a follow up phone call within 24-48 hours. Kern recommends patients avoid weight-bearing or other activity of the arm for 2-4 hr after sheath removal.

Current guidelines say "All patients, especially those having same-day discharge post-PCI, should be contacted by a CCL team member within 24–48 hr of the procedure to ensure that no complications have occurred, medication adherence is reinforced, and to answer any questions the patient or caregiver may have.... There are no ambulation restrictions with radial access, but patients should avoid weight-bearing or other activity of the arm for 2–4 hr after sheath removal." **See:** SCAI expert consensus statement: "2016 best practices in the cardiac catheterization laboratory"

321. **When you attempt to pull the 6 Fr. radial sheath the patient experiences pain and the sheath cannot be easily withdrawn. Before further attempts to pull the sheath you should:**
a. **Inject 1-2 ml of 1% lidocaine through the sheath**
b. **Inject 2 mg verapamil through the sheath**
c. **Inject 100 mg nitroglycerin IV**
d. **Inject 10 mg fentanyl IV**
e. **Apply cold compress over the sheath**

ANSWER: b. Inject 2 mg verapamil through the sheath (or nifedipine). These Ca channel blockers act to vasodilate the artery. Verapamil 1 mg and 200-400 mg of lidocaine are normally given in the initial cocktail. Warm compresses and 30-50 mcg of fentanyl may be given, not 10 mg.

Kern says, "Some spasm during sheath withdrawal is common. One should tell patients that removal of the sheath will be associated with discomfort. The sheath is taken out fast (but gently); usually the duration of discomfort (if any) is short. Despite all precautions, if radial artery spasm occurs or persists, the operator should consider the next suggestions. One does not allow the patient to experience significant pain. Analgesics and sedation should be administered. If spasm is severe and the sheath is stuck, the following actions can be undertaken:
1. 10 mg p.o.
2. More analgesia and sedation
3. Warm compresses over the forearm to relax the spastic artery
4. Nitroglycerin 200 µg i.a.; repeated if necessary
5. Verapamil 2 mg i.a. (Diltiazem can also be used)
If this does not work, one should wait for an hour and try again. During this time, proper sedation and deep analgesia (morphine) should be maintained. If nothing helps, an axillary block might be required to relax the radial artery. One should never apply excessive force. This might result in rupture or avulsion of the radial artery. Ultimately the vascular surgeon can be consulted to remove the sheath."
See: Kern, chapter on "Arterial and Venous Access"

3C. Hemostasis - Femoral Artery

322. At the conclusion of a diagnostic right femoral arterial (RFA) catheterization the catheter has been removed, the sheath flushed, and the ECG leads removed. You notice the patient has some minor bleeding around the sheath site. The patient needs to be moved to a holding area where you will pull the sheath. How should he be moved to the gurney?
 a. Have the patient remain on his back, crawl over using his unaffected left leg.
 b. Hold the patient's groin at the sheath insertion site while 4 assistants body lift him on a draw sheet.
 c. Apply the mechanical compressor and then have 4 assistants body lift him using a draw sheet
 d. Refuse to move the patient until hemostasis is achieved. Insist on holding pressure on the cath table!

ANSWER b. Hold the patient's groin at the sheath insertion site with a pinching motion while 4 assistants body-lift him on a draw-sheet or transfer-board to the gurney.

Refusing to move the patient is admirable, but it will not endear you to the doctor doing the next case who has to wait to get started.
See: Personal experience

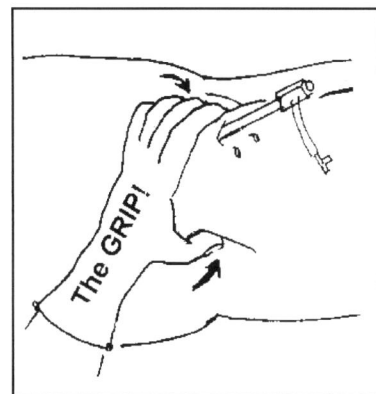

"Pinching" holding method

323. Which of the following instructions are acceptable to give a patient following a femoral artery access procedure? (Select 3 from below.)
 a. Press on the wound if you have to cough
 b. Drink lots of fluids
 c. You may have the bed raised to a slight sit-up position.
 d. You may get up to go to the bathroom
 e. Call the nurse if you need to move your contralateral leg

ANSWERS: a, b, & c. The fourth answer - **You may get up to go to the bathroom** - is NOT correct. Patients are kept in bed with the leg immobilized for 6-8 hours post cath. Patients must call the nurse for a bedpan, and MUST NOT GET UP or the arterial puncture wound may break open.

The person holding pressure and establishing hemostasis usually has the responsibility of teaching the patient how to care for his puncture wound. Instructions should include:
 • **PRESS ON THE WOUND IF YOU HAVE TO COUGH, laugh, or move.**
 • **DRINK LOTS OF FLUIDS:** Patients are instructed to drink lots of fluids, because the contrast is a diuretic and may dehydrate them.

- **YOU MAY HAVE THE BED RAISED TO A SLIGHT SIT-UP POSITION.** But, do not raise your head. This strains the abdominal muscles around the wound.
- **DON'T MOVE OR LIFT YOUR RIGHT LEG.**
- **FEEL GENTLY AROUND THE WOUND OCCASIONALLY FOR WETNESS.** If it starts bleeding you'll be the first to know. Call the nurse immediately.

See: Grossman, chapter on "Percutaneous Approach." **Keywords**: Post cath no bathroom

324. After an uncomplicated diagnostic coronary arteriogram on a patient that received no anticoagulation, how long should you manually compress the femoral artery after pulling a 5 F femoral artery sheath?
   a. 8-10 min
   b. 10-15 min
   c. 15-20 min
   d. 21-30 min

ANSWER a. 8-10 min. These hold times vary from lab to lab, but hold times on patients with no anticoagulation and 4-5 F catheters can be very short. Watson say, "If the patient has not received any anticoagulation and proper technique is followed,...arterial sheaths of 4-5 F, hemostasis may be achieved in under 10 minutes; for 6-8 F, 10-15 minutes of manual compression is generally sufficient..." Note that Kern says holding pressure should be 20-45 min after PCI, depending on sheath size, ACT, and ease of control of bleeding.
See: Watson, chapter on "Hemostasis" **Keywords**: Hold 5 F <10 min

325. When should the femoral artery sheath be removed from a patient with acute coronary syndrome (ACS) who has received LMWH during the heart cath?
   a. As soon as ACT <180 sec
   b. As soon as ACT <120 sec
   c. 8 to 12 hrs after last dose
   d. 2 to 3 hrs after last dose

ANSWER c. 8 to 12 hrs after last dose
   SCAI standards say: "Sheaths can be safely removed 8 to 12 hr after the last dose of acute coronary syndrome therapeutic LMWH.... ACT is generally not useful with LMWH..."
   "For bivalirudin, sheath removal and manual compression can occur at 2 hr post cessation of infusion in patients with normal renal function. In patients with a creatinine clearance <30 mL/min or those on dialysis, ACT should be checked and sheaths removed once the value is <180 sec." **See:** SCAI expert consensus statement: "2016 best practices in the cardiac catheterization laboratory"

Diagnostic Techniques: D5 - Vascular Access, Scrub & Hemostasis   177

326. After successful PCI and satisfactorily pulling a 5 F femoral sheath you should hold manual pressure for _____ post-cath, and then the patient should lie flat in bed for _____.
   a. 5-10 min, 1-2 hours
   b. 10-20 min, 1-2 hours
   c. 5-10 min, 4-6 hours
   d. 10-20 min, 4-6 hours

ANSWER: d. 10-20 min, 4-6 hours. Kern says, "After an appropriate period of compression (15-20 minutes), the patient is returned to his or her room. For sheaths of 5 F to 6 F, recovery usually requires 4 hours or more of bed rest.... With small-diameter catheters (i.e., $\leq$ 5 F), shorter times (< 2 hours) can be used." Grossman says, "Pressure is gradually reduced over the next 10 to 15 minutes....bed rest with the leg straight for 4 to 6 hours." The patient does not have to lie flat the whole time. The head of the bed may be elevated slightly, 30 -45 degrees. **See:** Kern, chapter on "Vascular Access" & Grossman, chapter on "Percutaneous Approach"

327. A patient has just finished having a right and left heart cath from the right leg. Both arterial and venous sheaths remain in the groin. The safest method (of Kern) to establish hemostasis for both vessels is to first remove the _____ sheath and apply pressure to that site for _____, and then remove the other sheath and hold pressure on _____ .
   a. Arterial, For 15 min, The vein for 10 min
   b. Arterial, For 10 min, Both of them for 5 min.
   c. Arterial, For 1 min,   Both of them for 15 min.
   d. Venous,   For 5 min,   The artery for 15 min.
   e. Venous,   For 10 min,   The artery for 10 min.
   f. Venous,   For 15 min,   Both of them for 5 min.

ANSWER a. Kern recommends first controlling each puncture separately. First remove the arterial sheath. Pull and hold it 15 min. Then pull the venous sheath and hold pressure on it for 5-10 min. This keeps venous access longer, should the patient need emergency medications. It also reduces the chance of an A-V fistula and allows one hand to be free to check pedal pulses. This is the safest method but total hold time is long (20-25 min.).

   Grossman mentions a method of holding both simultaneously with different hands. He recommends positioning your left hand over both puncture sites. First pull the arterial sheath then after 5 minutes, if there are no complications, pull the venous sheath and apply gentle pressure with your right hand positioned directly over the venous puncture site. Since venous blood flows in the opposite direction you need to hold pressure below the puncture site. Remember that venous pressure is much less than arterial, so compression pressure is much less. Continue to hold both of them together another 10 minutes. This makes a total hold time of 15 minutes.

   Some experienced techs have developed a method of holding both vessels simultaneously with one hand. **See:** Kern, chapter on "Vascular Access" and Grossman, chapter on "Percutaneous Approach." **Keywords:** Pulling two sheaths arterial hold 15 min., then venous for 10 min.

328. The recommended way to pull the sheath and hold manual pressure while establishing hemostasis on the femoral artery post-cath is to hold pressure _____ the skin puncture site with _____ pressure.
  a. Just above, 2-3 fingers digital
  b. Just above, heel of the hand
  c. Just below, 2-3 fingers digital
  d. Just below, heel of the hand

ANSWER a. Just above the skin puncture site with 2-3 fingers digital pressure., Most authors recommend that pressure be held with the 2-3 left middle fingers, with the index finger just superior to the skin puncture site. The index finger compresses the arterial puncture, while the middle (and ring) fingers compress the artery upstream to occlude the artery. This requires a strong left hand and fingers. Finger pressure is more focused than the heel of the hand and makes it easier to see any bleeding.

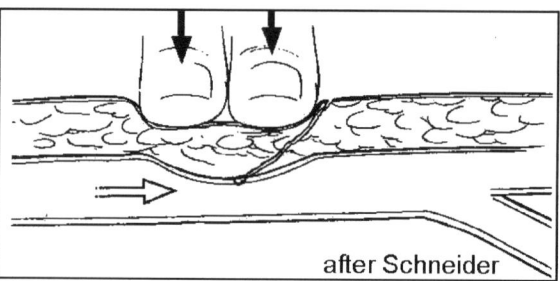
Holding pressure just above puncture site

Notice that the needle track starts at the skin, but travels at an angle superiorly down to the artery. If you push directly on the skin puncture you will not see bleeding. If you press below the skin puncture site, you will not compress the needle track.

Ragosta says, "With the sheath still in place, the arterial pulse is palpated above the sheath insertion site using the middle and index fingers of the left hand. The sheath is slowly removed with compression applied above the site using the left hand....[but not excessive pressure which might strip a clot from the sheath]. Compression should be applied with enough force to prevent bleeding; initially, this usually obliterates the distal pulse. Pressure should be slowly relieved to allow the palpation of the distal pulse [with the right hand on a foot artery] yet still maintain hemostasis. Usually, 10 to 20 minutes of compression is required to achieve hemostasis in an unanticoagulated patient with a 6 to 8 Fr sheath. In patients who received anticoagulation with heparin, an activated coagulation time of less than 180 seconds is required before manual compression is performed."
See: Ragosta, chapter on "Vascular Access and Hemostasis" **Keywords:** Holding finger pressure above puncture site

329. You are holding pressure post femoral PCI on a patient with bounding arterial pressures. Heparin was administered at the start of the case. Now the ACT is 125 sec. You must press very hard with your fingers to stop bleeding at the site; so hard that you can no longer feel the pedal pulse. The leg shows a mottled coloration. You should:
  a. Continue with intense pressure for 5 minutes. It is vital to stop the bleeding.
  b. Temporarily ease up on the pulse every minute, to allow a few seconds of faint pedal pulse
  c. Ease up on your pressure to allow a continuous faint pedal pulse even though there is some femoral bleeding
  d. Administer protamine to reduce the ACT and bleeding

ANSWER: b. Temporarily ease up on the pulse minute, to allow a few seconds of flow with a faint pedal pulse. Mottling of the limb is a sign of ischemia. This is an ideal case to use a vascular closure device if hemostasis cannot be achieved with pressure. ACT has fallen to an acceptable level (Grossman recommends ACT<160 seconds before pulling the arterial sheath). You need to give the leg an occasional "drink" to prevent ischemia and allow normal healing at the puncture site.

Kern says, "Manual compression technique: To remove the sheath, the operator places left-hand fingers over the femoral artery, an inch more cranial (toward the patient's head) than the skin incision. The operator applies gentle pressure and removes the sheath, taking care not to crush the sheath and "strip" clot into the artery. Allow a small spurt of blood to purge the track of retained thrombi. Then apply firm downward pressure for 15 to 20 minutes (5 minutes of full pressure, 5 minutes of 75% pressure, 5 minutes of 50% pressure, and 5 minutes of 25% pressure). Patients receiving antiplatelet treatment may need more compression time.

"During compression, the pedal pulses are checked every 2 to 3 minutes. A diminished pulse is acceptable during brief full-pressure application, but the distal pulses should not be obliterated completely. If the pedal pulse is absent during compression, the pressure over the artery should be decreased periodically to allow distal circulation. Complete artery occlusion prevents clotting factors and platelets from being deposited at the arterial wall puncture site."

"Firm three-finger pressure should control most femoral bleeding. A rolled gauze pack may be placed over the artery to the groin, and pressure applied with the palm of the hand. Standing on a short stool at bedside permits the operator's upper body weight to be used for pressure application. In patients with low cardiac output, mitral stenosis, or cardiomyopathy with a small pulse pressure, the femoral artery can easily be obliterated. In these patients, the distal pulses should be checked more frequently and less pressure should be applied to the groin."

See: Cath Lab Digest, Kern, "Back to Basics: Femoral Artery Access and Hemostasis," Issue 10 - October 2013

330. You are about to establish hemostasis following RFA catheterization. Prior to pulling the sheath you should position your _____
   a. Left index finger just superior to the skin puncture.
   b. Left index finger on the skin puncture site.
   c. Left middle finger just inferior to the skin puncture.
   d. Right index finger just superior to the skin puncture.
   e. Right index finger on the skin puncture site.
   f. Right middle finger just inferior to the skin puncture.

ANSWER a. Left index finger just superior to the skin puncture.

You don't want to be on top of the puncture because bleeding cannot exit the wound, and will contribute to hematoma. You don't want to use your right hand because you'll need that to feel the pedal pulses. With your fingers feel the hard sheath in the artery.

By holding pressure just above the skin puncture you are able to observe the wound for bleeding and hold pressure at the location where the needle enters the artery. Both the needle and the sheath enter the artery is 1-2 cm superior to the skin wound. This is because needle usually enters the artery at 45 degrees. **See:** Kern, chapter on "Vascular Access."

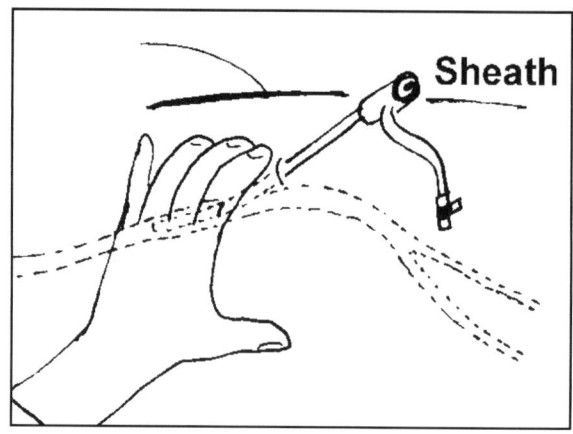
Finger position for Hemostasis

331. After antegrade femoral intervention on the peroneal artery, the sheath is pulled and hemostasis established. To accomplish this the ANTEGRADE puncture site should normally be held with:
   a. 2-3 fingers proximal to the puncture
   b. 2-3 fingers distal to the puncture
   c. Broad heel of the hand directly over the puncture
   d. Both hands, 2 fingers proximal and 2 fingers distal to the puncture

ANSWER **d. Both hands, 2 fingers proximal and 2 fingers distal to the puncture**. Schneider says, "Antegrade femoral artery puncture requires a two-handed technique. One hand is placed proximal to the inguinal ligament to apply pressure over the distal external iliac artery to decrease the head of pressure flowing through the punctured segment and to diminish any oozing into the retroperitoneal space. The goal is not to occlude arterial flow, even temporarily. The other hand places point pressure over the area of arterial puncture just distal to the inguinal ligament. The distal hand can also assess the pulse and ensure that the pressure exerted by the proximal hand is not significant enough to stop flow." **See:** Schneider, chapter on, "Puncture Site Management" **Keywords:** Antegrade puncture, 2 handed pressure holding

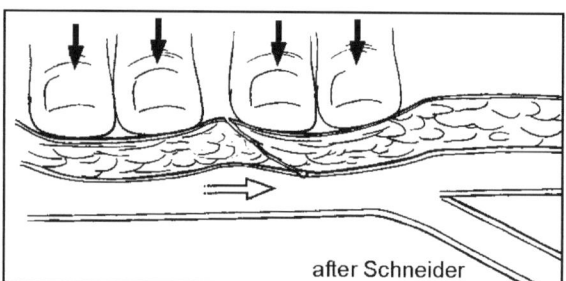
Holding pressure proximal and distal

332. When pulling a 4 F sheath, how much pressure should be exerted on the femoral artery, after initial bleeding has been stopped (according to Grossman)?
   a. As hard as you can push the entire time
   b. As hard as you can push for 5 min, then taper off
   c. Just enough to obliterate the pulse - so no pulse is felt in the foot for 5 min, then taper off
   d. Just enough so a faint pulse is felt in the foot for 5 min, then taper off

ANSWER d. After the initial bleeding has stopped press just hard enough so a faint pulse is felt. Kern recommends that a 20 minute arterial pressure hold be divided into 4 five minute periods - each held with diminishing pressure.
- **0-5 MIN: HOLD** firm steady pressure with the middle 3 fingers of your left hand. Compress the artery firmly but ease up enough so you can just barely feel faint pedal pulses with your right hand. (This takes practice and a strong left hand.)
- **5-10 MIN: HOLD** with 75% force used in the 1st 5 minutes. The pedal pulse should be stronger.
- **10-15 MIN: HOLD** with 50% force.
- **15-20 MIN: HOLD** with 25% force. Full pedal pulses.

Finally slowly lift your index and other fingers. Peek at the wound for bleeding or swelling (hematoma). If any is seen continue holding pressure for 5-10 more minutes - longer if there are bleeding problems or larger sheaths are used.

Sometimes, full compression of the artery is necessary to control bleeding. If the pulse MUST be temporarily cut off completely, allow distal circulation periodically by easing up for a few seconds. Give the ischemic leg a drink of fresh blood every few minutes.

The best pressure is steady. Never remove pressure suddenly or disturb the deep tissues until the initial thrombus plug has developed in the artery. **See:** Kern, chapter on "Vascular Access" **Keywords:** Initial hold pressure = just enough to feel faint pedal pulse

3D. Hemostasis - Radial Artery

333. When you attempt to pull the radial artery sheath it is tight in the vessel and painful to move. Which of the following medications may facilitate sheath removal? (Select 3 from below.)
   a. Inject nitroglycerin IV 20 mcg
   b. Give additional versed IV 10 mg
   c. Give additional fentanyl IV 100 mcg
   d. Inject lidocaine into the sheath 20 mg
   e. Inject verapamil into the sheath 2.5 mg

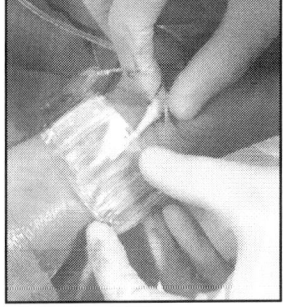

ANSWERS: c, d & e.
Injecting nitroglycerin IV, 20 mcg is not correct. The normal IA dose is 200 mcg. Neither is the versed dose correct - normal is 0.5-1.0 mg.
Almany & O'Neill say, "[Radial artery] Sheath Removal and Hemostasis:
 • Verapamil [IA]- pre-removal it aids in sheath removal by decreasing radial A. spasm.

- Nitroglycerin [IA] - It probably is less successful at arterial vasodilation. Many physicians include 200 mcg of nitro. in their radial cocktail, or administer IV nitro.
- Lidocaine - Given by some operators intra-arterial prior to sheath removal to decrease pain. Given in aliquots up to 20 mg.
- Sedation - Similar to drugs given during femoral line removal. Some operators find fentanyl 50-100 mcg extremely effective" **See:** Almany & O'Neill, online: "Radial Artery Access for Diagnostic and Interventional Procedures."

Dr. Venkatesan says, "The arterial cocktail consists of combination of Nitroglycerin (200 mcg), Xylocaine (50 mg), Verapamil (5 mg) and Heparin(5000 IU). Ideally spasmolytic cocktail should be given before the sheath is introduced immediately after puncture. As the drugs have to contact the arterial wall. If the cocktail is given after introduction of the sheath one of the following may be done: ...Pull back the sheath when injecting the drug or use a side holed sheath."

See: https://drsvenkatesan.com/2009/04/16/is-radial-artery-size-more-impartant-than-allen-test-in-planning-radial-coronary-angiogram/
See: http://www.accumedsystemsinc.com/resources/radial_artery_access_manual.pdf

334. **Certain types of PCI cases favor use of the radial approach over the femoral approach. Which type of patients tend to have fewer bleeding problems & better outcomes with the radial approach as compared to the femoral access approach?**
a. Chronic total occlusion cases
b. Left main disease cases
c. Triple vessel CAD cases
d. Acute STEMI cases

ANSWER: d. Acute STEMI cases.

Current standards say, "The use of radial access for primary PCI in STEMI potentially affords the greatest opportunity to improve outcomes compared to femoral access. Patients presenting with STEMI are frequently placed on aggressive anticoagulant and anti-platelet therapies that increase their risk of vascular access site complications. The prespecified STEMI subgroup from the randomized RIVAL (Radial V. femoral for coronary intervention) study showed an association between radial access and reduced mortality compared with femoral access." **See:** Best Practices for Transradial Angiography and Intervention: A Consensus Statement From the Society for Cardiovascular Angiography and Intervention's Transradial Working Group, by Rao, et al., Core Curriculum, Catheterization and Cardiovascular Interventions (2013)

Topol says, "Because of its extremely low vascular-site complication rates, the transradial approach to PCI is clearly the method of choice in the setting of PCI with highly active anti-thrombotic regimens [such as STEMI] and early or rescue PCI after thrombolysis." **See:** Topol, chapter on "Transradial PCI for major reduction in bleeding complications."

335. After a PCI you have pulled your patient's radial artery sheath and tightened/inflated the wrist band gradually to the point where pulsatile bleeding at the access site just stops. The index finger shows a pulsatile arterial plethysmographic waveform with normal O2 sat. But, when you occlude the ulnar artery the pulsatile waveform disappears and O2 sat

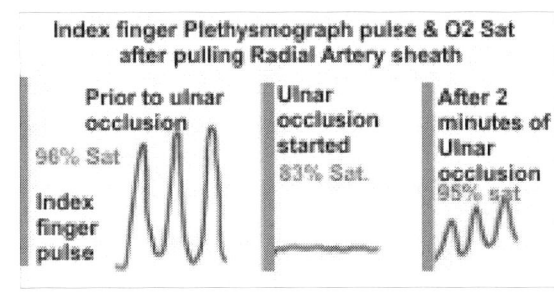

drops. When both pulse and O2 sat. return slowly (by 2 minutes) as shown. This is _____ .
a. Barbeau class A, indicating normal radial flow
b. Barbeau class B, a partially occluded radial artery
c. Barbeau class C, patent radial hemostasis
d. Barbeau class D, an occluded radial artery

ANSWER: c. Barbeau class C, patent radial hemostasis. Type C Barbeau pattern is shown, where both plethysmograph & oximetry indicate radial artery patency. The artery is considered occluded only when there is NO pulsatile radial flow by 2 minutes and NO return of normal O2 saturation.

Mukherjee says, "The Barbeau classification: Four patters of the Allen test, as detected by plethysmography with temporary occlusion of the radial artery."
A: Normal "positive Allen test, showing no significant diminution of the waveform immediately after radial occlusion.
B: The initial postocclusion waveform is present but diminished, and returns to a full excursion within two minutes.
C: Phasic waveform is seen within two minutes
D. There is no flow detected by plethysmography in class D even after two minutes of arterial occlusion.

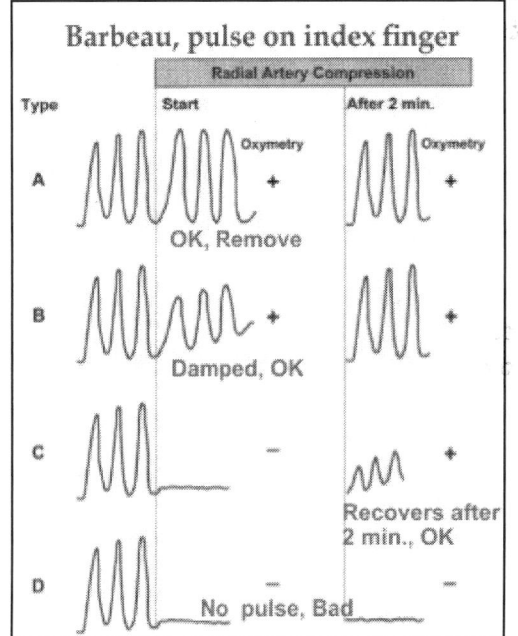

"Oximetry is expected to demonstrate saturation of 90% or greater with a waveform present. Note that patients with a type C response, presumably after recruitment of collaterals, will frequently exhibit a type B response if the test is repeated early." **See:** Mukherjee, et al., Cardiovascular Catheterization and Intervention, chapter on "Vascular Access and Closure", 2010

336. After pulling the radial artery sheath the pressure band should be applied tightly enough so that no pulsatile bleeding occurs at the site but continuous radial blood flow remains. This is termed:
a. Barbeau optimal occlusion
b. Partial radial occlusion
c. Patent hemostasis
d. Hemostatic flow

ANSWER: c. Patent hemostasis is best done with the reverse Barbeau technique. This is analogous to holding pressure by hand on the CFA. It should be applied just hard enough to stop bleeding yet allow pulsatile flow down the artery. This prevents blood stagnation which might lead to arterial occlusion or distal tissue damage. Thus, the artery should be "patent" (open) but not bleed (hemostasis).

Patel says, "At the end of the procedure, the catheter is removed. A hemostasis band is placed on the wrist with the sheath still in place. Our preference is the TR Band (Terumo Interventional Systems). The balloon is inflated with 15 cc of air after being secured firmly over the access point and sheath. The sheath is then removed. The balloon is then deflated slowly 1 cc at a time until there is bleeding at the access site, then 1 cc of air is replaced into the balloon. This is done to obtain "patent hemostasis" and decrease the risk of radial artery occlusion. Occluding the ulnar artery and confirming there is still a waveform present can also confirm patent hemostasis."
See: Patel, Radial Artery Access: The Basics, Vascular Disease Management, 2017

337. When applying a hemostasis band during radial artery hemostasis, you should apply enough pressure to stop bleeding and:
a. Occlude the radial artery
b. Occlude flow through the palmar arch
c. Assure flow through the radial artery
d. Assure flow through the palmar arch

ANSWER c. Assure flow through the radial artery (and the ulnar artery). After applying the hemostasis band you can assure radial flow by briefly occluding the ulnar artery manually and observing the pulse oximeter and plethysmograph. Remember there is a palmar arch in the hand connecting radial and ulnar flow. If both are occluded there will be no arterial flow to the hand - bad. So, occluding the ulnar and getting a pulse proves good radial flow. This is termed a reverse Barbeau test.

Company literature says, "Warning: Do not apply occlusive pressure using the D-stat Radial. Arterial damage and thrombosis may result. Check pulses frequently to maintain arterial flow, and loosen the retention strap as necessary." **See:** D-Stat Radial hemostatic band instructions for use at:
http://vasc.com/wp-content/uploads/2013/07/D-Stat-Radial-Topical-Hemostat-IFU-US-42-0447-01-rU.pdf

One study showed superiority of the Terumo TR Band™ Hemostasis Device over occlusive bands on long term radial artery occlusion. PTCA.org says, "A new study, conducted by Dr. Samir B. Pancholy of Mercy Hospital in Scranton, Pennsylvania, shows that the concept of "guided compression" in transradial procedures can reduce radial artery occlusion by 56%, especially when facilitated by the use of the TR Band™ Hemostasis

Device." See: http://www.ptca.org/news/2008/1111_RADIAL.html

338. In passing the Judkins catheter from the radial artery the operator finds it difficult to pass around the carotid and innominate arteries and into the arch. You should recommend to the physician operator: (Select 2 answers.)
   a. Move the patient's arm toward the head
   b. Have patient take a deep breath
   c. Have patient cough repeatedly
   d. Change to an Amplatz catheter
   e. Change to a movable core guide wire

ANSWERS: a & b. Move the patient's arm toward the head & have the patient take a deep breath. Kern says, "For all catheter advancement from the arm approach, there may be a sharp caudal turn near the origin of the carotid artery. To facilitate passage in to the central aorta, the patient should be instructed to inspire deeply while the operator advances the guidewire and catheter. The operator also may pull the patient's arm straight and extend it toward the head at a 90-degree angle with the chest wall and repeat the maneuver." See: Topol, chapter on "Arterial and Venous Access, Equipment Used"

339. For a bilateral heart cath the operator used a single wall needle and easily obtained arterial and venous access. However, after vascular access your patient had a severe vasovagal reaction, converted with IV atropine. After the case you are instructed to pull both sheaths. Which sheath would you pull first?
   a. Venous sheath first and hold pressure on that site for 5 min.
   b. Venous sheath first and hold pressure on that site for 15 min.
   c. Arterial sheath first and hold pressure on that site for 15 min.
   d. Arterial sheath first and hold pressure on that site for 30 min.

ANSWER: c. Arterial sheath and hold pressure on that site for 15 min. Grossman also agrees saying, pull the arterial sheath first and hold, then pull the venous and hold 5 min. See: Grossman, chapter on "Percutaneous Approach"
   Kern agrees saying, "Preservation of venous access for the first 15 minutes of arterial compression may provide a useful means of treating a vagal reaction...." But, he recommends the opposite, pulling the venous sheath first if there is a chance of an AV fistula. This could occur in a double wall stick, where the arterial needle punctures both artery and vein. See: Kern, chapter on "Arterial and Venous Access"

3E. Hemostasis - Vascular Closure Devices

340. Identify the arterial hemostatic closure device labeled #1 in the diagram.
a. Starclose (Abbott Corp.)
b. AngioSeal (St. Jude Medical)
c. Perclose (Abbott Corp.)
d. Duett (Vascular Solutions)

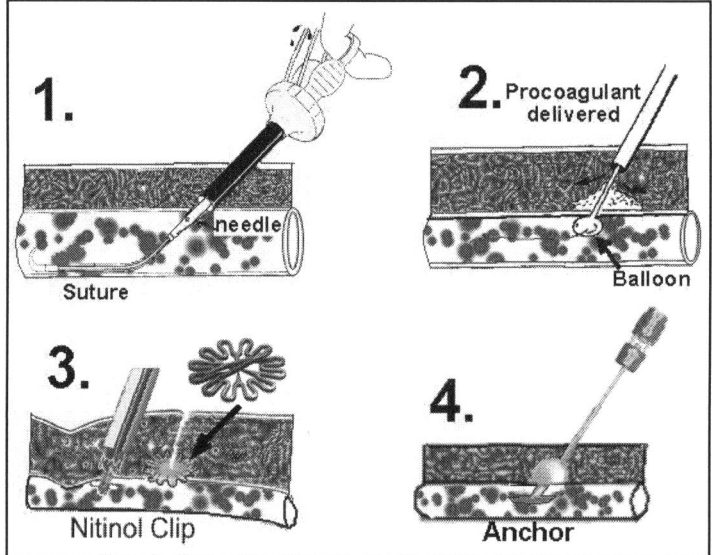

Four types of percutaneous closure devices

ANSWER c. Perclose (Abbott Corp.) All of these devices provide more positive closure of the arterial puncture site after catheterization.
1. Perclose (Abbott Corp.) sutures and ties the arteriotomy.
2. Duett (Vascular Solutions). A compliant balloon-on-a-wire is first inflated within the artery, pulled into contact with the end of the sheath, and pulled back against the inside of the puncture site to tamponade bleeding. The sheath is then withdrawn roughly 1 cm and you inject thrombin and collagen into the soft-tissue tract.
3. Starclose nitinol clip device (Abbott). Four small flexible wings expand and locate the vessel wall. When released nitinol tines on the clip grasp the edges of the arteriotomy and draw them together, much like a purse-string suture. The arterial wall "puckers up" and pulls together in the center of the star, closing the arterial puncture site on the vessel.
4. AngioSeal (St. Jude Medical) positions a rectangular absorbable "anchor" against the inside wall of the artery and uses an attached suture to winch down a small collagen plug down against the outside of the artery. **See:** Grossman, chapter on "Percutaneous Approach" **Keywords:** 4 hemostatic closure devices
See: http://www.invasivecardiology.com/articles/clinical-experience-circumferential-clip-based-vascular-closure-device-diagnostic

341. Match the hemostatic closure device #2 (extravascular collagen) to its description and company.
a. FemoStop (Radi)
b. EVS-Angiolink (Medtronic)
c. Angio-Seal (St. Jude)
d. Perclose (Abbott)

ARTERIAL ENTRY SITE
1. Suture mediated
*2. Extravascular collagen
3. Staple mediated
4. Passive pressure

ANSWER c. Angio-Seal (St. Jude) uses the anchor on the inside arterial wall to winch a collagen plug outside the arterial wall .
  a. **FemoStop (Radi)** .   .   4. Passive pressure
  b. **EVS-Angiolink (Medtronic)**.   3. Staple mediated
  c. **Angio-Seal (St. Jude)** .   2. Extravascular collagen
  d. **Perclose (Abbott)**   ..   1. Suture mediated
See: Ragosta, chapter on "Vascular Access and Hemostasis" **Keywords:** ID closure devices

342. **The Perclose hemostatic closure device uses:**
  a. **Absorbable suture**
  b. **Nonabsorbable suture**
  c. **Four suture needles**
  d. **One suture needle**

ANSWER b. Nonabsorbable suture is permanent because the suture is a nonabsorbable monofilament or polyester. It uses 2 needles attached to this suture material. These 2 needles are pulled from inside the vessel, back around the device foot, into a sheath, and out of the body. The needles drag a suture with them that takes a stitch in the arterial wall. You then use a knot pusher to tie a knot in the suture and push it down to the arteriotomy closing it permanently. Watson terms perclose "the gold standard" closure device. **See:** Watson, chapter on "Hemostasis and Vascular Closure Devices" **Keyword:** Perclose permanent

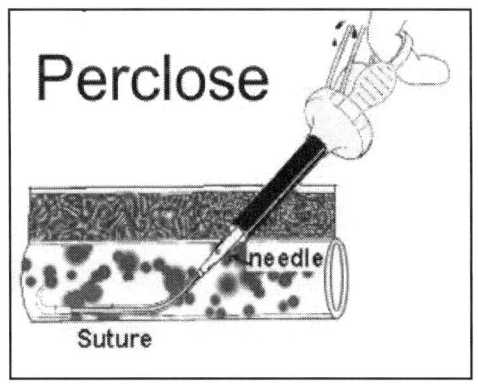
Hemostatic closure device

343. **The Syvek NT and Chito-Seal are:**
  a. **Collagen based closure devices**
  b. **Balloon based closure devices**
  c. **Mechanical compression devices**
  d. **Topical hemostasis accelerators**

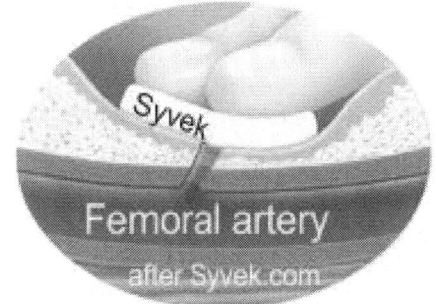

ANSWER d. Topical hemostasis accelerators that are completely external and applied with digital pressure during manual compression. They leave no foreign material behind. The Syvek NT Patch is composed of a bio-polymer isolated from marine algae. Instead of applying pressure above the needle stick, apply the patch on the stick.
    The Chito-seal is a wound dressing with an active clotting ingredient made from marine chitin molecules.
See: Watson, chapter on "Hemostasis and Vascular Closure Devices" **Keywords:** Syvek

344. After pulling a sheath you apply a procoagulant infiltrated pad or a gelatin sponge to the puncture site under hand-held pressure. It uses a:
a. Manual compression pad
b. Topical hemostasis pad
c. Vascular closure device
d. Passive vascular closure device

ANSWER: b. Topical hemostasis pad. Topical agents that stop bleeding may include chitosan, polysaccharides, glucosamine, or thrombin. They reduce the time of hemostasis and ambulation. See: Use of the SafeSeal Hemostasis Patch Following Coronary Intervention, by Rocco & Narins, CLD, Nov 2008

345. The thrombogenic materials in Chito-seal and the Syvek Patch are made from:
a. Thrombin
b. Marine algae
c. Crustacean shells
d. Polysaccharide (MPH)

ANSWER: c. Crustacean shells. Chito-Seal & Clo-Sur P.A.D. are made from chitin, a natural hemostatic agent extracted from crustacean shells. Its positively charged ions helps attract and bind red blood cells. The Syvek Patch comes from marine algae. SafeSeal and Stasys are made from polysaccharide (MPH).

346. From these arteriograms on 4 patients, why is Patient #1 NOT a good candidate for a femoral artery vascular closure device (VCD)?
a. Peripheral artery disease
b. Puncture above inguinal ligament
c. Puncture into PFA or SFA
d. Aortic bypass graft with small arteries

ANSWER a. Peripheral artery disease. Note the irregular outline of the RFA indicating severe PVD.
MATCH ALL CORRECT ANSWERS BELOW.

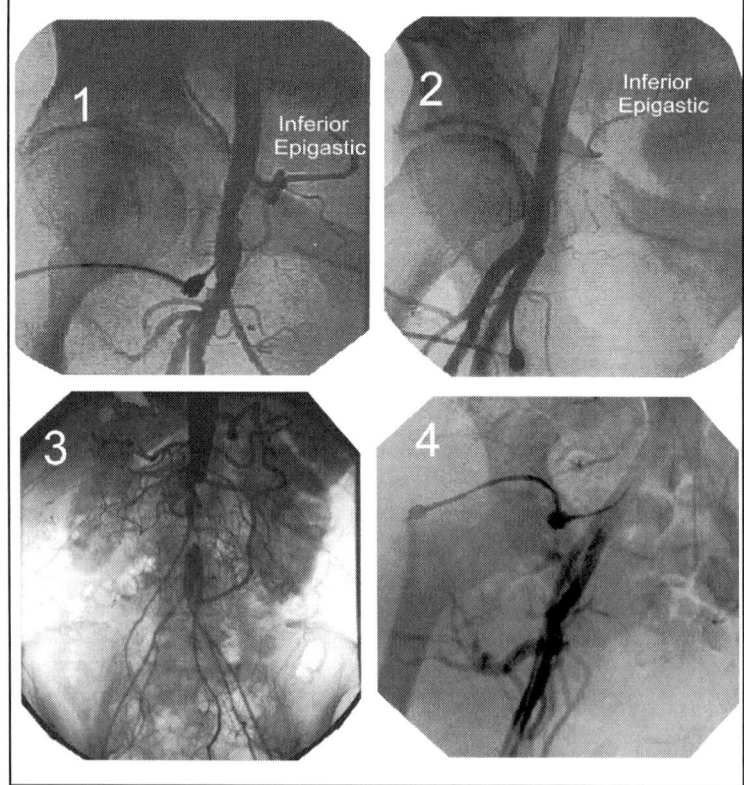

Femoral angiograms on 4 poor candidates for VCD

1. Peripheral artery disease - severe peripheral vascular disease (PVD)
2. Puncture into profunda or superficial femoral artery- TOO LOW
3. Aortic bypass graft - small leg arteries. Descending AO occlusion. Go radial.
4. Puncture above inguinal ligament and inferior epigastric artery - TOO HIGH.

Dauerman says, "Should all patients get a VCD? No—those with severe femoral arterial disease and sheath insertion above the inferior epigastric artery may have a higher risk with VCD than manual compression. Should most patients undergoing femoral arterial access get a VCD? For diagnostic cases, the answer may be "yes" based upon both decreased complication rates and improved time to ambulation. For PCI patients, contemporary data support a neutral effect [jury still out] on complications in the setting of ongoing concerns regarding device costs." Safety of VCD has not been established in: Patients on warfarin, inflammatory disease, morbid obesity, thrombolysis, access via vascular graft, significant PVD, uncontrolled hypertension, ipsilateral venous sheath, femoral artery calcium, small femoral artery size, if the puncture is through the posterior wall or if there are multiple punctures.

See: http://www.onlinejacc.org/content/50/17/1617.full Dauerman, J Am Coll Cardiol, 2007; 50:1617-1626, doi:10.1016/j.jacc.2007.07.028 **Keywords:** Poor candidates for closure devices severe PVD, Ca, high or low punctures, etc.

3F. Hemostasis - Bandaging and Patient Teaching

347. What type of dressing is recommended over the femoral artery puncture site after 15-20 minutes of manual pressure on an obese hypertensive female patient?
a. Band-aid
b. 3 inch "Elastoplast" stretch pressure dressing
c. Encircling inflatable pressure bandage
d. "Compressar" mechanical clamp

ANSWER a. Band-aid or similar small dressing. Kern says "In obese, hypertensive, or elderly female patients and patients with aortic insufficiency it may be difficult to obtain hemostasis. In some patients (e.g. those who are obese or who have large thighs), more than 500 ml of blood can be lost before the patient or nurse identifies the problem. For this same reason a large opaque occlusive dressing over the puncture site is **NOT** recommended." Large opaque dressings cover the wound making frequent site inspection difficult. You need to observe any swelling and bleeding immediately and "jump on it."

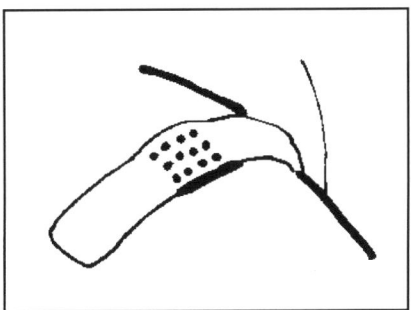
Band-aid dressing

Research suggests results are similar between the two bandaging methods. For this reason, many hospitals have stopped using expensive and cumbersome arterial pressure dressings. They just cover up the problem.

See: Kern, chapter on "Vascular Access" **Keywords:** Hematoma prone patients use band-aid dressing

348. In teaching a patient to care for his femoral artery puncture site following angiography, which instruction below is correct?
   a. "Never press on the wound for any reason - even if you have to cough. They break open easily."
   b. "Never touch the bandage. These arterial puncture sites break open easily."
   c. "Don't sit up by yourself. But the nurse may elevate your bed to a slight sit up position."
   d. "Occasionally raise your head to look down at your groin to see if it's bleeding. If it is call the nurse."

ANSWER c. "Don't sit up by yourself. But the nurse may elevate your bed to a slight sit up position."

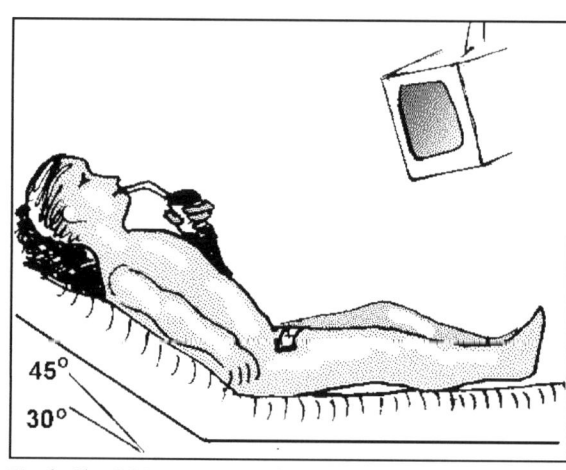

Bed tilt OK - post cath

   A. **NO: It is GOOD** to teach the patient to gently press on the wound if they have to cough, move around, or laugh. This applies pressure to prevent vessel rupture at the puncture site.
   B. **NO: It is GOOD** to teach the patient to feel gently around the wound for wetness (bleeding). Then, if it feels wet - press on it and call the nurse.
   C. **YES:** Grossman says "Although the patient should be instructed to not move the leg for several hours following the catheterization procedure, this does not mean that the patient must lie flat during this time. Elevation of the head and chest to 30-45 degrees by the electrical or manual bed control, without muscular effort by the patient, greatly increase the patient's comfort and will not increase the risk of local bleeding." New flexible sheaths are available that bend up to 60 degrees without kinking. This may allow patients to safely sit up more comfortably in bed.
   D. **NO: It is BAD** for a patient to raise his head for any reason. This pulls the abdominal muscles and may break open the puncture site.
      Other important instructions include:
      • Stay in bed.
      • Keep the affected leg straight.
      • Call a nurse if there is bleeding or chest pain.
      • Drink plenty of fluids.

See: Grossman, chapter on "Percutaneous Approach." **Keywords:** Post-cath instructions - to raise bed 45 degrees is OK.

Diagnostic Techniques: D5 - Vascular Access, Scrub & Hemostasis 191

349. What post cath instructions should be given to a patient following a radial PCI?
   a. Bed rest for 4-6 hours with pressure bandage in place
   b. Bed rest for 1-2 hours with finger and arm exercises encouraged
   c. Immediate walking OK, but avoid arm weight bearing for 2-4 hours
   d. Immediate walking and arm exercises are encouraged, early discharge

ANSWER: c. Immediate walking OK, but avoid arm weight bearing for 2-4 hours.
   SCAI standards say: "There are no ambulation restrictions with radial access, but patients should avoid weight-bearing or other activity of the arm for 2-4 hrs after sheath removal." **See:** SCAI expert consensus statement: "2016 best practices in the cardiac catheterization laboratory"
   Kern says "If late bleeding occurs (this is rare), give the patient instructions on using the fingers to compress the puncture site. In addition, instruct the patient to limit lifting any item more than 10 pounds for the next 3 days."

350. When applying a TR band the green marker should be placed:
   a. Just above brachial puncture site
   b. Distal to skin puncture site
   c. Directly over the skin puncture site
   d. Proximal to skin puncture site

ANSWER: d. Proximal to skin puncture site. Position the TR band marker on the center of balloon, at the site of the arterial entry (usually 1/4 inch above (proximal to) skin entry site, depending on depth of artery). Ensure the Terumo logo is closest to the patient's little finger. The velcro is applied tightly. The inflatable bladder is then inflated with 15 ml of air. The sheath is then pulled out of the artery. If hemostasis is not achieved, the band is inflated with a larger volume of air.
See: http://www.terumois.com/products/closure/tr-band.html

3G. Hemostasis - Post Cath Patient Care

351. After transfemoral coronary angiography patients are instructed to:
   a. Ambulate early
   b. Drink 1-2 quarts of fluid
   c. Eat only nonfat high-fiber foods
   d. Eat only a light no-salt diet

ANSWER b. Drink 1-2 quarts of fluid. Contrast begins to be washed out of the blood stream by the kidneys immediately. It has a strong diuretic effect, making the patient need to urinate.
   This half gallon of fluid is to compensate for the diuretic effect of the dye, as well as wash it out of the vascular system. It promotes excretion of dye by the kidneys and thus dilutes the toxic effects of dye on the heart and other organs.
   After transfemoral arterial catheterization, patients should be at bed rest with their leg

straight for several hours. They should not be encouraged to ambulate early, for fear of breaking open the puncture site.
See: Grossman, chapter on "Percutaneous Approach." **Keywords:** Post cath → drink 1-2 quarts fluid

352. **A large volume of IV fluids may be given to patients post angiography because it:**
   a. Promotes excretion of dye by the kidneys
   b. Promotes metabolic breakdown of dye by liver
   c. Hydrates the tissues to reduce chance of pulmonary edema
   d. Increases blood volume and cardiac output

ANSWER a. Promotes excretion of dye by the kidneys. Patients who cannot drink the half gallon of water suggested post-cath need to be hydrated by IV. The increase in vascular fluid is to compensate for the diuretic effect of the dye, as well as wash it out of the vascular system.
   However, this may be harmful to patients with a history of heart failure. They generally have too much fluid already. Excess fluid may tip them over into pulmonary edema.
See: Grossman, chapter on "Percutaneous Approach." **Keywords:** Post cath → hydrate with IV fluid to promote dye excretion

353. **Within 30 minutes after returning a heart catheterization patient to the ward, the patient's right leg becomes pulseless, cool, pale, and painful. The floor nurse's first action should be to:**
   a. Elevate the extremity
   b. Cool the extremity with ice packs
   c. Wait 5-10 minutes to see if spasm resolves
   d. Call the catheterizing physician
   e. Call a vascular surgeon

ANSWER d. Call the catheterizing physician. These signs and symptoms indicate that femoral artery occlusion is likely. The catheterizing physician should be notified immediately. Initial therapy is to anticoagulate the patient to prevent further embolization and clot extension with a heparin infusion. Definitive treatment is surgical removal of the clot, usually with Fogarty catheters. Other emergency therapy includes: Pain control with narcotics and keeping the patient very warm to relieve arterial spasm.
See: Hurst and Logue, chapter on "Vascular Disease." and **See:** Underhill chapter on "Vascular Diseases." **Keyword:** Rx for arterial occlusion = heparin

REFERENCES

Baim, D. S and Grossman W.., Cardiac Catheterization, Angiography, and Intervention, 7th Ed., Lea and Febiger, 2006
Burton, R.W., Microbiology for the Health Sciences, J.B. Lippincott Co., 1988
Cummins, R. O., Ed., *Textbook of ADVANCED CARDIAC LIFE SUPPORT*, American Heart Association, 1994

Daily, E. K., and Schroeder, J. S., *Techniques in Bedside Hemodynamic Monitoring*, 4th Ed., C. V. Mosby Company, 1989

Grollman, "Does Use of Vascular Introducer Sheath Obviate need for Catheter Exchanges over a Guidewire?" editorial in <u>Catheterization and CV Diagnosis</u> 23:1-2

Gruendemann and Meeker, Alexander's Care of the Patient in Surgery, CV Mosby Co., 1987

Hurst, J. W., and Logue, R. B., et. al., *THE HEART Arteries and Veins*, 3rd Ed., McGraw-Hill Book Co., 1974

Johnsrude, I. S., Jackson. D. C., Et. al., *A Practical Approach to Angiography*, 2nd Ed., Little, Brown and Co., 1987

Kandarpa, K., *Handbook of Cardiovascular and Interventional Radiologic Procedures*, 1st Ed., Little Brown and Co., 1989

Kern, M. J., Ed., The Cardiac Catheterization Handbook, 4th Ed., Mosby-Year Book, Inc., 2003

Ragosta, Michael, Cardiac Catheterization, Saunders, 1st Edition, 2008

Schneider, Endovascular Sills, Guidewire and Catheter Skills for Endovascular Surgery, 2nd Edition, Marcel Dekker, Inc., 2003

Snopek, A. M., *Fundamentals of Special Radiographic Procedures*, W. B. Saunders, 1992

Tilkian, A. G., and Daily, E. J., *Cardiovascular Procedures, Diagnostic Techniques and Therapeutic Procedures*, C. V. Mosby Company, 1986

Torres, Basic Medical Techniques and Patient Care for Radiologic Technologists, J.B.. Lippincott Co., 1989

Underhill, S. L., Ed., *CARDIAC NURSING*, 2nd Ed., J. B. Lippincott Co., 1989

OUTLINE: Vascular Access & Hemostasis

5. GENERAL
   a. Lifelines
      i. ECG
      ii. IV
   b. Antegrade = cathing with flow
   c. Retrograde = cathing against flow
   d. Transthoracic - Transseptal - Translumbar
   e. Coronary approaches
      i. Seldinger (Femoral puncture)
      ii. Sheath (Femoral puncture)
      iii. Sones (Brachial cutdown)
      iv. Sheath (Brachial Puncture)
   f. Right Heart Cath approaches
      i. Cutdown
      ii. Percutaneous Sheath
   g. Use of Rt. Ht. Catheters
      i. Flush continuously (const. flow device & constant IV gravity drip
      ii. Double flush catheter
      iii. Flush manually & gently every few minutes
      iv. Never flush against resistance (clot?)
      v. Remove air bubbles (especially if suspected shunt)
      vi. Change sterile dressings daily
      vii. Change catheters and tubes every 2-3 days
   h. Left Heart Cath approaches
      i. Seldinger
      ii. Sheath
      iii. Cutdown
   i. Rationale for arterial catheterization
      i. Pressure measurement/monitoring
      ii. Blood Gases
      iii. Arteriography
      iv. Ventriculography
      v. Cardiac Outputs (Fick)
      vi. IABP
   j. Lidocaine administration.
      i. 25 gage subcutaneous wheal
      ii. deep injections, aspirating 1st
      iii. Withdraw, readvance, and inject many times
      iv. Locating vessel with lidocaine needle
      v. Marking the location
      vi. Allergic reactions to Local Anesthetics.
      vii. Lidocaine 1%
      viii. Other (-caines)
      ix. Avoiding allergic reactions
      x. Signs/symptoms
      xi. Treatment
6. SELDINGER
   a. LHC by the percutaneous method.

- i. Selection of equipment
- ii. J, movable, Benson
- iii. Arterial puncture
    - (1) Locating artery
    - (2) 11 blade stab
    - (3) single / double wall needle
    - (4) Identify needle bounce
    - (5) Depress needle on withdrawal
    - (6) Difficulty puncturing
- iv. guide wire use and care
    - (1) floppy end only
    - (2) soften in needle/cath
    - (3) never force
    - (4) hold wire when wiping
    - (5) keep hold of guide during cath insertion
    - (6) wipe bloody wires
    - (7) store in heparinized saline
- v. catheter use and care
    - (1) drawback and flush every 3 minutes
    - (2) flush pig vigorously
    - (3) never inject all solution in (air)
    - (4) oozing around catheter (larger size)
- vi. Steps in Seldinger technique
    - (1) Needle insertion into a vessel
    - (2) Insertion of a wire through the needle
    - (3) Removal of the needle over the wire
    - (4) Insertion of the catheter over the wire
    - (5) Remove wire, leaving catheter
- vii. Sheath insertion techniques
    - (1) Needle insertion into a vessel
    - (2) Insertion of a wire through the needle
    - (3) Removal of the needle over the wire
    - (4) Insertion of the sheath and dilator over the wire
    - (5) Remove wire and dilator, leaving sheath
    - (6) Insert catheter preloaded with wire
- viii. Rt. Ht. Cath. by percutaneous method
    - (1) flush sidearm with saline
    - (2) may monitor pressure from sidearm
    - (3) Needle, sheath and Catheter selection
    - (4) prophylactic pacer, BBB
    - (5) flush (Heparinized?)
    - (6) continuous flow device
    - (7) PACs., PVCs
    - (8) Venous spasm
    - (9) passing obstructions, Tricuspid, PA,
    - (10) possibility of perforation
    - (11) wedge maneuvers
    - (12) adequacy of wedge
    - (13) use of guide wires with swan (.025")
    - (14) pressures
    - (15) blood samples
    - (16) Cardiac Outputs
        - (a) Thermodilution
        - (b) Fick
    - (17) suture down catheter
    - (18) antibiotic ointment
    - (19) dressing, suturing
    - (20) If patient to remain on ward, setup continuous flow device and pressure bag
    - (21) guide wire use and care
        - (a) floppy end only
        - (b) soften in needle/cath
        - (c) never force
        - (d) hold wire when wiping
        - (e) keep hold of guide during cath insertion
        - (f) wipe bloody wires
        - (g) store in heparinized saline
    - (22) catheter use and care
        - (a) drawback and flush every 3 minutes
        - (b) flush pig vigorously
        - (c) never inject all solution in (air)
    - (23) oozing around catheter (larger size)

7. CUTDOWN
   a. anatomic landmarks
      - i. Antecubital vein
      - ii. nerves & veins
   b. LHC by cutdown (Sones):
      - i. Heparinization/ flush
      - ii. Catheter selection
      - iii. inability to enter LA
      - iv. arterial spasm
      - v. Catheter selection
      - vi. use of guide wires
      - vii. arteriotomy
          - (1) Skin lateral incision (15 blade)
          - (2) Longitudinal tissue incisions
          - (3) blunt dissection
      - viii. Elastic tags/ties around artery
          - (1) Release prox./tighten distal on - NOW!
      - ix. closing / suturing
      - x. Embolectomy
      - xi. Flushing wound with Povidone Iodine
      - xii. pulse check
      - xiii. post cath orders
   c. RHC by cutdown
      - i. #15 blade incision
      - ii. blunt dissection
      - iii. ligature
      - iv. tying off vein

8. ARTERIAL SITES
   a. arterial puncture sites
      - i. Femoral Art.
      - ii. Axillary
      - iii. Brachial
      - iv. Radial

9. VENOUS SITES

a. Femoral vein
   b. Subclavian v.
   c. Internal Jugular
   d. External Jugular
   e. Antecubital vein (Arm)
10. CATHETER HANDLING TECHNIQUES
   a. Flushing and care of catheter before
   b. Control of both ends in one hand
   c. Catheter insertion - Seldinger
   d. Torquing and manipulating
   e. flushing an angiographic catheter
      i. vertical (tip down), draw back first
   f. Catheter exchange
   g. Pulling catheter
11. GUIDEWIRE HANDLING TECHNIQUES
   a. Never use a kinked or defective guide wire.
   b. Use "J" wires in tortuous vessels
   c. Insert floppy end only
   d. NEVER force guide wires.
   e. Stop, withdraw, inspect and report when resistance is felt
   f. Precautions during deep cannulation of selective vessels
   g. Minimize manipulation time (< 3 min prevents clots)
   h. Control movable core wires from body of wire.
   i. Do not control from the movable handle. THEY PULL OUT!
   j. Pin at skin, when removing cath over wire
   k. DON'T ACCIDENTALLY PULL WIRE OUT!!!
   l. Never let Dr. advance catheter and wire into patient without assistant controlling stiff end of wire. DON'T Loose wire in patient!
   m. Soften tip of movable-core guides before it enters vessel. STIFF, STRAIGHT TIPS CAN PUNCTURE.
   n. Never exchange larger for smaller catheters (BLEEDING AROUND DILATED PUNCTURE SITE)
12. SHEATH HANDLING AND INSERTION TECHNIQUES.
   a. Flushing and turning off stopcock
   b. Sizing to catheter
   c. Introduction: sliding down, rotation in
   d. Removal of dilator & wire
   e. Preloading catheter
   f. Catheter insertion
   g. Sheath removal
13. CATHETER EXCHANGE
   a. "Over the wire" (leave wire in the vessel)
   b. "with the wire" (remove both wire and catheter together)
   c. "Without the wire" (no wire used)
   d. "Monorail" (alongside the wire)
14. HEMATOMA
   a. Difficult patients to hold pressure
      i. Obese patients or those with large thighs
      ii. Hypertensive patients or those with bounding aortic regurgitation
      iii. Elderly patients especially women
      iv. Patients who have undergone prior puncture
      v. Patients who suffer from coagulopathy or are on anticoagulants
      vi. Patients with peripheral atherosclerosis (Calcified arteries)
   b. Types of Hematoma
      i. Hematoma
      ii. retroperitoneal bleed
      iii. false aneurysm
         (1) Use of Ultrasound to Dx
         (2) Use of Compressor to close neck of false lumen
      iv. AV fistula
      v. Femoral thrombus
   c. Care of Hematoma
      i. Continue pressure to stop bleeding
      ii. Sandbags
      iii. Circle the swollen area with a pen
      iv. "Mashing out" a hematoma
         (1) prevent infection
         (2) easier monitoring of new hematoma
   d. venous sites
      i. Femoral vein (easiest to control)
      ii. Subclavian vein (most difficult)
      iii. Internal jugular vein
      iv. external jugular vein
   e. Arterial sites
      i. Grading pulses (0 to +4)Femoral artery (above the femoral head in each groin)
      ii. Popliteal artery (posterior aspect of leg behind each knee)
      iii. Dorsalis pedis artery (on the anterior aspect of the foot between the first and second metatarsal.)
      iv. Posterior tibial artery (behind or posterior to the medial malleolus ankle bone.)
15. PULL SHEATH or CATHETER
   a. Remove Pt. to holding area
   b. Inspect and feel sheath in artery
   c. Pull steadily, let little blood spurt
   d. Arterial Sheath/catheter
   e. Venous Sheath/catheter
   f. Both Arterial and venous sheaths
16. TECHNIQUES OF HOLDING PRESSURE
   a. Position to hold pressure
   b. Hold above arterial puncture to stop bleeding (below venous site)
   c. Don't cut off pulse (after initial closure)
   d. Hold steadily, not letting up 15-20 min.
   e. Methods of applying pressure
      i. 3 fingers
         (1) pinching (thumb on hip)
      ii. heel of hand
      iii. Compressor
      iv. Inflatable Cuff
      v. Weight and/or straps
   f. Peek at wound at 15 min. - if bleeding - hold 10 more minutes

- g. Time to hold pressure
  - i. 0-5 MIN: HOLD firm steady pressure with the middle 3 fingers of you left hand. Compress the artery firmly but ease up enough so you can just barely feel faint pedal pulses with your right hand.
  - ii. 5-10 MIN: HOLD with 75% force used in the 1st 5 minutes.
  - iii. 0-15 MIN: HOLD with 50% force.
  - iv. 5-20 MIN: HOLD with 25% force. Full pedal pulses.
17. BANDAGING AND PATIENT TEACHING
    - a. apply sterile dressing
      - i. Elastoplast
      - ii. band-aid
      - iii. other
    - b. instruct patient re. wound care
      - i. PRESS ON THE WOUND IF YOU HAVE TO COUGH, Laugh, or move around.
      - ii. DRINK LOTS OF FLUIDS: Patients are instructed to drink lots of fluids, because the contrast is a diuretic and may dehydrate them.
      - iii. DON'T SIT UP BY YOURSELF. The nurse may elevate your bed to a slight sit up position.
      - iv. DON'T MOVE OR LIFT YOUR RIGHT LEG. (affected leg)
      - v. FEEL GENTLY AROUND THE WOUND FOR WETNESS OCCASIONALLY. If it starts bleeding call a nurse.
      - vi. Do not raise your head to look down at your groin. Call the nurse for

HOLDING ARTERIAL

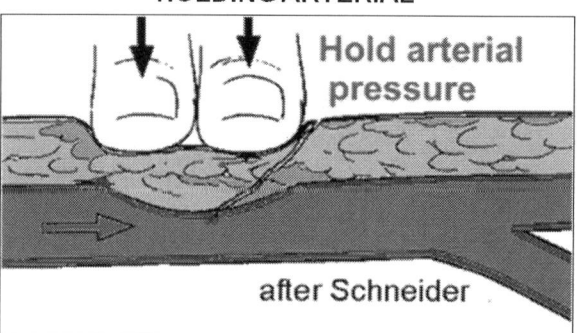

HOLDING ANTEGRADE

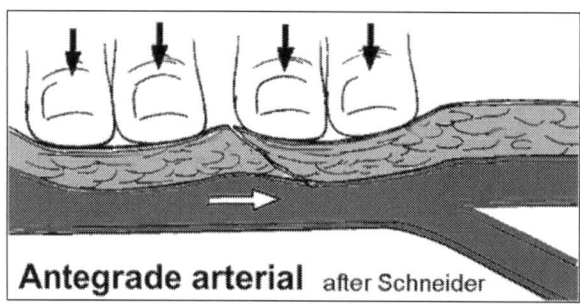

HOLDING VENOUS

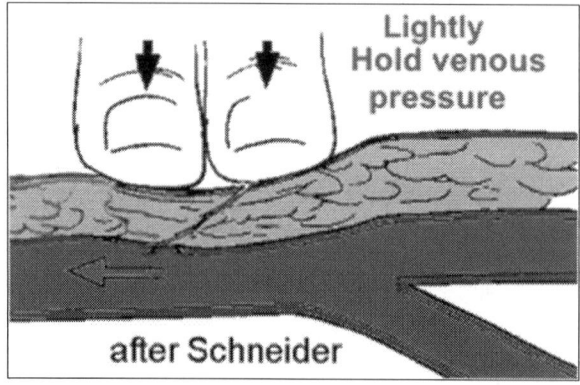

Right Heart Catheterization

INDEX: D6 - Right Heart Catheterization
1. Equipment . . . . p. 197 - Know
2. Insertion Techniques . . . p. 201 - Know
3. Hemodynamics . . . . p. 210 - Know
4. Myocardial Biopsy Equipment . p. 223 - Know
5. Chapter Outline . . . . p. 230

1. Equipment

354. Swan-Ganz right heart catheterization is most justified in patients with:
a. Cardiogenic shock
b. Chronic heart failure
c. Acute coronary syndrome
d. Acute STEMI

ANSWER a. Cardiogenic shock. Chatterjee says, "The randomized clinical trials in patients with acute coronary syndrome, noncoronary high-risk patients (including noncardiac surgical patients and patients with sepsis and ARDS), and patients with chronic heart failure have established that its routine use is not necessary and may be associated with increased complications, including death. However, it is still necessary in patients with cardiogenic shock, for the differential diagnosis of pulmonary arterial hypertension, and for diagnosis and treatment of uncommon causes and complications of heart failure."

"In patients with severe chronic heart failure requiring inotropic, vasopressor, and vasodilator therapy, hemodynamic monitoring is essential. For heart and lung transplantation workup, hemodynamic monitoring is always necessary... [They are] frequently overused in critical care units, resulting in many complications, including mortality. The prospective randomized trials have reported that in the majority of clinical circumstances, the routine use of balloon flotation catheters is not indicated."
See: Kanu Chatterjee, The Swan-Ganz Catheters: Past, Present, and Future: A Viewpoint, Circulation. 2009;119:147-152

355. Standard femoral Swan-Ganz catheters are _____ cm long.
a. 100 cm.
b. 110 cm.
c. 120 cm.
d. 150 cm.

ANSWER b. 110 cm. These catheters must traverse the long distance from the groin or arm to the distal lung bed. PAW catheters for use in the internal jugular (IJ) and subclavian veins can be 70 cm long because of the much shorter distances they must traverse. **See:** Baim and Grossman, chapter on "Percutaneous Approach." **Keywords:** Swan-Ganz is 110 cm. long

356. The quadruple-lumen thermodilution Swan-Ganz catheter is used to measure cardiac output. CO is normally accomplished with injection of cool or iced saline into the _____, while the thermistor measures the blood temperature in the ____.
  a. RA, RV
  b. RA, PA
  c. RV, PA
  d. PA, AO

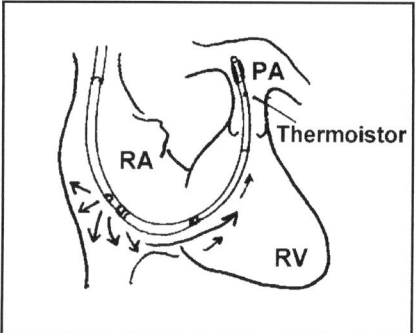

ANSWER b. RA, PA. The cold saline is injected into the RA through the proximal Swan-Ganz port. The thermistor is near the distal tip of the catheter in the PA. As the cooled blood passes it the temperature time curve is recorded/integrated to measure CO.
See: Baim and Grossman, chapter on "Percutaneous Approach" Keywords: Thermodilution CO inject RA sample PA

Inject RA - Sample PA

357. Several special types of thermodilution (TD) balloon floatation catheters have been developed. The type labeled #3 in the box has unique characteristics of:
  a. 2 RV electrodes, 3 RA electrodes
  b. A built in RV thermal heating element
  c. Oximetry for continuous mixed venous O2
  d. A rapid response thermistor, two intracardiac electrodes, and a multi-hole RA opening

SPECIAL TYPES OF TD CATHETERS
1. Pacemaker Thermodulution
2. Fiber optic Thermodilution
3. Thermodilution Ejection Fraction
4. Thermodilution / for continuous CO measurement

ANSWER d. A rapid response thermistor, two intracardiac electrodes, and a multi-hole RV opening. A spray of cold solution into the RV assures mixing of the iced thermal indicator. Beat-by-beat temperature changes in the PA are used to calculate RV ejection fraction.

MATCH EACH TD CATHETER TO IT'S CHARACTERISTICS:
  1. Pacemaker Thermodilution: 5 electrode RA & RV pacing. These 5 electrodes can provide atrial, ventricular or AV pacing or sensing. Another form of "pacing Swan" is the Paceport catheter. It has an RV port that will pass a "Chandler" pacing wire into the RV for emergency pacing.
  2. Fiber Optic Thermodilution: Besides TD it has a fiber optic oximeter that directs a beam of light at the PA blood, and then samples its color. This allows continuous mixed venous monitoring.
  3. Thermodilution Ejection Fraction: It provides intracardiac electrodes in the RA & PA for sensing V complexes. It has a special multi-hole injectate opening that creates a spray of cold solution into the RA. This assures mixing of the iced thermal indicator used to accurately measure PA temperature. Beat-by-beat temperature

changes are used to calculate RV ejection fraction (averages 40%). The thermistor has a rapid response time.
   4. **Thermodilution / For Continuous CO Measurement**: This is a new product containing a built in thermal element for the RV portion of the catheter. It provides 7.5 W of energy to heat the surrounding blood. The thermistor located in the PA measures the rise in temperature and correlates it to blood flow. **See**: Darovic, chapter on "PA Pressure Monitoring."

358. Long term PA monitoring lines should be connected to a "CONTINUOUS FLUSH DEVICE" which at 300 mmHg infusion pressure will deliver approximately:
   a. 1-2 ml flush/min
   b. 5-10 ml flush/min
   c. 3-5 ml flush/hour
   d. 20-40 ml flush/hour

ANSWER c. 3-5 ml flush/hour. These continuous flush devices have made extended hemodynamic monitoring possible. At this low flow rate catheters can be kept open while simultaneously measuring pressure through the transducer. By squeezing the device or pulling the "pigtail" valve - rapid flush occurs. This high volume flow is used to rapid flush new tubing or the PA catheter. **See**: Daily, chapter on "PA Monitoring."

359. For a pressure transducer to be accurately zeroed and calibrated it must be:
   a. Bubble free
   b. Open to air
   c. Closed on both ends
   d. Open to the catheter

ANSWER b. Open to air. The zero reference point must be set with one stopcock open at a mid-chest reference point. This air-zero adjusts the recorder baseline. If a baseline is set while the transducer has any residual pressure trapped within it, the baseline level will incorrectly read zero mmHg. Resulting pressure measurements will all be too low. Bubbles in a transducer are also a NO-NO. But small bubbles only affect the dynamic response - damping and resonance. **See**: Kern, chapter on "Hemodynamics."

360. You are assisting a new cardiologist do a right heart cath on a cyanotic child. Before inflating the balloon he asks you "What should I use to inflate this balloon?" You should answer_____.
   a. "Air"
   b. "CO2"
   c. "Sterile saline"
   d. "50%-50% contrast and saline"

ANSWER b. CO2 is 20 times more soluble in blood than air. If the balloon breaks or leaks in the right heart it will be more quickly absorbed. Since cyanotic shunts move across the septum in a R-L direction, some of the gas may pass through the R-L shunt. If it does embolize into the left heart it might lead to a dangerous arterial embolism or stroke. Get the CO2 from a CO2 tank off the table.

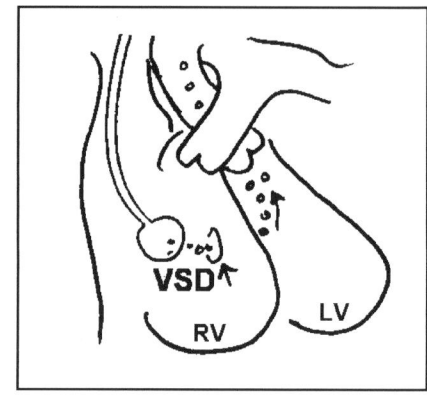
Bubbles crossing shunt

O2 gas is heavier than air, so let it bleed into a glass or basin through a sterile tube on the table. Then fill the balloon syringe by aspirating CO2 from the bottom of the glass. Use this to inflate the balloon. One problem with CO2 is that it diffuses rapidly through rubber so you may have to replenish the CO2 frequently.

Never inflate a Swan-Ganz balloon with any fluid, especially contrast! Its high viscosity may prevent you from removing it through the tiny catheter lumen. **See:** Baim and Grossman, chapter on "Percutaneous Approach" **Keywords:** Cyanotic kid → use CO2 in Swan

361. This is a pulmonary artery monitoring setup. Identify component #2 shown attached to the transducer.
  a. **Blood sampling stopcock**
  b. **Transducer zeroing stopcock**
  c. **Quick flush device**
  d. **Dead ender**

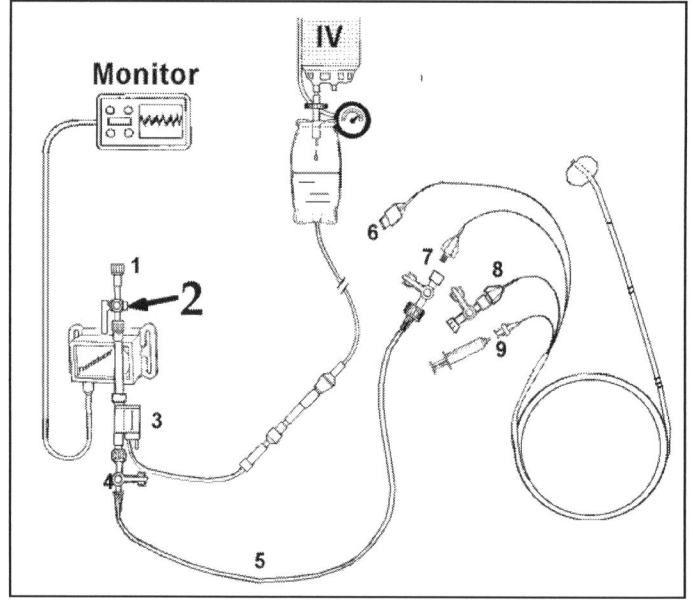
Swan-Ganz monitoring line

ANSWER b. Transducer zeroing stopcock is normally attached to the top of the pressure transducer. This allows you to purge the bubbles from the transducer as they float upward. Monitor zeros should be set to mid-chest level when the stopcock is closed, dead-ender removed & the zeroing stopcock is opened to air at mid-chest level..
1. Dead ender
2. Transducer zeroing stopcock
3. Quick flush device
4. Stopcock
5. Pressure tube
6. Thermistor connector
7. Distal (PA) port
8. Proximal (RA) port
9. Balloon inflation port

See: Darovic, chapter on "Pulmonary Artery Pressure Monitoring"

362. **Which statement regarding the set-up of long term hemodynamic monitoring equipment is most correct?**
    a. The system should only be flushed with saline to remove air bubbles at the time of set-up, prior to connection to the patient
    b. The pressure cuff on the IV solution bag must be maintained at 200 mmHg
    c. All stopcock side-arm ports should be replaced with closed (dead-ender) caps
    d. A properly inflated pressure cuff on the IV solution bag, along with an in-line continuous flush device, provides a continuous flow rate of 10-20 ml/minute

    ANSWER c. All stopcock side-arm ports should be replaced with closed (dead-ender) caps. This prevents accidental opening to air which could allow contamination or blood leakage. Systems should be flushed whenever air bubbles or blood are present. Air bubbles should be vented up and out of the transducer. Blood should be flushed through the catheter back to the patient. The pressure cuff on the IV solution bag must be maintained at 300 mmHg not 200. Normal continuous flow rates are 3-5 ml/hr not 10-20 ml/minute.
    See: Darovic, chapter on "Pulmonary Artery Pressure Monitoring"

363. **A patient with low EF, LBBB and probable AS comes to your lab for a bilateral heart catheterization. Which of the following would you prepare?**
    a. Transseptal equipment
    b. A temporary pacemaker
    c. Cardiac resynchronization therapy
    d. Apply Hands-off defibrillation pads due to high incidence of VF and VT

    ANSWER: b. Insertion of a temporary pacemaker prior to right heart catheterization. Patients may develop RBBB if the RBB is irritated during catheter passage through the RV. If the patient has pre-existing LBBB, complete heart block may ensue, requiring pacing via a temporary pacer, paceport catheter, or a pacing Swan. **See:** Darovic, chapter on "Pulmonary Artery Pressure Monitoring" **Keywords:** BHC in patient with LBBB= insert temp pacer

2. Insertion Techniques

364. **How are IV Swan Ganz catheters usually inserted?**
    a. Percutaneously over a guide wire (Seldinger technique)
    b. Through a sheath (which was inserted via Seldinger technique)
    c. Through a large bore needle inserted into the femoral vein
    d. Via a cutdown (on an antecubital vein)

    ANSWER b. Sheath. The Swan-Ganz catheters are put in through a venous sheath slightly larger than the catheter to allow room for the balloon. The sheath itself is put in by the Seldinger technique (needle - guidewire - catheter directly through skin).

Modern balloon catheters are rarely inserted by the cutdown method. Cutdown techniques are more prone to infection. Swan-Ganz catheters should NOT be inserted by the Seldinger percutaneous method, because the soft rubber balloon may be damaged by pressure from the tissues.
See: Baim and Grossman, chapter on "Percutaneous Approach" **Keywords:** Insert Swan-Ganz catheters via venous sheath

365. **When inserting a Swan-Ganz catheter the balloon should be inflated in the:**
   a. **Sheath**
   b. **Femoral vein**
   c. **IVC-RA**
   d. **RV**
   e. **PA**

ANSWER c. IVC-RA. The balloon should not be inflated until it reaches the large vena-cava or RA. If inflated in the sheath or small vein it may rupture the balloon or damage the vessel. In an average sized adult the RA is usually reached after inserting the catheter 15-20 cm from the internal jugular (I.J.) vein or 30 cm from the femoral vein. The inflated balloon then floats downstream with the RA-RV-PA blood flow. **See:** Baim and Grossman, chapter on "Percutaneous Approach" **Keywords:** Inflate Swan balloon in RA

366. **Grossman recommends passing the Swan-Ganz catheter from RA to RV by gentle forward and backward motion and clockwise rotation of the catheter, while the patient takes a deep breath. If these maneuvers fail to pass the tricuspid valve after several attempts Grossman recommends:**
   a. **Reducing the catheter size**
   b. **Injecting contrast to outline RV anatomy**
   c. **Insertion of J-guide wire through the catheter**
   d. **Adding another 0.5 ml of air to the balloon**

ANSWER c. Addition of a J-guide will stiffen the catheter making it more maneuverable. Most Swan-Ganz catheters will allow a .025 wire through the distal lumen. The wire itself may pass the valve, in which case it may be used as a track for the catheter. Other tricks are: to stiffen the catheter with iced saline, replace the catheter, torque the catheter, or withdraw a small amount of air from the balloon (to more easily pass the valve).
See: Baim and Grossman, chapter on "Percutaneous Approach" **Keywords:** Use guide wire through Swan-Ganz

367. According to the markings shown, this Swan-Ganz catheter has been inserted _____ cm into the femoral vein. Its distal tip is probably located in the _____.
   a. 20 cm, RA
   b. 40 cm, RV
   c. 60 cm, PA
   d. 80 cm, PAW

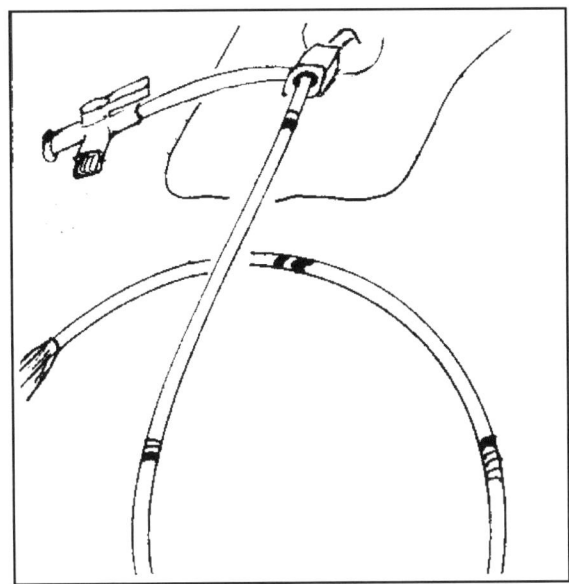
Swan-Ganz inserted into Femoral Vein

ANSWER c. 60 cm, PA. These depth ring markers appear every 10 cm on the shaft of the catheter. They are read with the large markings being 50 cm each, similar to the V in Roman numerals (e.g. VI = 5+1 = 6). This diagram shows one large mark and 1 small ring, or 50 + 10 = 60 cm. The RA is usually entered after passing 30 cm from the femoral route (15 cm from jugular, and 40 cm from the right arm vein.) Advancing another 30 cm should put the catheter tip through the RV into the PA. Check the pressure monitor to see if the tip is still in the RA. If so, the catheter may be coiling in the RA. Deflate the balloon, pullback, and start the insertion again. A small guide wire may occasionally be needed to enter the RV. **See:** Baim and Grossman, chapter on "Percutaneous Approach" **Keywords:** # Swan markings, 70 cm depth = PA

368. A Swan-Ganz catheter has been inserted into the internal jugular vein of a CCU patient in an attempt to obtain PA wedge pressures. The balloon was inflated and the catheter advanced 70 cm. Pressure wave forms remain as shown. What should be done?
   a. Inflate the balloon, advance another 20 cm.
   b. Deflate the balloon, withdraw to 20 cm then re-inflate balloon and re-advance catheter
   c. Pull catheter back to 30 cm, flush catheter with iced saline, insert guidewire for stiffness, and re-advance catheter
   d. Deflate the balloon, withdraw to 40 cm then re-inflate balloon and re-advance catheter

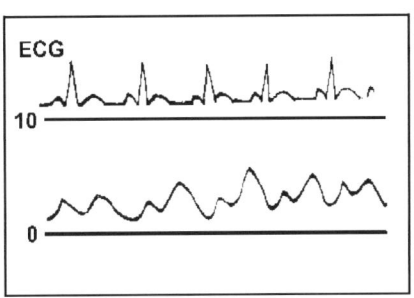
Pressure through Swan

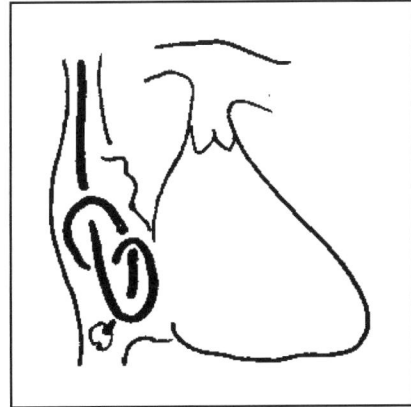
Swan coiling in RA

ANSWER b. Deflate the balloon, withdraw to 20 cm then re-inflate balloon and re-advance catheter. The catheter tip is still in the RA as indicated by the continuous RA pressure. It is **COILING UP** because it should have reached the RV at about 40 cm and the PA by 50 cm depth. Unless the catheter bend is pointed in the right direction it may not pass the tricuspid valve. Several attempts may be needed to work the catheter into the PA wedge position. This table shows the approximate depth where a Swan-Ganz catheter should reach the various right heart chambers. Note that the internal jugular (I.J.) and the subclavian site is much closer to the heart. The arm site is furthest from the heart. In all cases by 70 cm the PA should have been reached.

SWAN-GANZ DEPTH FROM INSERTION SITE TO VARIOUS CHAMBERS

Chamber	Internal Jugular	Femoral Vein	Right Arm Vein
RA Chamber	15-20 cm.	30 cm.	40 cm.
RV Chamber	40	50	60
PA Chamber	50	60	70

See: ACLS, chapter on "Invasive Monitoring Techniques."

369. You are advancing a Swan-Ganz catheter into an elderly lady with a dilated right heart. With balloon inflated the catheter passes easily from the IVC and RV but won't pass into the PA. Additional maneuvers include:
a. Deflating the balloon
b. Rapid pushing and pulling on the catheter
c. Have her hold her breath
d. Have her turn onto her left side
e. Have her inhale deeply and cough

ANSWER: e. Inhale deeply causes a negative pressure in the thorax, which increases venous return. This may cause enough increased flow to float the balloon through the tricuspid valve. Grossman says, "Having the patient take a deep breath and cough during advancement is often of assistance in achieving a wedge position....If needed, either pulmonary artery can be catheterized by appropriate manipulation or careful introduction of a curved J guide-wire, but extending guidewires into the thin walled pulmonary arteries should be avoided unless absolutely necessary." PA puncture is a dreaded complication.
See: Grossman, chapter on "Percutaneous Approach"

370. On the second day of pulmonary artery catheter monitoring, an RV waveform is observed from the distal catheter port. Which one of the following is the most appropriate action?
a. Advance the catheter 10 cm with the balloon deflated
b. Switch monitoring lines to the proximal port of the catheter
c. Inflate the balloon with 1.5 ml air and withdraw the catheter
d. Inflate the balloon with 1.5 ml air and advance the catheter
e. Leave in RV, you can still get PA systolic pressure from RV

ANSWER d. Inflate the balloon with 1.5 ml air to make a soft tip. Then advance the catheter until the PA wedge waveform appears, and deflate the balloon. Check the waveform to assure it is in the PA. You do not want to insert the catheter deflated, because the hard catheter tip may lodge in and damage the RV or PA wall (remember the trabeculations in the RV). Neither, do you want to leave the tip in the RV because it causes PVCs and ventricular arrhythmias.

371. **The most stable place to leave a right heart monitoring catheter positioned is with the tip in the:**
a. RA
b. RV
c. PA
d. PAW

ANSWER c. PA. Most monitoring catheters are left in the PA position because it produces fewer arrhythmias than the RA (PACs) or RV (PVCs). After obtaining a PA wedge the balloon is deflated to prevent obstruction of blood flow, and the catheter is pulled back out of wedge so in cannot damage the lung. Monitoring Swan-Ganz catheters may be left in the PA position long term. **See:** Baim and Grossman, chapter on "Percutaneous Approach" **Keywords:** PA most stable position

372. **Identify the structure or catheter shown in this aortic angiogram labeled #1.**
a. **Swan-Ganz thermodilution catheter**
b. **Pigtail catheter**
c. **Right coronary artery**
d. **Left coronary artery**
e. **Aortic insufficiency jet**

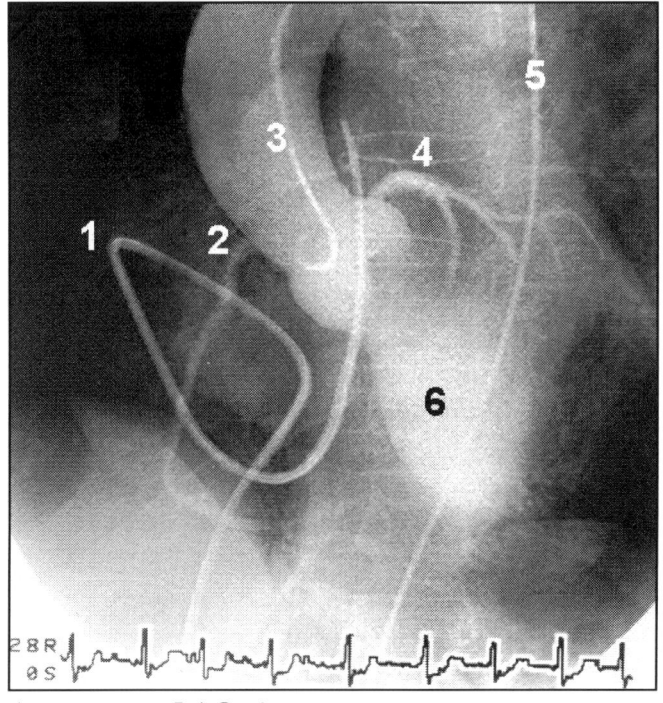

Aortogram - LAO view

ANSWER a. Swan-Ganz thermodilution catheter. Note the balloon is deflated on the end so it is not visible. The catheter passes through RA, RV and PA. **OTHER STRUCTURES SEEN ARE:**
1. Swan Ganz IVC-RA-RV-PA (loop coiled in RA)
2. Right coronary artery
3. Pigtail catheter in ascending AO
4. Left coronary artery
5. Pigtail catheter is descending AO
6. AI jet regurgitating backwards through aortic valve

See: Braunwald, chapter on "Radiology." **Keywords:** Swan, angio showing in heart with AI, LV angio

373. An ICU patient has a balloon-tipped flow-directed catheter positioned in his PA via the internal jugular vein. But, the catheter no longer moves into PA wedge position when inflated. In order get PAW tracings you should:
   a. Add an additional 1 cc of air to the balloon
   b. Rapid flush the catheter with the continuous flow device
   c. Put on sterile gloves, cut the sutures around the catheter and insert it a few cm
   d. Grab the catheter through the sterile sleeve and insert it a few cm

ANSWER d. Grab the catheter through the sterile sleeve and insert it a few cm. after inflating it. Flow-directed catheters often migrate over time. Catheters cannot be inserted into the sheath once sterile conditions no longer prevail. You can advance the catheter only if a sterile sleeve was put on the sheath before the catheter was inserted under sterile conditions.
See: Baim and Grossman, chapter on "Percutaneous Approach" **Keywords:** Unable to wedge → advance cath using sterile sleeve

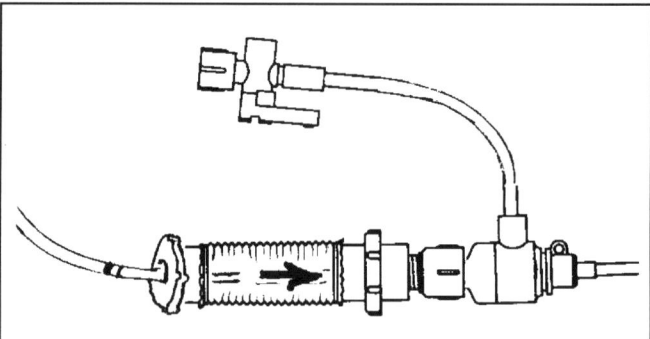
Insert using sterile sleeve

374. This PA view shows a multipurpose catheter inserted via a right arm vein. It will not advance into the PA and pressure mean is only 4 mmHg. The catheter is probably in the ___.
   a. Pericardium
   b. RV outflow tract
   c. Coronary sinus
   d. LA via ASD

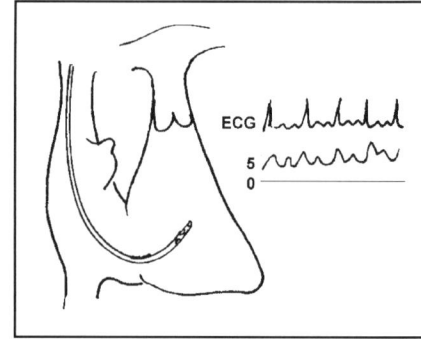
PA view - MP cath & pressure

ANSWER c. Coronary sinus. It is common to malposition right heart and pacemaker catheters in the coronary sinus. It appears to be in the RV in the PA view. But once the fluoro arm is turned to the lateral view the catheter is obviously posterior to the RV. The CS runs between the LV and LA on the inferior-posterior wall of the heart.
  The catheter should be pulled back into RA and reinserted through the tricuspid valve.
See: Johnsrude, chapter on "Cath. and Pulm. Angiog."
Keywords: Right heart catheter in CS

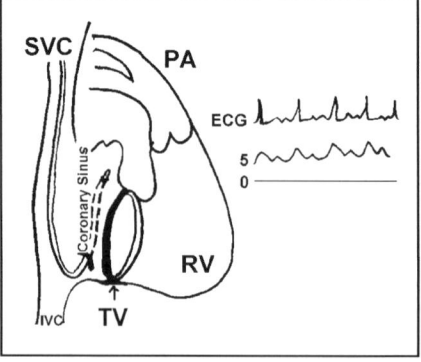
Lateral view - MP cath. in CS

375. What type of INVASIVE electrophysiology PROCEDURE uses electrical energy to BURN an area of myocardium breaking an electrical pathway to stop an arrhythmia?
  a. CABG
  b. HIS study
  c. Ablation
  d. Heart block
  e. Atherectomy

ANSWER c. Ablation. The "EP Lab" uses ablation energy (burning or freezing) to break adverse electrical pathways which lead to tachy-arrhythmias. The classic adverse pathway is found in WPW where a accessory bundle bypasses the AV node leading to rapid heart rates. A catheter placed near the pathway can burn it with radio-frequency energy (as found in a Bovie).
See: Baim and Grossman, chapter on "Electrophysiology." **Keywords:** Ablation defined

376. What is the most common complication of right heart catheterization?
  a. RV rupture
  b. Ventricular arrhythmia
  c. Right bundle branch block
  d. Inability to pass pulmonic valve

ANSWER: b. Ventricular arrhythmia. Kern says, "The most common complication of right-sided heart catheterization is arrhythmia resulting from mechanical catheter stimulation of the right ventricular outflow tract (RVOT), which can lead to ventricular tachycardia (VT), atrioventricular (AV) block or, rarely, right bundle-branch block. Significant but transient ventricular arrhythmias occur in 30% to 60% of RHC procedures and are self-limited (not requiring treatment). The arrhythmia is terminated when the catheter is readjusted. Sustained ventricular arrhythmias have been reported, especially in unstable patients or those with electrolyte imbalance, acidosis, or concurrent myocardial ischemia. In patients with left bundle-branch block, a temporary pacemaker may be necessary if right bundle-branch block occurs. Clinical trial data do not support the routine use of PAC in patients with heart failure. No studies have examined the clinical utility of PAC in acute myocardial infarction or cardiogenic shock." **See:** Kern, chapter on Hemodynamics

377. A 70-year-old lady with pulmonary hypertension has a Swan-Ganz monitoring catheter placed during her bilateral heart cath. She suddenly develops coughing, massive hemoptysis, and dyspnea. What complication is likely?
  a. Pulmonary infarction
  b. RV infarction
  c. PA rupture
  d. PA dissection

ANSWER: c. PA rupture. Grossman says, "Rupture of the pulmonary artery is also rare, but care must be taken not to use stiff-tip guidewires in these thinner-walled vessels. Patients typically develop massive hemoptysis of bright red blood and respiratory distress. This requires tamponade of the proximal pulmonary artery, embolization of the bleeding branch, and placement of a double-lumen endotracheal intubation to protect the uninjured lung." **See:** Baim and Grossman, chapter on "Percutaneous Approach" **Keywords:** PA rupture = hemoptysis

378. **Which of the following statements regarding pulmonary artery rupture is most correct?**
   a. Withdraw the PA catheter if a wedge is obtained with balloon inflation of >1.25 ml of air.
   b. If possible, have the patient cough every two hours to avoid catheter migration
   c. Avoid placing the patient in a lateral position after catheter placement
   d. Minimize or avoid PAOP measurements; monitor the PAedp instead of PAOP if pressure values are close.

ANSWER d. Minimize or avoid PAOP (wedge) measurements; monitor the PAedp instead of PAOP if pressure values are close. This avoids frequent inflation and wedging of the balloon, which can lead to PA weakening and rupture. The PE-EDP is normally within 4 mmHg of the wedge and LV-EDP. When re-wedging inflate the balloon slowly.
   If it wedges with low volumes (<1.25 ml of air) stop injecting air. It may "over-wedge." Then, after deflating the balloon, the catheter position should be withdrawn.
See: Darovic, chapter on "Pulmonary Artery Pressure Monitoring"

379. **To help prevent pulmonary artery rupture when wedging a Swan-Ganz catheter:**
   a. Check the pulmonary artery occlusion pressure frequently
   b. Withdraw PAC slightly if a PAOP waveform is obtained with inflation of <1.25 ml air
   c. Advance PAC slightly if a PAOP waveform is obtained with inflation of <1.25 ml air
   d. Always use 1.5 ml air to inflate the balloon for a PAOP

ANSWER b. Withdraw PAC slightly if a PAOP waveform is obtained with inflation of <1.25 ml air. You want the catheter to wedge with <1.5 ml of air. But, if the wedge air volume is <1.25 the hard catheter tip may be exposed. Darovic says: "The following guidelines should prevent damage or rupture of the pulmonary artery:
   1. Do not advance the catheter with the balloon deflated.
   2. Slow balloon inflation while continuously observing the PA waveform. Inflation is stopped immediately when the PA trace changes to a wedged pressure trace.
   3. Do not inflate the balloon with fluid.
   4. Keep the wedging time and the number of balloon inflation/deflation cycles to a minimum. If a close pulmonary artery diastolic/wedge pressure relationship exists, pulmonary artery diastolic pressure may be used to assess left atrial pressure.

5. Position the catheter tip in a central pulmonary vessel so that the full or nearly full recommended inflation volume produces the wedge waveform.
6. Avoid excessive catheter manipulation.
7. Avoid irrigating the pulmonary artery lumen under high pressure. ... The damped tracing may be due to spontaneous wedging, and forced irrigation may produce rupture of the pulmonary artery."

See: Darovic, chapter on "Pulmonary Artery Pressure Monitoring"

380. Which 3 of the following statements regarding PA catheter insertion are true? (Select 3 below.)
 a. Following vessel puncture, to assure venous access, SaO2 analysis of a withdrawn blood sample should be <95%.
 b. Use a Paceport Swan in patients with LBBB.
 c. The major risk of internal jugular cannulation is carotid artery puncture.
 d. Air embolism is of concern at the time of guidewire and catheter insertion.
 e. Use 50% contrast & saline to inflate the balloon

ANSWERS: b, c, & d
The SvO2 (not SaO2) must be less than 85% to be sure you are in the vein. Unlike arterial access, venous access is non pulsatile. Patients may develop RBBB if the RBB is irritated during catheter passage through the RV. If the patient has pre-existing LBBB, complete heart block may ensue, requiring pacing via a paceport catheter, a pacing Swan or external transcutaneous pacing. The carotid artery is close to the internal jugular. Take precautions against air embolism by placing the patient in the Trandelenburg position. Balloon is inflated with air.
See: Darovic, chapter on "Pulmonary Artery Pressure Monitoring"

381. Which of the following may be included in the immediate treatment of pulmonary artery rupture? (Choose 3 from below.)
 a. Discontinuation of anticoagulation
 b. Placing patient in lateral position with unaffected side down
 c. Selective bronchial intubation
 d. PEEP ventilation

ANSWERS: a, c, & d.
 a. Discontinuation of anticoagulation - YES
 b. Placing patient in lateral position with unaffected side down - NO. You would want the unaffected side up to prevent blood aspiration into good alveoli.
 c. Selective bronchial intubation - YES
 d. PEEP ventilation - YES. Positive pressure breathing helps push blood out of alveoli back into the capillary.

Darovic says: "Any condition that produces chronic pulmonary hypertension (mitral valve disease, COPD) increases the risk of vascular damage or rupture, because the enlarged pulmonary arteries allow the catheter to wedge more peripherally.... Patients with vascular rupture may present with minimal blood-tinges sputum. At the other end of the clinical spectrum, massive hemoptysis may quickly lead to shock and death.... If minor damage is incurred and the patient's condition is stable, conservative management with close observation as well as reversal of anticoagulation, if relevant, may suffice. With significant, active bleeding, the patient should be placed with the affected side (usually right) down to prevent spillage of blood into the uninvolved lungs. Control of the airway, ventilatory support, and circulatory support are primary goals. The application of PEEP also may tamponade hemorrhage. Although the simple removal of the pulmonary artery catheter may help in patient stabilization, emergency thoracotomy with resection of the involved lung lobe may be required."

See: Darovic, chapter on "Pulmonary Artery Pressure Monitoring"

382. Which statement regarding thrombus formation on Swan-Ganz catheters is most correct?
   a. **All intravascular monitoring catheters are thrombogenic.**
   b. **Heparin should be added to the IV solutions of all patients with a PA catheter.**
   c. **Catheters occluded by thrombus should be flushed vigorously with saline to clear the catheter.**
   d. **Thrombus begins to form on catheters only after 3 to 5 days in the vessel**.

ANSWER a. All intravascular monitoring catheters are thrombogenic. Even heparin does not guarantee they will not clot. However, many physicians are not using heparin for right heart cath or PA monitoring. And, if a catheter does become clotted, do NOT flush the catheter into the circulation. That causes an embolus.

Darovic says: "Any catheter in the vascular system can promote thrombus formation, particularly in patients who have prolonged circulatory failure.... Prevention of catheter thrombus formation requires consideration of anticoagulation in hypercoagulable patients if pulmonary artery pressure monitoring is prolonged or if catheter insertion is known to have been traumatic."

See: Darovic, chapter on "Pulmonary Artery Pressure Monitoring"

3. Hemodynamics

383. Identify 4 methods used to tell if a balloon catheter is truly wedged (PAW).
   a. **As seen on fluoro the balloon stops bobbing**
   b. **Distinct systolic waves are seen on the pressure trace**
   c. **The mean pressure is lower than PA**
   d. **O2 sat exceeds 95%**
   e. **Flush the catheter to assure it is not damped PA**

ANSWERS: a, c, d & e.
   a. YES: As seen on fluoro the balloon stops bobbing. This bobbing is seen with the catheter in the PA and the balloon inflated. As the balloon wedges itself in the distal PA it ceases to bob in and out with RV contraction.
   b. NO: Distinct systolic waves are NOT seen on the pressure trace. That is a PA pressure. What you see are two distinct small waves:
       1. The "a" wave - associated with atrial contraction
       2. The "v" wave which is an atrial filling wave associated with bulging of the AV

valve back into the atrium at the end of systole.

c. **YES:** The mean pressure is lower than PA. PAW is normally around 10 mmHg whereas PA mean is usually around 15 mmHg.

d. **YES:** O2 sat exceeds 95%. This is highly saturated blood pulled backwards through the pulmonary capillary bed. Remember to discard 5-15 ml of blood which is the approximate dead space between the balloon and the capillary bed.

e. **YES:** Flush the catheter to assure it is not damped PA. A stiff end-hole catheter actually gives more accurate wedge pressures than the balloon catheter and are more similar to LA pressure waveform.

Kern says, "Rules for obtaining an accurate PCWP that agrees with LA pressure are as follows:

1. Position the catheters correctly and verify position through waveform, oximetry (oxygen saturation >95%), and fluoroscopy. The wedged position of the catheter is confirmed by an oxygen saturation sample >95%. Note: Obtaining this saturation uncontaminated by low-saturation PA blood can be challenging because of the volume of low-saturation blood that must be discarded before wedge blood is collected. Use of a large-bore catheter and saline flushing during antegrade movement into the pulmonary capillary wedge (PCW) position can help with obtaining accurate oxygen saturation measurements.
2. Confirm that PCWP is not a damped PA pressure by using a precise A and V waveform timed against the ECG or LV pressure. Use a stiff, large-bore, end-hole catheter and connect it to the pressure manifold with stiff, short pressure tubing. The system should be thoroughly flushed and bubble free.
3. For mitral valve area (MVA) determinations, correct for the time delay (i.e., phase shift the PCWP v wave to match the LV down stroke) in pressure gradient calculations. However, it is important to note that this time delay does not correct for the damping of the PCW tracing that occurs due to its distal position relative to the LA."

See: Kern, chapter on "Hemodynamics"

384. **Which of the following formulas is used to calculate pulmonary arteriolar vascular resistance units?**
a. PVR = CO / $(\overline{PA-LA})$
b. PVR = $(\overline{LA-PA})$ x CO
c. PVR = CO / $(\overline{AO-RA})$
d. PVR = $(\overline{PA-LA})$/ CO

ANSWER d. PVR = $(\overline{PA-LA})$/CO. The numerator of the PVR equation is the difference between mean pressures across the lung bed (PA-LA) or (PA-PAW). The denominator is the flow across the lung bed (Pulmonary Blood Flow) - normally the cardiac output (unless a shunt is present). A way to remember this formula is to relate it to Ohm's law: R=Voltage drop/flow of current. Note that the lines over the pressures in the formulae indicate the chamber "mean" or "average" pressure level. **See:** Baim and Grossman, chapter on "Clinical Measurement of Vascular Resistance." **Keywords:** Systemic vascular resistance calculation.

385. Read the following RV pressure on range X40.
a. 20/-2/0
b. 22/0/6
c. 22/6/10
d. 23/-2/4

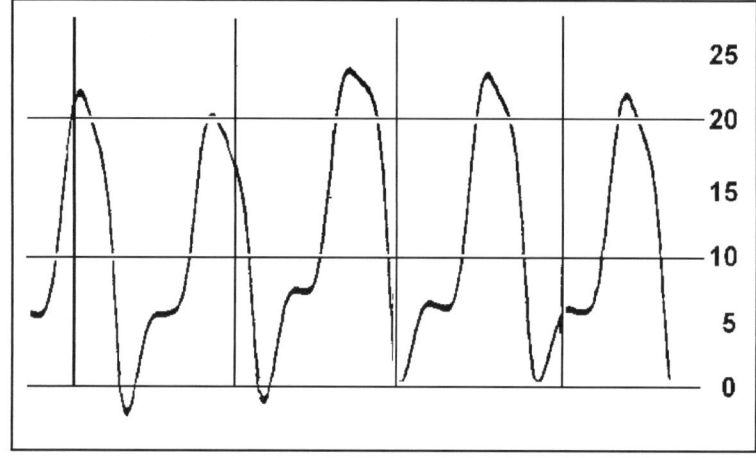
RV Pressure 0-40 scale

ANSWER b. 22/0/6. Systolic peaks average 21 mmHg. Early diastolic is zero or below zero (never read as negative). EDP is 5-7 mmHg. Understand how to read atrial, ventricular and arterial pressures.
See: Kern, chapter on "Hemodynamics." **Keywords:** Read RV pressure

386. Read the LA pressure tracing below in mmHg.
a. 10/32/15
b. 20/32/20
c. 32/10/15
d. 32/20/20

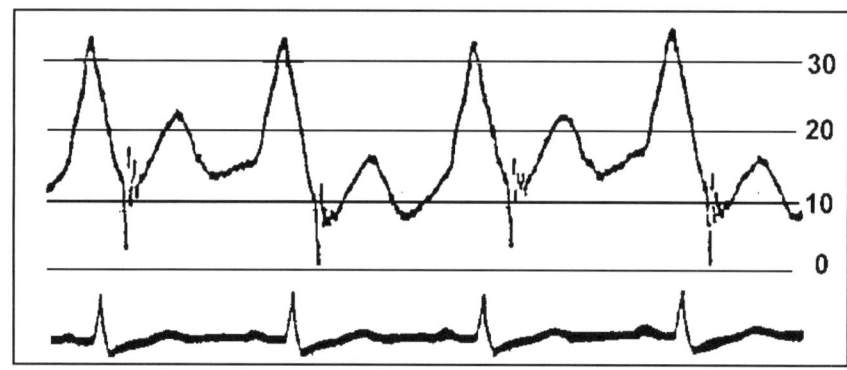
PAW pressure recorded x 40 (no transmission-time delay)

ANSWER d. 32/20/20 mmHg. Read A/V/mean on all atrial pressures.
The large A waves follow immediately after the p on the ECG, indicating atrial contraction. The V is lower between 18 and 22 mmHg. It follows the "T" wave. You have to estimate the mean pressure between peaks and valleys (it is not the average of "a" and "v" waves). There is virtually no delay in this LA pressure recording, with the "a" wave immediately following the "p" wave. Wedge pressures are typically delayed so that the "a" wave follows the "p" wave by 0.10 to 0.15 sec which places it following the QRS complex. Note the high frequency tricuspid closure artifact as it snaps down on the catheter.
See: Kern, chapter on "Hemodynamics." **Keywords:** Read PAW pressure

USE THIS PRESSURE TRACING FOR THE NEXT 2 QUESTIONS.

387. This pressure sequence shows a Swan-Ganz catheter passing from:
a. PAW, PA, to RV (pullback)
b. PAW, RV, to RA (pullback)
c. RV, PA, PAW (advance)
d. LV, AO, LA (pullback)

388. This patient has abnormal pressures indicating:
a. Tricuspid stenosis
b. Pulmonic stenosis
c. Mitral stenosis
d. Pulmonary hypertension

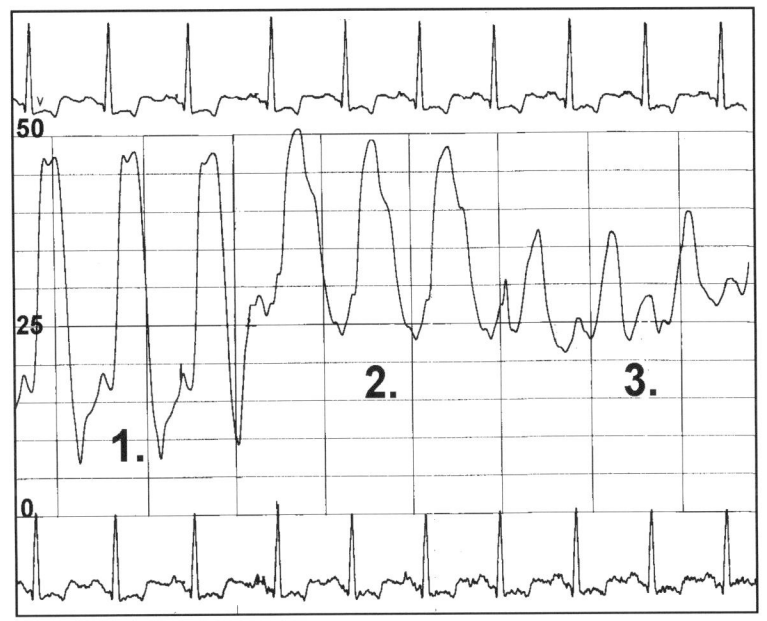

Right heart pressures recorded x 50

BOTH ANSWERS ARE LISTED BELOW CONSECUTIVELY.

387. ANSWER c. RV, PA, PAW (advance). The Balloon catheter was floated through the RV (#1), across the pulmonic valve into the PA (#2), and finally into PA wedge position (#3). Note how the first pressures resemble a square wave, and the PA a triangle wave. The RV and PA systolic pressures match. PA diastolic and wedge pressures match. The final tracing shows a sine wave pattern with a small "a" and large "v" waves. **See**: Kern, chapter on "Hemodynamics." **Keywords**: RV, PA, PAW insertion, pressure waveforms

388. ANSWER d. Pulmonary hypertension. RV and PA systolic pressures are high at 45-50 mmHg. This is far higher than the normal systolic of 25 mmHg. Mean wedge pressure is 32 mmHg. This elevated wedge pressure indicates probable congestive left heart failure. But, the high wedge has backed up into the right heart, causing pulmonary hypertension. The elevated RV-EDP of 17 mmHg indicates that the left heart failure has backed up into the right heart, causing its failure as well. Although not shown on this tracing, this patient had severe aortic stenosis.
See: Kern, chapter on "Hemodynamics." **Keywords**: Pulmonary hypertension

389. The normal blood oxygen saturation in the right heart is:
a. 20-40 %
b. 50-70 %
c. 70-80 %
d. 90-100 %

ANSWER c. 70-80 % is the normal range of SvO2 (Systemic venous O2). Venous saturation varies with metabolic state and disease. But at rest the normal is around 75%. With venous saturations higher than this, suspect a L-R shunt. And if SvO_2 is lower than 70%, suspect a low cardiac output or tissue hypoxemia.
See: Kern, chapter on "Hemodynamics." **Keywords**: Normal SvO2

390. A Swan-Ganz catheter is correctly placed in the PA. To obtain the PAW pressure inflate the balloon _____.
   a. Slowly until it suddenly pops open (usually <1 cc)
   b. Slowly until the pressure configuration changes from PA to PAW
   c. Quickly to the rated balloon volume (usually 1.5 cc)
   d. Quickly, then insert the catheter into the sheath 20 cm

ANSWER b. Slowly until the pressure configuration changes from PA to PAW. A Swan-Ganz properly positioned in the PA does not need to be inserted to move the catheter into wedge position. When the balloon is inflated it should pull the catheter tip into the lung bed and wedge itself. You don't have to push a Swan-Ganz catheter, they "float."

Dr's. Swan and Ganz state in Grossman's text: "To avoid damage to the pulmonary vessel wall and recording inaccurate pressures, *it is imperative that inflation of the balloon for obtaining wedge pressure be performed gradually under continuous monitoring of the pulmonary artery pressure and that the inflation of the balloon be stopped when the change from pulmonary artery to pulmonary wedge pressure configuration is noted.*"
See: Baim and Grossman, chapter on "Percutaneous Approach" **Keywords**: Stop inflating Swan-Ganz catheter when wedge pressure develops

391. Prior to pulling back a Swan-Ganz catheter to record PA-RV pressures you should _____.
   a. Inflate the balloon
   b. Deflate the balloon
   c. Flush the distal lumen of the catheter
   d. Flush the proximal lumen of the catheter

ANSWER b. Deflate the balloon. If you pull back an inflated balloon catheter across a valve, you may damage that valve. The balloon should be "up" when inserting and "down" when withdrawing the catheter. It won't hurt to flush the distal lumen through which your pressures are coming. It will reduce damping. But it is not necessary at this time.
See: Baim and Grossman, chapter on "Percutaneous Approach"
Keywords: Deflate balloon when withdrawing

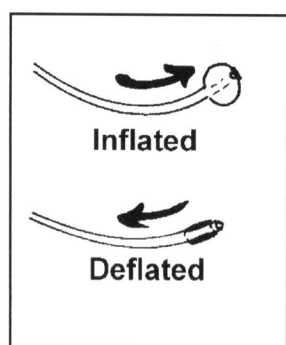

Balloon up - insert, Down - withdraw

392. What normal cardio-vascular chamber is indicated by the pressure recorded at #3 on the diagram?
   a. RA
   b. RV
   c. PA
   d. PAW

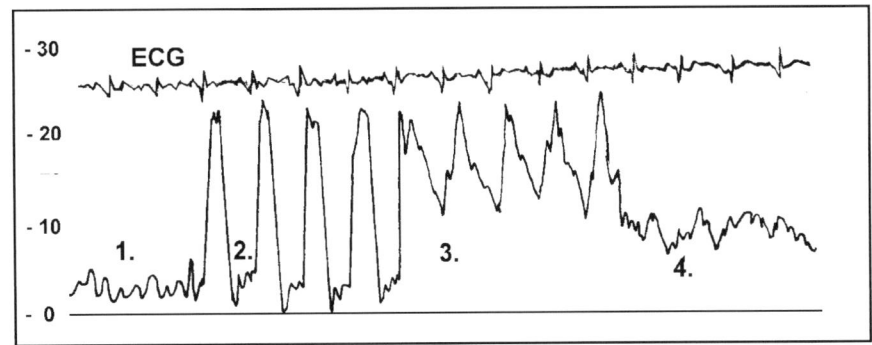
Cardiac cath "Insertion" pressures, recorded x 40

ANSWER c. PA. This sequence shows normal pressures recorded as a Swan-Ganz catheter floats into the right heart.
CORRECTLY MATCHED ANSWERS ARE:
   1. = **RA** (0-5 mmHg) systemic venous pressure
   2. = **RV** (25/5 mmHg) ventricular square waveform
   3. = **PA** (25/10 mmHg) arterial triangular waveform
   4. = **PAW** (5-10 mmHg) pulmonary venous pressure reflecting LA

See: Baim and Grossman, chapter on "Percutaneous Approach" **Keywords:** Identify Swan flow through pressures➔ RV

393. PA wedge pressure is an indicator of _____ filling pressure.
   a. RV
   b. PA
   c. LV
   d. CVP

ANSWER c. LV. Wedge pressure is important for two reasons: LV preload and pulmonary edema. First it measures the LV filling pressure (LV preload = PAW mean) and is an important index of LV function. It looks through the pulmonary capillary bed into the LA and when the mitral valve is open (diastolic filling) into the LV.

Second, PAW measures the pressure in the capillaries of the lung. This "hydrostatic" cause of pulmonary edema is common in congestive heart failure. Increased wedge pressure transfers fluid from the capillary into the interstitial space and alveoli leading to pulmonary edema and dyspnea.
See: Baim and Grossman, chapter on "Percutaneous Approach" **Keywords:** PAW ➔ LV filling pressure

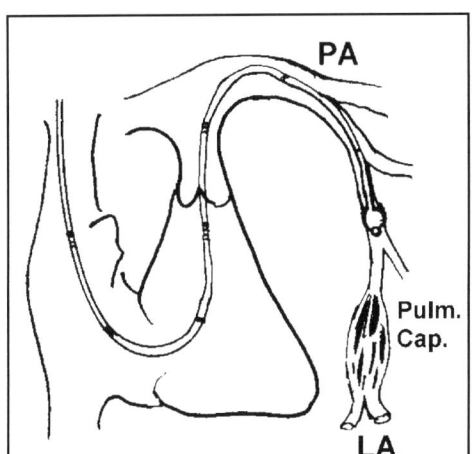
PA "Wedge" pressure

216 ◂◂ Diagnostic Techniques: D6 - Right Heart Catheterization ▸▸

394. In a Swan-Ganz catheter PULLBACK what cardiac pressures are normally recorded? In order they are _____, _____, _____.
 a. LA-LV-AO
 b. LV-AO-PA
 c. PA-RV-RA
 d. PAW-RV-PA

ANSWER c. PA-RV-RA. Knowing pullback pressure sequences is essential to knowing what is being recorded next on the hemodynamic monitor. Since the Swan-Ganz can only be inserted antegrade (with the flow) it must be pulled back from PAW-PA-RV-RA. Be sure the balloon is deflated - record PA, then RV, then RA.

Other cardiologists prefer to record pressures on the "way in" - as soon as they enter a chamber. This "push through" sequence then would be RA, RV, PA, PAW. The rationale for doing "push through" pressures as opposed to "pullback" pressures is utility. These cardiologists believe they should get as much information as possible on the way in because, should an emergency occur (e.g., arrhythmia), one may need to pull out quickly. **See:** Daily, chapter on "PA Pressure Monitoring." **Keywords:** Recording sequence, pullback

USE THIS PRESSURE TRACING FOR THE NEXT 2 QUESTIONS.

395. Identify the right heart chambers shown on this X50 pullback recording.
 a. RA-RV
 b. PA-RV
 c. PA-PAW
 d. PAW-PA

396. What pressure is recorded at #1 in the diagram?
 a. Mean RA
 b. Mean PAW
 c. Phasic RA
 d. Phasic PAW

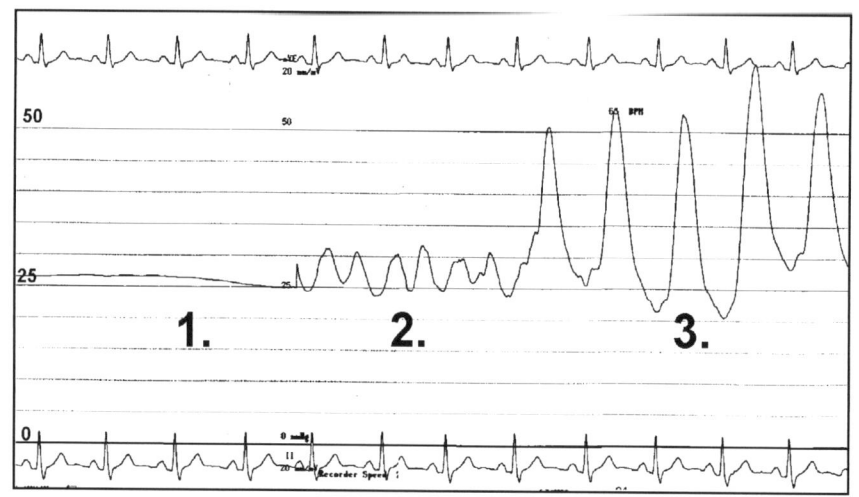
Rt. Ht. Pullback pressure

BOTH ANSWERS ARE LISTED BELOW CONSECUTIVELY:
395. ANSWER d. PAW-PA. This is what you will see when a Swan-Ganz balloon is deflated from the wedge position, or any catheter is pulled back from wedge. The pressure changes from venous PAW (#2) to PA (#3). It changes from a low sinusoidal shaped venous pressure to a triangular shaped arterial pressure. The pressure levels normally increase from a PAW of 10 mmHg to a PA of 25/10 mmHg. These pulmonary pressures are elevated and go from a PAW of 27 mmHg to a PA of 60/25/70 mmHg.

See: Baim and Grossman, chapter on "Percutaneous Approach" **Keywords:** ID pullback tracing from PAW to PA

396. ANSWER b. Mean PAW. With the recorder set to record mean pressure this very damped pressure records its average over time. Modern recorders now calculate and display the digital mean pressure. So, recording this damped "mean" pressure (shown at #1) is now seldom done. **RECORDINGS SHOWN ARE:**
  1. Mean PAW pressure displays the time average.
  2. PAW pressure displays all peaks and valleys Here "a" and "v" =30 mmHg.
  3. Phasic PA pressure shows systole and diastole. Here 55/25 mmHg.

See: Baim and Grossman, chapter on "Percutaneous Approach" also, see simulation: https://www.youtube.com/watch?v=Di7CHR4fmog

397. The cardiac silhouette is shown in the PA X-ray view on different patients with normal anatomy. What cardiac chambers/vessels does the catheter shown at #3 pass through?
  a. IVC - RA - RV - PA
  b. IVC - RA - RV - PA - LPA wedge
  c. AO - LV
  d. IVC - RA - (Transseptal Puncture) - LA - LV
  e. FA - AO - RCA
  f. SVC - RA - RV - PA
  g. IVC - RA - RV
  h. BA - AO - RCA (Sones)
  I. SVC-RA (Swan-Ganz)

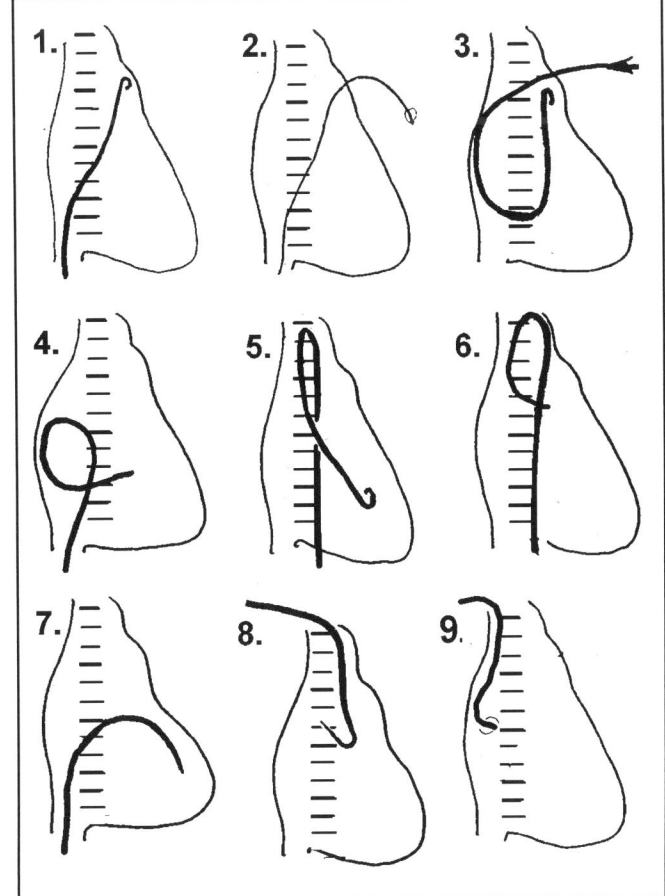

PA view of caths in normal patients

ANSWER f. SVC - RA - RV - PA. Note that right heart catheters always enter at the patient's right cardiac border to the right of his spine (SVC-IVC), whereas retrograde aortic catheters enter on the left side of the patient's spine (descending AO). The patient's left cardiac border is made up of the aortic knob on top, pulmonary bump, and LV outlines. Catheters leaving the PA or entering the AO must pass through their respective knob/bump.
CORRECTLY MATCHED ANSWERS ARE:
1. IVC - RA - RV - PA (Grollman Cath)
2. IVC - RA - RV - PA - LPA wedge (Swan-Ganz)

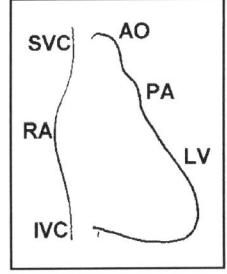

Heart silhouette

3. SVC - RA - RV - PA (Pigtail)
4. IVC - RA - RV (Multipurpose)
5. AO - LV (Pigtail)
6. FA - AO - LCA (Judkins)
7. IVC - RA - (Transseptal puncture) - LA - LV (Brockenbrough)
8. BA - AO - RCA (Sones)
9. SVC-RA (Swan-Ganz)

See: Johnsrude, chapter on "Cath. and Pulm. Angiog." **Keywords:** ID catheter positions in normal heart.

398. The cardiac silhouette is shown in the PA X-ray view on different patients with abnormal anatomy. What cardiac chambers/vessels does the catheter shown at #1 pass through?
  a. IVC - RA - RV - PA - (PDA) - desc. AO
  b. AO - LV - LA - LPV
  c. SVC - RA - RV - (VSD) - LV - LA - RPV
  d. IVC - RA (ASD) - LA - LV
  e. IVC - RA - (ASD) - LA - LPV
  f. SVC - RA - (ASD) - LA - RPV
  g. SVC - RA border (Cardiac Tamponade)
  h. IVC - RA - RV - (VSD) - LV - AO Arch
  I. SVC-RA-RV-(VSD) - LV - AO

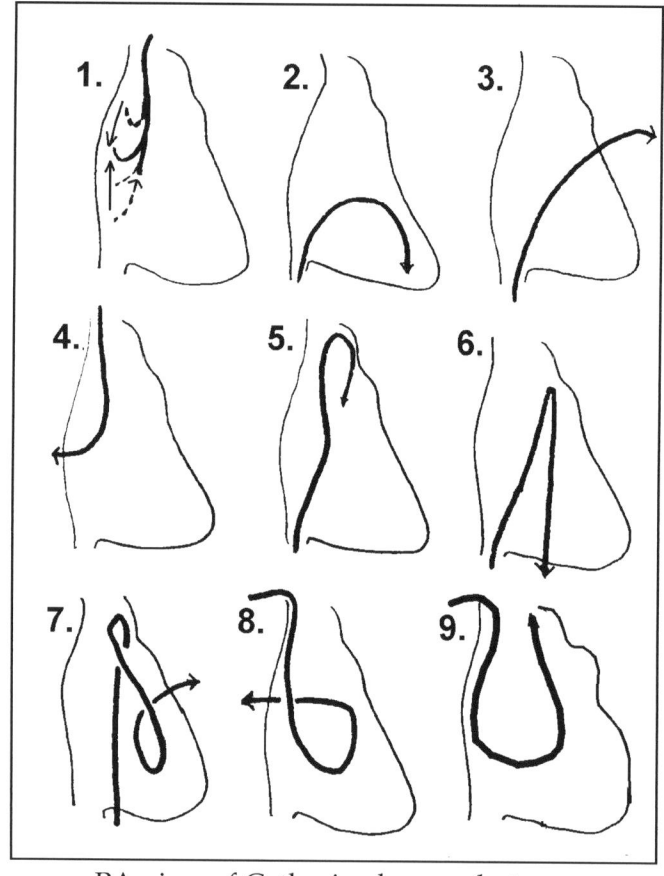

PA view of Caths. in abnormal pts.

ANSWER g. SVC - RA border (Cardiac Tamponade). Be able to match all answers. **CORRECTLY MATCHED ANSWERS ARE:**
  1. **SVC - RA** border. Cardiac tamponade is seen because catheter tip does not reach the patient's right cardiac border. The RA wall is normally thin, and tamponade fluid is indistinguishable from blood and myocardium on fluoro.
  2. IVC - RA (ASD) - LA - LV (Similar to transseptal cath.)
  3. IVC - RA - (ASD) - LA - LPV (Passes through cardiac border below PA bump (bifurcation) so this must be in the LA exiting a left pulmonary vein.
  4. SVC - RA - (ASD) - LA - RPV (From RA inferiorly through ASD into and out the right pulmonary vein.)
  5. IVC - RA - RV - (VSD) - LV - AO Arch. (From RA to RV and inferior through VSD into LV and up into AO.)

6. **IVC - RA - RV - PA - (PDA) - desc. AO** (Standard right heart cath which enters the patent ductus arteriosus and moves inferiorly down descending AO.)
7. **AO - LV - LA - LPV** (The L. signature of a full left heart cath. with catheter entering mitral valve retrograde into LA and left pulmonary vein. Difficult to perform. Judkins could do it with a pigtail catheter!)
8. **SVC - RA** - RV - (VSD) - LV - LA - RPV (Right heart cath which crosses a VSD posteriorly then crosses the mitral valve retrograde. Then out the right pulmonary vein - HARD!)
9. **SVC - RA - RV - (VSD) - LV - AO**

See: Johnsrude, chapter on "Cath. and Pulm. Angiog."

399. When using an O2 monitoring Swan-Ganz, which one of the following statements about abnormal central venous O_2 saturation (SvO_2) is most correct?
a. SvO2 values <0.60 indicate threatened tissue oxygenation
b. SvO2 values >0.80 indicate adequate or increased tissue oxygenation
c. SvO2 values <0.60 indicate low oxygen consumption
d. SvO2 values >0.80 indicate increased oxygen consumption

ANSWER a. SvO2 values <0.60 indicate threatened tissue oxygenation. This low venous saturation suggests low cardiac output (wide A-V difference) and poor tissueoxygenation. Darovic says: "SvO2 monitoring is a sensitive indicator of the oxygen supply/demand balance. When the SvO2 values fall to less than 50 percent, the patient should be rapidly assessed for conditions that increase oxygen demand.... Acute changes in the patient's oxygen supply/demand balance may be simply and safely assessed in the clinical setting by two technologies. First, continuous SvO2 monitoring [via Swan-Ganz fibreoptic catheters] ... Second, pulse oximetry can be used with cardiac index and hemoglobin values to estimate the amount of oxygen delivered to the body cells."

See: Darovic, chapter "Continuous Monitoring of Mixed Venous Oxygen Saturation (SvO_2)"

400. When using an SVO2 monitoring Swan-Ganz an SVO2 <40% sat. suggests that:
a. L-R shunt is likely
b. The catheter tip is against the wall
c. Blood is shunted to core tissues
d. O2 is relatively unavailable to tissues

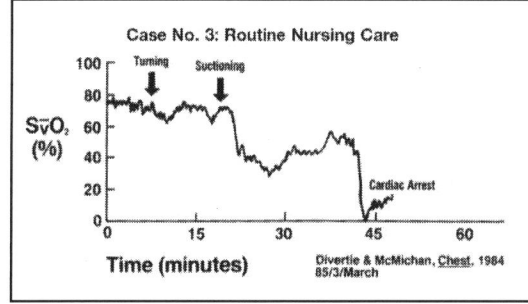

ANSWER: d. O2 is relatively unavailable to tissues. Edwards literature says, "Abnormal SvO2 Values: The normal range for SvO2 is 60 – 80%. If the SvO2 value is normal, then the clinician may assume that there is adequate tissue perfusion. If SvO2 falls below 60%, a decrease in oxygen delivery and/or an increase in oxygen consumption should be suspected. When SvO2 falls below 40%, the body's ability to compensate is limited, and oxygen is relatively unavailable for use by the tissues." Note the graph showing SVO2 monitoring of a patient whose SVO2 fell to 40% and shortly succumbed .

See: http://ht.edwards.com/resourcegallery/products/swanganz/pdfs/svo2edbook.pdf

401. Patients with acute inferior wall myocardial infarction are most likely to need an RV assist device when they have a low:
a. CVP
b. FFR measurement
c. Wedge pressure
d. Arterial pulse pressure
e. Pulmonary artery pulsatility index

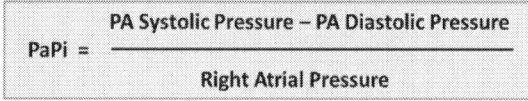

ANSWER: e. A low pulmonary artery pulsatility index (PaPI).
PAPi is the PA pulse pressure /RA pressure ratio. So, lower the PA pressure and higher the CVP or RA pressure the higher the risk of RV failure and need of an RV assist device (Impella RP). Thus, a patient with a PA pressure of 20/10 with a CVP of 10 would have a PAPi of 1.0 which is dangerously close to the limit of 0.9 indicating RV failure.

Protectedpci.com says: "Risk Stratification in the Setting of Acute Inferior Wall Myocardial Infarction...The presence of RV dysfunction increases the risk of CS (coronary syndrome), high-grade AV-conduction block, and higher mortality. The pulmonary artery pulsatility index (PAPi) is a hemodynamic measurement index which helps predict severe RV dysfunction during acute inferior wall myocardial infarction (IWMI), aiming to identify subjects requiring a percutaneous RV assist device (RVAD).... Invasive hemodynamic measurement with the PAPi may identify patients with severe RV dysfunction while predicting in-hospital mortality risk and the need for mechanical circulatory support... A PAPi <0.9 is highly specific and highly sensitive in identifying RV dysfunction" **See:** https://www.protectedpci.com/utility-papi-risk-stratification-setting-acute-inferior-wall-myocardial-infarction/

402. What does central venous pressure (CVP) directly assess? (Select 2 below.)
a. RV function
b. LV function
c. Fluid volume status
d. Myocardial **contractility**
e. **Vascular resistance**

ANSWER a & c: (RV function and fluid volume status.) To measure CVP, a catheter may be placed in the SVC or a Swan-Ganz catheter may be monitored from the RA port. CVP or RA pressure directly measures right heart preload and RV function. The RV filling pressures will be elevated in right heart failure (assuming no tricuspid disease). Darovic says: "The central venous pressure measurement also can be used to assess and manage intravascular volume status because pressure in the great thoracic veins generally correlates with the volume of venous return. The amount of blood that returns to the heart is normally ejected by the heart. Therefore, in patients with hypovolemia, a decreased CVP measurement is associated with a decreased cardiac output, whereas patients with volume overload typically have increased CVP and cardiac output."

CVP can indirectly monitor LV function, but only in normal young people. The frequent disparity between right and left heart function in critically ill patients requires a

Swan-Ganz catheter so that each side of the heart can be evaluated independently.
PAPulsatility Index (PaPI) evaluates for LV failure and need of RV assist.
See: Darovic, chapter on "Monitoring Central Venous Pressure"

403. Which of the following is most likely to be associated with hypovolemia?
   a. Increased central venous pressure
   b. Decreased RV end-diastolic pressure
   c. Increased PA occlusion pressure
   d. Decreased heart rate

ANSWER b. Decreased RV end-diastolic pressure which is usually the same as the RA or CVP pressure. Darovic says: "Progressive intravascular volume losses produce greater decrements in right atrial pressure and CVP. Patients with acute, profound hemorrhage may have measurements as low as minus 8 to minus 10 mmHg." In acute decompensated hypovolemic shock vasoconstriction increases to maintain BP, skin is cool & pale, along with signs of tachycardia, lactic acidosis, and hypoxemia.
See: Darovic, chapter on "Monitoring the Patient in Shock"

404. Which one of the following statements about the pulmonary artery occlusion pressure (wedge) is most correct?
   a. The pulmonary artery occlusion pressure is measured through the most proximal catheter port
   b. Inflation of the balloon momentarily stops the flow of blood and creates a static column of blood between the tip of the catheter and the left atrium
   c. The PAOP waveform always contains 3 positive waves (a, c, v)
   d. During inflation of the balloon the pulmonary artery pressure changes to a right ventricular waveform

ANSWER b. Inflation of the balloon momentarily stops the flow of blood and creates a static column of blood between the tip of the catheter and the left atrium. This static column transmits the LA pressure back to the catheter tip. Since LA is the filling pressure of the LV, wedge tells us about the LV filling pressure and LV function. The PA occlusion pressure (wedge) is measured through the distal catheter port, as it is directed into the pulmonary capillary bed. The wedge waveform will show A and V waves, but commonly no C wave is visible, because it merges with the a wave.
See: Darovic, chapter on "Pulmonary Artery Pressure Monitoring"

405. Which one of the following statements about the pulmonary artery occlusion pressure (PAOP or wedge) waveform is most correct?
   a. To measure the wedge the value of the "A" wave is averaged
   b. The peak "A" wave best approximated LV-EDP
   c. The "A" wave is found just before the QRS complex
   d. Inflate the balloon with no more than 1.5 ml of sterile saline

ANSWER a. To measure the pulmonary artery occlusion pressure the value of the "A" wave is averaged. Find the "A" wave following the QRS. Although the "A" wave is caused by atrial contraction, the time delay through the lungs and catheter make it appear after the QRS. The wedge should be measured with the balloon inflated with air, not saline.

To measure the PAOP, take the average "A" wave. It is ½ the distance between the "A" peak following the QRS and "X" descent between A & V waves. Here is how it's measured: add the top of a representative "A" wave to the bottom of that "A" wave ("X" or "X_2" trough). Then divide that sum by 2, to get the "MEAN 'A' wave." The mean 'A' wave is then midway between the top and bottom of the A wave. Because it is so seldom seen, this measurement ignores any "C" waves. Ahrens says, "*The primary method to ensure that all clinicians are consistently reading waveforms correctly is for all interpreters of waveforms to locate the A wave and determine its mean...*"

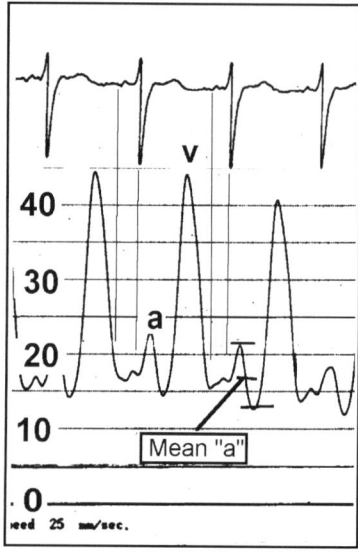

Mean a in PAW tracing x 50

The end expiratory point is the most consistent point to read all hemodynamic values. **See:** Ahrens, chapter on "Normal Pulmonary Capillary Wedge and Central Venous Pressure." **Keywords:** LV-EDP best approximated by mean A wave

406. Which 3 of the following statements about measurement of the pulmonary artery occlusion pressure are most correct? (Select 3 below.)
   a. The Swan-Ganz balloon should remain inflated for at least 45 seconds to insure an optimal seal within the pulmonary artery
   b. To deflate the balloon draw negative pressure on the syringe
   c. "Overwedging" can occur with excessive balloon inflation
   d. The wedge pressure is lower than the mean pulmonary artery pressure
   e. Never pull the inflated Swan-Ganz back through a valve

ANSWER c, d & e. "Overwedging" can only occur with excessive balloon inflation, the wedge pressure is always lower than the mean pulmonary artery pressure and never pull and inflated balloon back (deflate 1st).

Darovic say of prolonged wedging or overinflation: "The balloon, which is compressed by the surrounding pulmonary artery, may 'herniate over' and pressurize the sensing tip of the catheter...." This give a false damped and increasing pressure reading. You should not leave the balloon inflated for over 15 seconds to reduce the risk of lung ischemia and PA rupture. You should not have to aspirate air from the balloon. Simply opening the balloon stopcock is enough. Air from the balloon is under slight pressure and will cause the balloon to empty by itself into the syringe. "An intact balloon offers a slight resistance to inflation that may be perceived by the examiner. In addition, when thumb pressure is removed from the plunger, it usually spontaneously moves back to the extended position."

The PAOP (wedge) pressure should always be lower than the mean PA pressure and usually the PA-EDP. The syringe should fill passively with 1.5 ccs of air. Undue suction could damage the rubber balloon. "Wedging of the catheter is associated with a dramatic change from the pulmonary artery waveform to a low amplitude tracing that relates to left atrial pulsations." **See:** Darovic, chapter on "Pulmonary Artery Pressure Monitoring"

407. Which one of the following statements about hemodynamic waveforms is most correct?
   a. Hemodynamic pressures rise during inspiration in a patient breathing spontaneously
   b. Hemodynamic pressures fall during inspiration in a patient receiving positive-pressure mechanical ventilation
   c. Hemodynamic pressures should be read at end-expiration in a patient breathing spontaneously
   d. Hemodynamic pressures should be read at peak-inspiration in a patient receiving positive-pressure mechanical ventilation

ANSWER c. Hemodynamic pressures should be read at end-expiration in a patient breathing spontaneously and when the patient is receiving mechanical ventilation. So end-expiration is always correct. The problem with mechanical ventilation is, end-expiration pressures tends to be at the bottom of the tracing, where it is normally at the top. Normal inspiration makes the pressures go down, while mechanical inspiration makes the pressures go up. **See:** Darovic, chapter on "Pulmonary Artery Pressure Monitoring"

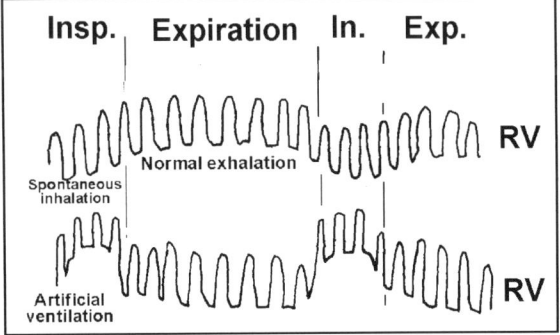
Effect of ventilation on cardiac pressures

4. Myocardial Biopsy Equipment

408. Which of the following are definitive indications for diagnostic myocardial biopsy? (Select 2 from below.)
   a. Cardiac transplant patient follow up
   b. LV hypertrophy associated with systemic hypertension
   c. RV hypertrophy associated with pulmonary hypertension
   d. Amiodarone toxicity
   e. Anthracycline cardiotoxicity

ANSWERS: a & e.
1. Cardiac transplant patient follow-up - YES
2. LVH may be caused by systemic hypertension - NO
3. RVH may be caused by pulmonary hypertension - NO
4. Amiodarone toxicity - NO. Amiodarone can cause pulmonary damage, not heart.
5. Anthracycline cardiotoxicity - YES. Anthracycline is a chemotherapy drug that also effects cardiomyocytes. Toxic amounts of anthracycline reduces LVEF and damages cardiac cells seen on histology. Definitive diagnoses of these conditions can only be

made with microscopic tissue analysis.

Kern says, "Monitoring cardiac transplant rejection and determining anthracycline cardiotoxicity are the only two definitive indications for endomyocardial biopsy. Other indications include evaluation for infiltrative cardiomyopathy, myocarditis that may benefit from immunosuppressive therapy, and occasionally, differentiation between restrictive and constrictive cardiomyopathies." See: Kern, chapter "Special Techniques."

409. Stiff shaft cardiac bioptomes are designed to gain access into the _____ via a _____ sheath:
  a. Internal jugular vein, short
  b. Internal jugular vein, long
  b. Femoral artery, long
  c. Femoral vein, long

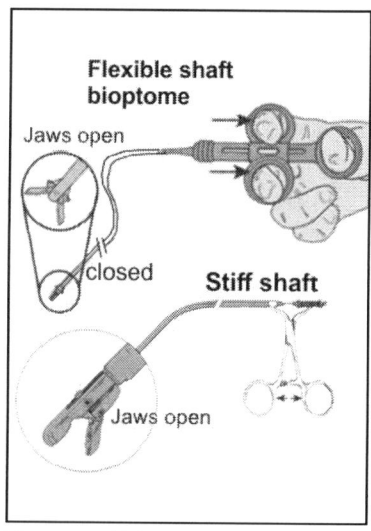

Types of bioptome

ANSWER a. Internal jugular vein, short sheath.
Kern says, "An 8-F short sheath is inserted into the right internal jugular vein by the standard Seldinger technique. A rigid, curved bioptome is inserted through the venous sheath and into the RA." [Then it is advanced closed, across the tricuspid valve into the RV.] "The operator should readily target the apical septum to avoid trauma to the tricuspid valve, which is abundant in chordae...." The femoral approach requires a long sheath and flexible shaft bioptome. See Kern, chapter on Special Techniques.

410. The RV biopsy from the femoral vein requires a _____ sheath that is advanced into the:
  a. Long (85-94 cm.) sheath advanced into the RA
  b. Long (85-94 cm.) sheath advanced into the RV
  c. Short (40-53 cm. sheath) advanced into the RA
  d. Short (40-53 cm. sheath) advanced into the RV

ANSWER b. Long (85-94 cm.) Sheath, into the RV
It has a double action 2 cup jaw operated with finger loops like a control syringe, squeezing closes the jaws.

Alverez says, "A modified Cordis bioptome ... or similar device with a long sheath is used for access from the right femoral vein. The femoral artery may be used as an access site for left ventricular biopsy. The right ventricular septum is the preferred initial site for EMB to minimize the risk of perforation. Fluoroscopic and/or echocardiographic guidance will be required to localize the site of biopsy." See: Catalina Sanchez Alvarez, Leslie T. Cooper, in Cardiology Secrets (Fifth Edition), 2018

411. The most common access for RV endomyocardial biopsy using stiff shaft devices is:
a. Femoral vein
b. Subclavian vein
c. Apical puncture
d. Internal jugular vein

ANSWER: d. Internal jugular vein from the neck is a straight shot down the SVC into the RV. Grossman says, "Right ventricular endomyocardial biopsy procedures are most commonly performed via the right internal jugular vein." This may be done under echocardiographic or fluoroscopic guidance. Kern reports advantages of echo guidance include: no radiation, can be performed in patient's room, and more accurate positioning of the bioptome. The floppy shaft bioptomes are designed for femoral vein access.
See: Grossman, chapter on Endomyocardial Biopsy" and Kern, chapter on "Special Techniques" **Keywords:** RV biopsy from IJV

412. From what part of the heart are intracardiac myocardial biopsy samples normally taken?
a. RV septum
b. RV outflow tract
c. Inferior RV wall
d. LV free wall

ANSWER a. The RV septum is the safest area from which to take a sample. Being part of the LV septum, it is the thickest part of the RV. Overzealous sampling may perforate the RV wall, leading to pericardial tamponade. 4-5 samples should be taken from the RV. It is not usually necessary to sample LV because most of the diseases diagnosed are diffuse and effect both chambers. In addition, Kern states that sampling from the RV outflow tract (near the pulmonic valve) and inferior wall should be avoided due to tricuspid valve chordae tendineae. **See:** Baim and Grossman, chapter on "Myocardial Biopsy" and Kern, chapter "Special Techniques."

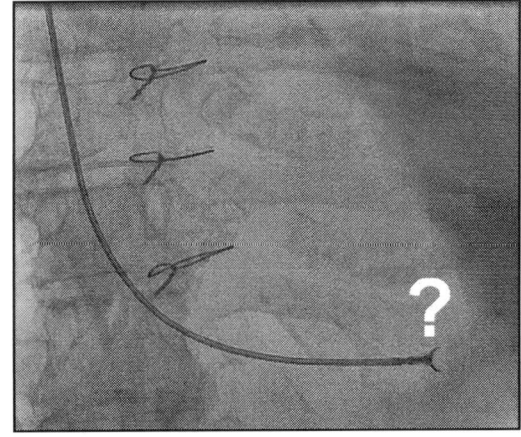
Biopsy of RV septum

413. What is shown in this procedure?
a. Liver biopsy
b. Pericardial centesis
c. RV septal biopsy
d. LV endocardial biopsy

ANSWER c. RV septal biopsy with stiff shaft bioptome jaws open - ready to take a sample. Access appears to be from the internal jugular vein.

414. How much heparin should a patient receive for <u>right heart</u> myocardial biopsy? How much for <u>left heart</u> biopsy?

	RT. HEART BIOPSY	LEFT HEART BIOPSY
a.	None,	None
b.	None,	5000 u
c.	5000 u,	None
d.	5000 u,	5000 u

ANSWER b. None for RV, 5000 u for LV. Heparinization encourages the bleeding from biopsy sites and pericardial tamponade into perforations. Grossman states "*We avoid right ventricular biopsy in any patient with a Prothrombin time greater than 17 sec, any patient who is heparinized or any patient with a clinical coagulopathy.* On the other hand, left ventricular biopsies are generally performed *with* systemic anticoagulation (heparin 5000 u), which is *not* reversed with protamine at the end of the procedure to minimize the risk of thrombus formation at the biopsy site."

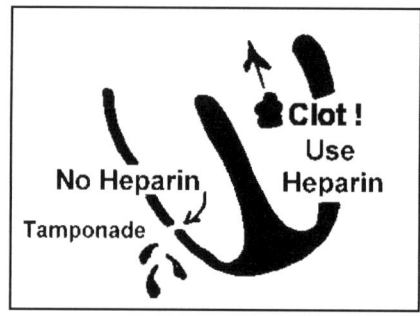
RV-No heparin, LV-yes

RT. HEART BIOPSY	LEFT HEART BIOPSY
None, -	5000 u

Bleeding from the right side is more serious than emboli (they will be filtered by the lung). Whereas, emboli from the left side are more serious (possibility of stroke).
See: Baim and Grossman, chapter on "Myocardial Biopsy" **Keywords:** No heparin for RV biopsy, 5000 u for LV biopsy

415. The main hazard of myocardial biopsy is:
a. Air embolism through the large sheath
b. Bundle branch or complete heart block
c. Coronary artery perforation and fistula
d. Infection at the biopsy site
e. Cardiac perforation

ANSWER e. RV perforation is the most dreaded complication since it can lead to fatal pericardial tamponade. The RV is only a few mm thick and with force any stiff catheter can perforate. That is why only septal wall samples are taken and heparin is not given with RV biopsy. Simple pericardial centesis usually cures the tamponade problem.

The other complications listed are also possible. This is a very safe procedure with approximately half the mortality of a left heart cath and coronaries (0.10% vs .05%). **See:** Baim and Grossman, chapter on "Myocardial Biopsy." **Keywords:** Main complication biopsy = perforation

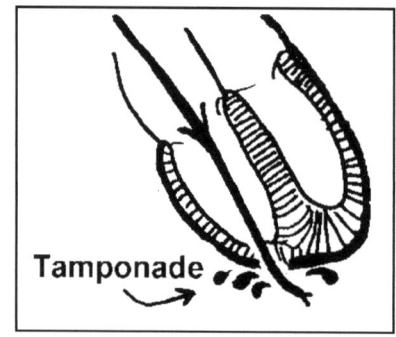
Bioptome RV perforation

416. A complication of myocardial biopsy is inadvertently puncture through the ventricular free wall. What lifesaving measure should be considered if hypotension develops following this procedure?
a. Thoracentesis
b. Pericardial centesis
c. Coronary artery bypass surgery
d. Aortic valve replacement surgery

ANSWER b. Pericardial centesis. If blood builds up in the pericardial sack, causing restriction of ventricular filling, pericardial centesis may be lifesaving. **See:** Baim and Grossman, chapter on "Percutaneous Approach." **Keywords**: With biopsy wall puncture - treat pericardial tamponade with pericardio-centesis

417. During endomyocardial biopsy Your patient suddenly develops severe hypotension . What complication is most likely to be responsible for this?
a. Air embolism and no-reflow
b. Embolism to brain and stroke
c. RV perforation and tamponade
d. Venous dissection with retroperitoneal bleed

ANSWER: c. RV perforation and tamponade. Grossman says, "The greatest risk to patients from the performance of endomyocardial biopsy is ventricular perforation. This may result in pericardial tamponade and death." Other associated complications include arrhythmias, heart block, pneumothorax, carotid artery or subclavian artery puncture, pulmonary embolism, nerve paresis, venous hematoma, and arterial A-V fistula. **See:** Grossman, chapter on "Myocardial Biopsy" **Keywords:** Complication RV biopsy=RV perforation

418. Myocardial biopsy samples for light microscopic analysis are placed in a solution of:
a. 10% formalin
b. 56% formalin
c. 5.0% glutaraldehyde
d. 50% glutaraldehyde

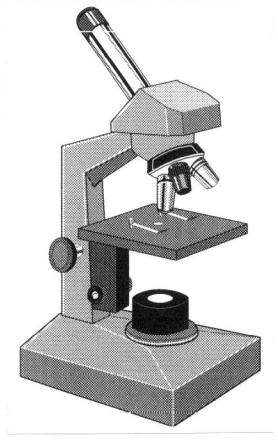

ANSWER a. 10% formalin (formaldehyde) preserves the sample. 2.5% glutaraldehyde solutions are used for electron microscopic analysis. **See:** Baim and Grossman, chapter on "Myocardial Biopsy." **Keywords**: Preserve biopsy samples in 10% formalin

419. Identify 3 histologic signs of cardiac transplant rejection found in myocardial biopsy samples.
   a. Interstitial edema and inflammation
   b. Erythrocyte hemolysis
   c. Lymphocyte infiltration
   d. Myocyte necrosis
   e. Hemolytic anemia

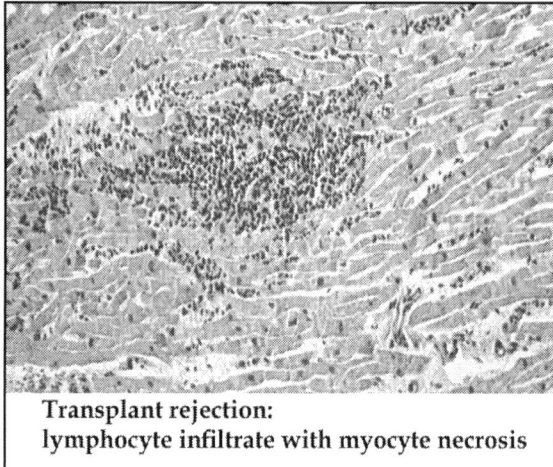

Transplant rejection: lymphocyte infiltrate with myocyte necrosis
http://www.ucsfcme.com/2012/slides/MMC13001/17.%20Teresa%20De%20Marco.pdf

ANSWERS: a, c, & d.
   a. Interstitial edema and inflammation - YES
   b. Erythrocyte hemolysis - NO. Erythrocyte hemolysis is rupture of red blood cells. It may occur in hypertonic solutions or mechanical valve turbulence (hemolytic anemia), but not with transplant rejection.
   c. Lymphocyte infiltration - YES
   d. Myocyte necrosis - YES
   e. Hemolytic anemia - NO. Hemolytic anemia is erythrocyte hemolysis found in mechanical heart valves that traumatize RBCs. Same as answer b.

Braunwald says, *"The most important feature of post-transplant biopsies is the detection of lymphocyte infiltration and the presence of myocyte necrosis."* That involves white blood cells (lymphocytes) rushing in to remove dying (necrotic) cardiac muscle cells (myocytes). The early stages of rejection also involve inflammation and edema of the transplanted myocardial cells. **See:** Baim and Grossman, chapter on "Myocardial Biopsy" and Braunwald, Heart Disease..., chapter on "Heart and Lung Transplantation." **Keywords:** Histologic signs of rejection NOT erythrocyte hemolysis

Right Heart Simulation

We suggest practicing with the University of Toronto right heart simulation as shown below. It is sponsored by Medtronic and shows various hemodynamics with various disease states and allows you to treat and see the results.
http://pie.med.utoronto.ca/edwards/

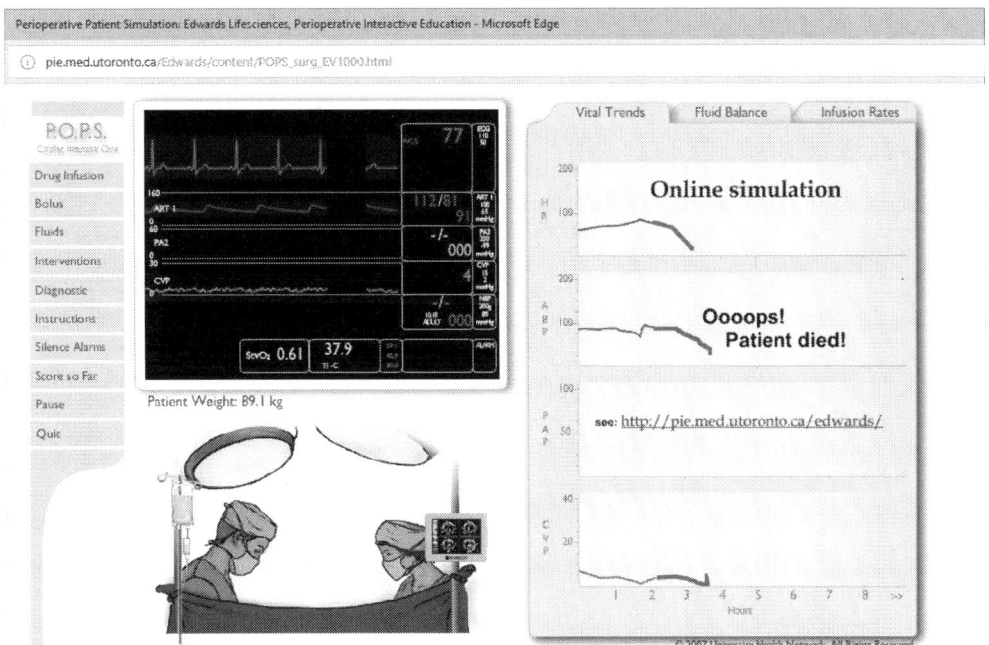

References

American Heart Association, Textbook of ADVANCED CARDIAC LIFE SUPPORT, American Heart Association, 2001

Baim and Grossman, *Cardiac Catheterization, Angiography, and Intervention*, 7th Ed., Lea and Febiger, 2006

Braunwald, Eugene, Ed., HEART DISEASE A Textbook of Cardiovascular Medicine, 5th Ed., W. B. Saunders Co., 1996

Kanu Chatterjee, The Swan-Ganz Catheters: Past, Present, and Future: A Viewpoint, Circulation. 2009;119:147-152

Crawford, Michael H., Current Diagnosis & Treatment in Cardiology, McGraw-Hill Co., 2007

Daily, E. K., and Schroeder, J. S., Techniques in Bedside Hemodynamic Monitoring, 4th Ed., C. V. Mosby Company, 1989

Darovic, G.O., Hemodynamic Monitoring: Invasive and Noninvasive Clinical Applications, 2nd Edition, W. B. Saunders Co., 1995

Johnsrude, I. S., Jackson. D. C., Et. al., *A Practical Approach to Angiography*, 2nd Ed., Little, Brown and Co., 1987

Kern, M. J., Ed., *The Cardiac Catheterization Handbook*, 6th Ed., Mosby-Year Book, Inc., 2016

OUTLINE: Right Heart Catheterization

6. EQUIPMENT
   a. RHC Indicated in cardiogenic shock
   b. Flow Directed Catheters
      i. Review Swan Ganz catheter construction and features
         (1) Monitoring Swan - 2 port
            (a) Distal - PA & wedge
            (b) Balloon port (with stopcock)
         (2) Thermo Swan - port, thermistor
            (a) Distal - PA & wedge
            (b) Balloon port (with stopcock)
            (c) Thermistor (Red cap)
            (d) Proximal - RA (blue for Ice water)
         (3) PA Watch catheter
            (a) includes additional RV monitoring port
         (4) J - curved Swan (from Subclavian)
         (5) S - curved Swan (from Femoral)
         (6) Femoral adult size = 110 cm length
   c. Guidewires - .025"
   d. Sheaths - 1 French size larger than catheter
   e. Continuous flow devices
      i. 3-5 ml/hr

7. INSERTION TECHNIQUES
   a. Review technique of Swan-Ganz insertion
      i. Flush ports
      ii. Test balloon
      iii. measure length to heart (30 cm from fem)
      iv. Observe pressures as inserting intrathoracic pressure phasic with resp.
      v. Inflate in thorax
         (1) Not in smaller veins (rupture?)
      vi. Inflate with Air
         (1) CO2 if R-L shunt present
         (2) Air embolism less traumatic
      vii. Depth markers (Roman numeral stripes)
      viii. Insertion Depth from Femoral vein
         (1) RA @ 30 cm
         (2) RV @ 50 cm.
         (3) PA @ 60 cm
   b. Precautions in Rt. Ht. Cath.
      i. palpate artery (to locate vein)
      ii. avoid nerves
      iii. avoid spasm
      iv. brisk "wiggling" movement of catheter
      v. Avoid Lidocaine in catheter
      vi. Nitroglycerine/paperverine
      vii. Reduce catheter size
      viii. Inadvertent arterial puncture
      ix. Valsalva enlarges vein (easier to stick)
      x. avoid arterial puncture
      xi. use small syringe
      xii. place small amt. Lido or Saline in
      xiii. Check blood color/pressure
      xiv. use oximeter if questionable
      xv. Verify cath position with X-ray
      xvi. flush continuously (const. flow device & pressure bag)
      xvii. double flush catheter
      xviii. flush manually & gently every few minutes
      xix. Never flush against resistance (clot?)
      xx. meticulously remove all air
      xxi. Change sterile dressings daily
      xxii. Change catheters and tubes every 2-3 days
   c. Peripheral and central access
   d. Central Venous cannulation sites
      i. Location
      ii. Indications
      iii. Relative contraindications
   e. Central Venous puncture Complications
      i. Venous air embolism
         (1) manifestations
         (2) prevention
         (3) occlude needle
         (4) Trendelenburg position, pillows
         (5) Use sheath with valve
         (6) Luer lok connections
         (7) Seal cath connections (dead enders)
         (8) Restrain pt. as necessary
         (9) don't allow IVS to go empty
   f. Diagnosis of Air embolism
      i. Ultrasound
   g. Therapy for of Venous Air embolism
      i. place in Lt. Trendelenburg position
      ii. Give 100% O2
      iii. Aspirate air via catheter
      iv. hyperbaric O2
      v. CPR- ACLS as necessary
   h. ARM VEIN CANNULATION
      i. Review RHC from arm vein by the Seldinger technique
      ii. technique
      iii. Tourniquet
      iv. Seldinger
      v. don't force/ withdraw, rotate, advance
      vi. Turn patients head
      vii. have pt. inspire deeply
      viii. partially inflate balloon
      ix. only enter well seen veins
   i. FEMORAL VENOUS CANNULATION
      i. Review anatomy of femoral area
      ii. NAVL
      iii. Femoral triangle
      iv. Rotate leg
      v. pred/drape/anesthetize
      vi. palpate FA - FV 1 cm medial

    vii. puncture
    viii. aspirate with 5 10 cc syringe with Lido in
    ix. Seldinger insertion
    x. Suture in sheath and catheter
   j. EXTERNAL JUGULAR CANNULATION
    i. Anatomy
    ii. Procedure
    iii. use of special J-tip guide
   k. INTERNAL JUGULAR CANNULATION
    i. Anatomy
    ii. procedure
    iii. Central approach
    iv. ant. medial approach
    v. Special precautions
    vi. air embolism
    vii. accidental puncture Carotids
    viii. accidental cannulation Carotid
    ix. Carotid pressure = neuro damage
    x. Doppler location method
   l. SUBCLAVIAN VEIN CANNULATION
    i. Positioning Pt.
    ii. Don't use rolled towel between scapulas
    iii. Turn pts. head contralaterally
   m. COMPLICATIONS OF SWAN-GANZ CATHETERIZATION
    i. Ventricular arrhythmia
    ii. Balloon rupture
    iii. V. Arrhythmia
    iv. Pulm. infarction
    v. Perforation of PA
    vi. Never remove inflation syringe
    vii. gradual inflation of balloon - up to but not over wedge
    viii. Knotting
    ix. Thrombosis
    x. Infection

8. HEMODYNAMICS
 a. take pressures going in RA- RV - PA - PAW
 b. "It is imperative that inflation of the balloon be performed gradually under continuous monitoring of PA pressure, and that inflation be stopped once wedge pressure is obtained
 c. Leave deflated catheter in Rt.. or Lt. PA
 d. Positioning wedge catheter
  i. inflate balloon in PA
   (1) Slowly until PAW waveform develops
   (2) Don't over wedge (rupture?)
  ii. advance if necessary
   (1) use of sterile sleeve
  iii. deep inspiration
  iv. Valsalva
  v. stiffening cath with cold saline infusion
  vi. insert .025 guide wire
  vii. change to different catheter if can't wedge
  viii. Deflate balloon when withdrawing
   (1) (can tear valves)
   ix. Inadvertent Coronary Sinus catheterization
 e. Wedge criteria
  i. Cessation of bobbing of cath tip on fluoro
  ii. appearance of "A" and "V" waves on tracing
  iii. O2 Sat >95% after withdrawing dead space
  iv. Flushing assures not damped PA
 f. Rt.. Ht. pressure monitoring.
  i. Pulm. congestion (elevated wedge)
  ii. LV diastolic and EDP pressures (preload)
  iii. Pulmonary vascular disease (gradient between PAedp and PAW)
  iv. Mitral regurgitation = large Wedged "V" waves
  v. Hemodynamically significant V waves.
  vi. end systolic atrial pressure waves at least 10 mmHg greater than the mean PAW (or 2 X wedge)
  vii. Associated with small stiff atrium which is filling with large amounts of blood during ventricular systole:
  viii. MR, MS, LV Failure, L-R shunt
  ix. Acute MR in noncompliant undilated LA
  x. V waves not necessarily large in MR
  xi. PAPi = (PA syst/PA diast.)/ RA mn
   (1) Low <0.9 = RV failure
  xii. Normal Rt.. Ht. pressures
  xiii. RA
  xiv. RV
  xv. PA
  xvi. PAW
 g. Identify Locations of catheter in normal Rt.. Ht. anatomy
  i. RA
  ii. RV
  iii. PA
  iv. PAW
 h. Identify Locations of catheter in abnormal Rt.. Ht. anatomy
  i. Coronary Sinus
  ii. ASD
  iii. VSD
  iv. PDA
  v. Pericardial Tamponade
  vi. Retrograde LA
 i. Systemic Venous O2 - SVO2
  i. Edwards SVO2 catheter
   (1) fiber optic O2 sat
  ii. Normal SVO2 70-80% sat
  iii. SVO2 < 60% low CO or O2 usage
  iv. SVO2 < 40 Critical - tissue ischemia

9. MYOCARDIAL BIOPSY
 a. EQUIPMENT
  i. Bioptomes
  ii. King - Requires Long Sheath
   (a) -disposable
   (2) Stanford - No sheath needed

                (a) -Short stiff and reusable
            (3) Kawai
                (a) -made by Terumo Co.
        iii. Sheath
            (1) Mullins
            (2) RV Biopsy
            (3) LV biopsy
        iv. Guidance
            (1) 2d Echo guidance of the bioptome
            (2) Fluoroscopic guidance
  b. INDICATIONS FOR BIOPSY
        i. graft rejection (heart transplant)
            (1) -interstitial edema and inflammation
            (2) -Lymphocyte infiltration
            (3) -Myocyte necrosis
        ii. cardiomyopathy
        iii. myocarditis
        iv. other
  c. MYOCARDIAL BIOPSY PROCEDURES
        i. Risks and contraindications for endomyocardial biopsy
            (1) bleeding disorders
            (2) thrombus dislodgement
        ii. RV & LV biopsy
            (1) preferably IV septum
            (2) RV not usually heparinized
            (3) LV usually heparinized
        iii. Approaches to biopsy
            (1) Internal jugular - RV
            (2) Femoral - RV
            (3) Femoral - LV
        iv. Precautions and risks of myo-biopsy
            (1) Perforation (0.3-0.5%)
            (2) Tamponade
            (3) Embolization (thrombus/air)
            (4) Arrhythmia
            (5) Bundle Branch Block
        v. Preservation solution
            (1) 10% formalin
            (2) 2.5% Glutaraldehyde
        vi. Handling of the biopsy samples
            (1) floating sample (fat?)
            (2) Number of samples taken = 3-5

Coronary Arteriography

INDEX: D7 - Coronary Arteriography
- 1. Equipment . . . . p. 233 - Know
- 2. Insertion Techniques . . p. 237 - Know
- 3. Hemodynamics & Damping . p. 246 - Know
- 4. Coronary Angiography . . p. 253 - Know
- 5. Other Coronary . . . p. 276 - Know
- 6. Chapter Outline . . . p. 280

1. Coronary Arteriography Equipment

420. This is a 2 stopcock manifold used for closed system coronary arteriography. Port #3 on the diagram is usually used for:
a. Catheter attachment
b. Pressure recording
c. Air zero
d. Contrast
e. Flush
f. Control syringe

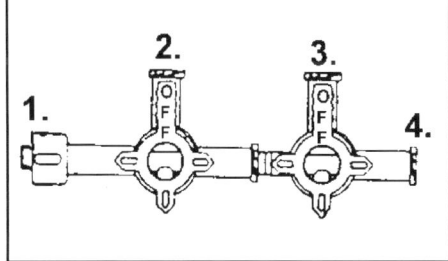
Coronary Manifold

ANSWER d. Contrast. Coronary arteriography requires frequent contrast injections. Having the contrast stopcock nearest your syringe is handy and saves time. The angiographer only turns one stopcock to fill the syringe and inject.

These closed systems allow the angiographer to fill and inject contrast repeatedly without having to remove the syringe. This minimizes the possibility of air embolism. If any bubbles are accidentally injected into the coronary system they could cause an "air lock" in the capillary bed possibly resulting in myocardial infarction.

MATCH ALL ANSWERS BELOW.
1. **CATHETER:** Judkins coronary most common.
2. **PRESSURE TRANSDUCER:** Air zero obtained from the transducer off the table.
3. **CONTRAST:** Line and bottle.
4. **CONTROL SYRINGE:** Also called a 3-ring syringe.

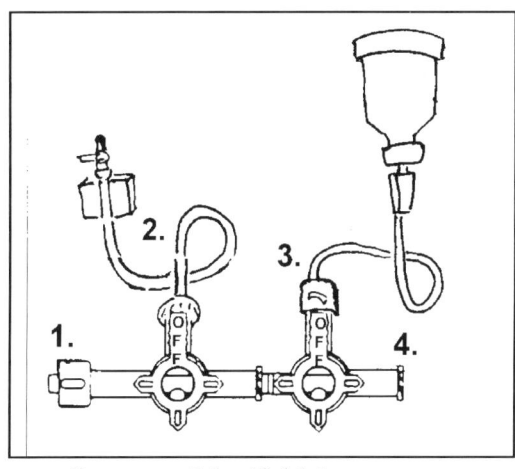
Coronary Manifold & contrast

See: Baim and Grossman, chapter on "Coronary Arteriography." **Keywords:** 2 stopcock manifold use of side ports → contrast

421. In the four-stopcock coronary manifold shown, identify the use of the side-port labeled #5 on the diagram.
a. Dye
b. Syringe
c. Waste bag
d. Transducer
e. Flush
f. Catheter

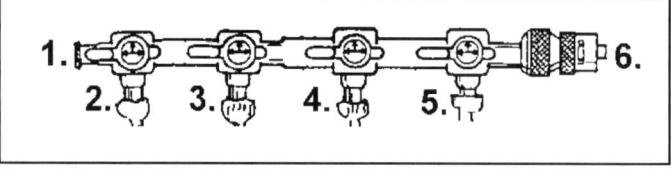
Four Stopcock Manifold setup

ANSWER d. Transducer.
BE ABLE TO MATCH ALL ANSWERS BELOW:
1. **SYRINGE:** A dye injection syringe is attached to this.
2. **WASTE BAG:** This empty IV sack is termed "waste". It receives the discarded blood and flush and prevents the cath team's exposure to blood born contaminants.

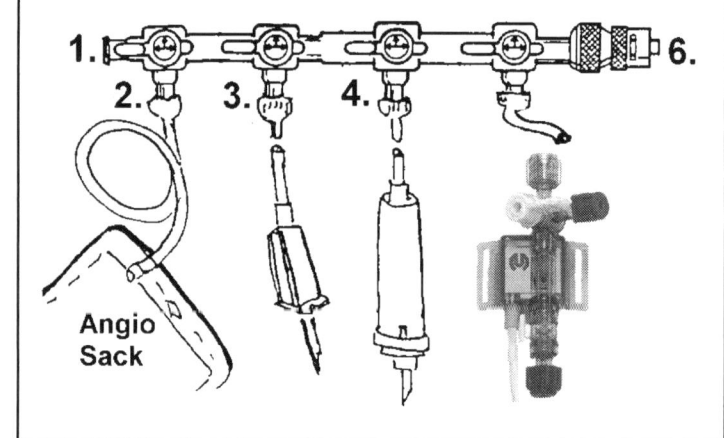
Four Stopcock Manifold setup

3. **DYE:** A dripless spike is used for dye to prevent air bubbles.
4. **FLUSH:** A macro drip spike is used for heparinized flush. This may also be connected to position #3. If pressurized flush is used it requires a special high pressure IV spike.
5. **TRANSDUCER:** Grossman recommends use of a micro-transducer here for high fidelity recording. Any movement or tipping of this transducer on-the-table will effect the zero level. For this reason an extension tube is often use to take the transducer off the table, but it may reduce the frequency response of the system.
6. **CATHETER:** A rotating adapter here allows torquing of the catheter without having to twist the manifold.
See: Baim and Grossman, chapter on "Percutaneous Approach."

422. What LEFT Judkins femoral coronary diagnostic catheter would be selected for the dilated aorta shown?
a. JR3.5
b. JR4
c. JL3.5
d. JL4
e. JL5

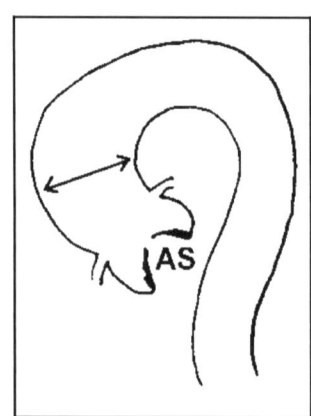
Dilated Aorta

ANSWER e. JL5 = Judkins Left coronary bend size is used for dilated aortas. The JL#4 is for an average sized aorta (4 cm bend diameter). Smaller bends are for smaller aortas or for superior angulation of the tip. Note in the middle diagram how the JR catheter angles superiorly. Larger bends are for larger aortas or for coronaries with inferior takeoff. **See:** Tilkian and Daily, chapter on "Tools for Catheterization." **Keywords:** Standard Left Judkins = JL4

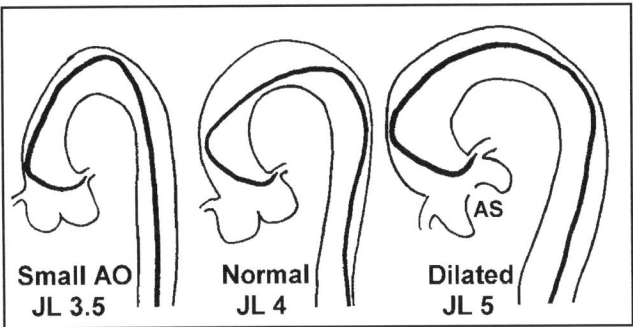

JL cath bend sizes in the Aorta

423. **In Judkins coronary catheters where is the bend size measured (e.g. JL5)?**
   a. **Tip of catheter to primary bend**
   b. **Tip of catheter to secondary bend**
   c. **Secondary bend to tertiary (3rd) bend**
   d. **Aortic root diameter**

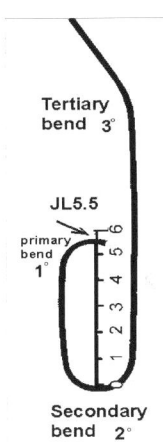

ANSWER b. Tip of catheter to secondary bend as shown. JL5 is 5 cm from tip to the 2nd bend. Both Right & Left Judkins are measured as shown between the tip (primary) and secondary bends. The JR3 is measured in cm from tip to second bend. The JR catheters have a 3rd or tertiary bend further up the shaft, while Judkins Left catheters do not. **See:** Baim and Grossman, chapter on "Coronary Arteriography."

424. **These coronary catheters resemble a family of ducks. What is the name of the largest of these catheters?**
   a. **Arani right coronary**
   b. **Arani left coronary**
   c. **Amplatz right coronary**
   d. **Amplatz left coronary**

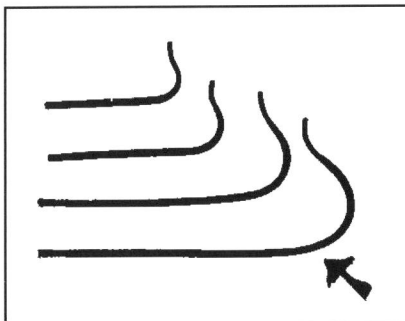

Family of coronary artery catheters

ANSWER d. Amplatz left coronary. When held up, the Amplatz shape resembles the head and bill of a "duck." The Left Amplatz coronary catheter is shown (AL). It must have a larger bend to reach across the aortic root. Whereas the right coronary catheters (AR) are smaller because the aortic arch directs the catheter along the right wall of the aorta as shown, into the RCA. The Amplatz catheter is considered to have a pre-shaped "Sones configuration" since the secondary curve sits in the aortic root like a "Sones" and arches up from the root. **See:** Company catalogs **Keywords:** Amplatz, largest → AL4

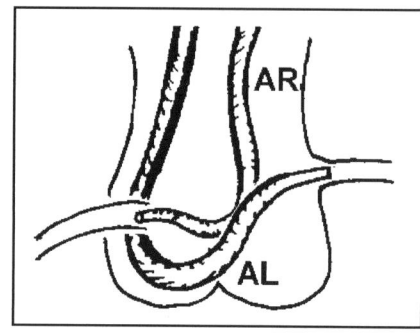
Rt. & Lt. Amplatz

425. Identify the diagnostic femoral coronary catheter bend labeled at #4 on the diagram.
   a. Amplatz Rt.
   c. Amplatz Lt.
   d. Judkins Rt.
   e. Judkins Lt.
   f. Internal mammary
   g. Multipurpose
   h. Jacky-radial

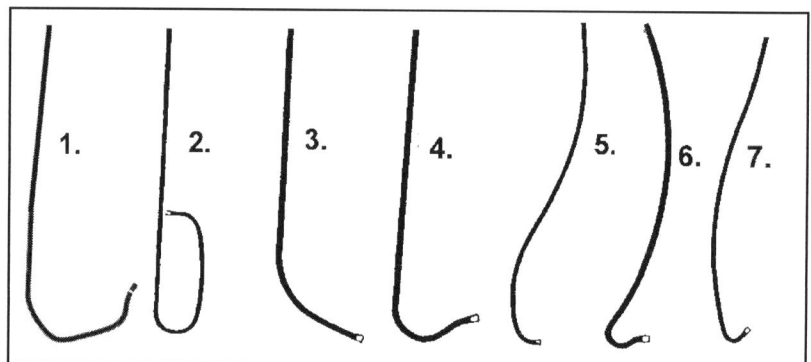
Common Femoral Coronary catheter bends

ANSWER a. Amplatz Rt. coronary. **BE ABLE TO MATCH ALL ANSWERS BELOW.**
   1. **JACKY UNIVERSAL RADIAL:** For both right and left coronary via radial approach. Similar to TIG Universal Radial catheter.
   2. **JUDKINS LT:** The "JL" catheters have a blunt reduced diameter tip with a 90° bend allowing it to enter the coronary ostium. The secondary bend provides backup support from the opposing aortic wall.
   3. **MULTIPURPOSE A2:** The "A" bend is like a hockey stick with a straight tip. The 2 refers to the two side holes (also has end hole).
   4. **AMPLATZ LT:** Single end hole braided steel catheter. Its duck bill shape fits the sinus of Valsalva.
   5. **JUDKINS RT:** Blunt reduced diameter tip with a 90° bend allowing it to enter the coronary ostium. The secondary bend is a gradual 30° that provides backup support from the opposing aortic wall.
   6. **AMPLATZ RT. (MODIFIED):** It is like the Amplatz Lt. except tighter curve radius. The Rt. and Lt. Amplatz catheters are usually displayed together. Then it is easy to distinguish the larger bends as Lt. Amplatz and the smaller as Rt. Amplatz.
   7. **INTERNAL MAMMARY:** Shaped much like a JR4 with a more acute primary bend. The hooked end allows it to hook in the LIMA and point inferiorly. It is also used for a superiorly directed RCA.
   See: Baim and Grossman, chapter on "Coronary Arteriography." **Keywords:** Types of

coronary catheters

426. Identify the coronary artery **BYPASS CATHETER** labeled at #4.
a. JR4
b. Internal mammary
c. Left coronary bypass
d. Right coronary bypass

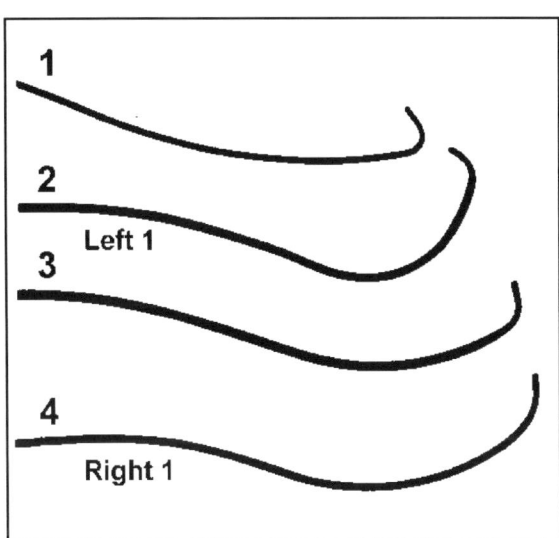
Coronary Bypass catheters

ANSWER d. Right coronary bypass catheter designed by Judkins. **BE ABLE TO MATCH ALL ANSWERS BELOW.**
1. **IMA** is like a JR catheter with a more angulated primary bend to hook into the internal mammary artery.
2. **Left coronary bypass** catheter. Similar to a cobra catheter. Designed by Judkins.
3. **Standard Judkins right** coronary catheter commonly used for bypass grafts.
4. **Right coronary bypass** catheter similar to the JR4 except with less angulated tip. Designed by Judkins.

See: King, chapter on "Angulated Views" and Co catalogs **Keywords:** Bypass catheters

2A. Insertion Techniques - Judkins Technique

427. How is the Judkins right coronary catheter manipulated into the RCA orifice? Initially position the tip of the JR4 _____ the RCA origin and then _____.
a. 2-3 cm above and pointing away from, torque clockwise 180 degrees.
b. 2-3 cm above and pointing towards, advance the catheter 2-3 cm.
c. at the same level pointing away from, torque clockwise 180 degrees.
d. 2-3 cm below and pointing towards, withdraw the catheter 2-3 cm.

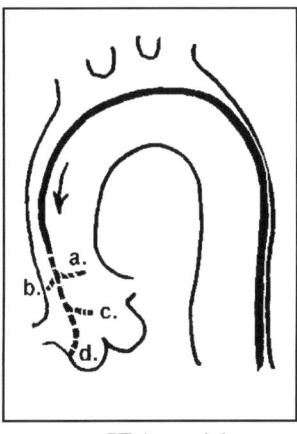
JR4 position

ANSWER a. Position the JR4 2-3 cm above and pointing away from the RCA then torque it clockwise 180 degrees. As this catheter is torqued in the aortic root, it sweeps the anterior aortic root. It springs forward in one motion - often jumping right into the RCA ostium. The secondary and tertiary (3rd) bends of the Judkins right catheter allow it to lie on the outside of the arch as it is inserted over the arch. Then when it is torqued and dives down, the secondary bend lies along the inside of the arch using it as a buttress support to direct the catheter tip towards the RCA.

See: Baim and Grossman, chapter on "Coronary Arteriography."

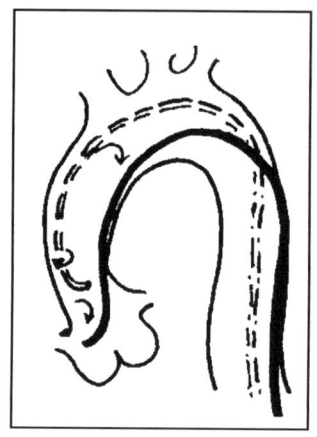
Torquing into RCA Os.

428. The problem the Judkins coronary catheter position at #4 on the diagram shows:
   a. Shepherd's hook tortuosity
   b. Too small a secondary bend size
   c. Too large a secondary bend size
   d. Selective conus injection
   e. Pressure damping

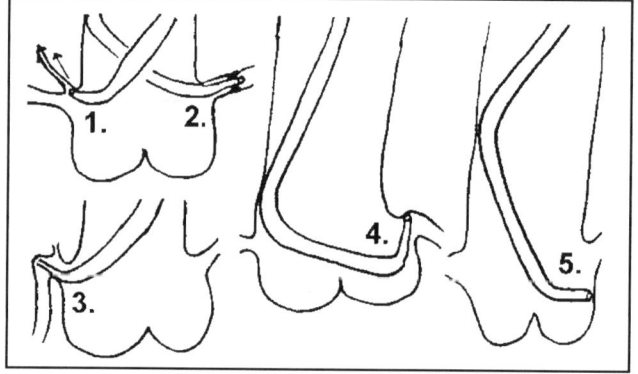
Poorly Positioned Coronary caths

ANSWER b. Too small a secondary bend size. **BE ABLE TO MATCH ALL ANSWERS BELOW.**

1. **SELECTIVE CONUS** injection: In ½ of all patients the conus has a separate origin near the RCA. It may be accidentally injected thinking it is the main right coronary artery. This could lead to a mistaken conclusion that the main RCA is occluded.
2. **PRESSURE DAMPING DUE TO WEDGING THE CATHETER** into a tight orifice or stenosis. This causes the pressure to damp out and may cause ischemia or infarction if occluded for too long. If necessary to do angiography from a damped catheter Judkins recommends pulling out within 10 seconds to prevent ischemia to the heart.
3. **SHEPHERD'S HOOK TORTUOSITY of the RCA MAY CAUSE DAMPING** or intimal dissection. This happens in PTCA where a wire and balloon catheter must pass a tortuous shepherd's hook. Because of the tight bend, they are difficult to maneuver around.
4. **TOO SMALL A SECONDARY BEND SIZE**: Note how the secondary bend is near the root. The catheter is almost doubled up. This directs the tip superiorly. Which may be OK if that is the takeoff of the artery.
5. **TOO LARGE A SECONDARY BEND SIZE**: Note how the secondary bend is high in the arch. And the tip points inferiorly. Not good for this superiorly directed left main.

See: Pepine, chapter on "Catheters...equipment." **Keywords:** Mal-positioned coronary catheters

2B. Insertion Techniques - Radial Artery Access

429. One disadvantage radial artery access has over femoral is:
a. Radial access is more difficult on obese patients
b. Radial causes more nerve damage
c. Radial has more arterial spasm
d. Radial bleeding may go unnoticed

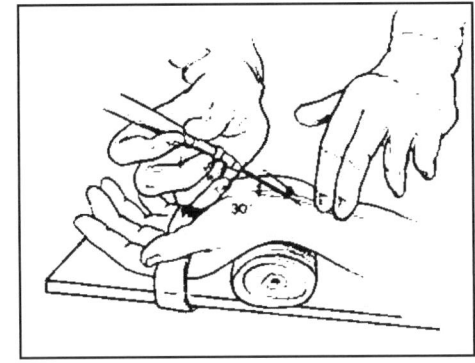
Radial artery access

ANSWER: c. Radial has more arterial spasm, although the advantages usually outweigh the spasm problem.
  Bilodeau says, "A major source of difficulty with the radial approach is vasospasm and subsequent patient discomfort that can occur with sheath placement and removal and with catheter manipulations.... The radial approach reduces access site complications, decreases length of hospital stay, and yields better outcomes at lower costs. The radial artery is superficial and easily compressible with no major nerves or veins in its vicinity, thereby reducing the risk of neuropathies or arteriovenous fistulas. Importantly, major vascular complications involving radial artery access are rare. Significant atherosclerosis of the radial and brachial artery is rare, so in this regard, transradial catheterization is particularly advantageous for patients with peripheral vascular disease or morbid obesity. In appropriately selected patients, repeat radial artery access can be performed safely and successfully....The radial approach is generally preferred by patients because of reduced periprocedural discomfort, decreased time to ambulation, and improved postprocedural quality of life. **See:** Bilodeau, et. al., "Transradial Basics", Endovascular Today, April 2010.
  See: http://www.cathlabdigest.com/articles/Transradial-Access-University-Miami

430. An obese acute MI patient is rushed to your cath lab. What type of arterial access would be best for this STEMI patient?
a. Left radial artery with Angiocath puncture through the anterior wall only
b. Right radial artery with Angiocath puncture through both walls
c. Common femoral artery with micropuncture needle puncture through both walls
d. Common femoral artery with micropuncture needle puncture through the anterior wall only

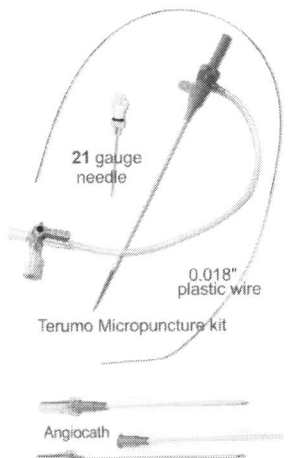

ANSWER: b. Radial artery with Angiocath puncture through both walls, because there will be less fat on the wrist for easier access and less chance of bleeding. Radial access is preferred on STEMI patients who are often loaded with antithrombotic drugs. The right radial is usually preferred over the left radial, because of most cardiologists are right handed and prefer to work on the patients right side. The Angiocath or 20 g needle with plastic cannula is used with a double wall stick after which the operator pulls the needle back to get access into the artery. Femoral sticks are usually single wall only, because it reduces the increased risk of bleeding and hematoma.

Topol says, "Because of its extremely low vascular-site complication rates, the transradial approach to PCI is clearly the method of choice in the setting of PCI with highly active anti-thrombotic regimens [such as STEMI] and early or rescue PCI after thrombolysis." **See:** Topol, chapter on "Transradial PCI for major reduction in bleeding complications"

Kern says: "There are two techniques for arterial puncture: the use of a micropuncture needle or the use of an Angiocath needle. The choice is really based on personal preference, although some data suggest that the Angiocath needle technique is easier to learn and decreases the time and number of attempts used to gain access. Using the micropuncture technique, the operator punctures the front wall of the radial artery only, whereas with the Angiocath technique, a through-and-through puncture must be used – whereby the needle is sent through the posterior wall of the radial artery. This is done to ensure access to the lumen and does not increase vascular complications as it might if the same approach were used for the femoral artery." **See:** Kern, chapter on "Arterial and Venous Access"

431. During a radial access PCI, large amounts of UFH were administered. At completion of the case, when should the radial artery sheath be pulled?
a. When the ACT falls below 150
b. Immediately after the procedure
c. After the vascular closure device is applied
d. After administration of the vasodilator cocktail
e. 90 minutes after applying the compression band

ANSWER: b. Immediately after the procedure as the compression band is applied. Because the radial artery is so close to the surface of the wrist, bleeding is easy to control. The amount of unfractionated heparin (UFH) and ACT level do not matter. The vasodilator cocktail is given at the beginning of the case, not the end.

SCAI standards say, "Hemostasis by manual compression for the radial access site is usually obtained with wristband compression devices. Sheaths are removed immediately after the procedure, regardless of anticoagulation status. The "patent hemostasis" [reverse Barbeau] technique should be used, performed by placing a pulse oximeter on the corresponding index finger [or thumb] and compressing the ulnar artery while lowering the hemostatic wristband compression pressure to the point where the plethysmographic waveform returns without pulsatile bleeding at the radial access site." **See:** SCAI expert consensus statement: 2016 best practices in the cardiac catheterization laboratory

Diagnostic Techniques: D7 - Coronary Arteriography   241

432. At the end of a radial PCI case the compression band is placed over the access site and tightened or inflated with 13 ml of air (TR band). The sheath is then pulled while you observe the site for bleeding. The compression band pressure is then adjusted using the reverse Barbeau technique and left in place for 3- 4 hours. You adjust the tightness of the band by slowly releasing band pressure:
a. Until Doppler flow begins in the palmar arch
b. Until the pulse disappears on a thumb plethysmograph
c. Until a pulse is seen on an index finger plethysmograph
d. Until the hand color pinks up and O2 sat rises above 95%

ANSWER: c. Until a pulse is seen on an index finger plethysmograph. You leave the wrist band at that pressure for 3-4 hours which allows patent hemostasis.

SCAI standards say, "Hemostasis by manual compression for the radial access site is usually obtained with wristband compression devices. Sheaths are removed immediately after the procedure, regardless of anticoagulation status. The "patent hemostasis" [reverse Barbeau] technique should be used, performed by placing a pulse oximeter on the corresponding index finger [or thumb] and compressing the ulnar artery while lowering the hemostatic wristband compression pressure to the point where the plethysmographic waveform returns without pulsatile bleeding at the radial access site." **See:** SCAI expert consensus statement: 2016 best practices in the cardiac catheterization laboratory

433. What drug cocktail may be given IA immediately after sheath insertion on transradial cases to prevent or reduce arterial spasm and forearm pain?
a. 5000 - 10000 units of heparin
b. Verapamil & nitroglycerine
c. Nitroglycerin and GP IIb/IIIa inhibitor
d. Adenosine & dipyridamole (Persantin)

ANSWER b. Verapamil & nitroglycerin. Ragosta says, "Complications of radial artery access are uncommon. The most frequent adverse event is forearm pain from radial artery spasm....Many operators locally administer a combination of drugs to prevent or reverse spasm provoked by instrumentation. The University of Virginia laboratory uses a cocktail of 1 mg verapamil combined with 100 mcg nitroglycerine in 10 mL heparinized saline. The entire 10 mL is administered as a bolus through the arterial sheath, and up to 10 doses may be used during a case. Others have used a mixture of 5 mg verapamil and 200 mcg nitroglycerine or administer topical nitrates over the site." **See:** Ragosta, chapter on "Vascular Access"

434. To reduce radial artery spasm and not significantly reduce BP what may be administered before pulling a radial sheath using a TR band?
a. Verapamil or nicardipine
b. Hydralazine or fenoldopam
c. Nitroglycerine or nitroprusside
d. Unfractionated or fractionated heparin

ANSWER: a. Verapamil or nicardipine are calcium channel blockers that prevent vasoconstriction, a common problem when removing a radial sheath. Nitro also prevents vasoconstriction but it has a great effect on the blood pressure.

435. Fifteen minutes ago after completing radial coronary arteriography, the sheath was pulled and a pressure band was applied to your patient's wrist. He was returned to the ward and states that he needs to go to the bathroom. You should tell him:
a. Stay in bed, we will have to put in a Foley catheter.
b. OK, but stay in bed, I will bring you a plastic urinal.
c. OK, get out of bed and go, just be careful of the wrist band
d. See if you can wait another 45 minutes, then we can take off the wrist band, and you can get up and go by yourself

ANSWER c. OK, get out of bed and go, just be careful of the wrist band.
Cohen says, "One of the most striking advantages of radial artery access is the free and immediate ambulation of the patient. "Transradial patients have a significantly shorter recovery period. They can get up right away and do not need assistance to go to the bathroom. Obviously, there is a decrease in nurse workload, patients go home sooner and the flow improves substantially." See: Dr. Cohen, et. al., Cath Lab Digest, Vol. 17, Sept. 01, 2009 http://www.cathlabdigest.com/articles/Transradial-Access-University-Miami

2C. Insertion Techniques: Other Methods

436. An Amplatz AL3 catheter tip is positioned at the origin of the main left coronary artery as shown. How can it be more deeply engaged?
a. Insert the catheter
b. Pull back the catheter
c. Rotate clockwise
d. Rotate counter-clockwise

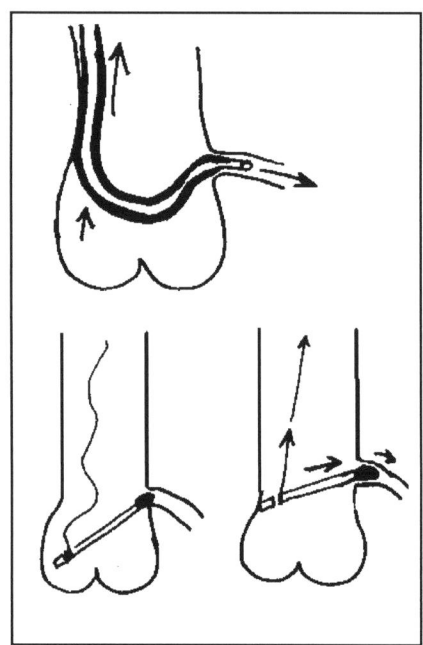

Deep Throat - Match stick analogy

ANSWER b. Pull back the catheter. This hooked (duck bill shaped) catheter tip design is inserted into the root as a "diving duck." In the root it will regain its curve. Pushing it down on the aortic cusps makes it arch up towards the coronary ostium. But, it will "deep throat" as you pull back the shaft of the catheter. Pulling more on the shaft will push the catheter tip deeper. This seems paradoxical, but can be explained by its strong "back up" against the right aortic wall. Another way to explain it is as follows:
Imagine a wooden match with the tip in the

coronary ostium and the other end tied to a string in the aortic root. Since the match is longer than the aorta is wide, as you pull the string, the match tip jams deep into the artery - "deep throats." *Never remove an Amplatz by just "pulling it out of the ostium.* This maneuver is especially hazardous with a stiff PTCA guider catheter.

To remove the deeply engaged Amplatz catheter the catheter body is ADVANCED. This sounds contradictory, but it works. This advance helps pull it out of the coronary artery by removing the backup support on the opposite wall. Then torque it to remove the tip from alignment with the coronary ostium and remove it. **See:** Baim and Grossman, chapter on "Coronary Arteriography." **Keywords:** To deep throat Amplatz → withdraw

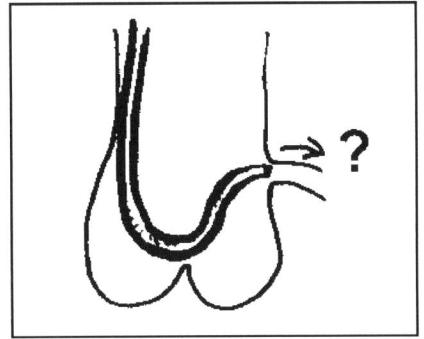
Advancing an Amplatz

437. **Which left coronary arteriography catheterization technique relies most heavily on "J-ing" and "torquing" in the aortic root, as shown?**
   a. Amplatz
   b. Multipurpose
   c. Judkins
   d. Dotter

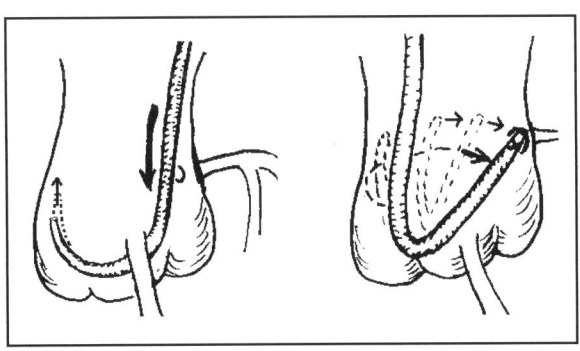
"J-ing" and "Torquing" catheter into Left Cor. Artery

ANSWER b. The multipurpose catheterization technique can be used from the groin to perform a full LV and coronary study. The multipurpose manipulations are similar to those in the Sones technique, except it uses the standard A-2 Multipurpose catheter through the femoral artery.

In the RAO view, the catheter is slid down the left coronary cusp and is J'd as it arches up the non-coronary cusp. Then the catheter is torqued until it flips to the right and the tip sits in the left coronary orifice. The catheter does not need to enter the left coronary artery completely. With the tip next to the LCA orifice (almost at right angles to it) it can still adequately inject the LCA. This is because of its 2 side-holes and large inner bore. **See:** Tilkian and Daily, CV Procedures, chapter on "Tools for Catheterization." **Keywords:** Single catheter method LV & Corns = Multipurpose & Sones

438. **Why is the patient commonly told to take a deep breath prior to coronary angiography injections?**
   a. A deep breath makes it easier to cough.
   b. A deep breath prevents Valsalva
   c. It moves the diaphragm out of the X-ray field
   d. It moves the catheter into a more selective position

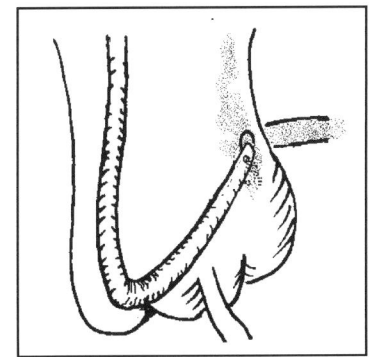
Multipurpose LCA

ANSWER c. It moves the diaphragm out of the X-ray field. The diaphragm and the spine are two dense structures that obscure X-ray penetration. Most oblique views move the heart off the spine. The deep breath lowers the diaphragm to remove it from the X-ray field.

Some patients bear down and Valsalva after taking a deep breath. This reduces venous return and coronary flow. One way to avoid the Valsalva is to have the patient continue taking in the deep breath slowly. Then their airway is always open and coronary flow will be normal. **See:** Baim and Grossman, chapter on "Coronary Arteriography." **Keywords:** Deep breath - moves diaphragm out of X-ray field

439. This is Grossman's graph showing the recommended rate of hand contrast injection during left coronary arteriography. What is the purpose of the rapid injection of dye at the end of the injection?
a. To adequately fill the vessel
b. To open up collateral or partially closed vessels
c. To prevent damping and clotting of the catheter
d. To overfill the vessel and see reflux into AO

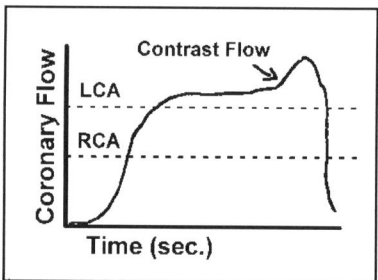

Rate of Coronary hand injection - fill the vessel completely then - - rapidly:

ANSWER d. Overfill the vessel to see reflux into AO. This will outline the coronary ostium and make ostial lesions visible. Grossman recommends that "The injection should be forceful enough to replace the blood contained in the involved vessel and cause slight but continuous reflux into the aorta. Too timid an injection allows intermittent entry of nonopaque blood into the coronary artery producing streaming... Too vigorous an injection may cause coronary dissection or excessive myocardial blushing, and too prolonged an injection may contribute to myocardial depression or bradycardia.

Injection velocity should build up gradually to match the rate of coronary flow and continue until the entire vessel is opacified and the distal vessels fill. If there is any question about the adequacy of reflux to visualize the coronary ostium a final burst of contrast may be given to eliminate any doubt about an ostial lesion. (That is the "extra reflux" bump near the end of the injection.) **See:** Baim and Grossman, chapter on "Coronary Arteriography." **Keywords:** rate of coronary angio. injection

440. If a pressure injector is used in coronary arteriography to inject the left coronary artery, it should be preset to a rate of:
a. Never use a pressure injector for coronaries
b. 300-400 psi
c. 1-2 ml/sec
d. 3-4 ml/sec

ANSWER d. 3-4 ml/sec. Grossman and Kern indicate that this is a safe way to inject coronaries and it eliminates the need for an assistant doing the injections. The angiographer can press the foot pedal to inject, manipulate the catheter, and "pan" by himself.

The flow rate needs to match the patient's normal coronary flow rate. But an average flow rate to start with in the LCA is 10 ml at 3-4 ml/sec. High pressure limit should be set to 150 PSI to avoid over-pressurizing the vessel. The RCA being smaller usually is set lower to 6 ml at 2-3 ml/sec. Note that the LCA flow and volume are almost double that of the RCA. Most labs still prefer to hand inject coronary artery arteriograms.

See: Kern, chapter on "Angiography." **Keywords:** Pressure injecting coronaries → 3-4 ml/sec

441. Internal mammary bypass grafts can be studied most easily from the _____ approach.
   a. Ipsilateral internal jugular
   b. Ipsilateral radial
   c. Contralateral internal jugular
   d. Contralateral radial

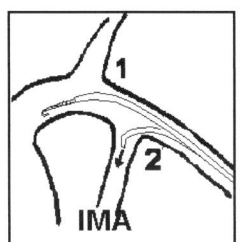

ANSWER b. Ipsilateral radial. Ipsilateral means "on the same side of the body." A term commonly used in vascular surgery. Since the internal mammary arises from the subclavian, a radial catheter goes right past it on the way into the aorta. But you have to enter the radial artery on the side where the IMA arises (ipsilateral). The guide wire must be manipulated into the left subclavian through an IMA catheter. Then the wire is withdrawn and the catheter pulled back slowly, attempting to hook the tip into the IMA. IMA's are more commonly approached from the femoral route, up the arch, to the subclavian, and IMA.

It is much more difficult to cath a RIMA from the left radial (contralateral). There is a technique described by Pepine using the Simmons sidewinder catheter. In this difficult maneuver the catheter must go down one subclavian, across the arch, and up the other subclavian to the "contralateral IMA."

See: Baim and Grossman, chapter on "Coronary Arteriography." **Keywords:** IMA study done on ipsilateral by radial approach

442. After all of a patient's internal mammary arteries are "used up" during coronary bypass, the gastroepiploic artery may be used as a single attached RCA graft. To catheterize a gastroepiploic artery bypass graft use a _____ catheter via the _____.
   a. Cobra, Superior mesenteric artery
   b. Cobra, Celiac artery and common hepatic
   c. JR4, Superior mesenteric artery
   d. JR4, Celiac artery and common hepatic

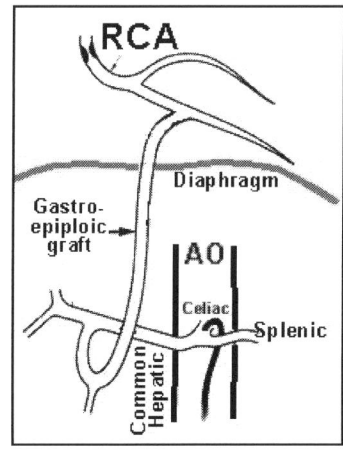

ANSWER b. Cobra, Celiac artery and common hepatic. A visceral catheter such as the Cobra is used with a .025" glidewire. The celiac artery must be catheterized, then the common hepatic (as opposed to the splenic) and then into the gastroduodenal artery. This artery may be dissected away from the stomach and tunneled through the

Gastroepiploic artery

diaphragm to reach the inferior wall of the heart and the PDA.
See: Baim and Grossman, chapter on "Coronary Arteriography." **Keywords:** Gastroduodenal artery

3. Coronary Hemodynamics & Damping

443. When attempting to catheterize the coronary artery, between test injections you should _____ .
a. Flush the catheter with heparinized saline
b. Insert a J-guide wire to minimize catheter tip trauma
c. Monitor catheter tip pressure for damping
d. Monitor catheter tip pressure for gradients

ANSWER c. Monitor catheter tip pressure for damping. When not injecting through the coronary catheter carefully monitor the tip pressure for damping. Although fluoroscopy and test injections tell you much about the position of the coronary catheter, tip pressure tells you about the physiology of what is going on there. When damping appears it indicates occlusion of the coronary orifice and obstruction to coronary flow. It is time to pull the catheter back. **See:** Baim and Grossman, chapter on "Coronary Arteriography." **Keywords:** Monitor for damping

444. During coronary arteriography "diastolic damping" or "coronary artery wedge", as seen in the diagram, is also termed:
a. Reduced frequency response
b. Increased frequency response
c. Arterialization
d. Ventricularization

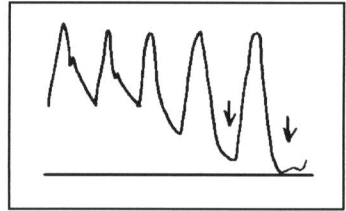
Diastolic damping

ANSWER d. Ventricularization. The normal triangular arterial waveform resembles LV - hence the term "ventricularization." However, there are major differences. Anytime the diastolic pressure falls below the normal diastolic level may be "ventricularization." The ventricularized systole may be lower than the LV systolic - especially if the catheter is in the RCA (RV capillary pressure is lower). Here the catheter is wedged into the coronary orifice. It occludes the coronary artery and cuts off blood flow, even though there is this dramatic waveform.

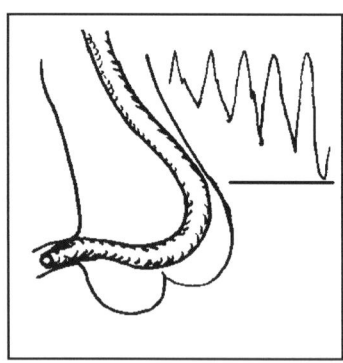
"Ventricularization"

Ventricularization reflects the ventricular pressure because the coronary capillaries pass through the LV myocardium that forcefully contracts on them.

Ventricularization is analogous to having a garden hose with a nozzle shut off - no flow; then driving back and forth over the hose with a car dramatically increasing the water pressure both upstream and downstream. Similarly, the coronary capillaries are being "smashed" by LV contraction. **See:** Baim and Grossman, chapter on "Coronary

Arteriography." **Keywords:** Coronary wedge = diastolic damping = ventricularization

445. These pressures seen on the monitor are taken through a JR4 catheter as it is manipulated into the coronary ostium. Identify the pressure pattern seen at #4 on the diagram.
a. Ventricularization
b. Reduced pressure damping
c. LV (retrograde across valve)
d. High frequency damping (incomplete damping) as from contrast in the catheter.

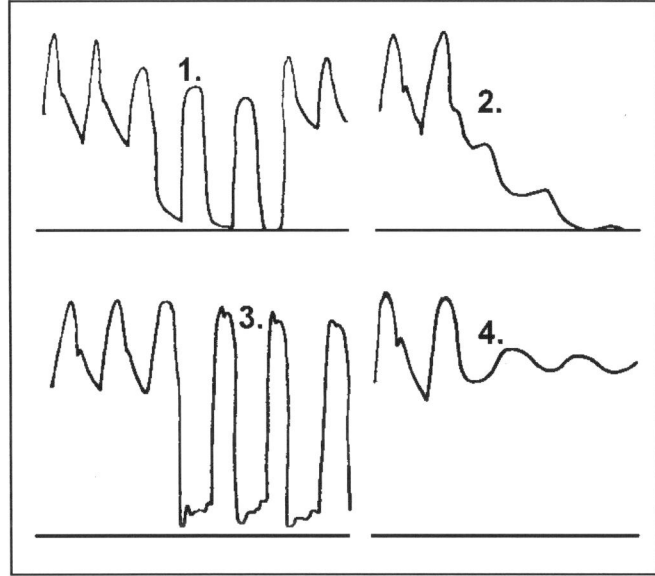

Types of coronary catheter DAMPING

ANSWER d. High frequency damping (incomplete damping) as from contrast in the catheter. **BE ABLE TO MATCH ALL ANSWERS BELOW.**
1. **VENTRICULARIZATION:** Arterial pressure mimics damped LV.
2. **REDUCED PRESSURE DAMPING:** Pressure falls off as the tip is occluded and does not transmit pressure to the transducer.
3. **LV (RETROGRADE ACROSS VALVE):** Catheter advanced across aortic valve into LV.
4. **REDUCED HIGH FREQUENCY DAMPING (CONTRAST):** Phasic pressure is smoothed out as the catheter lumen size is reduced due to clot, partial occlusion, or viscous fluid such as contrast or blood in the lumen.
See: Baim and Grossman, chapter on "Coronary Arteriography." **Keywords:** Coronary wedge = diastolic damping = ventricularization

446. You are monitoring the pressures during coronary arteriograms, and you note the ECG and the aortic pressure drop as shown in the diagram. What would you say to the catheterizing physician?
a. "V. tach. on ECG"
b. "Ventricularization"
c. "Zeroes please"
d. "Damping"

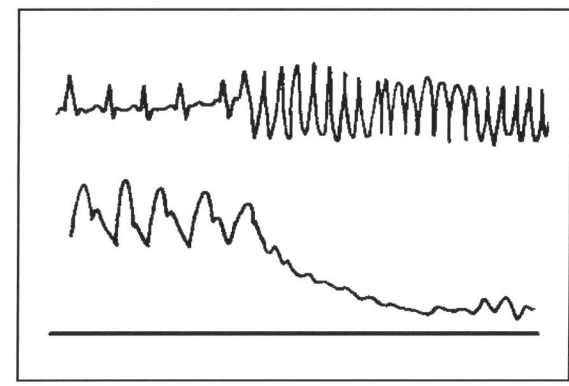

Monitoring ECG and coronaries

ANSWER a. This rapid V. Tach. is termed "Torsade De Pointes." It is a particularly lethal form of V. Tach which leads to V. Fib. Any very rapid ventricular tachycardia, like this may cause cardiac arrest. Note the BP on the diagram falls to zero. The patient will only remain conscious for 10 seconds. Instruct the patient to COUGH REPEATEDLY to prolong his conscious state. Then prepare the emergency treatment, which is immediate defibrillation. Let the patient go "out", then shock him. If the patient remains conscious then follow the less emergent "Conscious V. Tach." algorithm.

The precordial thump is now only recommended in VF/VT when a monitor and defibrillator are NOT available.
See: ACLS **Keywords:** Monitoring V. Tach./Fib

447. During right coronary angiography with contrast a patient's ECG becomes asystolic in all leads and the BP falls dramatically. Initial therapy should be to:
 a. Have the patient repeatedly cough
 b. Have the patient Valsalva
 c. Thump his chest
 d. Defibrillate

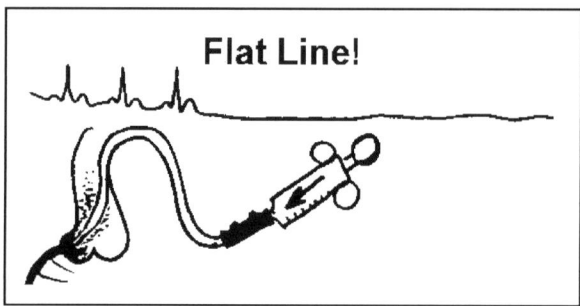
Asystole during RCA angiography

ANSWER a. Have the patient repeatedly cough. The cough should be taught to all patients undergoing coronary arteriography. Have them cough repeatedly whenever there is cessation of blood flow. It is a form of self induced CPR. Patients may remain conscious for several minutes coughing repeatedly that would otherwise have gone unconscious.

Also, the cough compresses the heart enough to squeeze out toxic dye from the coronaries and bring in fresh blood to the heart. Usually the ECG resumes and the patient comes back with a bradycardia and then normal sinus rhythm.

Sones had his first coronary arteriogram patient cough when he went asystolic. The cough brought him around. It has been an effective tradition ever since.

Defibrillation will not convert a patient in asystole (unless it is "fine VT"). There is no reentry loop to "convert." Atropine premedication may prevent bradycardia or short periods of asystole. **See:** ACLS, chapter 1. **Keywords:** Cough

448. Why might a patient go "asystolic" following RCA contrast injection?
 a. SA and AV nodal ischemia
 b. Toxic effect of iodine on epithelium
 c. "Deep throated" catheter-induced spasm
 d. Secondary adenosine liberation into right heart

ANSWER: a. SA and AV nodal ischemia and dye toxicity from the RCA injection can stop the automaticity of these nodes. There is no oxygen in contrast. Prolonged injections can deprive the SA and AV nodes for long enough to result in ischemia and dysfunction leading to asystole. One study bubbled O2 through contrast before injecting. It helped.
See: Grossman, chapter on "Complications.." **Keywords:** SA & AV node ischemia=asystole

449. You are monitoring the ECG and pressures during coronary injection with Renografin 76. With these depressed ST segments and pressure changes you should tell the catheterizing physician:

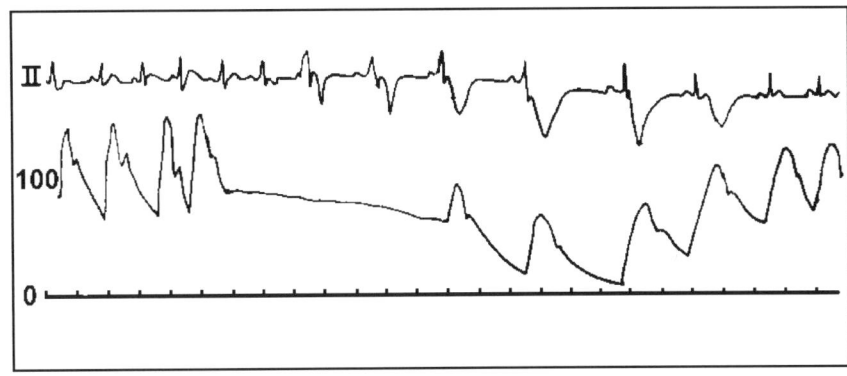

Lead II, ECG & pressure changes during coronary angio.

a. Nothing. It is a typical left coronary injection.
b. Nothing. It is a typical right coronary injection.
c. "Damping."
d. "Ventricularization."

ANSWER b. Nothing. It is a typical right coronary injection. Not used much anymore high osmolar contrast with RCA injection the ST segments depress markedly in the inferior leads. The flat pressure line occurs because the pressure stopcock is closed during injection. Mild transient hypotension and bradycardia are typical of RCA injection. Remember the SA and AV nodes usually arise from the RCA. Note that the pressure seems to be returning towards normal. Most experienced practitioners expect these transient ECG and pressure changes. So don't get too excited unless the BP doesn't come back within 15-20 seconds. These changes can be minimized by using the more expensive low-osmolar or non-ionic contrast materials.
See: Baim and Grossman, chapter on "Coronary Arteriography." **Keywords:** RCA injection → ST depression, bradycardia, mild hypotension

450. What should you closely monitor during contrast injections during coronary arteriography?
a. ECG & AO pressure changes
b. ECG & venous pressure changes
c. O2 saturation & AO pressure changes
d. O2 saturation & venous pressure changes

ANSWER: a. ECG & AO pressure changes as in the previous question. Different ST segment changes occur depending on which coronary artery is injected. Also, observe the ECG for heart rate changes (bradycardia) and arterial pressure changes (hypotension). These changes are more exaggerated than the mild changes seen with newer non-ionic and low-osmolar contrast agents. **See:** Baim and Grossman, chapter on "Coronary Arteriography." **Keywords:** Ionic dye, watch ECG & AO pressure

451. What type of angiography is probably being done here using Renografin 76? Note the elevated ST segments and pressure changes.
  a. Left coronary artery
  b. Right coronary artery
  c. Native IMA
  d. Bypass graft to PDCA

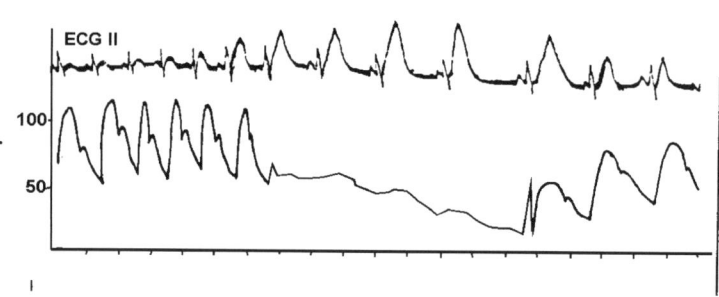

ECG & Aorta during coronary angiography

ANSWER a. With left coronary artery (LCA) injection the ST segments peak markedly in the inferior leads when using low-osmolar contrast. Mild transient hypotension and bradycardia are typical of these coronary angiographic injections. During contrast injection, when the stopcock is turned mid- tracing, no pressure is recorded. After injection stops the pressure seems to be returning towards normal. Most experienced practitioners expect these transient ECG and pressure changes. So don't get too excited unless the BP doesn't come back within 15-20 seconds. These changes can be minimized by using the more expensive low-osmolar or non-ionic contrast materials.
See: Baim and Grossman, chapter on "Coronary Arteriography." **Keywords:** LCA injection → ST elevation, bradycardia, mild hypotension

452. Which of the following are TRUE about coronary artery pressure damping? (Check 3 below.)
  a. Damping may cut off blood flow to an area of heart.
  b. Damping may lead to coronary artery spasm due to irritation of the artery.
  c. Damping may lead to tipping up a plaque in an ostial lesion.
  d. Damping may lead to clot formation in the catheter tip.
  e. Damping is allowed with side-hole catheters

ANSWERS: a, b, & c.
a. TRUE: CUTS OFF BLOOD FLOW TO THE HEART: When the catheter occludes the coronary orifice it cuts off blood flow to that area. This may lead to ischemia, injury, arrhythmia, etc.
b. TRUE: MAY CAUSE CORONARY ARTERY SPASM: Irritation of the coronary ostia (especially the right coronary) makes it prone to spasm. Nitroglycerin may help.
c. TRUE: MAY TIP UP A PLAQUE IN AN OSTIAL LESION: Damping means you are occluding the coronary orifice. If the orifice is tight anyway and has an atherosclerotic lesion as in ostial lesions, the catheter tip contact may tip a plaque leading to coronary occlusion.
d. FALSE: LEADS TO CLOTS FORMING IN THE CATHETER TIP: This is possible but not commonly seen. Contrast itself acts as an anticoagulant, so clotting seldom happens in coronary catheters which are flushed frequently. But, catheter occlusion may lead to clot formation especially in long-term small-bore catheters which are not flushed frequently.
e. FALSE: Although the pressure damping may disappear, you are no longer monitoring coronary pressure, and you may dissect. Actually if the damping remains with a side-hole

catheter, you probably have a clot in your catheter obstructing catheter pressure and flow. **See:** Baim and Grossman, chapter on "Coronary Arteriography."

453. Coronary artery damping is far more common when catheterizing the RCA. Which of the following are reasons why the RCA more commonly damps? (Select 3 from below.)
   a. The RCA is smaller in size than the LCA
   b. The RCA is more prone to spasm
   c. The JR4 catheter has a smaller inside diameter
   d. The conus artery is often mistaken for the RCA
   e. The RCA has more smooth muscle than the LCA

   ANSWERS: a, b, & d.
a. YES: The RCA is smaller in size than the LCA. This makes the catheter occlude the orifice easier.
b. YES: The RCA is more prone to spasm. The first inch of the RCA seems prone to spasm that can narrow the RCA size and make the catheter occlude easier.
c. NO: The JR4 catheter has the same inside diameter (not smaller) as the JL4.
d. YES: The conus artery is often mistaken for the RCA. It often arises from a separate origin in the right coronary cusp. It is a small artery which is easily damped.
e. NO. There is no additional smooth muscle in the RCA.
See: Baim and Grossman, chapter on "Coronary Arteriography." **Keywords:** RCA damping more common because...

454. This patient's JR4 diagnostic coronary catheter always damps when inserted into the coronary orifice. How can selective coronary angiograms still be taken with this catheter?
   a. It is too dangerous to do RCA selective injections.
   b. Do aortic root flood injection with a pigtail catheter.
   c. Do quick selective injections, then immediately pull out.
   d. Cut a side hole in the diagnostic catheter to remove damping.

ANSWER c. Do quick selective injections then immediately pull out. Note the diagram which shows ventricularization followed immediately by coronary angiography and immediate pullout of

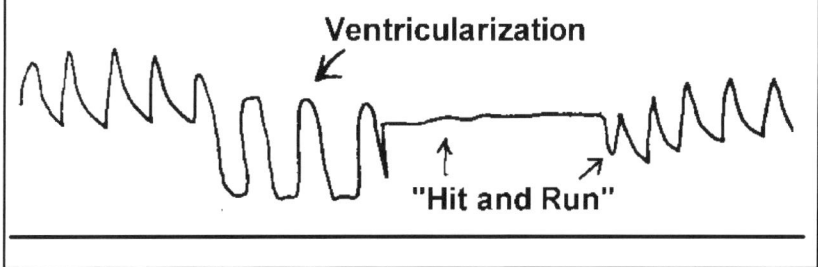

Damped pressure with injection and quick pullout

the catheter - "Hit and Run." An alternative method is to do cusp injections, where the catheter tip does not enter the coronary orifice.
a. NO: IT IS TOO DANGEROUS TO DO RCA SELECTIVE INJECTIONS - Grossman says if you are cautious and quick you can continue with selective injections.

b. NO: Aortic root flood injections are non-selective, use lots of dye and do not adequately visualize the individual coronary arteries.

c. YES: DO QUICK SELECTIVE INJECTIONS THEN IMMEDIATELY PULL OUT - make cautious small injections in the damped position and pull the catheter out immediately after each injection. *Never make vigorous injections in a damped vessel. It may dissect the vessel and lead to severe complications!* **CUSP INJECTIONS** may also be done - injecting with the catheter tip in the sinus of Valsalva, but not actually in the vessel. This usually allows enough contrast to adequately opacify the vessel.

d. NO: CUT A SIDE HOLE IN THE DIAGNOSTIC CATHETER TO REMOVE DAMPING - This works in a PTCA guider catheter, but not with a diagnostic catheter. Cutting a side-hole only masks the pressure, making it look like aortic pressure while the tip pressure is still damped.

See: Baim and Grossman, chapter on "Coronary Arteriography."

455. Which diagnostic test uses a pressure wire to measure the ability of the coronary vascular bed to maintain coronary perfusion pressures distal to a stenosis during maximum vasodilation?
a. Pressure Gradient Ratio (PGR)
b. Hyperemic Pressure Ratio (HPR)
c. Fractional Flow Reserve (FFR)
d. Coronary Flow Reserve (CFR)

ANSWER c. Fractional Flow Reserve (FFR) is the ratio of distal to proximal pressures during hyperemia. Normally the coronary pressures should be the same as you move the wire down an artery. But, when you cross a lesion a gradient will occur. This is accentuated by adenosine, which increases the flow and the gradient. The ratio of distal to proximal pressures is the FFR. Don't confuse this with coronary flow reserve (CFR) which measures hyperemic flow using the Doppler flo-wire. **See:** Braunwald, chapter on "Coronary Blood Flow and Myocardial Ischemia"

456. What does this FFR recording indicate about the LAD lesion tested?
a. .78 lesion is critical (treat)
b. .78 lesion is not critical
c. .82 lesion is critical (treat)
d. .82 lesion is not critical

ANSWER d. 0.82 lesion is not critical if the FFR is above 0.80. The lower distal pressure mean bottoms out at 78 mmHg with adenosine. The AO

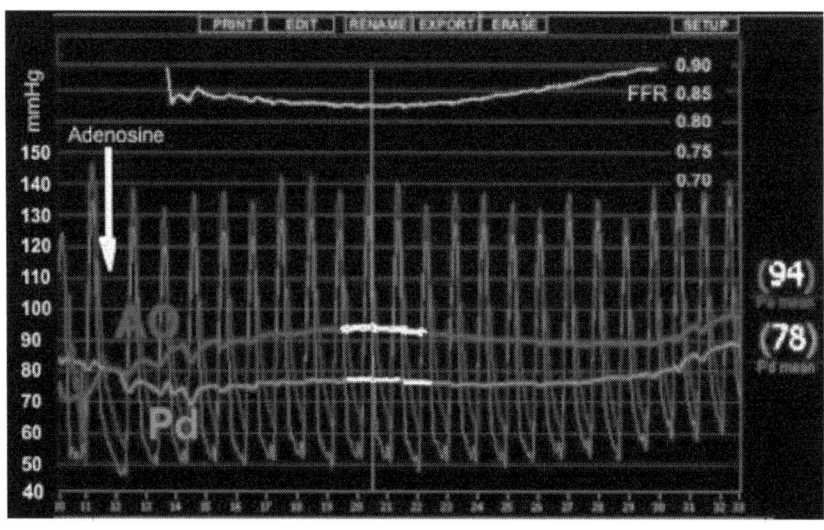

mean at the tip of the guider catheter at that time is 94 mmHg. The ratio of the 2 pressures is the FFR = 78/94 = 0.84 which is above the 0.80 cutoff for normal. The yellow line on top shows the instantaneous FFR, with 0.82 being the lowest. This suggests that the lesion crossed is physiologically insignificant and need not be treated. Note that zero supression is applied to the pressure scale, to make the zero line 40 mmHg. This effectively amplifies the pressures and makes them easier to read.

4. Coronary Angiography

457. Which left coronary artery is nearest the backbone in most oblique X-ray views?
a. LAD
b. LAO
c. Circumflex
d. PDCA

ANSWER c. Circumflex. Since the LAD and circumflex coronary vessels appear overlapping in angiography, it is often difficult to distinguish the LAD from the circumflex coronary artery. Anatomically the circumflex runs around the base of the heart near the backbone. In all oblique views the *"The CIRCUMFLEX is nearest the backbone, and the LAD nearest the sternum."* So the trick of distinguishing the circumflex is to find the backbone. The trick in finding the LAD is finding the sternum. In RAO views the backbone appears on the left. In LAO views it is on the right side of the frame. **See:** Braunwald, chapter on "Coronary Arteriography." **Keywords:** Coronary views, circumflex nearest backbone

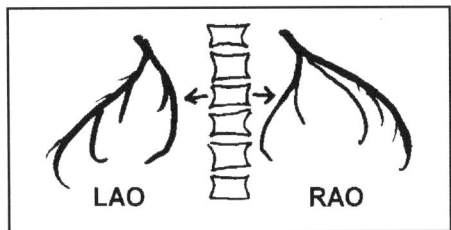
Circumflex nearest Backbone

458. How should you orient yourself to angulated coronary angiographic views? Orient yourself as if you are looking _____.
a. From the X-ray tube
b. Through the II or flat plate detector
c. From the feet of the patient
d. Through the patient's eyes

ANSWER b. As if looking through the image intensifier. For example, if you shoot an LAO caudal view. This angiogram is a short axis view, and viewed as if you were at the apex of the heart looking down the LV "barrel." In LAO caudal the image intensifier (I.I.) is positioned above the LV apex, left oblique and caudally. It is as if the I.I. were a "tube" you look through into the heart. What you see through the "tube" is what the angiogram shows. **See:** Baim and Grossman, chapter on "Coronary Arteriography." **Keywords:** View angulated

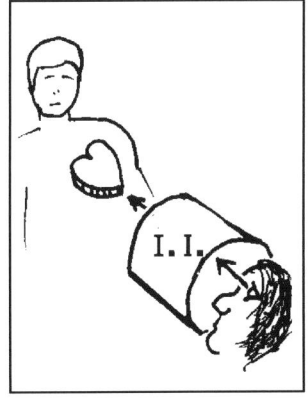
Viewing through I.I.

angiograms as if looking through the I.I.

459. What is the best radiologic view to image the diagonal -
LAD bifurcation as shown.
a. 30 degree LAO, 20 degree cranial
b. 30 degree LAO, 20 degree caudal
c. 30 degree RAO, 20 degree cranial
d. 30 degree RAO, 20 degree caudal

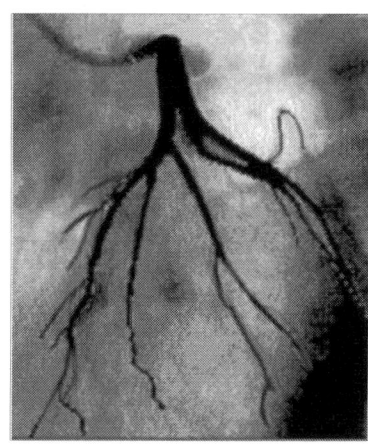
Diagonal - LAD bifurcation

ANSWER a. 30 degree LAO, 20 degree cranial. When selecting imaging views select ones which are perpendicular to the plane being imaged. Since the diagonals fan out across the anterior lateral wall, LAO-cranial is perpendicular.

Most LAO views of the left coronary system are shot with cranial angulation. These views are perpendicular to the long axis of the heart. An exception to this rule is the "spider view" which is an LAO caudal view.

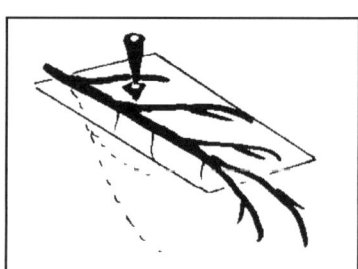
Cranial RAO for LAD - Diag. bifurcation

Left Cor. Imaged	Best Angio View
LCA orifice	20 deg. LAO
Circ. branches	30 deg. RAO / Caudal
Distal LAD	30 deg. RAO / Caud. or Cr.
Prox. LAD / Diag.	30 deg. LAO / Cr.
Bifurcation LAD/Cx.	30 deg. LAO / Cr. or (caud.-spider)
Bifurcation LAD/Cx.	20 deg. RAO / 15 Caud.

See: Pepine, chapter on "Coronary Arteriography."

460. In an individual with a horizontal heart what fluoroscopic angulated view best defines the area where the left main coronary artery bifurcates into the LAD and circumflex coronary arteries?
a. Cranial RAO
b. Cranial LAO
c. Caudal RAO
d. Caudal LAO

ANSWER d. Caudal LAO. The horizontal heart may have LAD - Circ. bifurcations in the horizontal plane. These are often poorly seen in standard views. The "spider" view is an angulated caudal view that can get under this plane. The anterior LV arteries clearly fan out as they course toward the viewer and down the heart toward the apex.

The heart may be made more horizontal by having

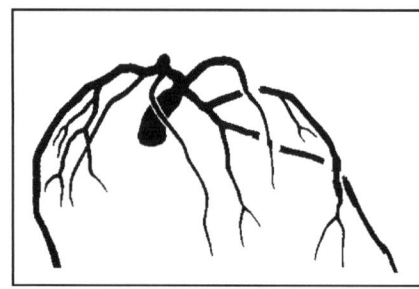
"Spider" view

the patient blow all the air out of his lungs. This raises the diaphragm and pushes the cardiac apex up - to a more horizontal position.
See: Baim and Grossman, chapter on "Coronary Arteriography." **Keywords:** Horizontal heart left main bifurcation → use spider view

BOTH QUESTIONS BELOW REFER TO THIS DIAGRAM.

461. Identify the location of the coronary lesion seen in this "spider" coronary arteriography view.
   a. Bifurcation of circumflex
   b. Bifurcation of LAD
   c. Proximal circumflex
   d. Distal LAD
   e. Distal diagonal

462. Identify the triangle seen at #5 in this "spider" view.
   a. Vein graft marker
   b. Kinked catheter
   c. Collateral to RCA
   d. Obtuse marginal artery
   e. Posterior descending artery

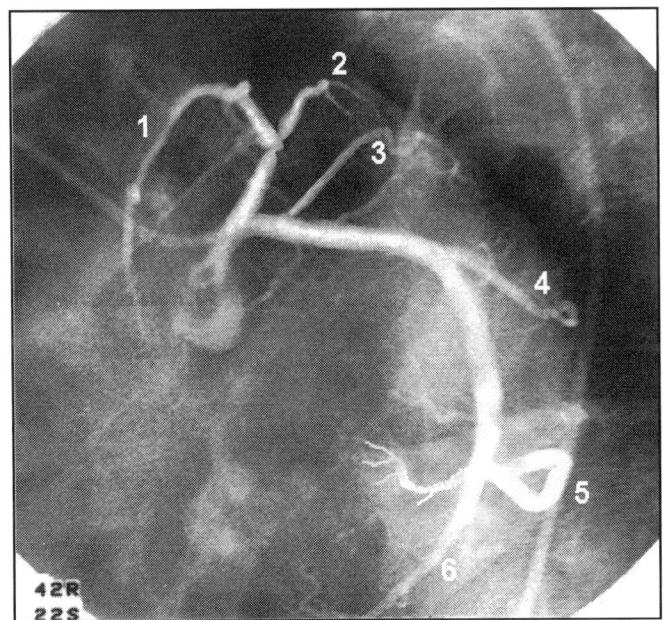
Spider View of LCA

461. ANSWER b. Bifurcation of LAD. The LAD is the large trunk arising vertically, in this view, from the main left coronary artery. As it bifurcates into mid-LAD and diagonal branches, the artery appears "pinched." This type of bifurcation lesion (type B) is moderately difficult to angioplasty because dilating one branch may occlude the other branch. A double wire or kissing balloon technique, where the other branch is protected, may prevent this. Note the three leaf clover appearance of this bifurcation lesion in the LAO cranial view. The circumflex branch is large. **BE ABLE TO MATCH ALL ANSWERS BELOW.** Arteries shown are:
   1. LAD
   2. DIAGONAL branch of LAD
   3. 1st obtuse marginal branch of circumflex
   4. 2nd obtuse marginal branch of circumflex
   5. 3rd obtuse marginal branch of circumflex
   6. Distal circumflex coronary artery

See: Baim and Grossman, chapter on "Coronary Arteriography."
Keywords: Spider view bifurcation lesion

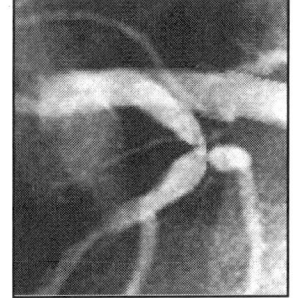
Cranial view with Bifurcation lesion

462. ANSWER d. Obtuse marginal artery. When an artery is directed toward the viewer in these "down the barrel" spider views, arteries may make unusual patterns, such as circles, triangles, or a bright dot. This is the large obtuse marginal branch of the large circumflex

coronary artery. The same patient is shown in the next question. Note the bifurcation lesion shown. This is seen better in the next diagram at #6. **See:** Baim and Grossman, chapter on "Coronary Arteriography." **Keywords:** Spider view bifurcation lesion

BOTH QUESTIONS BELOW REFER TO THIS DIAGRAM.

463. What coronary view is shown in this left coronary arteriogram?
  a. RAO cranial
  b. RAO
  c. RAO caudal
  d. LAO
  e. LAO caudal

464. Estimate the percent stenosis of the lesion shown at #2?
  a. 50%
  b. 75%
  c. 90%
  d. 99%

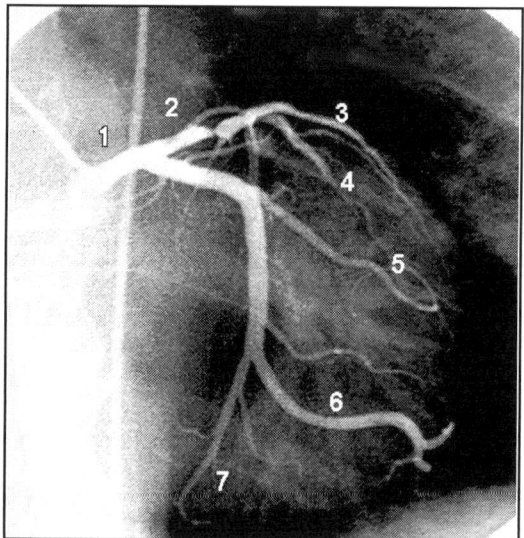

Left Coronary artery angiogram

463. ANSWER c. RAO caudal. Note that the apex points to the right (RAO) and the backbone is on the left. In this view, the heart apex is directed superiorly, and the circumflex system is seen beneath the LAD indicating a caudal view.
BE ABLE TO MATCH ALL ANSWERS BELOW.
  1. Main left coronary artery
  2. LAD
  3. Distal LAD
  4. 1st diagonal branch
  5. 1st obtuse marginal branch
  6. 3rd obtuse marginal branch of circumflex
  7. Distal circumflex coronary artery, in AV groove
See: Baim and Grossman, chapter on "Coronary Arteriography." **Keywords:** ID RAO caudal view

464. ANSWER d. 99%. The lesion is so tight only a thread of contrast is able to pass. These lesions are also termed "sub-total." The other half of this bifurcation lesion is obscured by the larger LAD artery.
See: Baim and Grossman, chapter on "Coronary Arteriography." **Keywords:** RAO grade 99% lesion of LAD

BOTH QUESTIONS BELOW REFER TO THIS DIAGRAM.

465. What type of catheter is being used in this angiogram?
   a. Judkins right coronary
   b. Judkins left coronary
   c. Amplatz right coronary
   d. Multipurpose

466. What defect is seen in this angiogram?
   a. Mainstem LCA lesion
   b. Subtotal diagonal lesion
   c. Proximal LAD occlusion
   d. Proximal circumflex occlusion

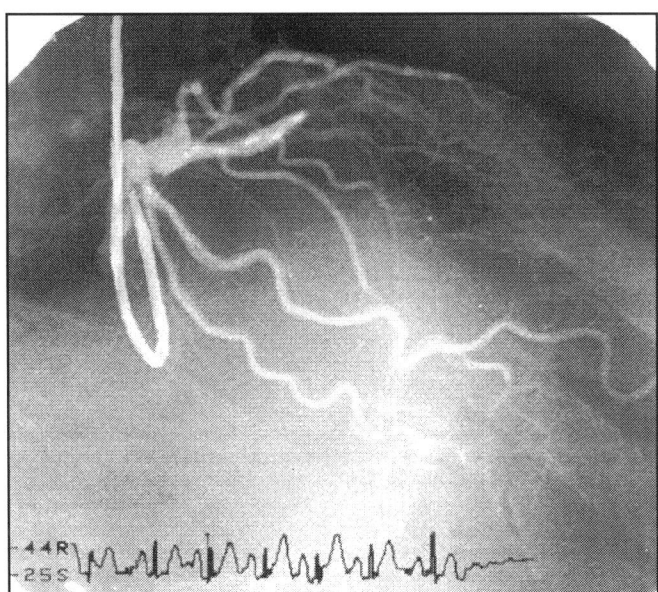
RAO cranial, Left Coronary artery angiogram

465. ANSWER d. Multipurpose or Amplatz Left coronary catheter. The catheter loop below the ostium is characteristic of a multipurpose or Sones catheter. The catheter is looped in the aortic root into a hook shape and the tip directed superiorly into the coronary ostium. **See:** Baim and Grossman, chapter on "Coronary Arteriography."
Keywords: Multipurpose catheter

466. ANSWER c. Proximal LAD occlusion. The stump of a large artery is seen pointing towards the apex. In this cranial view the diagonal branches are rotated up behind the blocked LAD. This RAO caudal view rotates the circumflex and diagonal arteries below the LAD. The LAD stump is clearly seen along the superior border of the LV in the RAO caudal view. There appears to be some collateral flow to the distal LAD. **See:** Baim and Grossman, chapter on "Coronary Arteriography."
Keywords: LAD occlusion

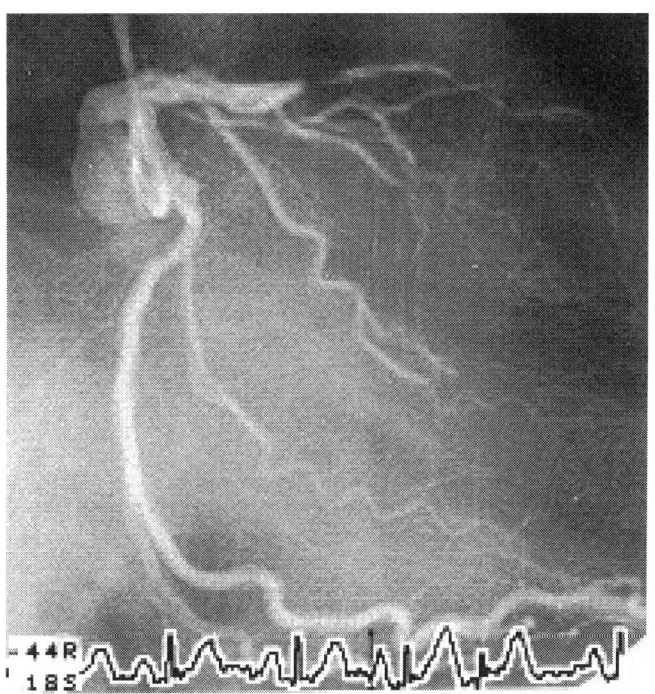
Multipurpose in LCA angio, 4° RAO caudal view

467. The coronary lesion shown on the diagram at #3 is:
a. LAD → RCA (PDCA) collateral
b. Circumflex → posterior lateral (RCA) collateral
c. Main stem stenosis
d. Circumflex stenosis
e. Diagonal stenosis
f. LAD stenosis

Coronary arteriogram

ANSWER e. Diagonal stenosis. This is a standard RAO left coronary arteriogram. **BE ABLE TO MATCH ALL ANSWERS BELOW.**
   1. Main stem stenosis
   2. Circumflex stenosis
   3. Diagonal stenosis
   4. LAD stenosis
   5. LAD → RCA (PDCA) collateral. The LAD can wrap around the apex like this to provide collateral to the PDCA (or vice versa). This LAD is thus supplying the entire ventricular septum. Since the LAD and main-stem LCA both have stenosis it would be very unusual to find the LAD helping the RCA like this. The RCA would be more likely to provide collateral to the LAD.
   6. Circumflex → Posterior lateral (RCA) collateral. The circumflex can grow collateral to the posterior lateral branches of the RCA (or vice versa).
See: Braunwald, chapter on "Coronary Arteriography." **Keywords:** Coronary lesions, RAO, RCA

468. The coronary lesion shown on the diagram at #1 is:
a. Acute marginal stenosis
b. PDCA stenosis
c. Posterior lateral stenosis
d. Conus → LAD collateral
e. Acute marginal → circ. collateral

ANSWER a. Acute marginal stenosis. This is a standard RAO right coronary arteriogram.
BE ABLE TO MATCH ALL ANSWERS BELOW.
   1. Acute marginal stenosis
   2. PDCA stenosis
   3. Posterior lateral stenosis

Coronary arteriogram

   4. Conus → LAD collateral. The conus coronary frequently collateralizes to the LAD across the RV outflow tract (or vice versa). Collateral vessels that develop usually grow in from another system supplying an adjacent area. The LAD is probably totally obstructed at the origin.

See: Braunwald, chapter on "Coronary Arteriography." **Keywords:** Coronary lesions: RAO, RCA

469. **The coronary lesion shown on the diagram at #3 is:**
a. Circumflex stenosis
b. LAD stenosis
c. LAD → PDCA division of RCA
d. Circumflex → posterior lateral branch of RCA collateral
e. LAD → PDCA branch of RCA collateral

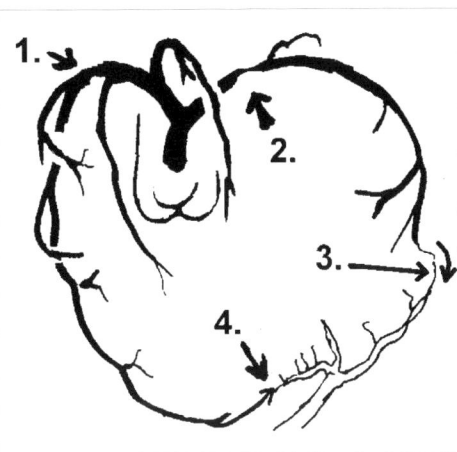
Coronary arteriogram

ANSWER d. Circumflex → posterior lateral branch of RCA collateral. This is a caudal LAO left coronary arteriogram (spider view). **BE ABLE TO MATCH ALL ANSWERS BELOW.**
1. LAD stenosis
2. Circumflex stenosis
3. Circumflex → posterior lateral branch of RCA collateral
   The circumflex travels toward the crux in the left AV groove. The posterior lateral branches of the RCA also travel in the AV groove. Where the both end is a natural place to exchange collateral circulations.
4. LAD → PDCA division of RCA collateral.
   The LAD runs to the apex in the anterior IV groove. The PDCA runs to the apex in the inferior IV groove. At the apex, where they both end, the LAD may grow collaterals over to help the starving RCA. You would expect to find a severely stenosed RCA when we do the right coronary arteriogram.
See: Braunwald, chapter on "Coronary Arteriography."

470. **A segment of LAD that occludes in systole and opens in diastole is termed a/an:**
a. Myocardial bridge artery
b. Myocardial tunnel artery
c. Coronary spasm
d. Epicardial coronary

ANSWER a. A myocardial bridge is contracting myocardium that encircles a coronary artery. It may pinch the artery, and obstruct it during systole. Then it may relax and open up in ventricular diastole. Significant myocardial bridges cause angina, especially during tachycardia - when diastolic coronary flow is limited. Surgery may relieve the problem.
See: Baim and Grossman, chapter on "Coronary Arteriography."

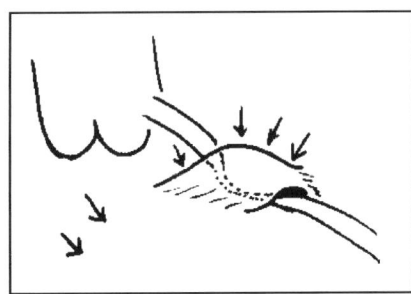
Myocardial Bridge

BOTH QUESTIONS BELOW REFER TO THIS DIAGRAM.

471. What coronary artery is receiving collateral circulation?
a. PDA
b. Acute marginal
c. Obtuse marginal
d. LAD
e. Circumflex

472. What coronary artery is labeled #5?
a. LAD
b. PDA
c. Acute marginal
d. Septal branches

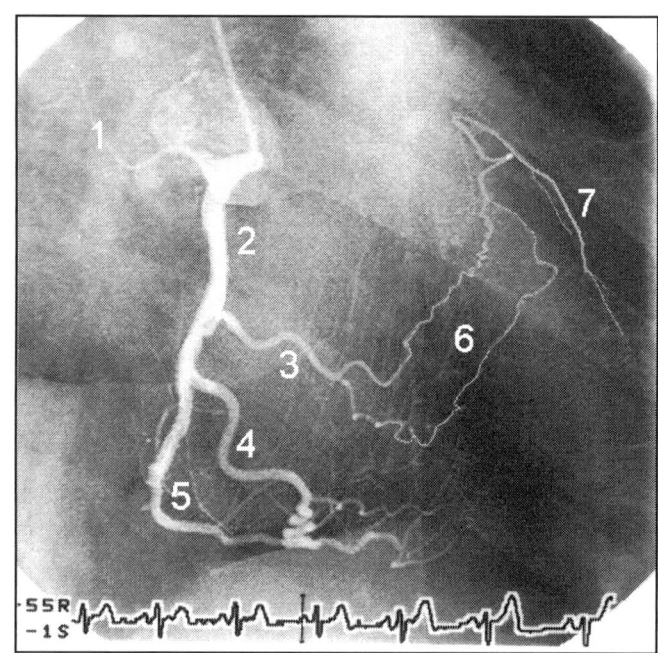

55° RAO coronary artery angiogram

471. ANSWER d. LAD. The LAD (7) is seen filling from large collaterals (6) from the RCA acute marginal branch (3). The LAD has a proximal occlusion. **BE ABLE TO MATCH ALL ANSWERS BELOW.**
    1. SA Node
    2. Proximal RCA
    3. 1st RV or acute marginal branch
    4. 2nd RV or acute marginal branch
    5. PDA (posterior descending coronary artery)
    6. Collaterals from 1st RV branch to LAD
    7. To distal LAD in anterior IV groove
See: Grossman, chapter on "Coronary Arteriography." **Keywords:** Collateral

472. ANSWER b. PDA. #5 labels the crux of the heart. The posterior descending artery makes a sharp turn here and descends in the inferior interventricular groove to supply the inferior aspect of the IV septum. Small but long septal perforators can be seen ascending to supply a major part of the IV septal supply.
See: Baim and Grossman, chapter on "Coronary Arteriography." **Keywords:** ID PDA of RCA

473. Identify the obstructed coronary artery receiving collateral flow in the coronary angiogram diagram labeled #3. Collateral flow is:
a. To the distal LAD via PDA branch of RCA.
b. To the distal RCA via the distal circumflex.
c. To the LAD via RCA septals.
d. To the OM branch of circumflex via diagonal.

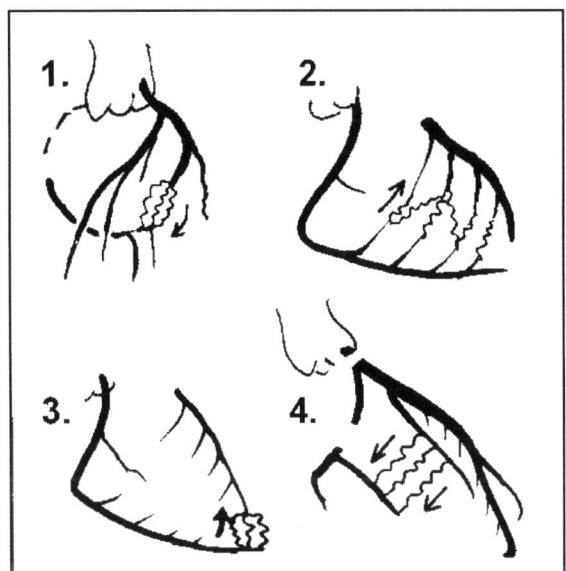

Collateral flow patterns

ANSWER a. To the distal LAD via PDA branch of RCA. **BE ABLE TO MATCH ALL ANSWERS BELOW.**
  1. TO THE DISTAL RCA VIA THE DISTAL CIRCUMFLEX:
    This LAO view shows the circumflex on the right of the diagram sends off a collateral network to the distal right coronary artery across the posterior lateral LV. The RCA appears totally obstructed.
  2. TO THE LAD VIA RCA SEPTALS:
    This RAO view shows the posterior descending branch of the RCA (bottom of diagram) sending off a collateral network feeding through the septum to the anterior LAD. The LAD appears totally obstructed.
  3. TO THE DISTAL LAD VIA PDA BRANCH OF RCA:
    This is an RAO view showing the obstructed LAD at the right. Note at the apex several tiny collateral channels arising from the distal posterior descending branch of the RCA. The right coronary is supplying the anterior wall of the heart via these collateral channels. The LAD appears totally obstructed.
  4. TO THE OM BRANCH OF CIRCUMFLEX VIA DIAGONAL:
    This RAO view shows the diagonal branch of the LAD (anterior) sending off a collateral network. These feed the obtuse marginal branch of the circumflex. The circumflex appears totally obstructed.
See: Baim and Grossman, chapter on "Coronary Arteriography." **Keywords:** Collateral

474. This patient has had coronary bypass surgery. His angiogram shows a/an:
a. IMA graft to LAD
b. IMA skip graft to Circ. and LAD
c. CABG skip graft to Circ. and LAD
d. CABG skip graft to diagonal and LAD

ANSWER d. CABG skip graft to diagonal and LAD. This is a standard RAO view of both coronary arteries. The dotted

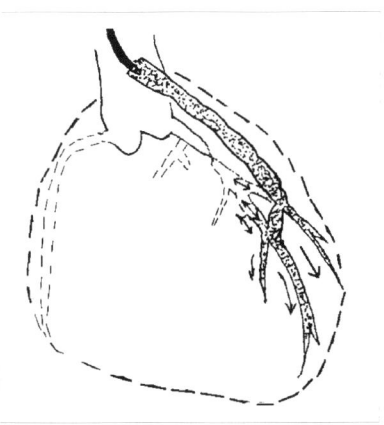

? Graft --→ to coronary

line is a CABG bypass from the aorta to the diagonal. Then it skips over to the LAD and supplies it also. The fresh blood from the aorta travels through the vein bypass distal to the stenosis in each vessel. You just have to identify the vessels.
See: Braunwald, chapter on "Coronary Arteriography." **Keywords:** CABG to Diag. & LAD

BOTH QUESTIONS BELOW REFER TO THIS DIAGRAM.

475. What type of bypass graft (CABG) does this patient have?
 a. IMA graft to LAD
 b. IMA skip graft to Circ. and LAD
 c. SVG skip graft to Circ. and LAD
 d. SVG graft to diagonal

476. The lesion seen in the graft is probably a:
 a. Stent
 b. Thrombus
 c. Bruise
 d. Plaque

BOTH ANSWERS ARE LISTED BELOW.

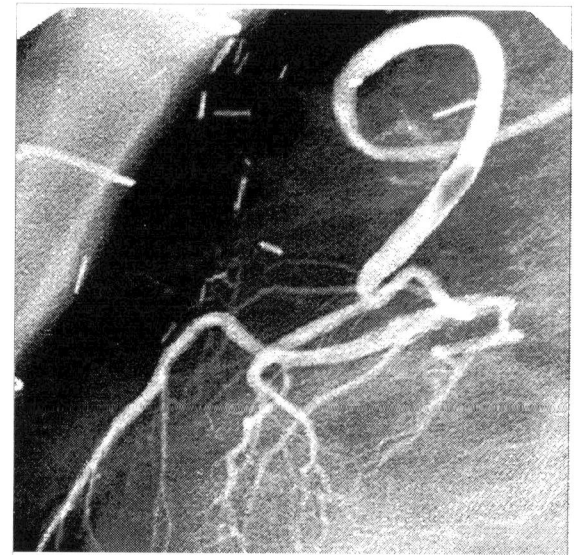
Post CABG coronary arteriogram

475. ANSWER d. SVG or saphenous vein skip graft to diagonal and LAD. This is a standard 45 degree LAO view of the bypass graft to the diagonal branch. The LAD fills from the diagonal branch.
   The JR4 catheter can be seen at the origin of the bypass. Fresh blood from the aorta travels through the vein bypass attached to the front of the aorta near the marker "staples." The vein bypass arches over the anterior wall of the heart. It anastomosis with the diagonal coronary artery distal to an unseen stenosis high in the LAD. This bypass was originally a "diagonal - LAD skip graft" where the "skip" portion to the LAD has clotted off. So blood from the graft must travel retrograde up the proximal diagonal artery to supply the LAD artery. Only the primary graft into the diagonal branch remains.
See: Braunwald, chapter on "Coronary Arteriography." **Keywords:** SVG to Diag.

476. ANSWER b. Thrombus. It appears to be a filling defect that displaces contrast. Since it seems to have definite borders it may be a thrombus. Bypass grafts are notorious for having thrombus and debris in them. These may embolize when angioplastied.
See: Braunwald, chapter on "Coronary Arteriography." **Keywords:** Bypass thrombus

BOTH QUESTIONS BELOW REFER TO THIS DIAGRAM.

477. What coronary lesion seen here needs immediate therapy?
a. Mainstem lesion
b. 80% proximal circumflex lesion
c. Filling defect in LAD
d. Hazy dissection in LAD

478. What coronary view and artery are shown at #5 in the diagram?
a. RAO, LAD
b. RAO, Circumflex
c. LAO, LAD
d. LAO, Circumflex

BOTH ANSWERS ARE LISTED TOGETHER BELOW.

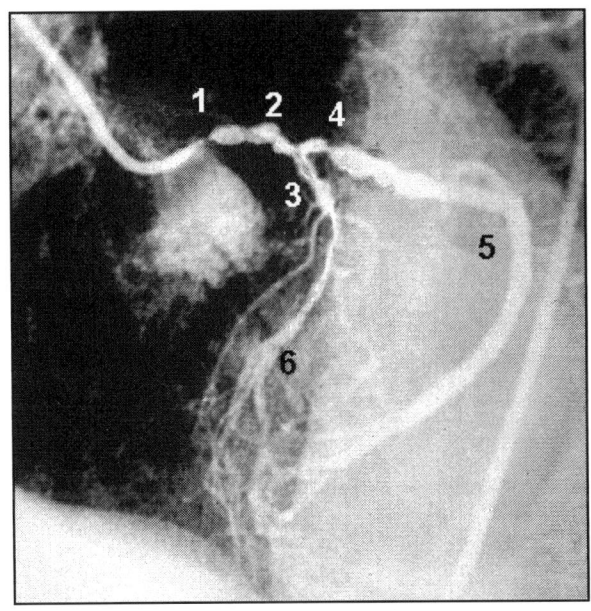

Post SVG coronary arteriogram

477. ANSWER a. Mainstem lesion. Main stem lesions of this type have a high mortality. They are too dangerous to angioplasty. Emergent bypass surgery is called for. These coronary arteries are ectatic, with many small saccular regions. A fresh clot is seen causing the filling defect at #3. See: Braunwald, chapter on "Coronary Arteriography."

478. ANSWER d. LAO, Circumflex. The catheter and backbone are seen on the right so the apex is pointing leftward. This makes this an LAO view (similar to #3 below). If you have difficulty locating the backbone, look for the catheter rising in the thoracic aorta. It is just to the left of the backbone. The artery labeled #5 is next to the backbone, so it is the circumflex coronary artery. See: Braunwald, chapter on "Coronary Arteriography."

479. What view of the LCA is labeled at #3 in the diagram?
a. Left lateral
b. 30° RAO
c. PA
d. 30° LAO
e. 60° LAO

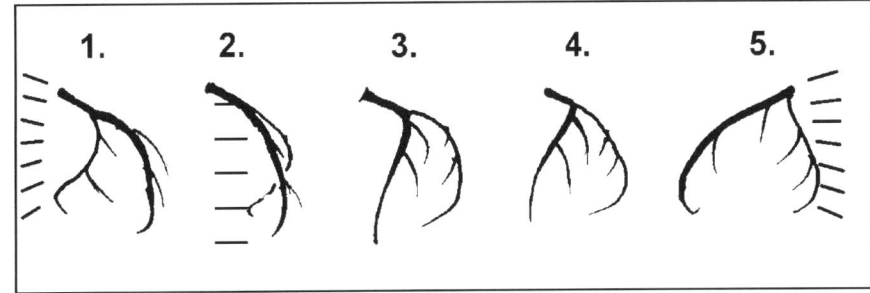

Non-Angulated (flat) views of LCA

ANSWER d. 30° LAO. This diagram shows five non-angulated views of the LCA. **BE ABLE TO MATCH ALL ANSWERS BELOW.**
1. **30° RAO:** LAD and apex to your right - long axis view.
2. **PA View:** The main-stem LCA shows well in the PA view. But, the LAD and Circ. overlap. Also, the backbone directly overlies the PA image. Thus, the PA view for the LCA is seldom used.
3. **30° LAO:** LAD and apex to your left. Note the excellent view of the main-stem LCA.
4. **60° LAO:** LAD and apex further to your left.
5. **90° LAO = Left lateral:** LAD and apex, further to your left. This view shows the widest separation of the LAD and Circ. Note that the right lateral is just a flipped image.

See: King, chapter on "Angulated Views." Keywords: ID angulated views LCA

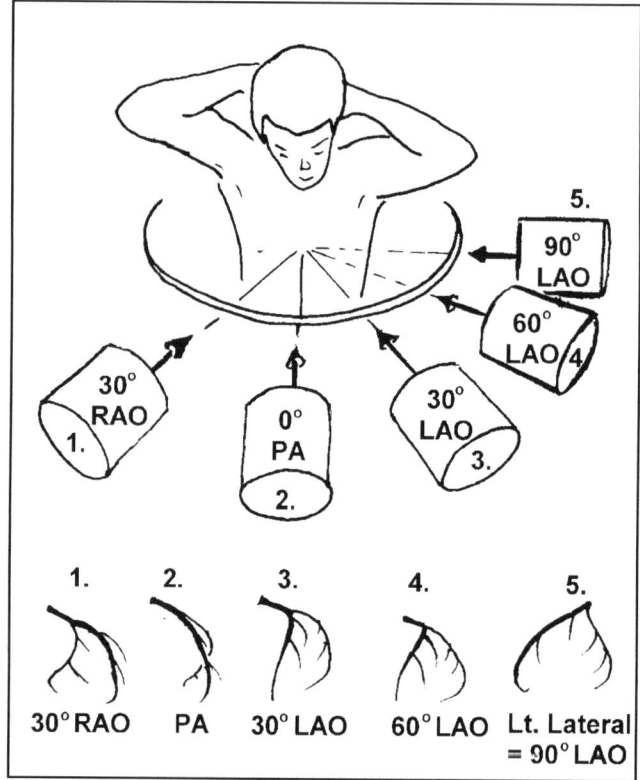

Image intensifier position, views of LCA

480. **When studying an unstable patient's left coronary artery, what angulated view is the "first view of choice" (according to Grossman)?**
   a. 0-10° RAO, 15-20° caudal
   b. 20-30° RAO, 15-20° cranial
   c. 30° RAO (flat)
   d. 30° LAO, 20-30° cranial

ANSWER a. 0-10° RAO, 15-20° caudal. Since you may only get one view Grossman recommends a "bread and butter view" which will give you the most information. It provides an excellent view of the area where most disease occurs - the left main bifurcation, the proximal LAD, and the proximal to mid circumflex artery.
See: Baim and Grossman, chapter on "Coronary Arteriography."
Keywords: Grossman's X-ray "view of choice" for unstable patients = 0-10° RAO, 15-20° caudal

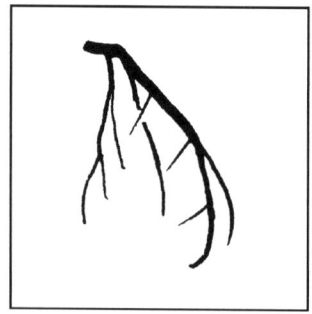

LCA View of choice

481. Which angulated view below is in the plane of the circumflex coronary artery and usually shows it in its largest circular, reverse "C" shape?

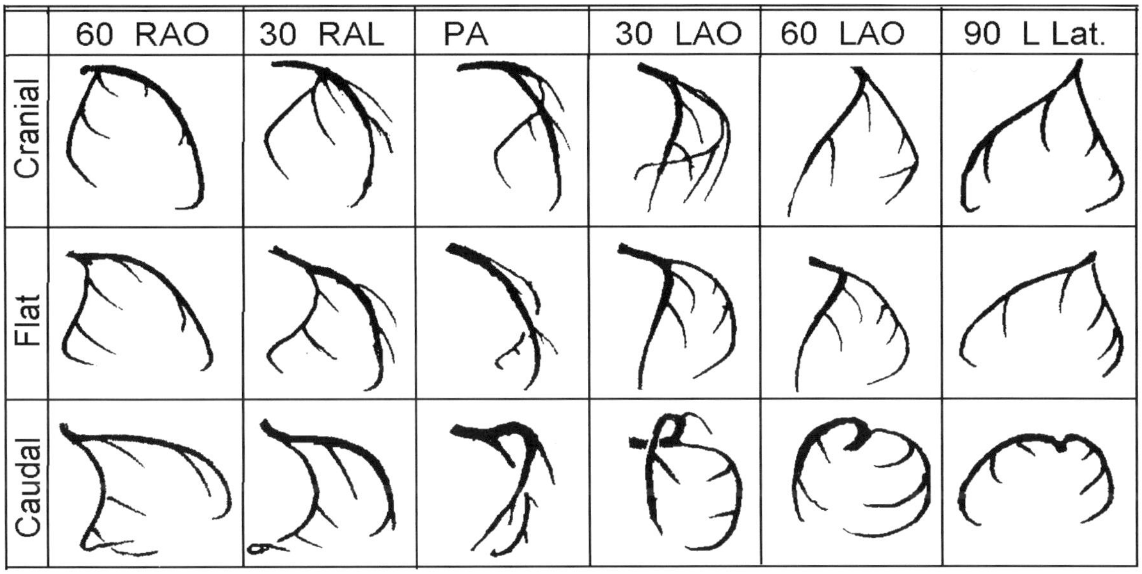

	60 RAO	30 RAL	PA	30 LAO	60 LAO	90 L Lat.
Cranial						
Flat						
Caudal						

a. PA cranial
b. 60° LAO caudal
c. 60° RAO cranial
d. 60° RAO caudal

ANSWER b. 60° LAO caudal. The short axis of the LV is the 60° caudal (spider) view. It looks down the barrel of the LV. This view is perpendicular to the plane of the circumflex artery, which curves around the barrel in the left AV grove. Note in the diagram below how the spider view shows the circumflex as a large reverse C shape. Note how most of the caudal views are best for the circumflex. **See:** Baim and Grossman, chapter on "Coronary Arteriography."

THE BEST LCA ANGULATED VIEWS

	60° RAO	30° RAO	PA	30° LAO	60° LAO	90° Lat.
Cranial		Mid & Distal LAD Septal & Diagonal LAD		Left Main Prox. LAD & Diag.		Distal LAD & Prox. Circ.
Flat			Origin Left Main			
Caudal		Left Main Bifurcation Prox. LAD & Circ View of choice*		SPIDER VIEWS Left Main, Prox. LAD & Prox. Circ.		

NOTE: *Grossman recommends the shallow RAO caudal view as his initial "view of choice" when studying unstable patients.

482. What defect is seen at #4 on the coronary angiogram shown?
a. LAD aneurysm
b. Circumflex aneurysm
c. LAD stent
d. Circumflex stent
e. Circumflex AV fistula

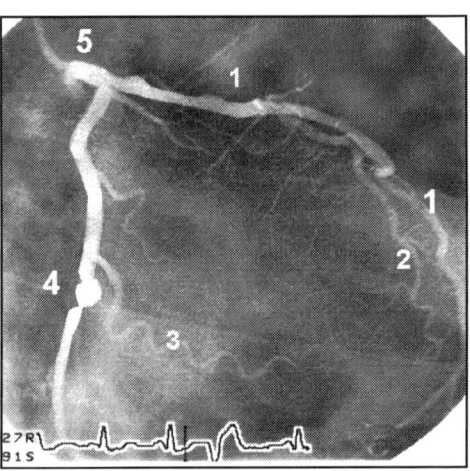

ANSWER b. Circumflex aneurysm. The circular structure is an aneurysm. Beneath it is an 80% stenosis.
VESSELS SEEN ARE:
1. LAD
2. Diagonal
3. Acute marginal
4. Circumflex (aneurysms & stenosis)
5. Main LCA

RAO view of Left Coronary Artery

See: Braunwald, chapter on "Coronary Arteriography." **Keywords:** Coronary aneurysm

483. The X-ray angulated view labeled #1 on the diagram at the right would result in a left coronary angiogram looking like diagram lettered ___ below.

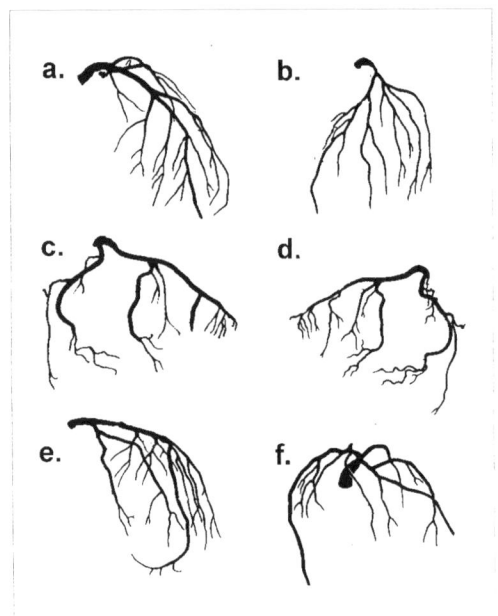

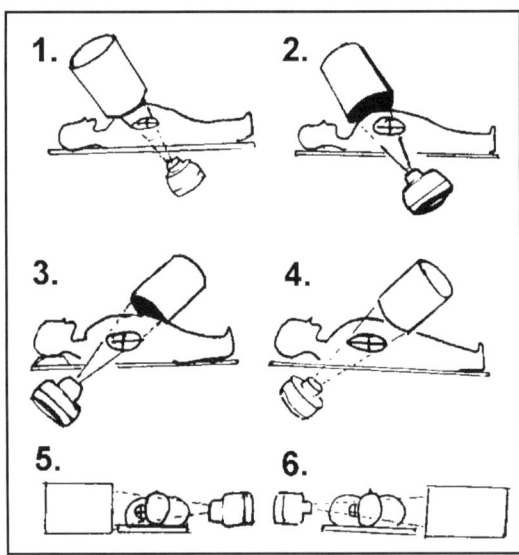

Resulting LCA angiogram

Different image intensifier & tube positions (angulated views for left coronary arteriography)

ANSWER a. RAO cranial. This diagram shows six angulated X-ray views of the LCA. Be able to match all.
   1. RAO CRANIAL: Image Intensifier (I.I.) positioned on patient's right side and tilted towards his head (cranial). Resulting angiogram shows LAD & apex to your right with the LAD and its branches well shown (diagonals & septals). Circumflex is

poorly seen behind LAD.

2. **LAO CRANIAL:** I.I. positioned on patient's left side and cranial. Resulting angiogram shows LAD and apex to your left. Fine view of LAD - Circ. bifurcation and diagonal branches between them.

3. **LAO CAUDAL = SPIDER VIEW:** I.I. positioned on patient's left side and caudal. Resulting angiogram shows LAD and apex to your left, circumflex to your right. This is the short axis view of the LV. You are looking down the LV barrel.

4. **RAO CAUDAL:** I.I. positioned obliquely to right and caudal. Proximal LAD shows clearly on top.

5. **LEFT LATERAL:** I.I. positioned on patient's far left side. Resulting angiogram shows LAD to your left, circ. to your right.

6. **RIGHT LATERAL:** A mirror image of #5 the other lateral. Since it gives no more information than the left lateral the right lateral is seldom shot.

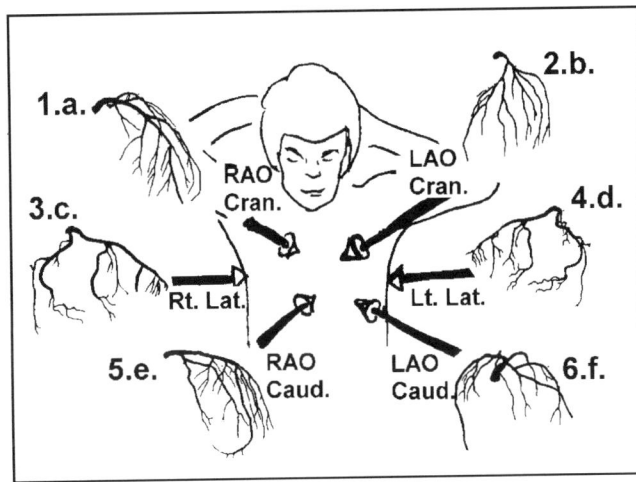

Angulate views of Left Coronary Arteriogram

See: King, chapter on "Angulated Views" **Keywords:** ID angulated views LCA

484. **What angulated view of the RCA is labeled at #1 in the diagram?**
   a. 30° RAO
   b. 30° RAO cranial
   c. 60° LAO cranial
   d. 60° LAO caudal (120° RAO cranial)
   e. Left lateral (90° LAO)

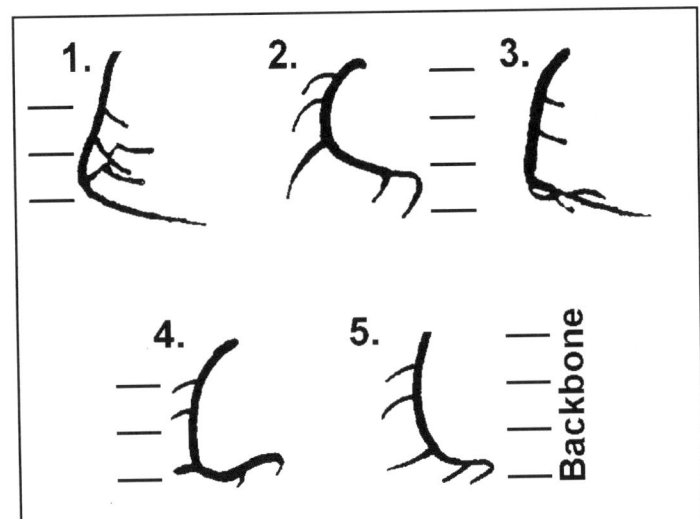

Identify the RCA Angulated views

ANSWER b. RAO cranial. Note that all the RAO views tend towards an "L" shape (RCA and PDA). All the LAO views tend towards a "C" shape (Main RCA). This diagram shows four angulated views of the RCA.

268 ◀◀ Diagnostic Techniques: D7 - Coronary Arteriography ▶▶

BE ABLE TO MATCH ALL ANSWERS BELOW.

1. **30° RAO CRANIAL:** The posterior lateral branches are rolled up above the PDA. Grossman recommends this as a screening view, because it is so good at separating the PDA from the post. lateral branches.
2. **60° LAO CRANIAL**
3. **30° RAO**
4. **60° LAO CAUDAL:** Kern terms this a 120° RAO CRANIAL because this is a 180° reversal of tube and I.I.
5. **LEFT LATERAL (90° LAO)** Most labs take very few angulated views of the RCA.

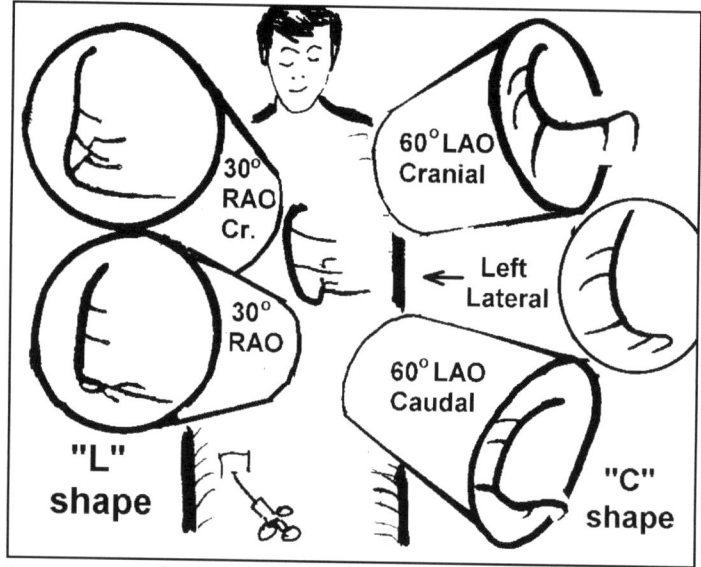

Image Intensifier Positions in angulated RCA views

See: King, chapter on angulated views   **Keywords:** ID angulated views LCA

---

485. What angulated view usually views the plane of the main RCA on edge, with the posterior lateral branches rolled down, well beneath the PDA?
   a. 30° LAO cranial
   b. 60° LAO caudal
   c. 30° RAO cranial
   d. 60° RAO caudal

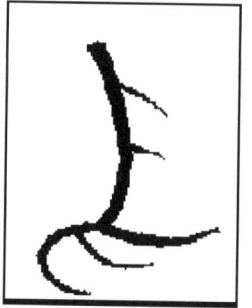

ANSWER d. 60° RAO caudal. The base of the heart is viewed on edge with the right ventricle in the long axis. Use of a caudal view allows you to look from below at the posterior descending artery, posterior lateral branches and the diaphragmatic surface. On the 18 RCA Angulated Views Table shown below, note in the 60 degree RAO caudal view how the RCA-PDA is L shaped, with the posterior lateral branches beneath the PDA. In steeper RAO views e.g. 80 degrees, the RCA forms a " J" shape, as it is seen from behind the base of the heart.

See: Grossman, chapter on "Coronary Arteriography."   **Keywords:** RCA caudal views

18 RCA ANGULATED VIEWS TABLE

	60 RAO	30 RAO	PA	30 LAO	60 LAO	90 Lat
Cranial						
Flat						
Caudal						

NOTE: Septals not shown & PDA exaggerated in size

THE BEST RCA ANGULATED VIEWS

	60° RAO	30° RAO	PA	30° LAO	60° LAO	90° Lat.
Cranial		PDCA & Crux Post. Lateral		Distal RCA Crux & PDCA		
Flat		Mid. RCA Post. Lateral Post. Descending		Prox. RCA RCA origin		Mid. RCA
Caudal				Prox. RCA Mid. RCA		

486. In order to perform a left internal mammary (internal thoracic) arteriogram a femoral catheter must pass though the:
a. Celiac axis
b. Innominate artery
c. Left vertebral artery
d. Left subclavian artery

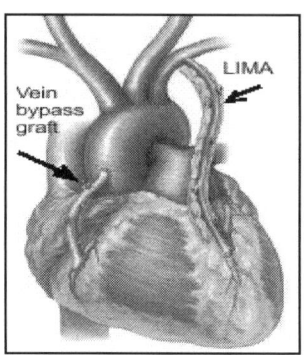
Bypass grafts

ANSWER d. The LIMA branches off the left subclavian. See diagram. The RIMA cath must pass through the innominate before getting to the right subclavian.
See: Baim and Grossman, chapter on "Coronary Arteriography." **Keywords:** LIMA - through the left subclavian

487. In this anterior oblique axial CT view of the base of the heart, what structure is shown at #5?
a. Ramus intermedius artery
b. Right coronary artery
c. Circumflex artery
d. LAD artery

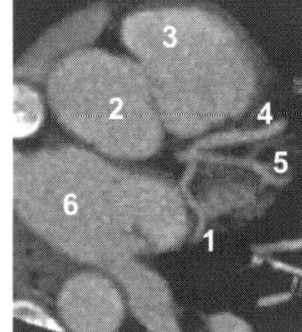
CT of heart

ANSWER: a. Ramus intermedius artery. CT angiography is revolutionizing cardiac imaging. This shows a cross section view with the 3 left coronary artery branches arising from the AO with a medianus or ramus intermedius arising between the LA and Circ.
#1 is LAD
#2 is AO
#3 is LA
#4 is Circ
#5 is Ramus
#6 is RA.

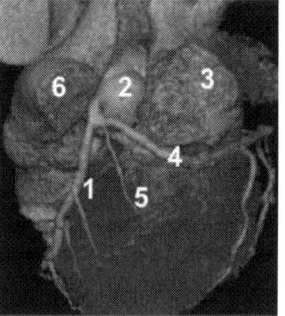
Reconstructed CT

In the reconstructed colored image (volume rendering format) it shows the surface of the heart with the left coronary epicardial arteries. Note at #5 the ramus intermedius branch between the LAD & CX. We expect more cardiac CT images to be on the RCIS exam in future. See: "Anatomy of the Heart at Multidetector CT" online at http://pubs.rsna.org/doi/pdf/10.1148/rg.276065747

PROCEDURE

488. To minimize the chance of CNS toxicity when attempting to catheterize the internal mammary artery bypass graft use ____.
   a. Low osmolar contrast
   b. Low concentration contrast (50%)
   c. Small slow hand injections
   d. High dose "Versed" premedication

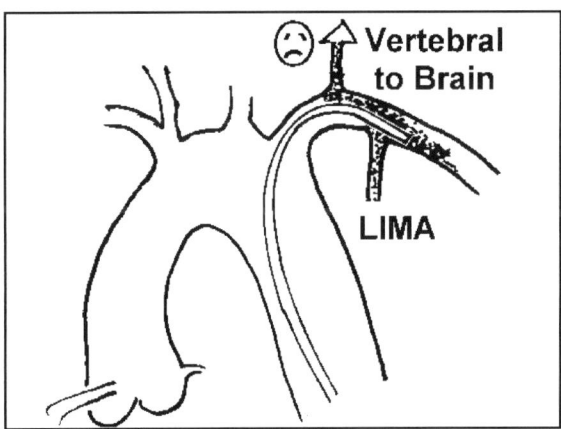

IMA - vertebral origin

ANSWER a. Low osmolar contrast. Since both the internal mammary and vertebral arteries arise from the subclavian artery, contrast may accidentally get into the brain via the vertebral artery. The low-osmolar and non-ionic contrasts are gentler on nervous tissue and much less toxic.

Injections into the intact IMA may cause pain and extreme burning sensations to the patient. Increased premedication and non-ionic contrast may make the patient more comfortable.
See: Baim and Grossman, chapter on "Coronary Arteriography." **Keywords:** IMA use low-osmolar contrast

489. What angiographic view is this? The fluoroscopic C-arm is angled so that the X-rays enters near the patient's left hip, and exits from the patient's right clavicular area as shown.
   a. Cranial RAO
   b. Cranial LAO
   c. Caudal RAO
   d. Caudal LAO

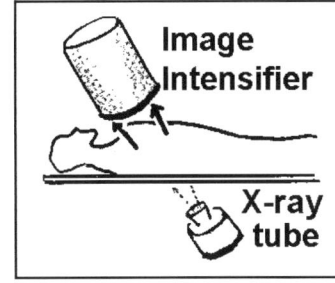

Angulated X-ray view

ANSWER a. Cranial RAO. The views are labeled by the position of the fluoroscope in relationship to the patient's anatomy. This is the same location that the X-rays exit the body. If it is near the right clavicle, then it is a right cranial oblique view. (Understand all X-ray views, RAO, LPO, right lateral...) **See:** Kern, chapter on "Angiography." **Keywords:** Cranial RAO

BOTH QUESTIONS BELOW REFER TO THIS ANGIOGRAM.

490. What major coronary artery defect is noted in this coronary angiogram?
   a. LAD aneurysm
   b. LAD to Circ. collateral
   c. Shepherd's crook
   d. Widow-maker

491. Which coronary artery needs PTCA?
   a. None - too risky
   b. Proximal LAD
   c. Distal circumflex
   d. RCA

BOTH ANSWERS LISTED TOGETHER BELOW.

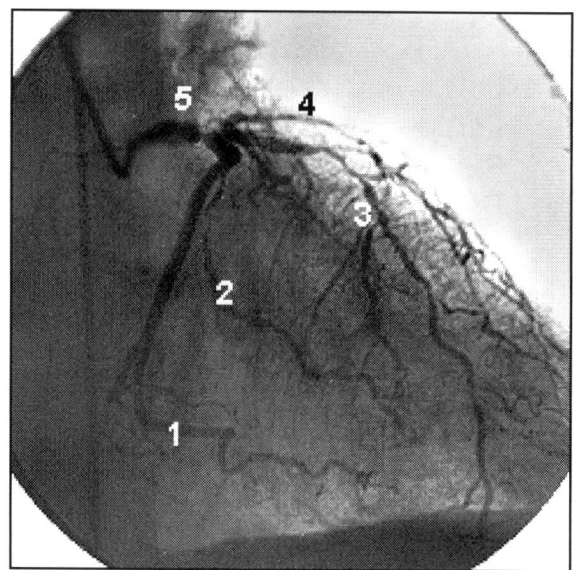
Coronary arteriogram

490. ANSWER d. Widow-maker. The main-stem left coronary has a tight stenosis at the bifurcation termed a "widow-maker" because of its high mortality. There is also a long proximal LAD lesion which needs grafting. CORRECTLY MATCHED ARTERIES ARE:
   1. Second obtuse marginal branch of circumflex
   2. First obtuse marginal branch of circumflex
   3. LAD
   4. Diagonal branch of LCA (note long proximal lesion)
   5. Main-stem LCA (note critical lesion)

See: Braunwald, chapter on "Coronary Arteriography" **Keywords:** Widowmaker, mainstem

491. ANSWER a. None - too risky. These lesions are usually too risky for PTCA and are sent to urgent CABG surgery. Braunwald says, "The only 'absolute contraindications' to angioplasty are the absence of a hemodynamically significant coronary stenosis, significant (>50% stenosis) left main coronary disease unprotected by at least one patent bypass graft, and (in the United States, at least) absence of on-site cardiac surgical support." **See:** Braunwald, chapter on "Coronary Arteriography." **Keywords:** Left coronary arteries, PTCA for widow-maker

Diagnostic Techniques: D7 - Coronary Arteriography 273

OTH QUESTIONS BELOW REFER TO THIS DIAGRAM.

492. This is a 30 degree RAO angiogram. What ECG monitoring lead would best monitor ischemic changes from the stenosed artery shown?
   a. I
   b. II
   c. aVF
   d. V2

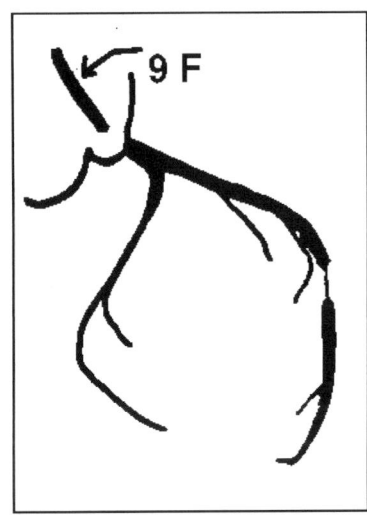
RAO Coronary angio.

493. This same coronary angiogram shows a 9 French JL4 - PTCA guider catheter. What size of dilatation catheter would you select to completely dilate the lesion shown?
   a. 2.0 mm. balloon
   b. 3.0 mm. balloon
   c. 4.0 mm. balloon
   d. 5.0 mm. balloon

BOTH ANSWERS ARE LISTED TOGETHER BELOW.

492. ANSWER d. V2 ECG lead is closest to the lesion and area of injury. The LAD normally supplies the anterior wall, so V leads will best monitor this segment. These leads are the same as those showing infarct patterns for specific LV segments. Position the V lead anteriorly out of the way of fluoroscopy and use lead wires that are radiolucent. Common Registry question.
See: Kern, chapter on "ECG in the Cath Lab." **Keywords:** V leads show anterior MI

493. ANSWER b. 3.0 mm balloon. Note that the 9F guider is the same diameter as the normal LAD segment just beyond the tight lesion. You know that each French size equals 1/3 of a mm. So 9F = 3 mm, and a 3 mm balloon would dilate the lesion completely. Understand all catheter and wire measurements.
See: Tilkian, chapter on "Tools of Catheterization."

494. This is an angiogram showing:
   a. Strong RCA dominance in RAO view
   b. Strong RCA dominance in LAO view
   c. Strong LCA dominance in RAO view
   d. Strong LCA dominance in LAO view

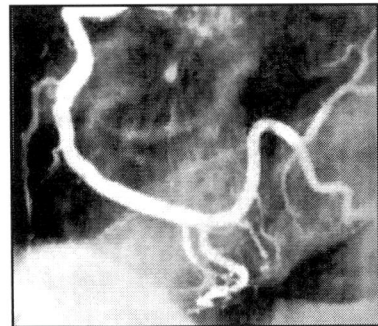
Coronary angio.

ANSWER b. Strong RCA dominance in LAO view. The apex is seen down and to the left with the backbone to the right. This is the main RCA forming a "C" configuration. The RCA is large with the posterior descending in the lower right corner. Branching from the PDA is a large posterior later branch seen in the left AV groove. This supplies the lateral LV which is normally part of the circumflex territory. **See:** Braunwald, chapter on "Coronary Arteriography"

495. This is an angiogram showing:
   a. Wrap-around LAD in PA view
   b. Wrap-around LAD in LAO view
   c. Collateral from RCA to Circ. in PA view
   d. Collateral from Circ to RCA in LAO view

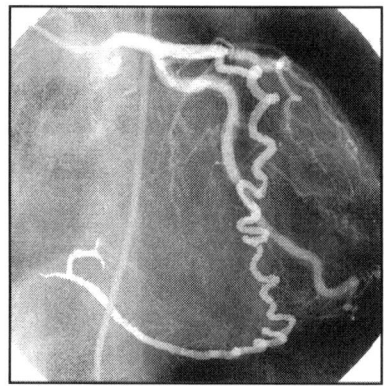
Coronary angio.

ANSWER a. Wrap-around LAD in PA view showing corkscrew LAD on the front of the heart, wrapping around the apex, feeding into the PDCA. Some septal and diagonal branches are evident. A large circumflex branch is seen behind the LAD. This is a strongly dominant left coronary artery. The backbone is evident on the left of the screen. There was also 30° caudal angulation on this PA view. The fistula could be occluded distally to block the shunt. There was a 30° caudal angulation on this PA view.
See: Braunwald, chapter on Corona ry Arteriography

496. In this 30 degree RAO cine angiogram, which coronary artery has a critical stenosis at the arrow?
   a. RCA - PDCA
   b. RCA 1st Septal
   c. LCA 1st Diagonal
   d. LCA 1st Obtuse marginal

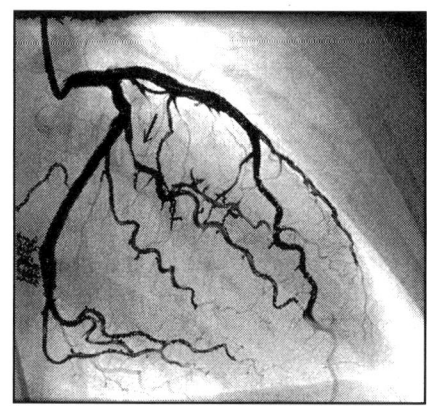

ANSWER: d. LCA 1st obtuse marginal branch of the circumflex is narrowed about 80%. The LAD is the large artery on the right and the circumflex on the left appears dominant. The circumflex has two branches supplying the lateral wall of the heart. Branches off the circ. are termed obtuse marginal branches. There is a tubular stenosis in the proximal 1st obtuse marginal. **See:** Kern, chapter on "Angiographic Data" **Keywords:** Obtuse marginal

497. In this RAO coronary angiogram, what is shown at the arrow?
   a. Large left atrial branch of circumflex
   b. Collateral from RCA to circumflex
   c. Saphenous vein graft filling entire left coronary artery
   d. Circumflex vein graft filling retrograde to AO

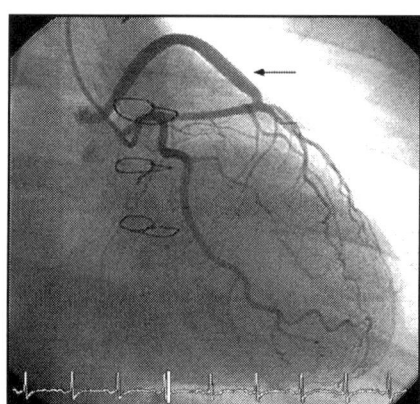

ANSWER d. Circumflex vein graft filling retrograde to AO. Note the left coronary catheter injecting into the left main. The saphenous vein graft fills from the proximal

circumflex and flows up and into the ascending aorta, where it may be partially obstructed. Normally, a vein graft flows antegrade from the AO distal to the obstructed coronary artery because pressure is higher in the AO than pressure below the stenosis. There often is competitive flow with small amounts of dye going retrograde into a graft, but, here flow appears to be reversed in the graft. Perhaps the LCA was Acist power-injected.
See: Kern, chapter on "Angiographic Data" **Keywords:** Retrograde flow up SVG

498. Which angiographic view is usually perpendicular to the left main coronary artery and shows it best?
a. 10-20 degree LAO
b. 30-45 degree LAO
c. 0-10 degree RAO
d. 30-45 degree RAO

ANSWER: c. 0-10 degree RAO. Kern says, "The AP view or shallow RAO displays the left main coronary artery (LMCA) in its entire perpendicular length." These shallow RAO views are also best to initially cannulate the LCA because the ostium is seen on edge.
See: Kern, chapter on "Angiographic Data" **Keywords:** Shallow RAO best for L. Main

499. In the LAO coronary angiogram, what branch is directed superiorly from the crux and labeled at #1?
a. SA node artery
b. AV node artery
c. 1ˢᵗ septal branch
d. Posterior lateral branch

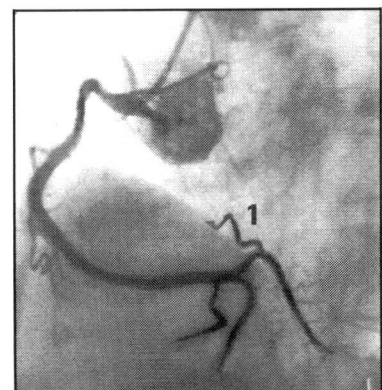

ANSWER: b. AV node artery arises from the distal RCA. This is normally at the crux where the RCA makes a U bend in the AV groove as it crosses the inferior IV septum. If this artery becomes ischemic AV block may occur. **See:** Kern, chapter on "Angiographic Data" **Keywords:** AV node artery

500. What does this RAO view show at B? (White arrows indicate direction of blood flow.)
a. Normal dominant RCA
b. Normal dominant LCA
c. Collateral from PDCA to CX
d. Collateral from conus branch to LAD
e. Collateral from acute marginal to CX

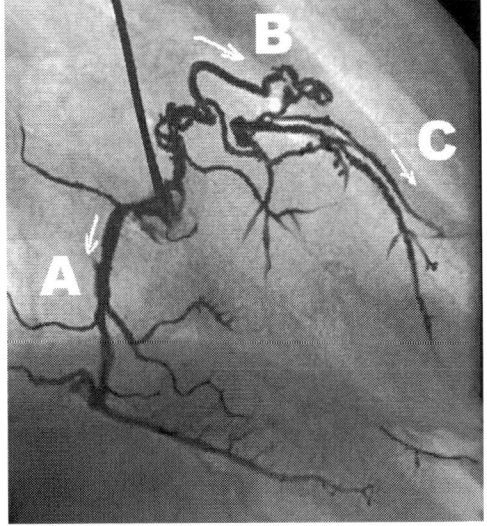

ANSWER: d. Collateral from conus branch to LAD. The large RCA (note the L shape at A) sends off a large bridging collateral across the conus area of the RV at B. It twists and turns, finally emptying into the LAD at C, which is probably occluded at the origin.

There also appears to be a portion of the circumflex artery filling from unseen collaterals in the lower right. **See:** Kern, chapter on "Angiographic Data" **Keywords:** Collateral

5. Other Coronary *(Note: Ergonovine testing was removed from RCIS in 2013)*

501. During coronary arteriography it is most essential to monitor_____ when using _____ contrast
a. ECG & BP, Low osmolar
b. ECG & BP, High osmolar
c. O2 Sat. & Respirations, High osmolar
d. O2 Sat. & Respirations, Low osmolar

ANSWER: b. ECG & BP, High osmolar, ECG & arterial pressure. Because these older dyes have high osmolarity they dramatically effect the heart when injected IC. Typical response is for the arterial pressure to fall for several seconds then come back. ST changes can also be dramatic (down for RCA injection, up for LCA). Observe the ECG for heart rate changes (bradycardia) and arterial pressure changes (hypotension). **See:** Todd book

502. What new noninvasive imaging and artificial intelligence method measures coronary FFR as shown in the upper color image?
a. Ultrasound color flow imaging
b. PET stress imaging
c. SPECT nuclear imaging
d. CT imaging with Heartflow

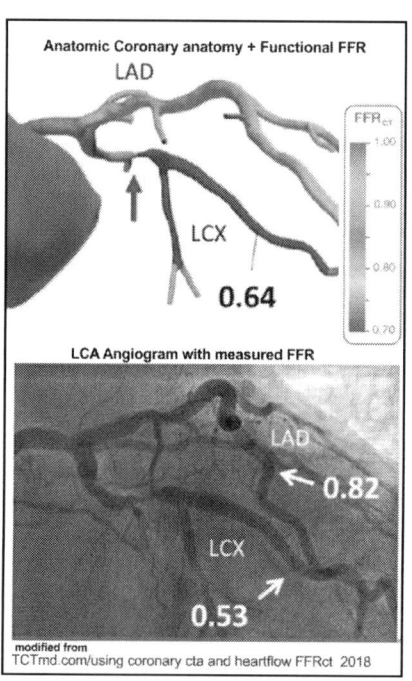

Answer d. CT imaging with Heartflow analyzes a CT scan with computational methods to derive the FFR at any point in the coronary tree. It is sometimes termed FFRCT. Heartflow company computes the FFR from the nonivasive CT angiogram and displays it on a color 3D image like the one shown. The lower image is a coronary angiogram on the same patient with measured FFR values showing close agreement.

DAIC magazine 2014 says: "The U.S. Food and Drug Administration (FDA) today cleared HeartFlow's FFR-CT (fractional flow reserve—computed tomography) software, which permits non-invasive evaluation of coronary artery blood flow in patients showing signs of coronary artery disease."

"The clearance may open a new era of coronary CT imaging, where a single scan can show blood flow with specific FFR flow rates for all segments in the heart. This may eliminate the need to perform diagnostic catheter angiography or to perform invasive catheter-based FFR tests. FFR-CT shows the exact area of blockages, the impact each has on flow and can help guide treatment and aid in interventional procedural navigation. Coronary CT experts predict the technology also may eliminate the need for myocardial perfusion nuclear imaging and other tests usually performed on patients presenting to emergency departments with chest pain." See: https://www.dicardiology.com/product/fda-clears-ffr-ct

503. What is the black spot at the arrows on this CT angiogram taken with single-energy myocardial perfusion imaging.
a. Apical cardiac myxoma
b. Apical LV aneurysm
c. Subendocardial LV apical myocardial infarction
d. Hypertrophic subvalvular stenosis

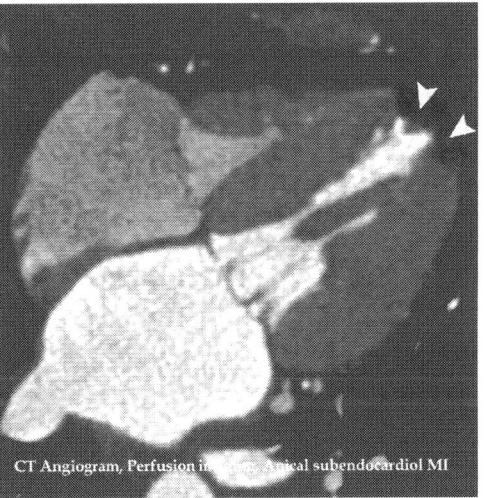

CT Angiogram, Perfusion — Apical subendocardial MI

ANSWER c. Subendocardial LV apical myocardial infarction shows as a black poorly perfused infarcted area in this 4 chamber view.

Varga-Szemes et al say, "Because of recent advancements in CT technology, coronary CT angiography (CTA) has become an integral part of the noninvasive diagnostic workup for the anatomic evaluation of the coronary arteries of patients with suspected CAD. According to the current appropriate use criteria, coronary CTA is the method of choice for the exclusion of significant coronary artery stenosis in patients with low and intermediate CAD risk profiles.... CT assessment of myocardial perfusion is based on the distribution of iodinated contrast material during its first pass through the myocardium. Because the contrast material's distribution is determined by the arterial blood supply, myocardial perfusion defects can be identified as hypoattenuating areas containing reduced amounts of contrast material. See, CT Myocardial Perfusion Imaging, AJR, 2015 also: https://www.ajronline.org/doi/10.2214/AJR.14.13546

504. During coronary angiography a patient may develop persistent angina. What therapy is usually given to the type of angina patient with signs listed in the box at #2 (angina unresponsive to nitroglycerin)?
a. Tridil
b. Popranolol
c. Nifedipine
d. Epinephrine
e. Temporary pacemaker

ANGINA COMPLICATIONS WITH
1. Angina lasting longer than 30 sec.
*2. Angina unresponsive to IC nitroglycerine
3. Angina with inappropriate SVT
4. Angina with persistent severe bradycardia
5. Angina with wheezing and allergic response

ANSWER c. Nifedipine, relaxes smooth muscle including coronary arteries.
BE ABLE TO MATCH ALL ANSWERS BELOW.
1. Angina >30 sec (Tridil IV or IC nitroglycerine)

2. Angina unresponsive to IC nitro (Nifedipine - Ca channel blocker)
3. Angina with SVT (Popranolol - beta blocker)
4. Angina with bradycardia (Temporary pacer)
5. Angina with allergic response (Epinephrine - catecholamine)
See: Kern, chapter on "Angiographic Data." **Keywords:** Meds for angio. complications

505. The effects of IV preop. meds. vary in rate of onset and elimination half life. Match the 4 sedatives/analgesics to their speed of action and class below.

a. Rapid onset, short acting benzodiazepine _____

b. Delayed onset, long acting benzodiazepine _____

c. Rapid onset, short acting synthetic narcotic _____

d. Delayed onset, long acting narcotic _____

1. Fentanyl citrate (Sublimaze)
2. Morphine sulfate (MS)
3. Diazepam (Valium)
4. Midazolam (Versed)

BE ABLE TO MATCH ALL ANSWERS BELOW.

1. Fentanyl citrate (Sublimaze) c. Rapid onset, short acting synthetic narcotic
2. Morphine sulfate (MS) d. Delayed onset, Long acting narcotic
3. Diazepam (Valium) b. Delayed onset, Long acting benzodiazepine
4. Midazolam (Versed) a. Rapid onset, short acting benzodiazepine

   Yaniga says: "Versed and Valium are benzodiazepines which are used for preoperative sedation and conscious sedation for invasive procedures. Valium is a long acting sedative and skeletal muscle relaxant... Versed is a short acting benzodiazepine which has amnesic as well as sedative effects...."

   Loebl says: "Fentanyl is a potent synthetic narcotic and analgesic resembling morphine.... It has short onset of action (almost immediate...) which lasts for 30 to 60 minutes after IV...administration. This makes it faster acting and of shorter duration than morphine." The potency of Fentanyl is up to 100 times that of morphine. **See:** Yaniga, chapter on "Analgesics, Anesthetic and Narcotic Medication"

506. Your patient has symptomatic and critical 65% diameter left main coronary stenosis. There is no collateral flow. The LAD and RCA also have significant stenoses. Current standards to improve survival recommend to:
   a. Send patient to ICU and get surgical consult
   b. Proceed with PCI on the most significant lesions
   c. Insert an Impella support device and send to early CABG surgery
   d. Insert balloon pump and proceed with bailout stenting of the left main coronary artery

ANSWER: c. Insert an Impella support device and send to early CABG surgery.
This is an unprotected critical left main lesion with 3 vessel disease.
   Kern says, "A commonly encountered and potentially critical problem is coronary angiography of patients who have LMCA stenosis, which is one of the few situations wherein the routine performance of angiography may be life threatening....After the left

coronary views are completed, right coronary angiography is performed. In symptomatic patients with RCA occlusion and a critical LMCA stenosis, abdominal aortography and insertion of an intraaortic counterpulsation balloon or percutaneous LV support device, intensive-care-unit admission, and early CABG surgery should be strongly considered." Most cardiologists now prefer the Impella to the IABP.

ACC, AHA, SCAI Guidelines 2011say:

IB CABG to improve survival is recommended for patients with significant ($\geq 50\%$ diameter stenosis) left main CAD.

IIB PCI to improve survival is reasonable as an alternative to CABG in selected stable patients with significant ($\geq 50\%$ diameter stenosis) unprotected left main CAD with: 1) anatomic conditions associated with a low risk of PCI procedural complications and a high likelihood of a good long-term outcome (e.g., a low SYNTAX score [≤ 22], ostial or trunk left main CAD); and 2) clinical characteristics that predict a significantly increased risk of adverse surgical outcomes (e.g., STS-predicted risk of operative mortality 5%)

IIIB PCI to improve survival should not be performed in stable patients with significant ($\geq 50\%$ diameter stenosis) unprotected left main CAD who have unfavorable anatomy for PCI and who are good candidates for CABG. See:
https://professional.heart.org/idc/groups/ahamah-public/@wcm/@sop/@smd/documents/downloadable/ucm_433501.pdf

507. What is robotic-assisted PCI?
a. **Cardiologist sits at a remote console that controls device movements**
b. **Cardiologist puts his head in a remote control station that controls 2 remote control arms used for device movement**
c. **Remote angio control and assistance from a distant expert in the field**
d. **Computer assisted algorithm to recommend appropriate PCI strategies and devices**

ANSWER: a. Cardiologist sits at a console that controls device movement. In robotic PCI, a robot that is controlled by a cardiologist who sits at a robotic console controls the guidewires. These can be manipulated to incredible degrees of precision and pass the area of blockage. The robot then is used to deliver stents to the diseased area and treat the blockages. Using robotics a specialized interventionalist could perform procedures from a distant location.

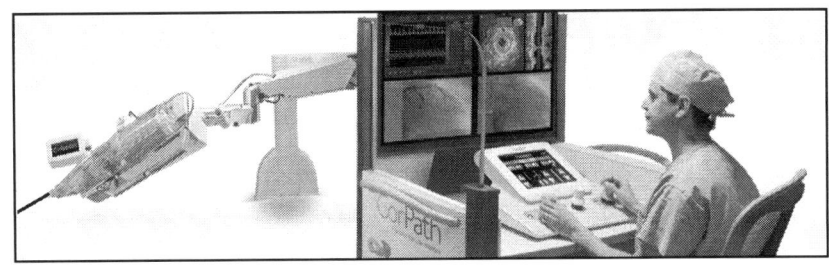

Corindus says advantages are: "Robotic-assisted control of coronary guide catheters, guidewires, and balloon/stent catheters. Radiation protection for the physician. Precise sub-millimeter measurement and 1 mm movement to position stents exactly where you need them."

See: www.corindus.com/corpath-grx

CardioThoracic Surgery

We recommend visiting the **CardioThoracic Surgery** web site to view angiograms and test yourself with their surgical question bank. Explore: Cardiac Radiology, Coronary Angiography, Angiography Simulator, Coronary Anatomy, Coronary Surgery & Question Banks.
See: https://www.cthsurgery.com

References:
Baim D. S. and Grossman W., Cardiac Catheterization, Angiography, and Intervention, 7th Ed., Lea and Febiger, 2006
Braunwald, et. al. Ed., Heart Disease, a Textbook of CV Medicine, 9th Ed., Saunders, 2012
Kern, M. J., Ed., *The Cardiac Catheterization Handbook*, 6th Ed., Mosby-Year Book, Inc., 2016
King, S. B. III, Yeung, Alan C, *Interventional Cardiology*, McGraw-Hill, 2007
Pappano & Wier (previously Berne and Levy), Cardiovascular Physiology, 10th Ed., Mosby Year Book, 2013
Pepine, J. C., and Hill, J. A., et. al., *Diagnostic and Theraputic Cardiac Catheterization*, 2nd Ed., Williams and Wilkins, 1998
Ragosta, Cardiac Catheterization, an Atlas and DVD, Saunders,1st Ed., Elsevier, 2010
Tilkian, A. G., and Daily, E, J, *Cardiovascular Procedures, Diagnostic Techniques and Therapeutic Procedures*, C. V. Mosby Company, 1986
Yaniga, Leslie, RCIS, *Cath Lab Pharmacology*, Smith Notes, 1998

OUTLINE: Coronary Arteriography

1. EQUIPMENT
   a. Catheters
      i. Amplatz Rt.& Lt.
      ii. Sizing for AO and coronary takeoff
      iii. Judkins Rt. & Lt.
      iv. Sizing for AO and coronary takeoff
      v. Internal Mammary
      vi. Multipurpose
   b. Guidewires
   c. Sheath
   d. Coronary Manifolds
      i. use of ports
         (1) Dye
         (2) Syringe
         (3) Waste bag
         (4) Transducer
         (5) Flush
         (6) Catheter
2. INSERTION TECHNIQUES
   a. Catheter manipulation
      i. Judkins Technique
      ii. JR3.5, 4, 5, or 6
      iii. Catheter sizing
      iv. Technique of rotating in Ao.
      v. JL3.5, 4, 5, or 6
   b. Catheter sizing
      i. dilated aorta, anterior take-off
   c. IMA graft technique
      i. From Femoral approach
      ii. From ipsilateral radial
   d. JUDKINS CORONARY ANGIO.
      i. Local anesthesia
      ii. Arterial access
      iii. Sheath
      iv. Catheter insertion with wire
      v. Preload and insert Pigtail
      vi. Pressures
      vii. AO, LV
      viii. LV Gram
      ix. post angio LVEDP
      x. Record pullback pressure
      xi. Shoot first Coronary
      xii. make catheter exchange
      xiii. Shoot second Coronary
   e. SONES TECHNIQUE
      i. Brachial cutdown
      ii. LV & coronaries
      iii. closing
      iv. Amplatz technique
   f. Multipurpose technique
      i. Schoonmaker/King catheter
      ii. single catheter technique
   g. Coronary Arteriography
      i. Rate of hand injection
      ii. overfilling vessel to see the Os.
      iii. Use of pressure injector
      iv. 3-4 ml/sec
   h. Cine equipment
      i. power requirements
      ii. panning table
      iii. grids
      iv. Image intensifier
      v. Cine camera
      vi. Cine film
      vii. Cine processing
      viii. Digital processing
3. HEMODYNAMIC CHANGES
   a. Contrast changes

- b. ECG
  - i. Bradycardia, T waves
  - ii. RCA inverts "T" waves
  - iii. LCA elevates "T" waves
  - iv. Arrhythmias
  - v. VT., V. fib., Asystole
- c. pressure changes
  - i. hypotension
  - ii. Damping
    - (1) cuts off blood flow
    - (2) may lead to cor. artery spasm
    - (3) may lead to tipping up a plaque
    - (4) "Hit and run" injection
  - iii. Ventricularization: Arterial Pressure Mimics Damped Lv
  - iv. Reduced Pressure Damping: Pressure Falls off
  - v. LV Retrograde Across Valve
  - vi. Reduced High Freq. Damping (Contrast)
4. ANATOMY
   - a. VIEWS
     - i. RAO - LAO
     - ii. Angulated Views
       - (1) LCA orifice   20 deg. LAO
       - (2) Circ. branches 30 deg. RAO / Caudal
       - (3) Distal LAD 30 deg. RAO/Caud./ Cr.
       - (4) Prox. LAD / Diag. 30 deg. LAO / Cr.
       - (5) Bifurcation LAD/Cx.   30 deg. LAO / Cr. or (caud.-spider view)
       - (6) Bifurcation LAD/Cx.   20 deg. RAO / 15 Caud.
     - iii. Dominance (Rt. or Lt.)
       - (1) depends on vessel to crux & PDA
   - b. CORONARY ANATOMY
     - i. Main Left coronary
       - (1) Ramus Medianus
       - (2) LCA
         - (a) LAD, Circumflex
         - (b) Septals, Diagonals
         - (c) Circumflex, obtuse Marginal
         - (d) Distal Circ. in AV groove
       - (3) RCA
         - (a) Conus branch
         - (b) SA node branch
         - (c) RV branches
         - (d) Acute Marginal
         - (e) PDA
         - (f) Septal branches (inferior)
         - (g) AV node
         - (h) Posterior Lateral (to LV)
     - ii. Bypass graft arteriography
     - iii. CABG, IMA
     - iv. Collateral circulation
     - v. common pathways
     - vi. Myocardial Bridge
   - c. PITFALLS IN CORONARY ARTERIOGRAPHY
     - i. Widowmaker lesion
     - ii. Early bifurcation
     - iii. spasm
     - iv. flow artifacts
     - v. eccentricity
     - vi. unrecognized occlusions
     - vii. Superimposition
     - viii. Myocardial bridging
     - ix. recanalization
   - d. ABNORMALITIES OF CORONARY CIRCULATION
     - i. Anomalies altering myocardial perfusion
     - ii. Anomalies not altering myo. perfusion
     - iii. Effect of stenosis on coronary flow
     - iv. Collaterals
     - v. Spasm
     - vi. Plaque morphology
     - vii. types of lesions
     - viii. risks associated with lesions
     - ix. Coronary bypass angiography
5. OTHER CORONARY
   - a. Premedication
     - i. Valium, versed
     - ii. Benadryl, Heparin
     - iii. Nitroglycerine, Atropine
   - b. Other Medications
     - i. Contrast material
       - (1) Renographin, Hypaque
       - (2) Nonionic
       - (3) Low osmolar
     - ii. Ergonovine - Methergine
       - (1) Provoke Spasm
       - (2) Reverse with Nitroglycerine IC
     - iii. Fibrinolysis
       - (1) Streptokinase IA, TPA
       - (2) Urokinase
     - iv. Findings pre & post SK
       - (1) Streptokinase IV
   - c. Digital coronary angiography
   - d. Quantitative Coronary angiography
   - e. FFR
   - f. CT coronary imaging
     - i. CT FFR., FFRct

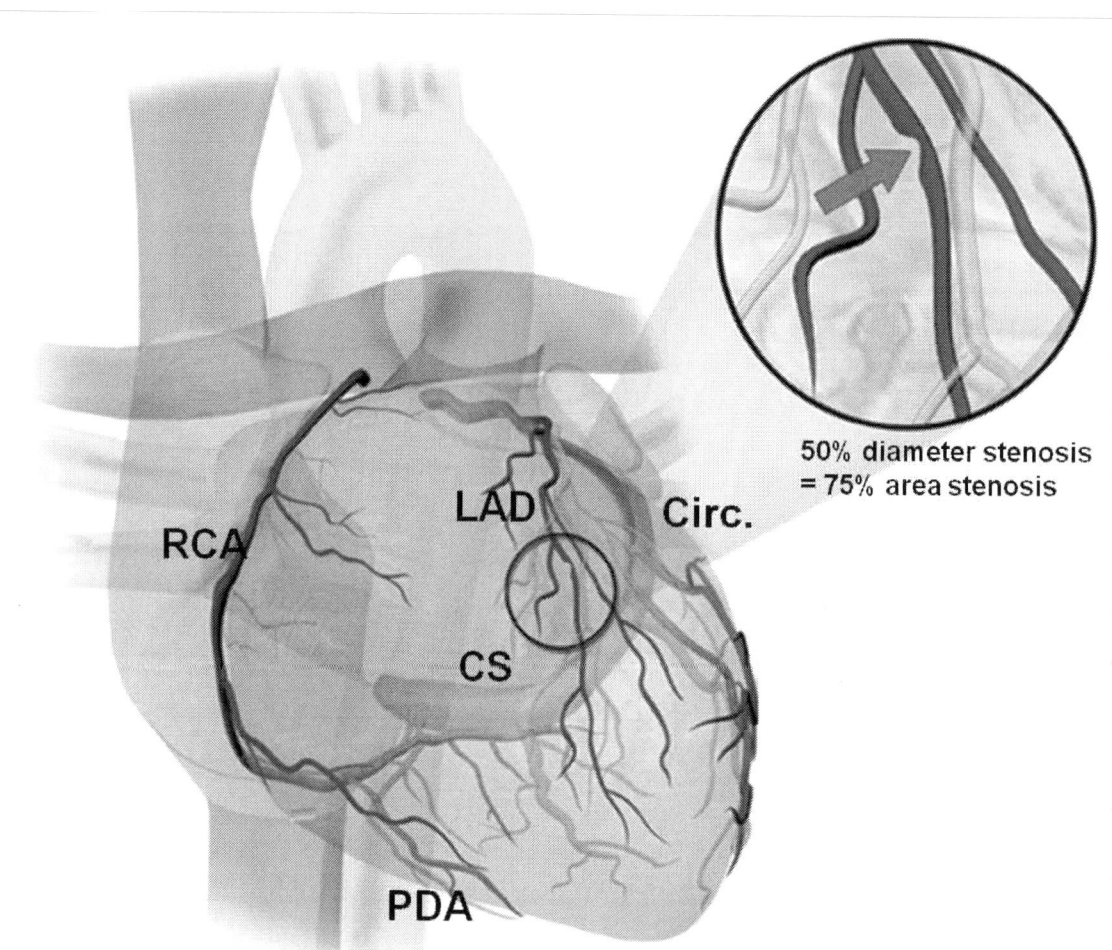

Modified from https://www.ehealthstar.com/conditions/coronary-heart-disease

Left Heart Catheterization

INDEX: D8 - Left Heart Catheterization
1. Equipment & Catheters . . . p. 283 - Know
2. Pressure Injectors . . . . p. 285 - Know
3. Contrast & Premedications . . . p. 289 - Know
4. Hemodynamics . . . . . p. 292 - Know
5. LV Angiography . . . . p. 298 - Know
6. LV Wall Motion . . . . . p. 305 - Know
7. LV Pathology . . . . . p. 313 - Know
8. Transseptal Heart Cath. . . . p. 317 - Know
9. Chapter Outline . . . . . p. 326

1. Equipment & Catheters

508. Identify the left heart and/or aortic angiographic flood catheter bend labeled #1 in the diagram.
   a. Pigtail
   b. Angled Pigtail
   c. Multipurpose A2
   d. Brockenbrough

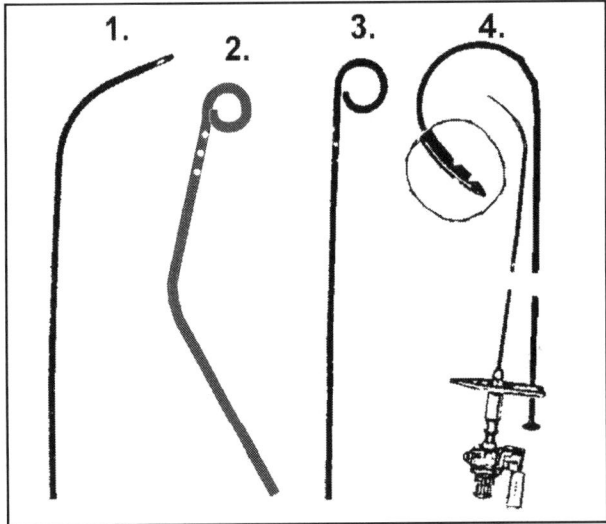

Left heart catheters

ANSWER: c. Multipurpose A2.
MATCH THE OTHER LEFT HEART CATHETERS IN THE DIAGRAM with the list below.
1. **MULTIPURPOSE A2:** Schoonmaker/King's all purpose catheter can be used for LV angiography and both right and left coronary arteries. Has 2 sideholes and end hole.
2. **ANGLED PIGTAIL:** LV flood catheter, 145 degree body angle to sit mid LV. The tip is curled like a "pig's tail."
3. **PIGTAIL:** An all-purpose flood catheter, very atraumatic. The tip is curled like a "pig's tail."
4. **BROCKENBROUGH:** This catheter crosses atrial septum after a transeptal puncture is made through fossa ovalis. The catheter is then advanced into the LA, across the mitral valve into the LV.

See: Kern, chapter on "Coronary Angiography and Ventriculography"

509. The angiographer wishes to cross the aortic valve retrograde on your patient with tight aortic stenosis. Which catheter and guide system would you suggest as a first choice?
a. Pigtail catheter and straight .038 inch wire
b. Pigtail catheter and curved tip Glide-wire.
c. JL4 catheter and .035 inch "J" wire
d. JL4 catheter and stiff Glide-wire

ANSWER: a. Pigtail catheter and straight .038 inch wire. Pigtail catheter is usually the first choice for attempting to cross the aortic valve with a stiff straight stainless steel wire. If the pigtail fails then try Judkins, Amplatz, or multipurpose catheters.

Stiff and straight stainless guide-wires can best be aimed at the orifice by advancing the wire wherever it vibrates in the high velocity AS jet. It's rather like blindly feeding a stick into an erupting volcano.

Kern says, "The AO valve is usually crossed using a 0.038-inch straight-tipped safety guidewire, extending the wire out of the catheter, straightening the pigtail, and directing the wire into the area of

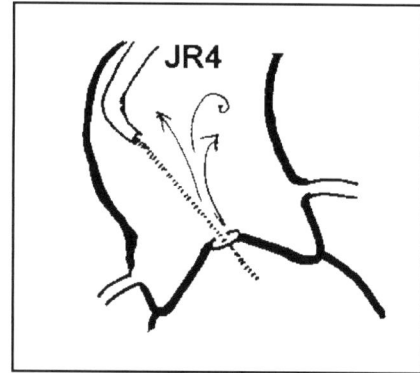

JR4 & .038 wire in AS

highest turbulence as detected by jet impact motion of the wire seen on the fluoroscopy monitor.... Other catheter choices for crossing the AO valve include the left and, occasionally, right Amplatz catheter, left and right Judkins catheters, multipurpose catheters, and specially designed catheters.... It should not require more than several minutes to cross an AO valve, even if severely stenosed, and if great difficulty is encountered, a trans-septal approach should be strongly and rapidly considered."
See: Kern, chapter on "Hemodynamic Data"

510. Which "universal" catheters have the most risk of kickback and myocardial perforation during ventriculography?
a. Omni, Halo or Royal Flush
b. Brockenbrough or Berman
c. Multipurpose or Jacky
d. Pigtail or angled pigtail

ANSWER c. Multipurpose or Jacky. The best flush catheters have multiple side holes to disperse the dye without kickback. Single end-hole catheters are the worse for this, because the catheter whip and kickback may inject contrast into myocardium. Even 2 side holes are not enough to prevent this problem. The Berman is a balloon floatation right heart flush catheter popular in pediatrics.

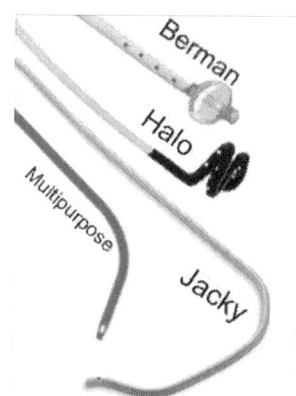

Kern says, "Radial Universal Catheters: Catheters used for coronary angiography from the radial approach are called generically 'universal catheters' because they can engage both the left and right coronary ostia. Among the most common is the 'Jacky catheter.' Although some operators perform ventriculography through universal catheters because there are side holes near the catheter tip, **we do not recommend this practice**. This end-hole LV catheter angiography can cause serious harm with poor catheter positioning. An operator can cause LV perforation with an end-hole catheter (e.g. an MP catheter) when the tip is against the LV wall and contrast is injected directly into or through the myocardium, followed by tamponade and cardiac arrest.... The Halo catheter is a novel 5-French catheter with a perpendicular helical tip with an inwardly and upwardly directed tip. The side holes are located on the helix and produce equivalent left ventriculograms with minimal ectopy because the contrast jets are directed inward and not to the myocardium." **See:** Kern, chapter on "Coronary Angiography and Ventriculography"

2. Pressure Injectors

511. The reason for "tapping" the pressure injector syringe just before performing an LV test injection is to:
 a. Assure a tight catheter - syringe connection
 b. Make sure you have drawn back blood into the injection syringe
 c. Test the integrity of the injection syringe
 d. Break loose any bubbles at the tip of the injection syringe

ANSWER d. Break loose any bubbles at the tip of the injection syringe. When a pressure injection is made, it is essential to get rid of all bubbles at the blood-dye interface and in the tip of the syringe. With the syringe tip pointed down first draw back a few cc of blood and then use a hemostat to "whack" the tip of the injection syringe. This breaks loose any unseen bubbles, visualizes them, and allows them to float to the top of the syringe where they will not be injected. This hemostat is then considered "contaminated" because it has touched a part of the syringe and injector which was nonsterile.
See: Grossman, chapter on "Cardiac Ventriculography." **Keywords:** "whacking" injection syringe → break loose bubbles

512. You are operating a Medrad pressure injector for left ventriculography. When connecting the catheter to the pressure injector the physician asks you to make a "running connection" to prevent bubbles. As the physician allows arterial bleeding from the catheter and starts to screw the catheter hub onto the injection syringe tubing you should:
 a. Check that the connection is tight
 b. Draw back blood from the catheter
 c. Tap the injector syringe with a hemostat
 d. Squirt a small amount of contrast from the injector

ANSWER: d. Squirt a small amount of contrast from the injector .
 Kern says, "Several techniques are used to establish a bubble-free system when connecting the catheter to the syringe. A running connection is a technique in which a small amount of contrast material is squirted out of the syringe while the catheter is being

connected to the syringe. Merging of the fluid streams of blood from the catheter and the forward flow of contrast material from the syringe prevents any large air bubbles from entering the system on connection." **See:** Kern, chapter on "Coronary Angiography and Ventriculography"

513. You are operating a Medrad pressure injector for left ventriculography. After the physician connects the catheter to the pressure injector tubing you should immediately:
a. Make a small LV test injection
b. Check that the connection is tight
c. Draw back blood from the catheter
d. Make control settings on the pressure injector

ANSWER: c. Draw back blood from the catheter

Kerns says, "After connection, the injector operator always aspirates more fluid (usually contrast material in the connector tube) into the syringe to ensure that no air bubbles are present. If air is present, it is expelled, and the clearing procedure is redone."

Kern says, "The practice of end-hole ventriculography often performed through a JR catheter with a hand injection for operator convenience has come under scrutiny as an inappropriate catheterization laboratory technique that should be abandoned....End-hole LV catheter angiography can cause serious harm with poor catheter positioning. An operator can cause LV perforation with an end-hole catheter (e.g. an MP catheter) when the tip is against the LV wall and contrast is injected directly into or through the myocardium, followed by tamponade and cardiac arrest.... The optimal catheter position for left ventriculography is one that avoids contact with the papillary muscles and is not positioned too close to the mitral valve, so that mitral regurgitation is not produced artificially."

"During contrast injection, the physician performing the ventriculogram should be holding the catheter with the right hand and the sheath with the left, preparing to withdraw the catheter if necessary, observing the physiologic monitor, and looking for problems, such as myocardial contrast staining, VT, or sudden hypotension. Rapid catheter withdrawal may be required." The technician operating the pressure injector should also be prepared to immediately stop the pressure injection if necessary. **See:** Kern, chapter on "Coronary Angiography and Ventriculography"

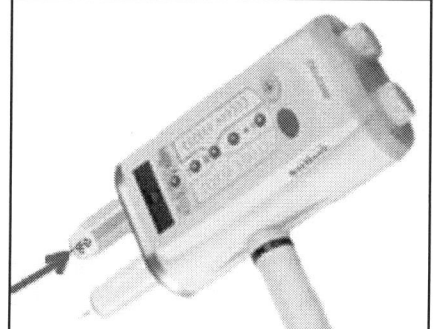

« Diagnostic Techniques: D8 - Left Heart Catheterization »   287

514. How should you inject the LV in patient #3 in the box? (Your hospital has a policy of using high-osmolar contrast for all "standard, low risk" cases.)
  a. Standard high-osmolar contrast at 10 ml/sec for 35 ml total
  b. Standard high-osmolar contrast at 15 ml/sec for 50 ml total
  c. Low-osmolar contrast at 10 ml/sec for 35 ml total
  b. Low-osmolar contrast at 15 ml/sec for 50 ml total

> **DOING LV-GRAM ON PATIENT WITH:**
>
> 1. Multipurpose catheter in an SOB patient with high wedge pressure
> 2. Pigtail in a patient with significant AR and elevated wedge pressure
> 3. **Multipurpose catheter in a small woman**
> 4. Pigtail catheter in a young athletic man with hyperkinetic ventricle

ANSWER a. Standard high-osmolar contrast at 10 ml/sec for 35 ml total.
MATCH THE OTHER NUMBERED PATIENTS WITH a suggested LV-gram.
  1. **Low-Osmolar Contrast** at 10 ml/sec for 35 ml total. Use low-osmolar contrast on sick hearts especially with low EF and SOB. Multipurpose catheters require lower injection rates because of the end-hole kickback problem.
  2. **Low-Osmolar Contrast** at 15 ml/sec for 50 ml total. Use low-osmolar contrast on sick hearts. Use high flow injections for AR or hypercontractile patients.
  3. **High-Osmolar Contrast** at 10 ml/sec for 35 ml total. Multipurpose catheters require lower injection rates because of the end-hole kickback problem. Ok for small female patients with no significant heart problems.
  4. **High-Osmolar Contrast** at 15 ml/sec for 50 ml total. Use faster flow rates and larger volumes for hyperkinetic hearts or all the contrast will be washed out of the heart before you get pictures.
See: Grossman, chapter on "Cardiac Ventriculography." **Keywords:** LV angio injection rates, volumes, low-osmolar contrast

515. Calculate the total injection time for the injector settings labeled #2 in the box (8 for 40).
  a. 2 sec
  b. 3 sec
  c. 5 sec
  d. 9 sec

> **INJECTOR SETTINGS**
> 1. 5 for 10 total
> 2. 8 for 40 total
> 3. 60 ml at 20/sec
> 4. 90 ml at 10/sec

ANSWER c. 5 sec. = (40 ml total Vol) / (8 ml/sec). The formula is Rate = Vol/Time or rearranged algebraically becomes Time = Vol/Rate. Note how unit cancellation gives the correct answer. Most technologists make the injector settings from two simple numbers like "**8 for 40**", where 8 is the rate and 40 is the total volume injected. The "**for**" means "**for a TOTAL VOLUME OF.**" It can also be stated as "40 ml at 8/sec" where 40 is the volume and 8 the rate. The "**at**" means "**at a RATE OF.**" Be able to match all answers.
CORRECTLY MATCHED INJECTOR SETTINGS ARE:
  1. 5 for 10 total =   2 sec   =   (10 ml total Vol) / (5 ml/sec)
  2. 8 for 40 total =   5 sec   =   (40 ml total Vol) / (8 ml/sec)
  3. 60 ml at 20/sec =   3 sec   =   (60 ml total Vol) / (20 ml/sec)

4. 90 ml at 10/sec = 9 sec = (90 ml total Vol) / (10 ml/sec)
See: Personal experience Keywords: Calculate injection time

516. For flood injections, which of the following would be a likely pressure limit setting on the power injector?
a. 10 atm
b. 120 psi
c. 900 psi
d. 5000 psi

ANSWER: c. 900 -1000 psi pressure limit will prevent catheter rupture during high pressure injection if the catheter becomes kinked or blocked. 2500 is too high and may rupture thinner catheters. If a catheter ruptures the most likely location is at the catheter hub where pressure is highest. **See:** Grossman, chapter on "Cardiac Ventriculography"
Keywords: high pressure limit 900-1000 psi

517. The "rate of rise" adjustment on power injectors is used in selective arteriography and LV grams to:
a. Reduce catheter whip
b. Reduce catheter rupture
c. Prevent air bubble injection
d. Optimize dye distribution in a vessel

ANSWER: a. Reduce catheter whip. Schneider says, "When selective arteriography is performed using specially shaped end-hole catheters, a rate rise is required to avoid the occasional high-pressure injection into the arterial wall [and catheter whip - similar to an unsecured garden hose turned on under high pressure].... Percutaneous arteriography in larger arteries, especially those with a high rate of flow, using small catheters would not be possible without a power injector." Although catheter whip is minimized in flood catheters because of the many side holes, a small rate-rise (0.05 - 0.2 second) helps stabilize these catheters as well.
See: Schneider, Endovascular Skills, chapter on "How to Get Where You are Going"

518. What is the most dangerous (but avoidable) risk associated with left ventriculography injection is:
a. Sustained arrhythmia
b. Intramyocardial staining
c. Air or thrombus embolism
d. Myocardial rupture and tamponade

ANSWER: c. Air or thrombus embolism. Grossman says, "The inadvertent injection of air or thrombus probably poses the greatest risk associated with ventriculography. The risk of air embolism should be avoidable by good technique in filling the injector and confirming a bubble-free hookup... The presence of thrombi on or within the catheter is minimized by frequent flushing of the catheter with a solution containing heparin when the ventriculographic catheter is first introduced and just prior to hooking up for the ventriculogram." **See:** Grossman, chapter on "Cardiac Ventriculography" **Keywords:** Air embolism during LV gram

519. Which of the following would most diminish the ability of quantitative LV-grams to accurately measure ejection fraction?
   a. Rapid injection rate, overfilling the chamber
   b. Catheter touching endocardium, frequent PVCs
   c. Catheter tip too close to semilunar valve, induced mitral regurgitation
   d. Catheter side-holes straddling tricuspid valve, inadequate opacification

ANSWER: b. Catheter touching endocardium, frequent PVCs. Catheter irritation causes PVCs. PVCs have reduced stroke volume and ejection fraction due to inadequate filling. Post PVC beats have increased stroke volume and EF due to excessive filling. They both mess up the accuracy of the LVgram and should not be measured. All the other catheter positions listed are poor as well, but do not necessarily effect SV and EF measurement. You need rapid injection for LV-grams, which does not overfill the chamber.
See: Kern, chapter on "Angiographic Data" **Keywords:** Don't quantify PVCs

3. Contrast & Premedications

520. Shortly after ventriculography high-osmolar contrast agents produce systemic _____ with a resultant transient _____ in arterial pressure.
   a. Vasodilation, drop in BP
   b. Vasodilation, rise in BP
   c. Vasoconstriction, drop in BP
   d. Vasoconstriction, rise in BP

ANSWER: a. Vasodilation, drop in BP although much diminished with low osmolar contrast..
   King says, "All contrast agents produce arterial vasodilation with a resultant decrease in systemic vascular resistance and a transient drop in arterial pressure shortly after administration. Vasodilation occurs more commonly with high-osmolality agents, high contrast agent volume use, and arterial (compared to venous) injection. Contrast agents also leads to an increase in intravascular volume, with agents of higher osmolarity having a greater effect. Ventricular filling pressures therefore rise following intravascular contrast media injection, which is an important consideration in patients with depressed left ventricular function and preexisting elevation of diastolic filling pressures." **See:** King, chapter on "Radiographic Contrast Media"
   Kern says, "Although uncommon with nonionic low-osmolar contrast media (LOCM), hypotension, bradycardia, and arrhythmias have been reported during injections. Therefore, the ECG and arterial pressure should be monitored continuously. Atropine, vasopressors, and antiarrhythmic agents should be available for prompt administration. Transient bradycardia or hypotension can be overcome with a brief forceful cough. Use of nonionic low-osmolality contrast agents has greatly reduced the incidence of bradycardia,

arrhythmias, hypotension, and the need for coughing during coronary angiography." **See:** Kern, chapter on "Coronary Angiography and Ventriculography"

521. What precautions should be taken while performing LV contrast injection, against contrast staining, induced arrhytmia and perforation of the LV endocardium? (Check 2 below.)
  a. Use large bore end-hole catheters
  b. Be ready to quickly pull catheter back
  c. Be ready to immediately stop injection
  d. Position the catheter tip near the mitral valve
  e. Use low pressure hand contrast injections

ANSWERS: b & c. Be ready to quickly pull catheter back and be ready to immediately stop injection. Kern says, "The practice of end-hole ventriculography often performed through a JR catheter with a hand injection for operator convenience has come under scrutiny as an inappropriate catheterization laboratory technique that should be abandoned....End-hole LV catheter angiography can cause serious harm with poor catheter positioning. An operator can cause LV perforation with an end-hole catheter (e.g. an MP catheter) when the tip is against the LV wall and contrast is injected directly into or through the myocardium, followed by tamponade and cardiac arrest.... The optimal catheter position for left ventriculography is one that avoids contact with the papillary muscles and is not positioned too close to the mitral valve, so that mitral regurgitation is not produced artificially."

"During contrast injection, the physician performing the ventriculogram should be holding the catheter with the right hand and the sheath with the left, preparing to withdraw the catheter if necessary, observing the physiologic monitor, and looking for problems, such as myocardial contrast staining, VT, or sudden hypotension. Rapid catheter withdrawal may be required." The technician operating the pressure injector should also be prepared to immediately stop the pressure injection if necessary. **See:** Kern, chapter on "Coronary Angiography and Ventriculography"

522. What chemical element in contrast material makes it radiopaque to X-rays?
  a. Calcium
  b. Iodine
  c. Barium
  d. Gadolinium

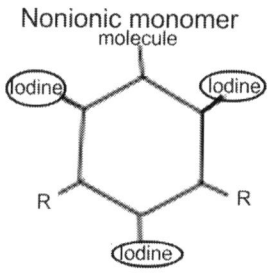

ANSWER b. Iodine. All vascular contrast media are organic compounds including the chemical element iodine on the benzene ring. It is a heavy metal which absorbs X-rays. This imparts its essential "radiopaque" quality. **See:** Grossman, chapter on "Angiography: Principles..." **Keywords:** Iodine in contrast = radiopaque

523. Older angiographic contrast agents such as Hypaque or Renografin commonly overload the blood volume of a patient in CHF. New contrast agents such as Ioxaglate (Hexabrix) and Iohexol (Omnipaque) do not increase the preload as much because of their:
a. Low osmolarity
b. Low Na+ and K+ content
c. Higher radio-opacity per cc
d. Increased ionization in solution

ANSWER a. Low osmolarity. The reason that these Low-Osmolar Contrast Media (LOCM) do not overload the blood volume is due to their low osmolarity (osmolality). Any high volume contrast injection suddenly increases the circulating blood volume. Besides the 30-40 cc of contrast added to the system, the high osmolarity of the contrast suddenly pulls plasma into the vascular space through osmotic action. It is analogous to eating a salty pork dinner. As a result, you retain water. Low-osmolar contrast media helps maintain normal fluid balance.
    The sudden increase in blood volume following LVgram dramatically increases preload and LV EDP. This may exacerbate a CHF patient's pulmonary edema.
See: Grossman, chapter on "Cardiac Ventriculography." **Keywords:** Less volume overload with low-osmolar contrast

524. A patient going for angiography has a history of previous allergic reactions to contrast media. All of the following premedications may be used to reduce the possibility of repeat reaction EXCEPT:
a. Cimetidone
b. Benadryl
c. Amrinone
d. Prednisone

ANSWER c. Amrinone is not for allergic reactions. It is an antiarrhythmic. Cimetidone, Benadryl and prednisone may be administered precath to patients with a history of allergy to contrast. This is also a primary indication to use low-osmolar contrast agents for all angiography. They are much less allergenic. **See:** Grossman, chapter on "Cardiac Cath..." **Keywords:** Previous allergic reaction premedicate with Benadryl, cimetidine, and prednisone

525. Patients in severe congestive failure should be "dried out" before LV angiography with _____ premedication.
a. Nitroglycerine/Tridil
b. Atropine/epinephrine
c. Benadryl/steroids
d. Diuretic/Lasix

ANSWER d. Diuretics such as Lasix will increase water elimination and "dry out" a patient's congested pulmonary system. This may help eliminate pulmonary edema following flood angiography caused by the sudden influx of contrast and plasma into the vascular space.

But the drying effect slows the elimination of contrast by the kidneys, and can worsen the toxic effects of contrast. So the cardiologist must use good judgement about balancing his patients fluid load. Low-osmolar contrast is recommended for CHF patients with elevated wedge or LVedp. **See:** Kern, chapter on "Angiographic Data." **Keywords:** Dry out a florid CHF patient with diuretics/Lasix

526. What helps patients with acute severe LV dysfunction and elevated wedge pressures undergo the hemodynamic stress of LV angiography?
a. Extra heparin
b. Steroids and Benadryl
c. Atropine and lidocaine
d. Nitroglycerin
e. Tell them to take a deep breath

ANSWER d. Either SL nitroglycerin, IV Tridel, or IV nitroprusside will protect the coronary circulation. Grossman states *"Failure to take a highly elevated pre-ventriculography pulmonary capillary wedge pressure seriously can lead to disastrous consequences, such as intractable pulmonary edema and even death."* Other protective strategies include:
• Using low-osmolar contrast
• Using DSA reduced volume injections.
See: Grossman, chapter on "Cardiac Ventriculography."
Keywords: # LV-gram with high wedge use a protective regimen of nitro.

4. Hemodynamics

527. What is the LV ejection fraction (EF) if the EDV=125 ml and the ESV=75 ml?
a. 40%
b. 50%
c. 60%
d. 75%
e. 80%

ANSWER a. 40%. Ejection Fraction (EF) is the ratio of blood ejected (Stroke Volume) per beat to the size of the diastolic ventricle.

A large ejection fraction usually shows a healthy vigorous myocardium.

SV = EDV - ESV
EF = (EDV-ESV)/EDV
EF = 100% x (SV/EDV)
EF = (125 ml - 75 ml)/125 ml = 50/125= 40%.

The contraction should be concentric with all points moving toward the center. This is called synergy. Myocardial ischemia and infarction all produce asymmetrical contractions termed asynergy.
See: Grossman, chapter on "Cardiac Ventriculography." **Keywords:** Calculate EF

528. A patient's LV angiogram shows apical hypokinesis during sinus rhythm. But following one PVC the compensatory beat shows significantly improved EF. This post-"PVC potentiation" of LV contractility suggests:
a. Reversible apical ischemia
b. Irreversible apical infarcted area
c. Recent LAD occlusion
d. Old LAD occlusion

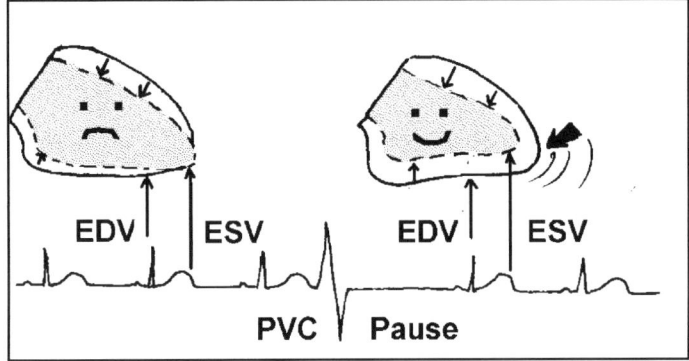
Post extra-systolic potentiation

ANSWER a. Reversible apical ischemia. Grossman says "Segmental dysfunction of the left ventricle can be caused by ischemia or infarction. Segments whose abnormal wall motion is caused by ischemia show improvement in systolic motion, whereas segments whose abnormal wall motion is due to infarction fail to improve. A single ventricular premature beat is introduced

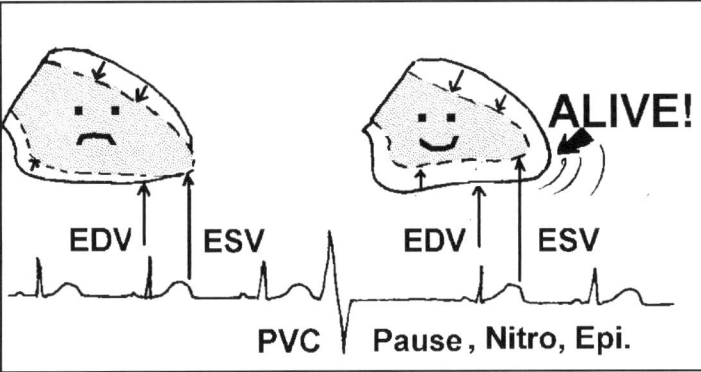
Post extra-systolic potentiation

during left ventriculography and is followed by a compensatory pause - then a potentiated beat. Segmental wall motion during one of the preceding sinus beats is compared to that of the post-extra-systolic beat. Left ventricles with asynergic wall motion during a preceding sinus beat which improves on the potentiated beat are ischemic, whereas those in which asynergy is similar on the preceding sinus beat and on the post-extra-systolic beat are infarcted."

This PVC may be introduced with a pacemaker or by irritating the ventricle while pulling back an RV catheter. Viable ischemic myocardium may also be evaluated on LV-gram post epinephrine, dobutamine, or nitroglycerin administration. As with post-extra-systolic potentiation, improved contractility indicates reversible ischemia.
See: Grossman, chapter on "Cardiac Ventriculography." **Keywords:** Post-PVC potentiation = reversible ischemia

THIS DATA GOES WITH THE NEXT 4 QUESTIONS. This patient has combined mitral stenosis and regurgitation.

529. Calculate the angiographic cardiac output (LVMF) of this patient. LVMF =
  a. 4.8 L/min
  b. 6.0 L/min
  c. 7.5 L/min
  d. 8.0 L/min

HEMODYNAMIC DATA on patient with MS & MR
- HR = 80 beats/min
- Thermodilution CO = 4.8 L/min

Quantitative LV angiography Data:
- EDV = 100 cc.
- ESV = 25 cc.

530. What is this patient's angiographic ejection fraction?
  a. 25%
  b. 45%
  c. 60%
  d. 75%

531. The same patient above has a thermodilution CO different from the angio CO because MR is present. What is the true regurgitant fraction?
  a. 15%
  b. 20%
  c. 48%
  d. 80%

532. Since the patient above has mitral stenosis and regurgitation, what is the forward flow through the mitral valve which should be used in the valve area calculation?
  a. 4.8 L/min
  b. 6.0 L/min
  c. 7.5 L/min
  d. 8.0 L/min

ANSWERS FOR ABOVE 4 QUESTIONS ARE LISTED TOGETHER BELOW.

529. ANSWER b. 6.0 L/min.
The formulas needed are:
- CO = SV x HR = LVMF
- SV = EDV - ESV = 100-25 = 75 ml.
- LVMF = 75 ml x 80 bpm = 6000 ml/min = 6.0 L/min

Note that LVMF is how much blood the LV pumps. This is not necessarily the CO since some blood may leak backward or be otherwise lost to shunts.
See: Kern, chapter on "Hemodynamics." **Keywords:** Calculate LVMF

530. ANSWER d. 75%. Stroke volume is EDV-ESV. This (angio. SV) is the difference between the largest (EDV) and the smallest (ESV) LV volume. Ejection fraction is the ratio of Stroke Volume / End Diastolic Volume. There is certain to be a question calculating EF because it is the most important measure of LV function. Become familiar with the terms involved and the calculations.
- SV = EDV - ESV = 100-25 = 75%
- EF = SV/EDV = 75/100 = .75 = 75%

See: Kern, chapter on "Hemodynamics." Keywords: Calculate EF

531. ANSWER b. 20% Regurgitation can be evaluated by subtracting the two measured cardiac outputs or stroke volumes.   Regurgitation/min = LVMF - TD CO
    Regurgitation = 6.0 - 4.8 L/min = 1.2 L/min
    (or Regurgitation/Beat = Angio. SV - TD SV.)
Calculate the thermodilution SV using the formula
    CO = SV x HR
Rearranging gives:
    SV = CO / HR = 4.8 L/min/80 bpm = 0.60 L = 60 ml/beat
Now: Regurgitation/Beat = SV_{angio} - SV_{TDCO}
    Reg./bt. = 75 - 60 = 15 ml/beat
Regurgitant fraction is the ratio of blood leaking back to that going forward. It can also be calculated on a per minute or a per beat method as above.
    RF = (Regurg./min) / (Largest CO) = 1.2 / 6.0 = .20 = 20%
    (or RF = (Regurg./beat) / (Largest SV) = 15 / 75 = .20 = 20%)
In this example with each beat 75 ml pumped by the LV, 60 ml goes out the AO and 15 ml leaks back. See: Kern, chapter on "Hemodynamics." Keywords: Calculate regurg. fraction

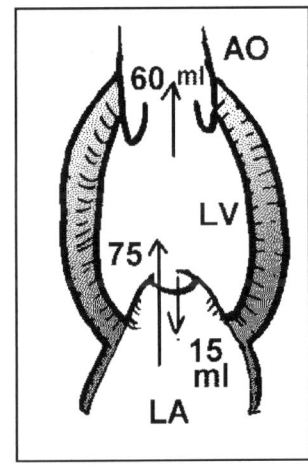
Stroke Vol in MS & MR

532. ANSWER b. 6.0 L/min. In every diastole 75 ml of blood passes forward through the mitral valve. True, 15 ml. leaks back, but all 75 ml causes the gradient. The 6.0 LVMF would therefore, be used in the valve area calculation - NOT the 4.8 thermodilution CO.
   The CO used in the Gorlin valve area formula must be the correct one. It varies with the combination of regurgitation and stenosis. Which CO is correct? You need to think about which flow is causing the gradient. If the stenosis and regurgitant are in the *same* valve then use LVMF (Angio CO). If the stenosis and regurgitation are in *different* valves use Fick or TDCO, e.g. in combined MR & AS (*different valves*) use the Fick CO to calculate the valve area. This is because in calculating AS valve area we need the flow across the AO valve in systole.
   The Fick CO does not include regurgitation as the LVMF does because it is measured in the lungs. If you get confused with all this, draw a picture like the one shown above to clarify the flows. Or calculate 2 valve areas, one for each CO and let the Drs. decide which they want. See: Kern, chapter on "Hemodynamics."
See online video: Dr. Bagnall, UK Endovascular Trainees, Left Ventricular Ejection Fraction - Mentice VIST-C Keywords: CO to calculate valve area

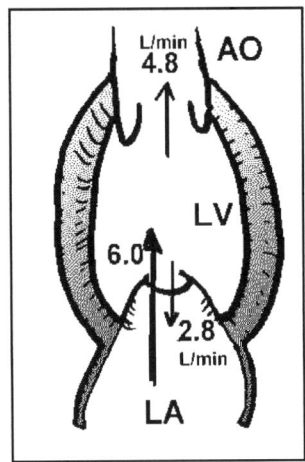
Flows in MS and MR

THIS PRESSURE TRACING RECORDED ON THE PATIENT ABOVE, SHOULD BE USED FOR THE NEXT 2 QUESTIONS.

533. What cardiac pressure level is recorded here with PA wedge to evaluate the end diastolic pressure level?
   a. RV
   b. RA
   c. LV
   d. AO

534. The LV end diastolic pressure measures _____ mmHg.
   a. 15 mmHg
   b. 22 mmHg.
   c. 26 mmHg.
   d. 42 mmHg.

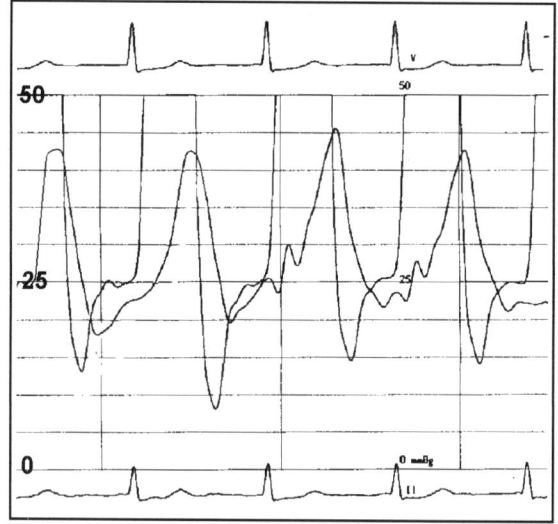

Ventricle & PAW Pressure, 0-40 scale

BOTH ANSWERS APPEAR TOGETHER BELOW.

533. ANSWER c. LV X50. Note that the LV systolic pressure curve is higher than the pressure scale, so the LV pressure goes off the top of the paper and "pegs" the recorder. The diastolic LV readings are made more accurately on this expanded scale. This LV tracing has a PA wedge recorded with it to evaluate for mitral stenosis. No gradient is seen, only the elevated PAW "v" waves of mitral regurgitation.
See: Kern, chapter on "Hemodynamics." **Keywords:** LV diastolic recording

534. ANSWER c. LV EDP = 26 mm Hg. LV-edp occurs at the end of ventricular filling. This occurs as the LV & LA pressures crossover each other and the mitral valve closes. It is also, measured at the peak of the R wave (actually .04 sec. after initial QRS deflection). Note how the R wave "points" to the LVedp. Use a ruler to draw a straight line up to the LV and read 25-26 mmHg. It can also be read at the point of rapid acceleration of the LV contraction wave. **See:** Kern, chapter on "Hemodynamics." **Keywords:** LVEDP measurement

535. The cutoff between normal and abnormal LV function is an EF of:
   a. 10%
   b. 30%
   c. 50%
   d. 70%

ANSWER c. 50%. EF is the most commonly used indicator of LV function and a good predictor of patient survival.
   50% is usually the cutoff for normal. Kennedy found that 94% of normal

individuals have an EF between 51% and 83%. **See:** Grossman, chapter on "Cardiac Ventriculography." **Keywords:** Normal EF > 50%

536. On the LV pressure curve (Wiggers diagram) identify the ventricular event shown at #6.
   a. The aortic valve closes
   b. Isometric relaxation
   c. The mitral valve opens
   d. Rapid diastolic filling
   e. Slow diastolic filling

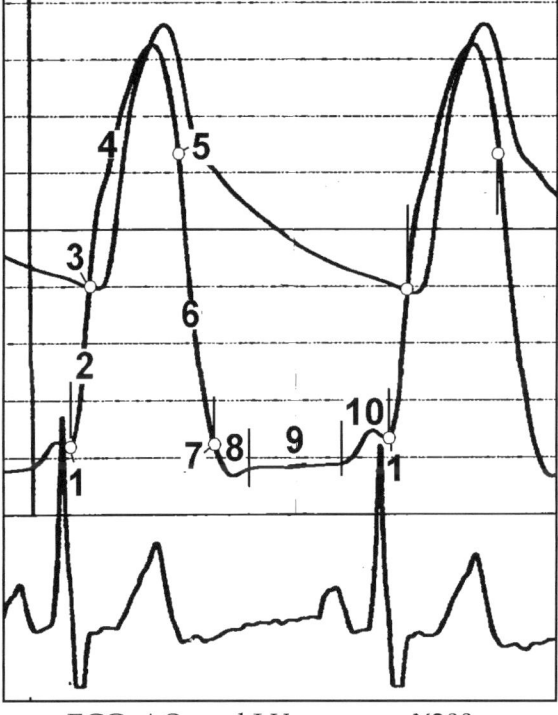

ECG, AO and LV pressure X200

ANSWER b. Isometric relaxation. **MATCH THE OTHER labeled waves with their name below.**
   SYSTOLE BEGINS at R WAVE)
   1. **MITRAL VALVE CLOSES:** QRS fires the ventricle, pressure begins to build up. When LV pressure > LA pressure the MV closes.
   2. **ISOMETRIC CONTRACTION:** The ventricle builds up pressure against closed valves.
   3. **AORTIC VALVE OPENS:** When the LV pressure exceeds the aortic pressure the aortic **valve opens. Note that all valve events are marked with a circle.**
   4. **SYSTOLIC EJECTION:** Occurs as blood flows out the aortic valve.
   5. **THE AORTIC VALVE CLOSES:** When AO pressure > LV pressure.
      DIASTOLE BEGINS
   6. **ISOMETRIC RELAXATION:** LV pressure falls to atrial level against closed valves.
   7. **THE MITRAL VALVE OPENS:** When LA pressure > LV pressures.
   8. **RAPID DIASTOLIC FILLING:** "Suction cup effect" as the LV sucks in atrial blood ("Y" descent wave).
   9. **SLOW FILLING:** Diastasis, or slow passive filling.
   10. **ATRIA CONTRACT:** Associated with "a" wave and "atrial kick".
See: Berne and Levy, chapter on "Cardiac Pump." **Keywords:** Wiggers, AO open

537. Following LV angiography, this LV-AO pullback pressure was recorded on X200. What abnormality is indicated?
a. None, this is normal pressure amplification in periphery
b. Aortic stenosis
c. Coarctation of aorta
d. Idiopathic hypertrophic subvalvular stenosis

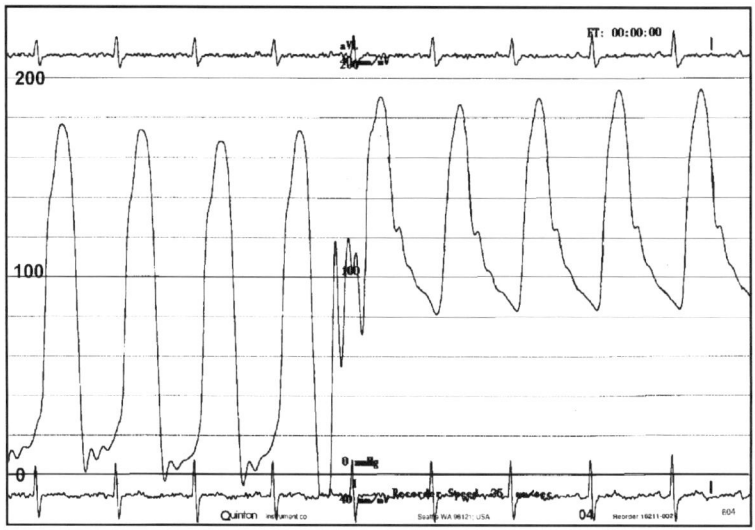
Abnormal LV-AO Pullback pressures

ANSWER a. No abnormalities are seen except the AO systolic is slightly higher than systolic LV, seemingly a hemodynamic impossibility. (AO pressure can't be higher or blood would flow backwards during systole). However, the further down the AO the catheter tip is withdrawn, systolic pressure increases due to wave reflections. The patient has systolic hypertension.
THIS IS NORMAL PRESSURE AMPLIFICATION IN PERIPHERY. Slightly higher systolic pressure is commonly seen when the catheter is pulled back into the descending AO. **See:** Grossman, chapter on "Pressure Measurements" **Keywords:** LV-AO pullbacks

5. LV Angiography

538. LV angiography is contraindicated in certain conditions such as LV thrombus, CIN, and elevated LVEDP. Most cardiologists don't do Lvgrams on patients:
a. When the ECG is normal
b. When LV function has recently changed
c. With acute coronary sydromes (STEMI & NSTEMI)
d. When echocardiography or CTA were done recently

ANSWER d. When echocardiography or CTA were done recently, because these LV studies usually are adequate or superior to LV angiographic analysis.
  SCAI standards 2015, "RECOMMENDATIONS FOR USE OF LEFT VENTRICULOGRAPHY: 1. Consider left ventriculography when left ventricular function or wall motion is unknown, or mechanical disruption is suspected and results of the study will help determine therapy. (Examples include acute coronary syndromes without prior noninvasive imaging, or when an acute change in clinical status suggests left ventricular function has recently changed.)
2. Perform left ventriculography selectively. Avoid it when an adequate alternative left ventricular imaging study has been performed.
3. Avoid left ventriculography in patients for whom it creates significant risk. Examples

include patients with renal insufficiency (when left ventriculography could increase the risk of contrast induced nephropathy), elevated end diastolic pressure (when left ventriculography could increase the risk of acute respiratory decompensation), known or suspected left ventricular mural thrombus, aortic valvular vegetation, and in those that have already received high levels of radiation exposure."See: Optimal Use of Left Ventriculography at the Time of Cardiac Catheterization: A Consensus Statement from the Society for Cardiovascular Angiography and Interventions, 2015

539. Your diagnostic heart cath patient has suspected double vessel CAD. He has left heart failure uncontrolled well with medication, a current wedge pressure of 48mmHg and an elevated creatinine level. For LV wall motion analysis you expect to use:
   a. 2D biplane echocardiography
   b. Doppler ultrasound wall analysis
   c. LV gram in RAO & LAO positions
   d. LV gram in AP & lateral positions

ANSWER: a. 2D biplane echocardiography. Doppler measures flow not wall motion.
   Kern says, "Left ventriculography, once an integral part of every cardiac angiographic procedure, has been reconsidered as often unnecessary in light of high-quality echocardiography for LV functional assessment.... Left ventriculography should be omitted in compromised patients not responding to conventional medical treatment for heart failure (i.e. with LV end-diastolic pressure >35 mm Hg) as well as in patients with chronic kidney disease or those at higher risk for contrast-induced nephropathy (diabetics, patients with proteinuria, or dehydrated/hypotensive patients) to limit contrast exposure." See: Kern, chapter on "Coronary Angiography and Ventriculography"

540. What diagnostic test is the new gold standard for measurement of LV volumes and global function?
   a. Magnetic Resonance (MRI/MRA)
   b. Computerized tomography (CTA/CCTA)
   c. Echocardiography
   d. LV angiography

ANSWER a. Magnetic Resonance (MRI/MRA). The only problem is it takes so long to do a study and the magnetism negates patients with metal objects (pacers, stents...).
   SCAI standards say, "Cardiac MRI is considered the gold standard for the measurement of left ventricular volumes and global function. A key role of cardiac MRI in left ventricular assessment has been for the validation of the accuracy of the competing modalities for left ventricular assessment. In clinical practice cardiac MRI is often relegated to the roles of clarifying the left ventricular ejection fraction after other modalities provide indeterminate results...."
   'CCTA allows accurate assessment of left ventricular function especially in individuals with normal ejection fraction and wall motion.... The very high spatial resolution of CCTA and the ability to perform post processing makes this the best technique for the assessment of complex LV geometric anomalies such as aneurysms or pseudo aneurysm. In this regard CCTA is far superior to cardiac MRI and the other competing modalities." See: Optimal Use of Left Ventriculography

at the Time of Cardiac Catheterization: A Consensus Statement from the Society for Cardiovascular Angiography and Interventions, 2015

541. For single plane quantitative angiography (Area-length method) the LV must be shot in the long axis _____ angiographic view.
a. 30 degree RAO
b. 60 degree RAO
c. 30 degree LAO
d. 60 degree LAO

ANSWER a. In the 30 degree RAO the heart's long axis is perpendicular to the X-ray beam. This is the standard view for the long axis which must be measured for LV volumes and ejection fraction.

SCAI standards say, "Left ventriculography is commonly performed in the right anterior oblique projection. This view allows the visualization of the anterior, apical, inferior, and high lateral walls. The left anterior oblique projection with steep cranial angulation allows visualization of the apical, lateral, and septal walls and ventricular septal defects." See: Optimal Use of Left Ventriculography at the Time of Cardiac Catheterization: A Consensus Statement from the Society for Cardiovascular Angiography and Interventions, 2015

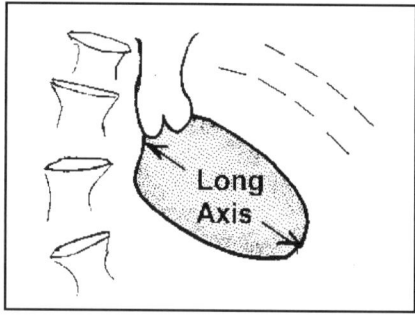

LV long axis = 30° RAO

542. For most accurate LV function (EF and wall motion analysis) the LV angiogram should ideally be done:
a. During deep inspiration
b. Prior to coronary arteriography
c. After inotropic drug administration
d. After nitroglycerin administration

ANSWER b. Prior to coronary arteriography. Grossman says, "Ideally it should be performed before coronary arteriography because of the depressant effect of radiographic contrast medium on LV function, which may last for up to an hour after injection." However, most centers do coronary angiography first, because LV function can always be evaluated by 2D echocardiography at a later date.
See: Braunwald, chapter on "Coronary Arteriography"

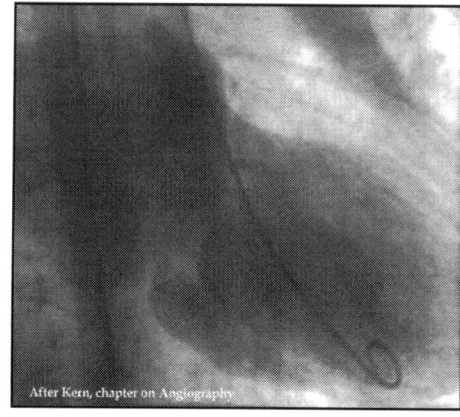

LV-gram, pigtail catheter

543. This _____ LV gram shows _____.
  a. LAO, mitral stenosis
  b. LAO cranial, mitral regurgitation
  c. RAO, mitral stenosis
  d. RAO cranial, mitral regurgitation

ANSWER d. RAO, mitral regurgitation. This is the LV long axis position which views the mitral valve on edge. Mitral regurgitation is seen as contrast leaking back into the LA through the mitral valve.
  Kern recommends the following projections:

Type of Valvular Regurgitation	Filming Projections	Site of Injection
Aortic	LAO, RAO	Aortic root
Mitral	RAO cranial, LAO (lateral)	LV
Tricuspid	RAO (shallow, lateral)	RV
Pulmonic	RAO, LAO, AP	Main PA
Type of Cardiac Shunt		
ASD	LAO cranial	PA
VSD	LAO cranial	LV
PDA	AP cranial	Aorta

See: Kern, chapter "Coronary Angiography and Ventriculography

BOTH QUESTIONS BELOW REFER TO THIS DIAGRAM.

544. The angiographic view of the LV labeled at #2 is the:
  a. Long axis view
  b. PA view
  c. Four chamber view
  d. Short axis view

545. What LV wall segments are not seen and cannot be evaluated with the LV angiographic view labeled #4?
  a. Anterior & inferior
  b. Apex and basal
  c. Septal and posterior lateral

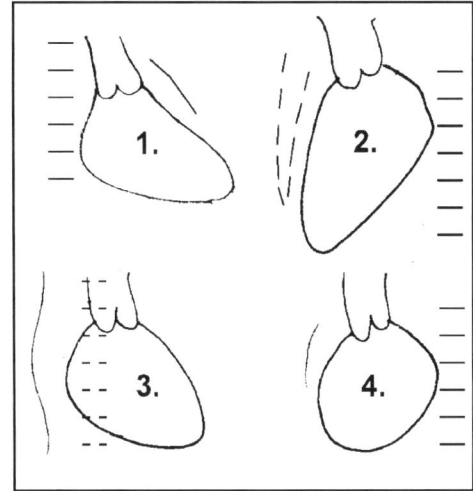

LV angio views

BOTH ANSWERS FOR THE DIAGRAM ABOVE APPEAR TOGETHER BELOW.
(Note, on diagram dotted lines are back wall of heart)

544. ANSWER c. Four chamber view cranial LAO. Note that in all LAO views the apex is to the left of the backbone. In all RAO views the heart is to the right of the backbone.

MATCH ALL LV-GRAM VIEWS WITH THEIR NAME BELOW.
1. **LONG AXIS VIEW:** 30-45° RAO view with apex to your right and backbone to your left. Mitral valve on edge. **This view is good for evaluating mitral valve and LV wall motion.**
2. **FOUR CHAMBER VIEW:** LAO with steep cranial is analogous to the echocardiographic 4-chamber view from the apex. It shows all 4 chambers by looking down onto the long axis from above. The IV septum is shown on edge. The RV shadow shows to the left of LV. This is the best view for VSD diagnosis.

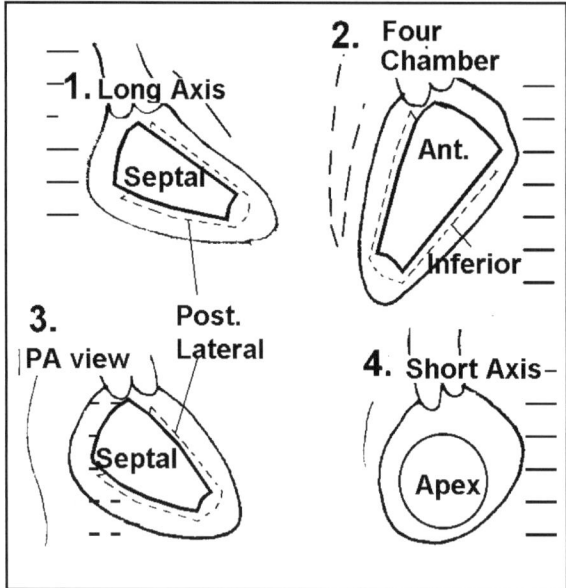

LV walls not seen in profile in these views

3. **PA VIEW:** Frontal view where the heart overlays the backbone.
4. **SHORT AXIS VIEW:** In this LAO caudal view, the LV appears as a circle. You are looking down the barrel of the LV with the mitral valve shooting right at you. The RV shadow shows to the left of LV. A good view for intra-chamber shunts.

See: Kern, The Cardiac Catheterization Handbook, chapter on "Angiographic Data."
Keywords: Views of LV - 4-chamber

545. ANSWER b. Apex and basal. Since the LV-gram is basically a shadow of the LV, the only segments seen to move are the edges. Just like you cannot see a squirrel's shadow on the trunk of a tree unless he is in profile on the side of the tree trunk. To see the walls in the center of image they must be visualized in a perpendicular plane. In the LAO caudal view (#4) the apex is buried in the center of the image and cannot be evaluated. However, the apex is well seen ion the RAO and LAO cranial views.

WALL SEGMENTS POORLY SEEN IN:
1. **Long axis 30° view:** septum and posterior lateral wall not seen.
2. **PA view:** septum and posterior lateral wall not seen.
3. **Four chamber LAO cranial view:** anterior and inferior wall not seen.
4. **Short axis LAO caudal view:** apex and mitral valve not seen.

These diagrams show the wall segments drawn on top of and beneath the LV image. This shows where they are. They just cannot be visualized in profile in this view.
See: Kern, The Cardiac Catheterization Handbook, chapter "Angiographic Data."
Keywords: LV wall segments NOT seen

546. What angiography best diagnoses a R-L VSD in a patient with extreme pulmonary hypertension?
 a. RV gram in RAO view
 b. RV gram in LAO view
 c. LV gram in RAO view
 d. LV gram in LAO view

ANSWER b. RV gram in LAO view. An RV injection would best show the shunt moving from RV-LV. The best view is LAO because the 2 ventricles do not overlap, and the shunt can be seen connecting the 2 adjacent chambers. Often cranial angulation is added to show the longer axis of the IV septum still on edge.

Usually VSDs create a L-R shunt, because of the much higher LV pressure. Then LV angiography is used to follow the shunt flow. Since this patient has extreme pulmonary hypertension, the normal L-R VSD has reversed into a R-L cyanotic shunt. So RV angiography is called for.
See: Kern, chapter on "Angiographic Data."

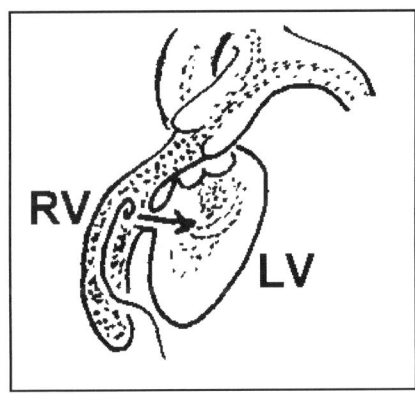
LAO RV-Gram, R-L VSD

547. Mitral valve prolapse is usually best seen in the _____ LV angio view, during _____.
 a. LAO, Systole
 b. LAO, Diastole
 c. RAO, Systole
 d. RAO, Diastole

ANSWER c. RAO, Systole. MVP and MR are best seen in the RAO view with the mitral leaflets on edge (although the LAO with steep cranial may also be used). The prolapse and/or MR are best seen during ventricular systole because that is when the closed mitral valve must hold back the LV pressure.

In prolapse the mitral leaflets are so enlarged they balloon back into the LA in systole. Mitral Valve Prolapse (MVP) is called by many names: Barlow's syndrome, floppy valve syndrome, ballooning mitral cusp syndrome, systolic click syndrome, hooded valve or redundant valve. Severe prolapse leads to mitral regurgitation. **See:** Underhill, chapter on "Acquired Valvular Heart Disease." **Keywords:** MVP, seen in RAO view in systole

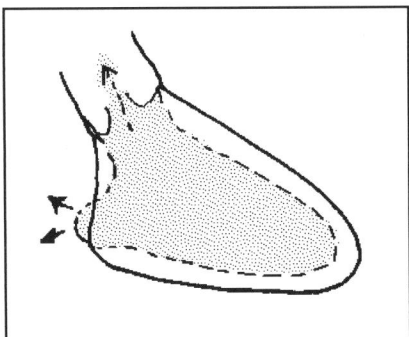
Mitral valve Prolapse

548. What angiographic view and injection site is generally best to diagnose the abnormality labeled #3 (ASD) in the box?
a. LAO, AO root injection
b. LAO cranial, PA injection
c. Steep LAO cranial, LV injection
d. PA cranial, aortic injection
e. RAO, LV injection

TO DIAGNOSE
1. Aortic dissection
2. Mitral valve regurgitation
*3. ASD
4. VSD
5. PDA

ANSWER b. LAO cranial, PA injection. Contrast flows through the lungs into the LA and through the shunt into the RA. The best view is generally perpendicular to the jet, and where chambers do not overlap. Inject in the upstream chamber where the jet originates. **MATCH THE OTHER CONDITIONS IN THE BOX** to a view & injection site below.
1. Dissection= 45°-60° LAO with AO ROOT INJECTION: The aorta is best seen perpendicular to the arch in the LAO view. The PA and RAO views are not as revealing because the ascending aortic arch overlaps the descending arch and the head vessels all overlie each other.
2. MR = 30° RAO with LV INJECTION: This views the mitral valve on edge so regurg. can be easily seen. The LAO view with cranial angulation may also be used.
3. ASD = 60° LAO CRANIAL with PA INJECTION. This is the 4 chamber view looking down the edge of the mitral valve and atrial septum. The PA injection will flow through the lungs into the LA. ASDs normally shunt from LA to RA.
4. VSD = 45°-60° LAO CRANIAL with LV INJECTION. The LAO view looks down the barrel of the LV with the ventricular septum on edge. Cranial LAO allows you to look down on the ventricular septum in its long axis so you can identify how close the jet is to the mitral valve (usually right under it). The VSD jet normally arises in the LV and shunts to the lower pressure RV. So LV injection is usually required.
5. PDA = PA CRANIAL with AORTIC INJECTION: Since the PDA enters the back side of the PA bifurcation cranial angulation helps get above the PA knob and visualize PDA the jet. PDAs normally arise in the AO and shunt into the lower pressure PA.
See: Kern, chapter "Angiographic Data." **Keywords:** Best LV angio view for VSD

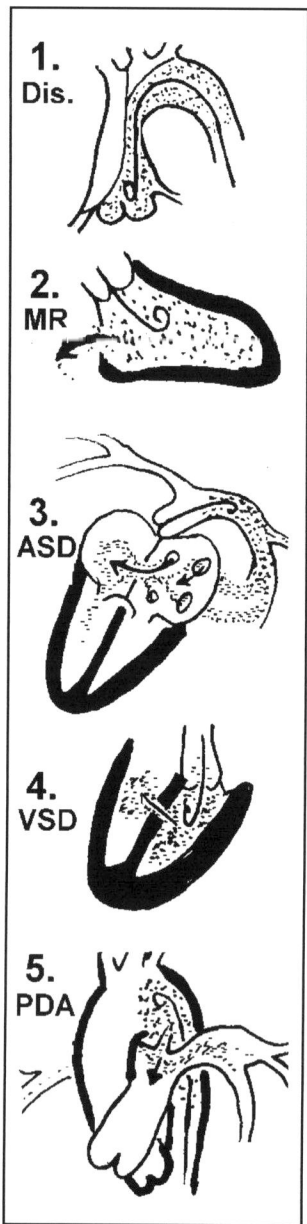

LV/AO angio.

549. Identify the severity and location of the valvular regurgitation from the LV gram labeled at #6.
   a. Mild AR
   b. Moderate AR
   c. Severe AR
   d. Mild MR
   e. Moderate MR
   f. Severe MR

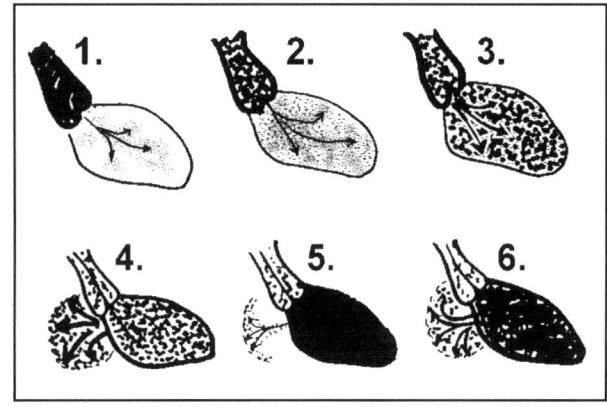
Angio: Valvular Regurgitation

ANSWER e. Moderate MR - based on the relative density of contrast in each chamber after 3rd cycle following contrast injection.
MATCH THE OTHER LABELED REGURGITATION ANGIOGRAMS to their severity rating below.
   1. MILD AR (also called 1+)
   2. MODERATE AR (also called 2+ to 3+)
   3. SEVERE AR (also called 4+) So much AO contrast is lost by the leak into LV, that the AO and LV appear equal in density.
   4. SEVERE MR (also called 4+) So much LV contrast is lost by the leak into LA, that the LA and LV appear equal in density.
   5. MILD MR (also called 1+)
   6. MODERATE MR (also called 2+ to 3+)
See: Kern, chapter "Angiographic Data." **Keywords:** Grading regurgitation

550. This ventriculogram shows:
   a. R-L VSD
   b. L-R VSD
   c. Aortic valve stenosis
   d. Pulmonary valve stenosis

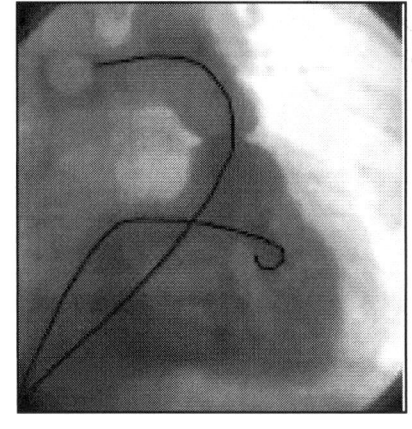

ANSWER: d. Pulmonary valve stenosis. This RV gram shows a pigtail catheter injecting in the RV, with contrast flowing into the pulmonary trunk. Note the pinched pulmonic valve. Also, note the inflated Swan-Ganz catheter in the distal right pulmonary artery. The LV will not be seen until several seconds later as contrast returns from the lungs. Normally, the balloon should not be inflated as seen here.
See: Kern, chapter on "Angiographic Data"

6. LV Wall Motion

551. Name the LV wall labeled #2 in the LV gram?
a. Mitral valve
b. Posterior lateral
c. Septal
d. Anterior
e. Apex
f. Inferior

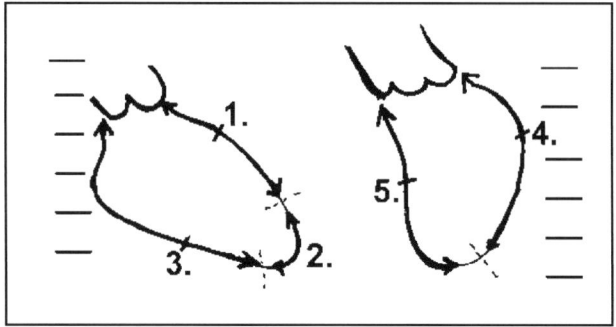
LV wall segments

ANSWER e. Apex, apical wall.
MATCH ALL LABELED LV WALLS TO THEIR NAME.
(Basal means near the base of the heart.)
1. ANTERIOR (RAO): Some authors break this segment into:
   a) Anterior-basal
   b) Anterior-lateral
2. APEX (RAO): Tip of LV
3. INFERIOR (RAO): Some authors break this segment into:
   a) Diaphragmatic
   b) Posterior basal
   c) Mitral valve
4. POSTERIOR-LATERAL (LAO): Some authors break this segment into:
   a) Supero-lateral = mitral valve (if steep LAO cranial)
   b) Infero-lateral
   c) Postero-lateral
5. SEPTAL (LAO): Between RV and LV. Some authors break this segment into:
   a) Septal-apical
   b) Septal-basal

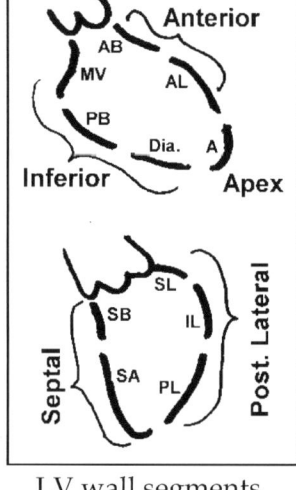
LV wall segments

See: Braunwald, chapter on "Coronary Arteriography." and SCAI Cardiac Cath database

552. Identify the major LV wall segment labeled at #5 in these standard LV views.
a. Apex (apical)
b. Inferior (diaphragmatic)
c. Posterolateral
d. Septal
e. Anterior

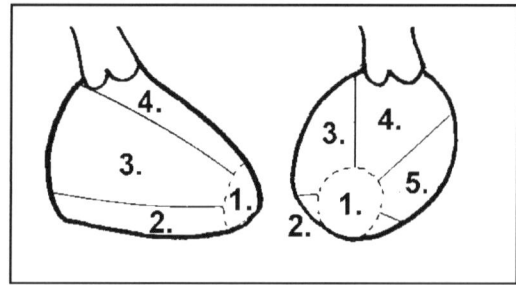
LV wall segments - RAO/LAO

ANSWER c. Posterolateral. Best seen on edge in LAO view.
MATCH ALL LABELED WALL SEGMENTS shown with their name below.
1. **APEX (APICAL):** Best seen on edge in the RAO view.
2. **INFERIOR (DIAPHRAGMATIC):** Best seen on bottom LV silhouette in RAO view.
5. **POSTERO-LATERAL:** Best seen on edge in LAO view.
3. **SEPTAL:** Best seen on edge in LAO view.
4. **ANTERIOR:** Seen only on top LV silhouette in RAO view.
   Note how the wall segments at the edge of each cardiac silhouette are seen on angio. The segments moving toward and away from you cannot be seen on angio (e.g. #3 septal wall in RAO). Also, some authors break these major segments down into 2-3 smaller segments (Shown in previous question). But if you know these 5 major segments you can always figure out the others (e.g. basal, apical). **See:** Braunwald, chapter on "Coronary Arteriography" (includes LV)

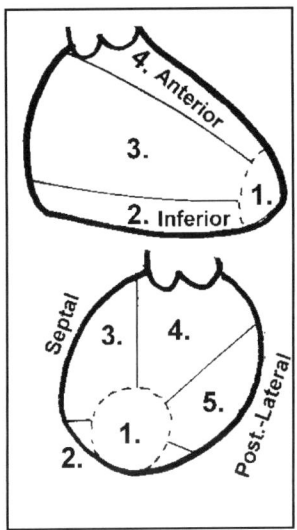

LV wall segments

553. Identify the LV wall motion abnormality labeled #2 in the drawing.
a. Septal hypokinesis
b. Septal dyskinesis
c. Inferior hypokinesis
d. Inferior dyskinesis

ANSWER b. Septal dyskinesis. **MATCH THE OTHER LABELED LV WALL MOTION ABNORMALITIES** with their name.
1. **INFERIOR HYPOKINESIS:** RAO view of diminished motion in an inferior wall.
2. **SEPTAL DYSKINESIS:** LAO view of aneurysmal motion in a septal wall.
3. **INFERIOR DYSKINESIS:** RAO view of aneurysmal motion in an inferior wall. This wall rarely bulges as shown, because the diaphragm seems to "splint" it from excessive paradoxical motion.
4. **SEPTAL HYPOKINESIS:** LAO view shows diminished motion high in a septal wall
See: Kern, chapter "Angiographic Data."

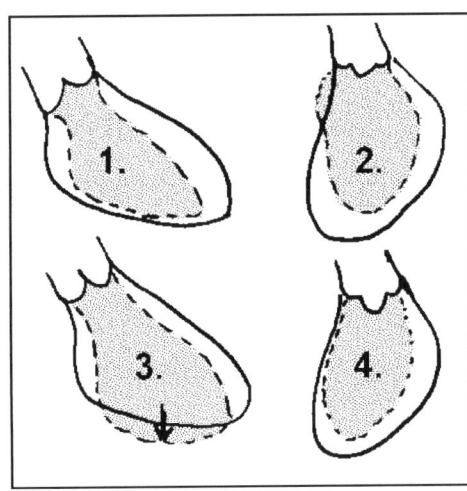

ESV (dotted) and EDV
LV Angiographic volumes

554. The systolic wall motion abnormality labeled at #3 would most likely be caused by _____ of the _____ coronary artery.
a. Infarction, LAD
b. Infarction, Circumflex
c. Ischemia, LAD
d. Ischemia, Circumflex

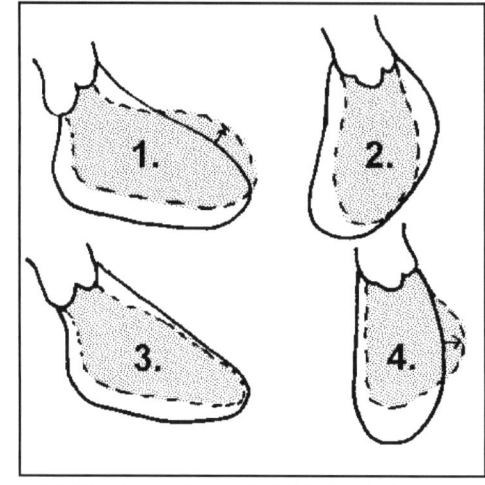

ESV (dotted) and EDV LV-Angio volumes

ANSWER c. Ischemia, LAD. The anterior wall hypokinesis shown in the RAO view is usually due to LAD ischemia. The LAD normally feeds the anterior wall and RCA normally feeds the inferior wall. Dyskinetic areas are usually infarcted with little salvageable myocardium. **MATCH THE OTHER LV WALL MOTION ABNORMALITIES**.
1. **INFARCTION, LAD:** The anterior wall dyskinesis shown in the RAO view is usually due to LAD infarction.
2. **ISCHEMIA, Circ.:** The posterolateral wall hypokinesis shown in the LAO view is usually due to circumflex ischemia.
3. **ISCHEMIA, LAD:** The anterior wall hypokinesis shown in the RAO view is usually due to LAD ischemia.
4. **INFARCTION, Circ.:** The posterolateral wall dyskinesis shown in the LAO view is usually due to circumflex infarction.

See: Grossman, chapter on "Cardiac Ventriculography."

555. These diagrams show the various patterns of LV systolic regional wall motion. The outer line is the EDV outline. The inner line is the ESV. What type of LV wall motion is shown at #3 on the diagram?
a. Normal
b. Akinetic
c. Dyskinetic
d. Local hypokinetic
e. Global hypokinetic
f. Asynchronous

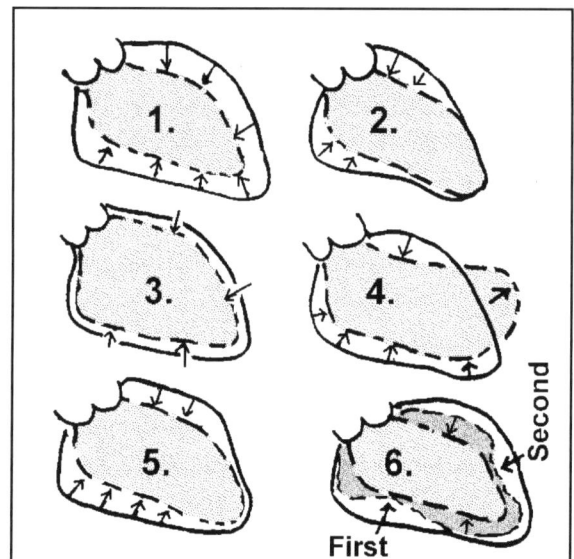

Superimposed ESV and EDV LV Angiographic volumes

ANSWER e. Global hypokinesis. **MATCH THE OTHER numbered diagrams.**
Types of asynergy shown are:
   1. **Normal:** EF is greater than 50%.
   2. **Akinetic:** No contraction in this area.
   3. **Global hypokinetic:** A diminished but visible motion of the entire LV. Often seen in

dilated failing hearts.
   4. **Dyskinetic**: A bulging or aneurysmal LV wall segment. Also termed paradoxical motion because it moves the wrong way.
   5. **Local hypokinetic**: A diminished but visible motion of part of the LV.
   6. **Asynchronous**: The LV wall does not beat synchronously. Part of the wall beats first - another part follows. This contractile pattern may be seen in bundle branch block.

See: Kern, chapter on "Angiography." **Keywords:** LV wall motion abnormalities, akinesis, dyskinesis, global hypokineses...

556. What coronary artery normally supplies the LV wall labeled at #2?
   a. PDA branch of RCA
   b. LAD septal branches
   c. Circumflex
   d. Distal LAD & distal RCA
   e. Proximal LAD & diagonal
   f. Distal LAD

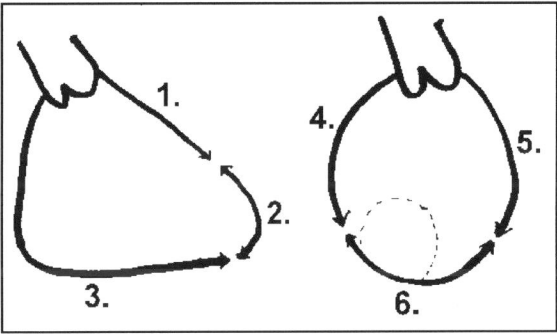
RAO LV-gram   LAO LV-gram

ANSWER f. Apex - distal LAD.
   MATCH THE OTHER LABELED LV WALLS with their name below.
   1. ANTERIOR WALL - LAD
   2. APEX - LAD
   3. INFERIOR WALL - PDA or RCA
   4. ANT. SEPTAL wall - LAD septals
   5. POSTEROLATERAL - Circ.
   6. APEX - Distal LAD (if wrap around LAD) - &/or inferior wall RCA, PDCA (if dominant RCA)

See: Pepine, chapter "Ventriculography"

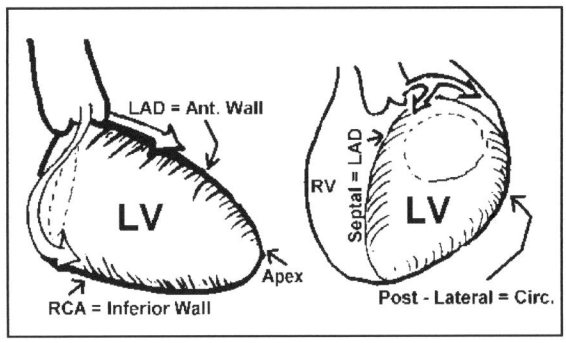
RAO LV-gram   LAO LV-gram

557. The coronary artery labeled at #5 normally supplies the _____ LV wall.
   a. Inferior
   b. Anterior IV septal
   c. Posterolateral
   d. Apex
   e. Anterior
   f. RA & RV

MAJOR CORONARY ARTERY
   1. LAD Septals
   2. Distal LAD
   3. LAD - Diagonals
   4. Circumflex - Obtuse marginals
   *5. Distal RCA - Post. Descending
   6. Prox. RCA, Acute Marg.

ANSWER a. Inferior LV wall and inferior IV septal wall

MAJOR CORONARY ARTERY
1. **LAD SEPTALS:** Anterior IV septum
2. **DISTAL LAD:** Apex (wrap around LAD)
3. **LAD - DIAGONALS:** Anterior wall
4. **CIRCUMFLEX - OBTUSE MARGINALS:** Posterolateral wall
5. **RCA - POST. DESCENDING:** Inferior wall & inferior IV septum
6. **Proximal RCA, Acute Marginals:** Supply right side of heart.

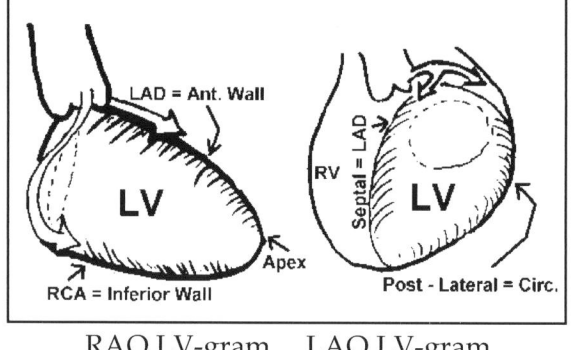

RAO LV-gram   LAO LV-gram

See: Pepine, chapter "Ventriculography" **Keywords:** # LV walls -supplying coronary

558. This 30° RAO LV wall-motion diagram uses the "100 chord centerline method" of Sheehan, Kennedy and Dodge. What LV wall motion abnormality is shown?
a. Anterior-apical akinesis
b. Anterior-apical hypokinesis
c. Anterior-apical dyskinesis
d. Inferior akinesis
e. Inferior hypokinesis
f. Inferior dyskinesis

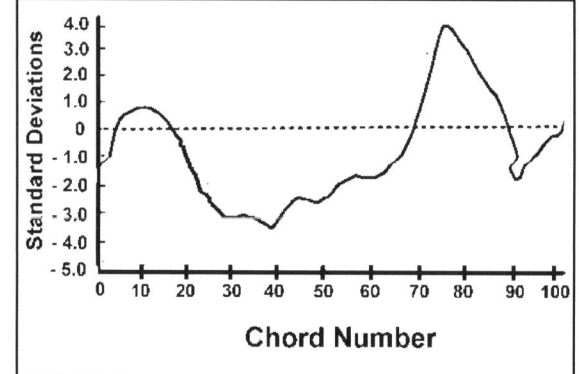

Normalized Segmental wall motion graph of Sheehan

ANSWER c. Anterior-apical dyskinesis. Sheehan's centerline method of wall motion analysis begins by superimposing the largest and smallest LV volumes as shown in diagram #1.

100 chords are then constructed perpendicular to, and evenly distributed along, a "centerline" (dotted) drawn midway between the EDV and ESV contours. Note anterolateral and apical akinesis and dyskinesis.

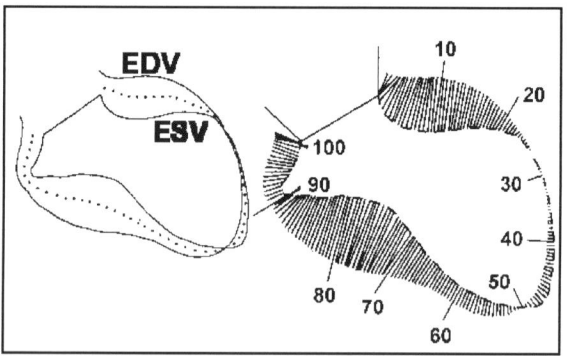

100 chord centerline method

Diagram 3 shows the 100 chords each reduced to a shortening fraction (chord length/LV circumference) and plotted along the horizontal axis. Dyskinetic motion is plotted as below zero (negative). Note how chords 30-50 show negative or dyskinetic motion. Chords 70-80 show compensatory hyperkinesis. The apex at chord 50 is the most dyskinesis. The dotted band shows the normal range of wall motion.

The diagram #4 shows chord fractional shortening re-plotted in "standard deviations" from normal. This relates the wall motion to normal. Normal is the flat dotted "0" standard deviation line.
See: Pepine, chapter "Ventriculography"
Keywords: Wall motion method of Sheehan

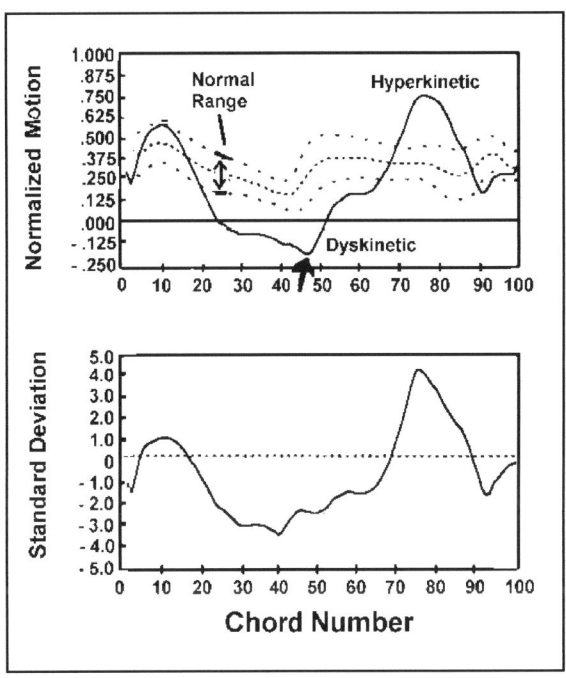
Normalized wall motion graphs

559. In a left dominant coronary artery system what LV wall will be affected by RCA myocardial infarction?
a. None, RCA supplies RV only
b. Inferior LV wall
c. Inferior septal wall
d. Posterolateral

ANSWER a. None (non-dominant). RCA supplies RV only. A dominant LCA system is only found in about 10% of normal people. Here the PDCA, inferior LV wall, and IV septum are supplied by the circumflex branch of the left coronary artery. The RCA which normally supplies this area only supplies the RV. So simple RCA occlusion results only in an RV infarction. However, the RCA is still important because it supplies the SA node pacemaker. **See:** Kern, chapter on "Angiography." **Keywords:** LAO LV angio, dominant RCA occlusion = RV infarct only

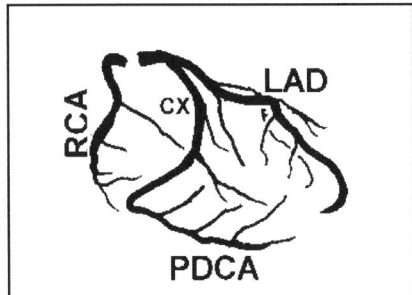
RCA in Left Dominance

560. What coronary artery obstruction would most likely cause the LV wall motion abnormality seen in this diagram?
   a. LAD
   b. Circumflex
   c. Diagonal
   d. RCA

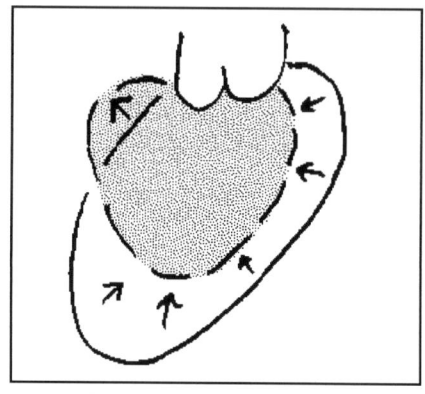
What coronary causes?

ANSWER a. Normally the LAD supplies the anterior 2/3 of the LV septum. This LAO view shows a dyskinetic high septal area indicative of LAD occlusion. The RCA normally controls the inferior 1/3. **See:** Kern, chapter on "Angiography." **Keywords**: LAO LV angio, septal wall dyskinesis

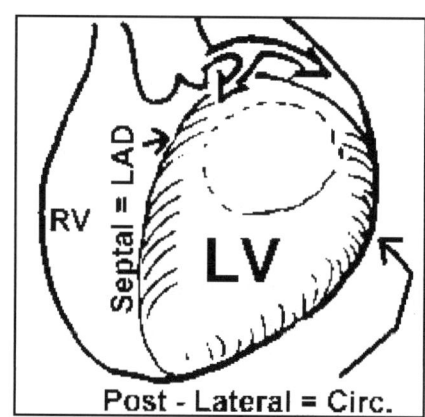
LAD feeds Septal wall

561. All the following LV wall segments are visualized in a 30 degree RAO LV angiogram EXCEPT:
   a. Septal, inferior
   b. Posterior, septal
   c. Anterior, inferior
   d. Inferior, posterior

ANSWER: b. Posterior, septal wall outlines are not seen in the RAO view as they are enclosed within the cardiac border behind the RV. Since an angiogram is a silhouette or shadow, any wall motion front to back is not seen. Any akinesis on these walls will not show, unless the LAO view is taken.
See: Kern, chapter on "Angiographic Data"
Keywords: RAO =inferior & anterior walls, not post. or septal walls

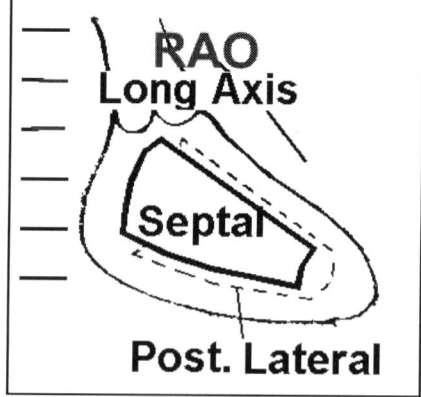

562. This LV gram shows:
  a. Apical dyskinesis
  b. Global hypokinesis
  c. Infero-basal dyskinesis
  d. Infero-apical-anterior akinesis

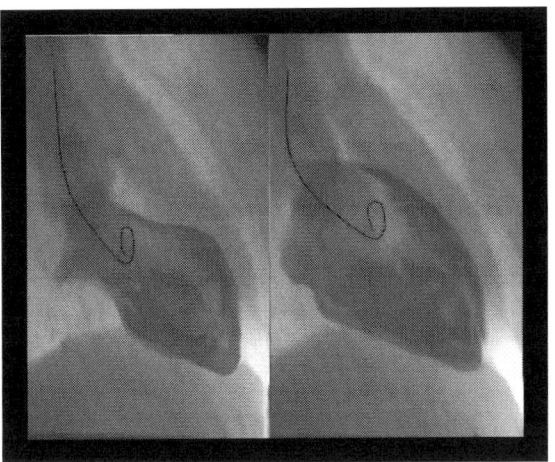

ANSWER: d. Infero-apical-anterior akinesis. The entire apex of the heart does not contract, including the inferior, anterior-lateral, and apical walls. The base of the heart is hyper-contractile to compensate for a probable apical infarction. **See:** Kern, chapter on "Angiographic Data"

563. This LVgram may be associated with:
  a. IHSS/HOCM
  b. Acute CX occlusion
  c. Acute RCA occlusion
  d. Acute LAD occlusion
  e. Prolapsing mitral valve

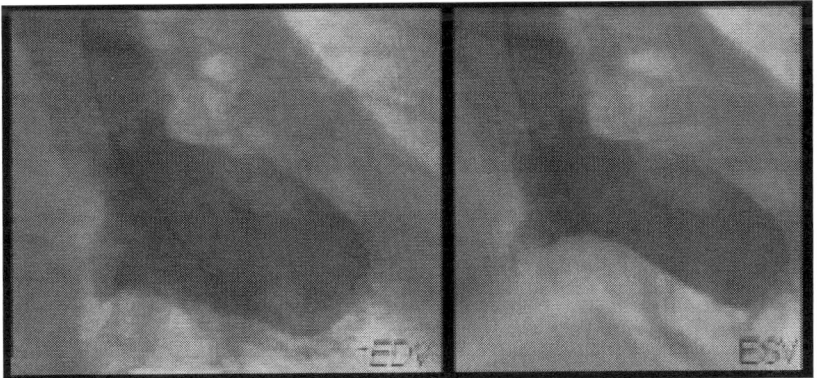

ANSWER: d. Acute LAD occlusion stuns and damages the anterior LV wall. Note that the anterior wall and apex are akinetic, while the inferior wall is hyperkinetic and contracting upward. This is to compensate for a probable anterior infarction.
See: Kern, chapter on "Angiographic Data" **Keywords:** LAD occlusion =anterior akinesis

7. LV Pathology

564. This LV angiogram is consistent with:
  a. Dilated cardiomyopathy (DC)
  b. Restrictive cardiomyopathy (RC)
  c. Subvalvular stenosis (IHSS-HOCM)
  d. Aortic stenosis (AS)

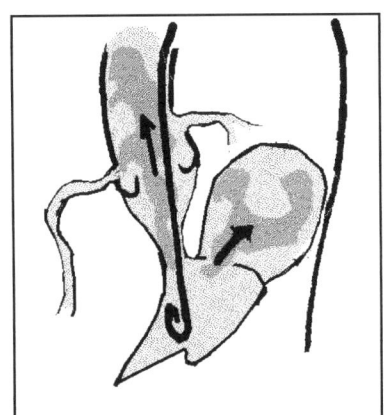

LAO LV gram

ANSWER c. In subvalvular stenosis or IHSS (Idiopathic Subvalvular Idiopathic Stenosis) or HOCM (Hypertrophic Obstructive CardioMyopathy) the LV septum is so thick that it impinges on the mitral valve and obstructs the outflow tract. A pressure gradient is often found within

the LV chamber at the constriction. This also deforms the mitral valve so that it may leak. This LV angio shows MR associated with the subvalvular obstruction. The view is a steep LAO with cranial angulation to profile the mitral valve. Know the hemodynamics of HOCM.
See: Grossman, chapter on "Cardiac Ventriculography."

565. Why is HOCM termed a *dynamic* LV outflow obstruction?
a. It causes both an aortic and mitral valve pressure gradient
b. It has a dramatic diastolic murmur
c. It is associated with multiple syndromes
d. It can be provoked with exercise

ANSWER d. It can be provoked with exercise. It is "dynamic" because the obstruction only occurs late in systole as the septum impinges on the LV outflow tract, and because the stenosis comes and goes. It can usually be brought on (provoked) with inotropic drugs and/or exercise. The obstruction causes a systolic ejection murmur similar to an AS murmur.
See: Grossman, chapter on "Profiles in Constrictive...Restrictive...Tamponade."

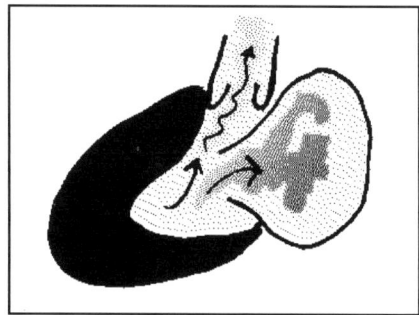

HOCM - IHSS

566. Which type of myopathy is shown in the diagram at #2?
a. Normal
b. Hypertrophic cardiomyopathy (HOCM)
c. Restrictive (RC) or congestive cardiomyopathy
d. Dilated cardiomyopathy (DC)

ANSWER b. Hypertrophic CardioMyopathy (HOCM or IHSS). For more information see chapter "B" of this published series.
MATCH ALL LABELED LVs with a myopathy below.

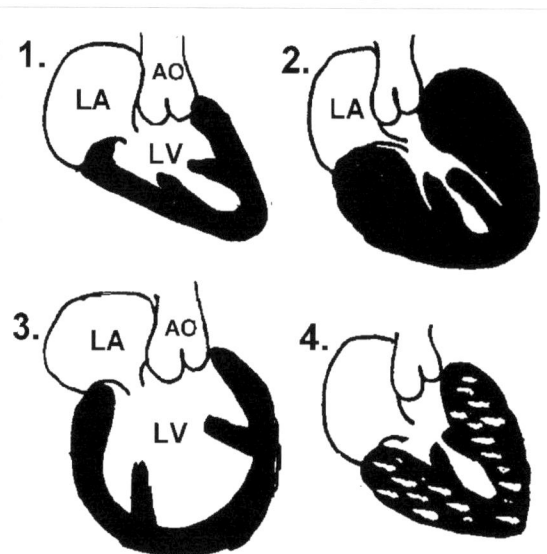

Types Cardiac Myopathy

1. **NORMAL**
2. **HYPERTROPHIC CARDIOMYOPATHY:** The IV septum is hypertrophied. Anterior leaflet is pulled up during systole and may obstruct LV outflow causing IHSS gradient.
3. **DILATED CARDIOMYOPATHY:** Formerly called congestive cardiomyopathy. This myopathy shows a dilated LV with no excessive thickening, systolic dysfunction and CHF.
4. **RESTRICTIVE CARDIOMYOPATHY:** Amyloidosis with stiff ventricle and impaired "diastolic filling." Elevated LV filling pressures.

See: Grossman, chapter on "Cardiac Ventriculography" and chapter on "Profiles in Constrictive...." **Keywords:** Types of cardiomyopathies.

567. Following a distal LAD occlusion a left ventricular wall thrombi may develop in the _____.
a. Posterolateral
b. Inferior wall
c. Anterior/apical wall
d. Anterolateral wall

ANSWER c. Anterior/apical wall. MI's are most common in the LAD which infarct the anterior and apical wall of the LV. Wherever an infarction causes an akinetic wall segment, a thrombus is likely to grow. These akinetic areas should be avoided with a LV catheter. If the angiographer breaks loose an attached clot, a stoke may result. **See:** Braunwald, chapter on "Acute MI."

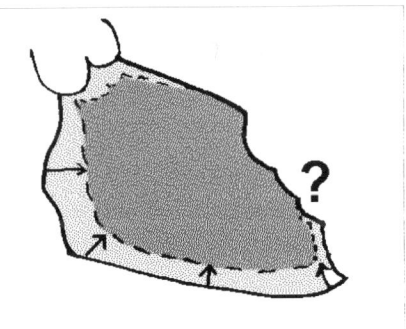

Anterior wall thrombi

568. The LV dilatation/hypertrophy pattern seen at #2 in the diagram is _____ and is usually a compensation for_____.
a. Normal
b. Dilation and hypertrophy, Volume overload
c. Hypertrophy, Pressure overload
d. Aneurysm, transmural infarction

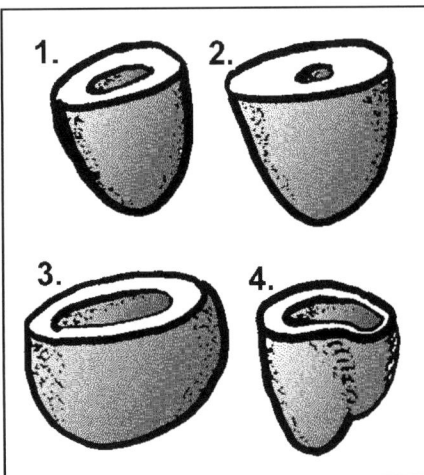

LV Hypertrophy-Dilatation patterns

ANSWER c. Hypertrophy, Pressure overload. **MATCH THE OTHER numbered diagrams to their LV pattern below.**
1. **NORMAL** LV chamber size to wall thickness ratio
2. **HYPERTROPHY due to pressure overload.** Increased LV pressure as seen in AS leads to a thick muscular LV. The LV wall is disproportional thickened.
3. **DILATION (And some hypertrophy) due to volume overload.** Increasing LV volume stretches the LV. The dilated LV has increased wall stress because of Laplace's law. So some hypertrophy must thicken the wall to keep the ratio of "wall thickness" to "LV radius" normal or it would continue to dilate like an aortic aneurysm. That is why you seldom see pure dilatation and thinning.
4. **ANEURYSMS DUE TO TRANSMURAL MYOCARDIAL INFARCTION:** The infarcted tissue is weakened and stretches with systolic pressure. They steal stroke

volume and waste the hyperkinetic contraction of the unaffected LV. If they don't rupture, LV aneurysms usually scar over and calcify. This reduces the dyskinesis.
See: Braunwald, chapter on "Pathology of Heart Failure."

569. A "false" or "pseudo" LV ventricular aneurysm is usually composed of bulging:
 a. Hyperkinetic LV apex
 b. Pericardium and clotted hematoma
 c. All three layers of myocardium
 d. Only one layer of myocardium

ANSWER b. Pericardium and clotted hematoma. These narrow necked thin aneurysms are usually results from rupture of a transmural MI. The aneurysm is composed of pericardium, hematoma, and clot. All this debris helps prevent LV rupture and cardiac tamponade. Some false aneurysms bulge in systole. Others seal off completely. If the narrow neck remains open, and the aneurysm bulges and enlarges, it may rupture.
See: Braunwald, chapter on "Acute MI." **Keywords**: False LV aneurysm

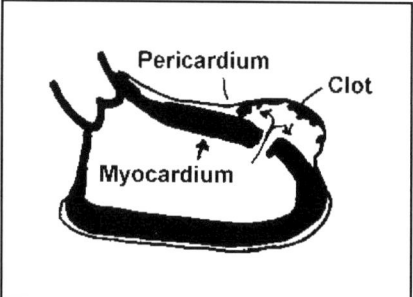
False Aneurysm

570. Aneurysmal LV walls which bulge in systole are termed:
 a. Akinetic
 b. Asyneresis
 c. Dyskinetic
 d. Hypokinetic

ANSWER c. Dyskinetic. A weakened LV wall can bulge in systole just like an aortic aneurysm. They are termed dyskinetic ("dys-" prefix means disordered or bad). It is also termed "paradoxical motion" because it moves the wrong way. Dyskinetic LV walls steal stroke volume from the heart and absorb the LV contraction. They are common immediately following myocardial infarction. They usually heal into a stiff akinetic scar which does not steal as much stroke volume. Open heart surgery can be done to excise or cut out the dead bulging aneurysm or scar to improve LV function. **See:** Medical dictionary **Keywords**: Dyskinetic LV

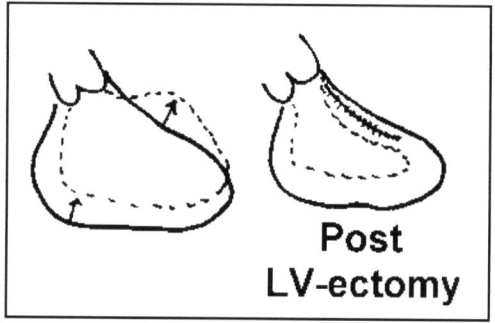
Dyskinetic LV

571. This LAO ventriculogram shows a/an:
a. VSD
b. R-L shunt
c. Aortic A-V fistula
d. Aortic regurgitation

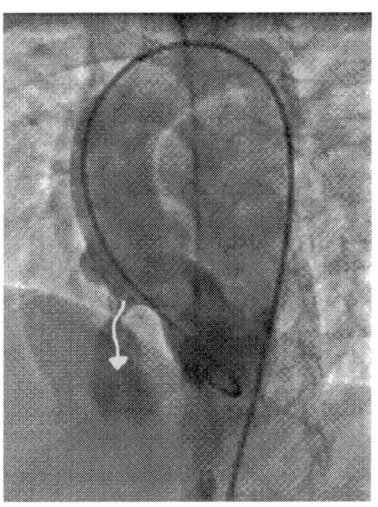

ANSWER: a. VSD with left to right shunt. Note the IV septum below the right aortic cusp, and contrast in the RV (shown on left). Contrast is flowing through a high VSD into the RV. Soon contrast will be seen flowing up and to the right through the PA into the lungs. VSDs like this may occur in adults after septal myocardial infarction. **See:** Kern, chapter on "Angiographic Data" **Keywords:** LV-gram of VSD

8A. Transseptal Heart Cath - Equipment

572. Identify the transseptal catheterization equipment labeled at #3 in the diagram.
a. Mullins sheath
b. Brockenbrough needle
c. Brockenbrough catheter
d. Bing stylet

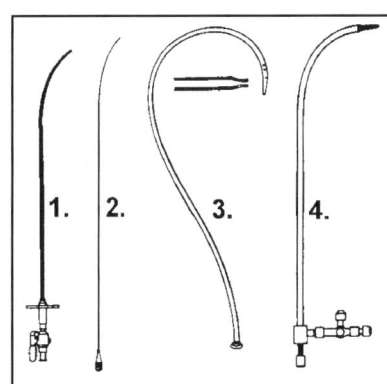

Transeptal equipment

ANSWER c. Brockenbrough catheter.
For more detailed information see chapter D1 on "Catheters."
1. **BROCKENBROUGH NEEDLE:** 70 cm needle to facilitate atrial septal puncture.
2. **BING STYLET:** A curved blunt obturator goes inside the needle.
3. **BROCKENBROUGH CATHETER:** A tapered tip, end and side-hole catheter to allow percutaneous entry and smooth passage through the atrial septum.
4. **MULLINS SHEATH and DILATOR:** This is a long Teflon sheath that can be advanced with its introducer catheter over the needle across the fossa ovalis and into the LA. **See:** Grossman, Cardiac Cath., Angiog., and Interventions, chapter on "Percutaneous Approach."

573. During the Brockenbrough transseptal catheterization several important measurements must be made between the needle flange and the catheter hub. The measurement labeled at #1 on the diagram is critical because it sets the tip of the_____ at the tip of the Brockenbrough catheter.
   a. Blunt stylet
   b. Brockenbrough needle
   c. Mullins sheath
   d. Guide wire

Transseptal setup, measurement

ANSWER a. Blunt Stylet. This is a critical measurement because the operator must know exactly when the tip of the stylet exits the catheter to prevent damage to atrial structures. It may not be seen on fluoroscope. **MATCH THE OTHER POSITION #2 with an answer below.**

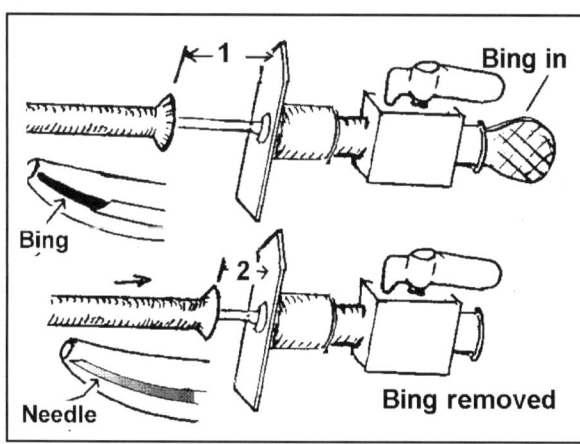

Bing stylet at tip - Needle at tip

   A. BLUNT (BING) STYLET: (Position #1) This is the first important measurement. Advance the needle and Bing TOGETHER until the Bing is at the catheter tip (position #1). This avoids abrasion or puncture of the catheter wall during needle advancement.
   B. BROCKENBROUGH NEEDLE: (Position #2) MOST CRITICAL measurement. When the obturator (Bing) is removed the needle is carefully advanced to the catheter tip. The operator must know exactly when the needle exits the catheter to prevent damage to atrial structures. It may not be seen on fluoroscope. From this point the needle may be advanced to puncture across the fossa ovalis and into the LA.
   C. MULLINS SHEATH: This would be another measurement to make if a Mullins sheath were used. The operator needs to know when the sheath has advanced over the needle enough to be in the LA
   D. GUIDE WIRE: The 145 cm guide wire is only used to place the catheter (and sheath if used) in the RA. Then it is removed. No measurements are necessary on the wire.

See: Grossman, Cardiac Cath., Angiog., and Interventions, chapter on "Percutaneous Approach." **Keywords:** Transseptal equipment: Brockenbrough, Mullins, Bing

574. A patient has a St. Jude aortic valve prosthesis. LV pressures may be most safely measured by:
a. Retrograde aortic catheterization (femoral approach)
b. Retrograde aortic catheterization (brachial approach)
c. Antegrade left heart cath (transeptal)
d. Apical LV puncture (direct transthoracic)

ANSWER c. Transeptal LHC.

St. Jude and other tilting disc valves are unsafe to cross retrograde. They may pinch and trap a catheter. The catheter may pass through the back side of the disk forcing it open. The problem occurs when the catheter is withdrawn. It may catch the disk and become trapped. Dr. Grossman recommends the transeptal method in these instances. The complication rate is 3-4% even in experienced hands.

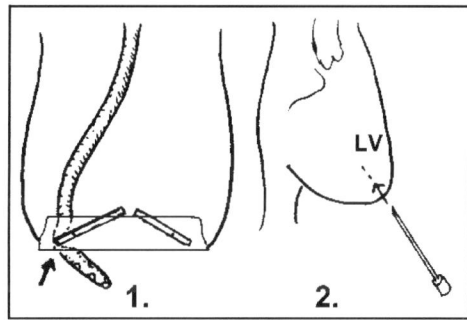
#1 St. Jude - #2 Apical stick

Direct apical puncture is usually used only when all other catheterization measures have failed. This is usually done with a 3" 18 gauge needle directly through the chest wall at the apex of the LV (PMI or Point of Maximum Intensity). A .035" guide wire is inserted, the needle removed and a small pigtail catheter introduced into the LV for pressure measurements and/or angiography.

TAVR may be done this way with an apical puncture. **See:** Grossman, chapter on "Percutaneous Approach." **Keywords:** Transseptal on St. Jude & tilting disc valves

575. When a Mullins sheath is used in transseptal heart catheterization, after successful transseptal puncture the sheath tip should:
a. Remain in the femoral artery
b. Remain in the RA
c. Be advanced into the LA with the dilator
d. Be advanced into the LV over the dilator, after the dilator has been successfully positioned in the LV

ANSWER c. Be advanced into the LA with the dilator. The long Mullins sheath should be advanced into the LA along with the dilator (catheter). This is done over the transseptal needle once it has been successfully placed in the LA. Correct positioning of the transseptal needle in the LA must be established by pressure, oximetry, and/or contrast injection. Then the transseptal needle is "pinned or fixed" to the patient, while the dilator and sheath are advanced as a unit across the septum.

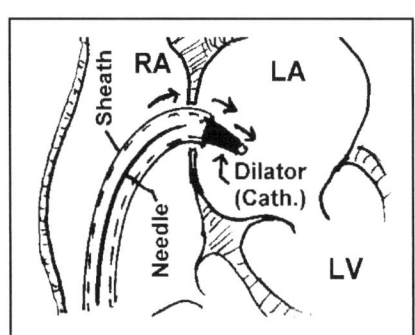
Advance Mullins Sheath

This is an "antegrade" passage following blood flow up the IVC - puncture across the atrial septum - into the LA - across the mitral valve - and into the LV. **See:** Pepine, chapter on "Review of

General Cath Techniques." **Keywords:** Mullins sheath positioned in LA

576. In performing transseptal catheterization all the following may be used EXCEPT:
  a. Brockenbrough needle
  b. Mullins sheath
  c. ICE guidance
  d. Multipurpose catheter
  e. Balloon floatation catheter

ANSWER: d. Multipurpose catheter is not used. Instead use a Brockenbrough catheter or balloon flotation catheter. "The technique for trans-septal catheterization using the Mullins sheath...Once the sheath is in the left atrium, the needle and dilator are withdrawn and the sheath is flushed carefully. Either a specially curved pigtail catheter (in patients with a normal mitral valve) or a CO2-inflated balloon floatation catheter (in patients with mitral stenosis) may be inserted through the sheath and passed [floated] into the left ventricle." Intracardiac echo (ICE) may be used to guide the needle during inter-atrial puncture. **See:** Grossman, chapter on "Percutaneous Approach"

577. What gauge/diameter is the long needle used for transseptal catheterization?
  a. 16 g. tapering to 18 g.
  b. 18 g. tapering to 21 g.
  c. 20 g. tapering to 22 g
  d. 22 g. and 70 cm long

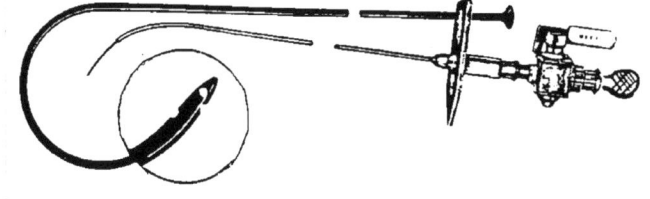

Brockenbrough catheter and long needle

ANSWER b. 18 gauge diameter which tapers to 21 gauge at the curved tip. The standard femoral Brockenbrough transseptal needle is 70 cm long. **See:** Grossman, chapter on "Percutaneous Approach" **Keywords:** Transseptal needle =18 g. tapering to 21 g.

8B. Transseptal Heart Cath - Techniques

578. Indications for transseptal left heart catheterization include all the following EXCEPT:
  a. Unable to cross tight aortic valve retrograde
  b. When the wedge pressure is unreliable in MR
  c. Mitral valvuloplasty
  d. LA myxoma

ANSWER d. LA myxoma or thrombus are contraindications to transseptal catheterization. The needle may disturb, fragment, or break off the tumor from the atrial septal wall. Embolism could result. The other distractors are indications for transseptal cath.
See: Grossman, Cardiac Cath., Angiog., and Interventions, chapter on "Percutaneous Approach" and Kern, chapter "Special Techniques"

579. **In transseptal catheterization of the left heart, the transseptal needle puncture should be made through the:**
a. Atrial appendage
b. Ventricular septum
c. Fossa ovalis
d. Ductus arteriosus
e. Ductus venosus

ANSWER c. The fossa ovalis (fossa ovale) is the thin atrial septal membrane which is the remnant of the foramen ovale the normal fetal ASD. This concave indentation in the septal wall is just below the aortic bulge that is termed the "limbus" or "limbic ridge."
  The transseptal catheter & needle puncture the atrial septum at the fossa ovalis and enter the LA.
See: Grossman, Cardiac Cath., Angiog., and Interventions, chapter on "Percutaneous Approach." **Keywords:** Transseptal puncture through fossa ovalis

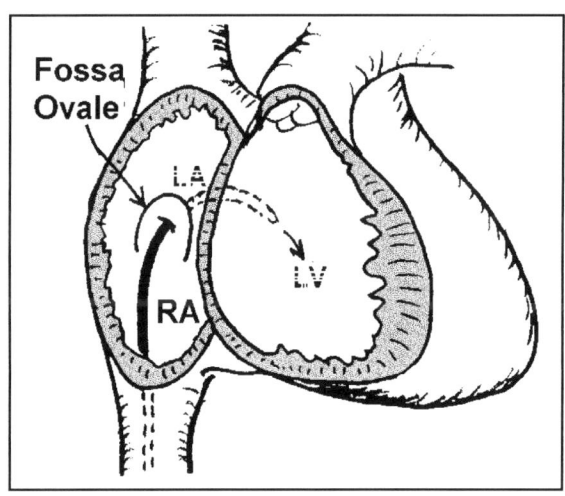

Transseptal puncture of septum

580. **What percentage of normal individuals have a "probe patent" atrial septum? In these individuals the transseptal catheter can be pushed into the LA without needle puncture across the atrial septum.**
a. None, only in patients with ASDs
b. 10-20%
c. 30-50%
d. 60-75%

ANSWER b. In 10-20% of normal individuals the transseptal catheter can be pushed across the fossa ovalis, without making a needle puncture. Remember that this "trap door" normally closes at birth due to higher LA pressure. In some individuals it just does not seal shut. Slight pressure on the fossa with the catheter may allow its easy passage into LA. Why use needle puncture if you don't have to?
See: Grossman, Cardiac Cath., Angiog., and Interventions, chapter on "Percutaneous Approach" and Kern, chapter "Special Techniques" and Pepine, chapter on "Review of General Cath Techniques."

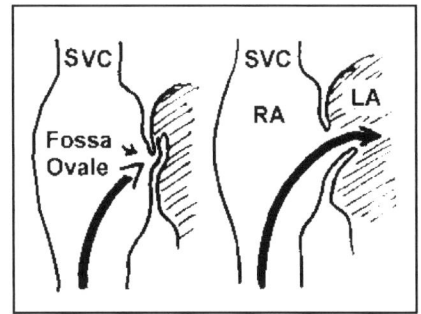

Probe-patent fossa Ov.

581. How should the transseptal needle be oriented, when advancing it into the LA? When viewed from the patient's feet the needle indicator should point towards the _____.
  a. 12:00 o'clock position
  b. 2:00 o'clock position
  c. 4:00 o'clock position
  d. 6:00 o'clock position

ANSWER c. 4:00 o'clock position. The pointer - indicator (hilt) on the Brockenbrough needle points in the same direction as the needle tip. This leftward and posterior direction positions the needle tip perpendicular to the atrial septum, and below the aorta. Kern states 45 degrees, not 4:00 o'clock.
See: Grossman, Cardiac Cath., Angiog., and Interventions, chapter on "Percutaneous Approach" and Kern, chapter "Special Techniques." **Keywords:** Needle pointed to 4:00 o'clock

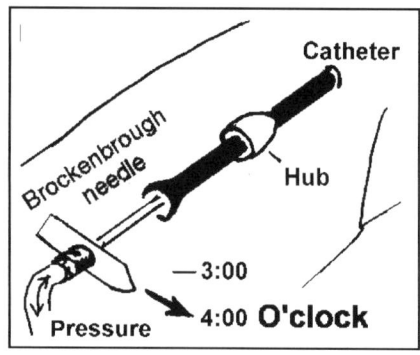

Brockenbrough needle position

582. An important anatomic landmark for transseptal puncture is the bulge of the ascending aorta in the atrial septum just superior to the fossa ovalis. The transseptal catheter is pulled down, over this ridge, then moves to your right into the fossa ovalis where the puncture is made. What is the name of this atrial septal ridge?
  a. Bachman's bundle (ledge)
  b. Coronary sinus ridge (ledge)
  c. Aortoseptal groove (tunnel)
  d. Limbus (limbic ledge)

ANSWER d. The limbus, limbic ridge or ledge is formed by the aortic root bulging into the atrial septum. It is just above the fossa ovalis where you need to puncture. When withdrawing the needle-catheter from SVC (shown as a dotted catheter) the needle

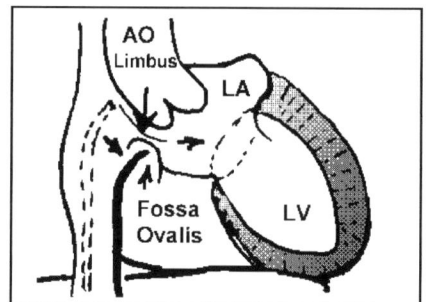

Aorta, Limbus, Fossa O

"trips" over the limbic ridge before "falling" into the depression of the fossa ovalis. In aortic stenosis the root may be dilated and displace the fossa ovalis antero-superiorly. Be careful to not puncture the limbus which is the aorta. It leads to tamponade.
See: Grossman, Cardiac Cath., Angiog., and Interventions, chapter on "Percutaneous Approach" and Clugston, CATHET. AND CV DIAGNOSIS, 26, 1992, "Transseptal Cath. Update 1992." **Keywords:** Limbic ridge, limbus

583. Following unsuccessful transseptal puncture how should the femoral catheter and needle be repositioned for another stab?
   a. Retract the needle into the catheter, reposition the catheter tip in the SVC.
   b. Retract the needle into the catheter, reposition the catheter tip in the mid RA.
   c. Remove the needle from the catheter, use a guide-wire to reposition the catheter tip in the SVC.
   d. Remove the needle from the catheter, use a guide-wire to reposition the catheter tip in the mid RA.

ANSWER c. Remove the needle. It is dangerous to torque the catheter in the RA with the sharp needle inside in the PA view. Replace it with a guide wire. Advance the wire and catheter into the SVC. Replace the wire with the needle protected by the catheter. Slide the catheter tip down the medial wall of the SVC, into the RA, over the limbic ridge (AO) and into the fossa ovalis. Only then should the needle be exposed.

Grossman says, "*One should never attempt to reposition the catheter-needle combination in the SVC in any other way, since perforation of the RA or atrial appendage is a distinct possibility during such maneuvers.*"
See: Grossman, Cardiac Cath., Angiog., and Interventions, chapter on "Percutaneous Approach." **Keywords:** Dangerous to manipulate needle-catheter together in RA

584. Transseptal heart catheterization is performed only from the _____ entry site.
   a. Right femoral arterial
   b. Right femoral venous
   c. Left femoral arterial
   d. Left femoral venous

ANSWER b. The right femoral vein is the only standard vascular entry for transseptal heart cath. Other venous entry sites may distort the needle position. This is an "antegrade" passage up the IVC, puncture across the atrial septum, into LA, across the mitral valve, and into the LV.

Grossman says, "Classically, trans-septal catheterization is performed only from the right femoral vein....With the advent of percutaneous mitral valvuloplasty and antegrade aortic valvuloplasty using the Inoue balloon, as well as the availability of improved equipment, trans-septal catheterization has again become a relatively common procedure." **See:** Grossman, Cardiac Cath., Angiog., and Interventions, chapter on "Percutaneous Approach."

585. Transeptal heart catheterization utilizes all of the following EXCEPT:
   a. Brockenbrough catheter
   b. Patient heparinization
   c. Right femoral vein puncture
   d. Pressure monitoring through transeptal needle

ANSWER b. Full patient heparinization is contraindicated for transeptal cath. Transeptal

324   ◄◄ Diagnostic Techniques: D8 - Left Heart Catheterization ►►

puncture should be done without heparin due to the possibility of accidental aortic puncture and tamponade. Some labs remove heparin from the table to avoid accidental heparinization of transseptal patients. Heparin may be added later if coronary or other additional studies are needed. **See:** Grossman, chapter on "Percutaneous Approach."

586. Your patient comes to the cath lab for evaluation of mitral stenosis (via transseptal cath) and CAD. How much heparin should the patient receive at the beginning of the case?
a. No heparin
b. 1000-2000 units of heparin IV
c. 3000-5000 units of heparin IV
d. 10,000 units of heparin IV

ANSWER a. No heparin is given initially. It would encourage pericardial tamponade across unsuccessful transseptal punctures. After unsuccessful Brockenbrough punctures the small tipped needle can be withdrawn into the catheter. The needle hole is small enough that is usually doesn't bleed.
   Heparin is withheld until the transseptal catheter is correctly positioned in the LA or LV. This late heparinization is essential when large valvuloplasty balloons are used. Then coronary arteriography with full heparinization can proceed.
See: Grossman, chapter on "Percutaneous Approach."until after successful puncture

587. During transseptal cardiac catheterization you are monitoring Brockenbrough needle pressure on X40. The cardiologist advances the needle and you note the waveform shown at #3. The most likely position of the needle tip is ___.
a. Aorta ___
b. LA ___
c. Pericardium ___
d. Myocardial wall ___

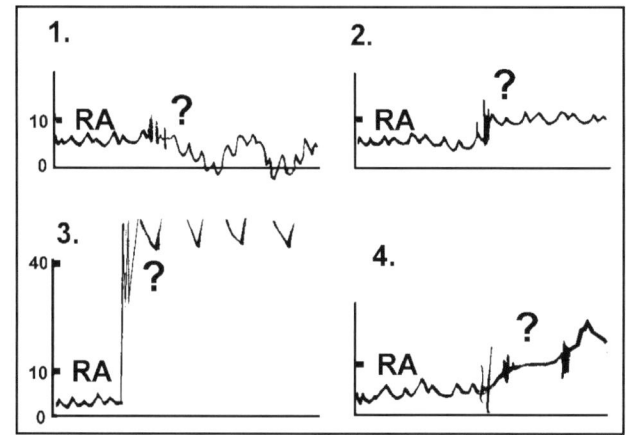
Brockenbrough needle monitored 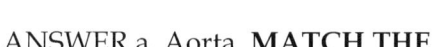Pressure

ANSWER a. Aorta. **MATCH THE OTHER WAVE-FORMS SHOWN** with the needle tip position below.
1. **PERICARDIUM.** As the needle crosses into the pericardium the pressure drops suddenly because of negative pleural pressure. This can lead to potential complication of tamponade. When the small needle tip is withdrawn it usually heals over. Do not advance the catheter. That just widens the hole, and tamponade is more likely.
2. **LA: GOOD!** That is what you want. LA pressure is 5-12 mmHg with "a" and "v" waves. This can be checked by drawing a small blood sample (it should be bright red) or by a contrast test injection through the needle.
3. **AORTA:** Aortic pressure is off the screen. This pressure monitoring is essential to see inadvertent aortic puncture. When the small needle tip is withdrawn it usually heals

over. Do not advance the catheter if the needle is in the aorta. That just widens the hole, and tamponade is likely. If bleeding does occur the Brockenbrough catheter can be used to plug the puncture site while the patient is taken to surgery. Pericardial centesis in the lab may be lifesaving.

4. **MYOCARDIUM: THIS** pressure appears damped because it is intra-myocardial, within atrial or aortic tissue. Small test injections (done by hand) may stain the myocardium, mark it, and make it more visible. With this, if the needle is found to be in the free it should be withdrawn. Advance only if it is within the interatrial septum or LA. **See:** Grossman, chapter on "Percutaneous Approach."

588. Mr. Jones has suspected aortic stenosis. Retrograde crossing of the aortic valve was impossible. During transseptal heart catheterization several unsuccessful transseptal needle advances have been made. Now, Mr. Jones becomes confused and lethargic. His BP is 80/40 mmHg and falling. RA pressure is 18 mmHg. Heart rate is 105 in sinus rhythm. The most likely therapy is:
a. IV dopamine and nitroprusside
b. Fluid administration and IV atropine
c. IV epinephrine and having Mr. Jones cough
d. Emergency valve surgery
e. Pericardial centesis

ANSWER e. Pericardial centesis. Pericardial tamponade is the most common serious complication of transseptal heart catheterization. Unsuccessful transseptal attempts may puncture the aorta or pericardial space allowing bleeding into the pericardium. This bleeding (tamponade) compresses the heart so that it cannot fill properly.

Cardiac tamponade may be a fatal complication if not recognized and promptly treated with pericardio-centesis. Here a needle and then a small catheter are placed within the pericardium, and the fluid drawn off. This simple lifesaving maneuver usually relieves the constriction immediately and establishes normal hemodynamics. **See:** Grossman, chapter on "Percutaneous Approach."

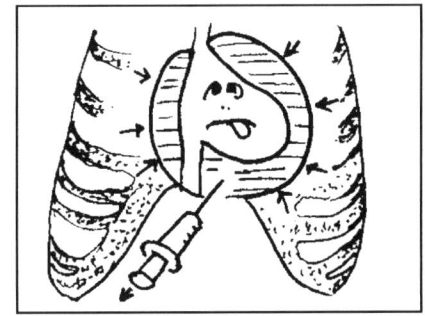

Transeptal puncture - induced Tamponade - pericario-centesis

Grossman says, "Classically, trans-septal catheterization is performed only from the right femoral vein....With the advent of percutaneous mitral valvuloplasty and antegrade aortic valvuloplasty using the Inoue balloon, as well as the availability of improved equipment, trans-septal catheterization has again become a relatively common procedure."
See: Grossman, chapter on "Percutaneous Approach"

589. PVC induced narrowing of the aortic pulse pressure and increase in the interventricular gradient (Brockenbrough-Braunwald-Morrow sign) is associated with:
a. Aortic stenosis (AS)
b. Constrictive pericarditis (CP)
c. Square root sign in ventricular pressures
d. Peripheral amplification of arterial pressure
e. Intraventricular pressure gradient (HOCM)

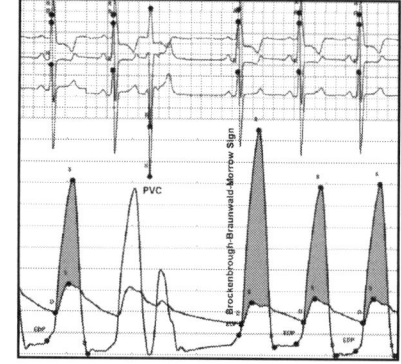
Brockenbrough sign

ANSWER: e. Intraventricular pressure gradient of HOCM. The Brockenbrough-Braunwald-Morrow sign is the post-PVC increase in LV-AO gradient due to trapping of the anterior mitral valve leaflet against the LV wall in systole. **See:** Braunwald, chapter on "Physical Assessment"

References
Baim D. S. and Grossman W., *Cardiac Catheterization, Angiography, and Intervention*, 7th Ed., Lea and Febiger, 2006
Braunwald, et. al. Ed., *Heart Disease, a Textbook of CV Medicine*, 9th Ed., Saunders, 2012
Kern, M. J., Ed., *The Cardiac Catheterization Handbook*, 6th Ed., Mosby-Year Book, Inc., 2016
Clugston, "Transseptal Cath. Update 1992", CATHETERIZATION AND CV DIAGNOSIS, #26, 1992
King, S.B. III and Douglas J. S. Jr., *Coronary Arteriography and Angioplasty*, McGraw-Hill, 1985
Johnsrude, I. S., Jackson. D. C., et al., *A Practical Approach to Angiography*, 2nd Ed., Little, Brown and Co., 1987
Pappano & Weir (previously Berne & Levy), *Cardiovascular Physiology*, 10th Ed., Mosby Year Book, 2013
Pepine, J. C., and Hill, J. A., et. al., *Diagnostic and Therapeutic Cardiac Catheterization*, 2nd Ed., Williams and Wilkins, 1994

OUTLINE: Left Heart Catheterization

1. Left Ventriculography
   a. May omitted if nonivasive studies adequate
   b. Often done after coronary angios
2. EQUIPMENT AND TECHNIQUES
   a. Special LV catheters
      i. Pigtail, Halo
      ii. Multipurpose, Jacky
      iii. Gensini
      iv. NIH, Eppendorf
      v. Sones
      vi. Lehman Ventriculography
      vii. Grollman
      viii. Brockenbrough / transseptal
   b. Positioning LV FLOOD catheters
      i. tip @ LV inflow
      ii. Catheter induced MR
      iii. Possibility of recoil
      iv. Apical irritation - PVCs
3. INJECTORS
   a. Construction / controls
      i. flow rate
      ii. Select appropriate inj. rate
      iii. Hyperkinetic ventricle
      iv. Low CO
      v. End-hole catheter (Recoil with MP)
      vi. Pigtail catheter
      vii. injection volume
      viii. delay time
      ix. film delay
      x. rate/linear rise
      xi. injection pressure limit - 1000 psi
      xii. syringe
      xiii. injection button - be ready to stop
      xiv. mechanical stop
      xv. electrical stop
   b. Filling injector
      i. Install syringe
      ii. open dye
      iii. attach straw
      iv. fill syringe
   c. Making safe injections
      i. Tilt and remove bubbles (tap)
      ii. attach Linden fitting to catheter
      iii. Running connection
      iv. withdraw blood
      v. Test injection
      vi. Make control settings

vii. Hold down inject button
viii. observe cine for problems
ix. staining endocardium
x. stop injection at 1st sign of trouble
xi. catheter recoil - risk of stain/perf.
xii. pt. reactions
  d. USE OF PRESSURE INJECTORS
    i. Catheter flow limits
    ii. LV size
    iii. Stroke volume
    iv. patient condition (CHF)
    v. staining & perforation
    vi. Pressure injections in sick patients
    vii. Elevated wedge/ LVEDP
    viii. Low Osmolar Contrast Media (LOCM)
    ix. Cost of Low Osmolar contrast
    x. reduced volume of contrast
      (1) 3 ml/Kg body weight
    xi. premedication to prevent allergic reaction
    xii. Loading contrast
      (1) Running connection
      (2) Draw back to eliminate bubbles
      (3) Turn down & tap syringe
    xiii. Contrast
      (1) Iodine content - absorbs Xrays
    xiv. Standard Contrast
      (1) Renographin, Hypaque, Angio-Conray
      (2) Cause vasodilation and transient hypotension
    xv. Low Osmolar - Nonionic
      (1) Isovue (nonionic)
      (2) Hexabrix (low osmolar)
      (3) Angiovist, Omnipaque, Other
4. TECHNIQUES
  a. Complications of LV angiography
    i. PVCs - mess up accurate EF
    ii. Dye toxicity
    iii. repeat LV grams 10 min apart
    iv. limit dose to 3 ml/Kg
    v. study pt. at optimal vascular volume
      (1) dry out CHF with Lasix
    vi. allergic reactions
    vii. minor common reactions
    viii. arrhythmia
    ix. staining - perforation
      (1) Position mid LV
      (2) No end hole only catheters
      (3) No MP or Jacky
    x. air/clot embolism
    xi. Uncompensated CHF
    xii. dry out (diurese patient)
    xiii. Protect coronary flow with Nitro premed.
  b. VENTRICULAR VOLUME ANALYSIS
    i. quantitative ventriculography:
    ii. fast/accurate/gold standard
    iii. assesses MR (LVMF FICK)
    iv. Forward flow for valve area if regurgitation present
    v. evaluate mass/hypertrophy of LV
    vi. 30 degree RAO Long axis LV gram
    vii. Post PVC potentiation = LV viability
5. HEMODYNAMIC CALCULATIONS
  a. QUANTITATIVE ANGIOGRAPHY
    i. EDV = largest LV volume
    ii. ESV = smallest LV volume
    iii. SV = EDV - ESV
    iv. EF = SV / EDV
    v. LVMF (angio. CO) = SV x HR
    vi. -normal EF > 50%
    vii. LV mass (measured from LV wall thickness)
    viii. Mass/vol ratio = LV mass/ EDV
  b. PRESSURES
    i. normal Left Ht. pressures
      (1) LA, LV. AO, Peripheral artery
    ii. Review abnormal pressures
      (1) AS, HOCM, AR, MS, MR
      (2) Constrictive, VSD
    iii. Read LV pressure (s/bd/ed)
      (1) Pressure pullback LV > Ao (Gradient?)
      (2) Reverse LV-Ao gradient (peripheral amplification)
6. LV ANGIO PROJECTIONS / VIEWS
  a. LV angio filming
    i. biplane - reduces contrast
    ii. single plane (RAO) cine
    iii. Area length measurement
    iv. diameter measurements
  b. Views for various lesions
    i. MR = RAO
    ii. VSD = LAO cranial
    iii. LONG AXIS VIEW: 30-45° RAO view
    iv. FOUR CHAMBER VIEW: LAO with steep cranial
    v. PA VIEW: Frontal view
    vi. SHORT AXIS VIEW: LAO caudal view
  c. PATHOLOGY SEEN IN LV GRAMS
    i. Best LV angio Views showing:
      (1) Aortic arch - LAO view best lays out
      (2) coronary artery take-off - LAO
      (3) Dissection= 45°-60° LAO with AO ROOT INJECTION
      (4) MR = 30° RAO with LV INJECTION
      (5) ASD = 60° LAO CRANIAL with PA INJECTION
      (6) VSD = 45°-60° LAO CRANIAL with LV INJECTION
      (7) PDA = PA CRANIAL with AORTIC INJECTION
      (8) RAO = Prolapse of Mitral valve
    ii. Grade severity of AR & MR
      (1) 1+ to 4+
7. LV SEGMENTS & WALL MOTION
  a. Wall motion analysis methods
    i. Centerline method (of Sheehan)
    ii. chord method
  b. LV gram diagnostic information:
    i. LV fn. CAD
    ii. Areas of infarct
    iii. AI, IHSS, MR, LV aneurysm, VSD
  c. LV WALL SEGMENTS

                i. Mitral valve
                ii. Posterior-Lateral
                iii. Septal
                iv. Anterior
                v. Apex
                vi. Inferior
        d. LV WALL MOTION - Coronary Supplying
                i. ANTERIOR WALL - LAD
                ii. APEX - LAD
                iii. INFERIOR WALL - PDA or RCA
                iv. ANT. SEPTAL wall - LAD septals
                v. POSTEROLATERAL - Circ.
                vi. APEX - distal LAD (if wrap around LAD) - &/or Inferior wall RCA, PDCA (if dominant RCA) motion
        e. ABNORMAL WALL MOTION
                i. asynergesis
                ii. akinetic
                iii. dyskinetic
                iv. asynchrony
                v. local hypokinetic
                vi. global hypokinetic
8. LV PATHOLOGY
    a. Myocardial Ischemia/Infarction
            i. Wall motion abnormalities (see above)
    b. Myocardial disease
            i. Dilated CardioMyopathy (DC)
            ii. Restrictive CardioMyopathy (RC)
            iii. Hypertrophic Obstructive CardioMyopathy (HOCM)
    c. Pressure/ Volume Overload
            i. Aortic Valvular Obstruction (AVO)
            ii. Dilation and hypertrophy, Volume overload
            iii. Hypertrophy, Pressure overload
            iv. Aneurysm, transmural infarction
    d. Valvular Regurgitation
            i. Mild, moderate, severe AR
            ii. Mild, Moderate, Severe MR
    a. LV Aneurysm
            i. True aneurysm
            ii. False aneurysm
    b. LV Thrombus
    c. VSD
9. GENERAL TRANSEPTAL
    a. ANATOMY
            i. Fossa Ovale
            ii. Limbic Ridge
            iii. Patent Foramen Ovale found in 10-20% of normals
    b. USEFULNESS OF TRANSEPTAL HEART CATH.
            i. If good 2D ultrasound, may omit
            ii. LA pressure most accurate (wedge?) in MR, MS
            iii. Best LA Angiogram
            iv. Safest LV entry in patients with:
                (1) prosthetic AO valve
                (2) tight AS
                (3) Distinguish IHSS from catheter entrapment
            v. Only way to detect pressure gradients between PCW and LA (PA edp - PCW Pulm. arteriolar gradient)
                vi. Mitral Valvuloplasty
                vii. Watchman plug implant
                viii. EP - AF ablation in LA
    c. INDICATIONS
            i. Unable to cross tight aortic valve retrograde
            ii. When the wedge pressure is unreliable in MR
            iii. Mitral valvuloplasty
            iv. If noninvasive LV studies inadequate
    d. CONTRAINDICATIONS
            i. giant RA
            ii. Atrial Myxoma
            iii. LA thrombus
            iv. cyanotic congenital disease
            v. anticoagulant therapy
            vi. severe chest deformity
            vii. inability to lie flat
    e. TRANSSEPTAL EQUIPMENT
            i. Brockenbrough needle
            ii. Bing stylet
            iii. Brockenbrough catheters
            iv. Mullins Sheath
            v. positioning across Atrial Septum
            vi. Measurements taken of catheter and needle
    f. TECHNIQUE -PROCEDURE
            i. Standard Seldinger cath from Rt. Fem. Vein
            ii. Exchange Rt. Ht. Cath. for Brockenbrough cath
            iii. Pass Brockenbrough needle into cath.
            iv. Connect needle to pressure monitor
            v. Record & monitor pressures via needle
            vi. Position needle tip in fossa Ovalis
            vii. Repositioning (Remove needle 1st)
            viii. Puncture into LA
            ix. Take pressures and blood sample
            x. When in LA advance catheter into LA over needle
            xi. remove needle
            xii. Record LA pressure
            xiii. Advance cath across Mitral valve
            xiv. Record LV pressure
            xv. Angiography
    g. TRANSSEPTAL CONSIDERATIONS
            i. Don't anticoagulate with heparin
            ii. Always done from Rt. Fem. Vein
            iii. Pressure Monitoring through Brockenbrough needle
            iv. ID Waveforms through needle
                (1) in Pericardium
                (2) in CS
                (3) in AO
                (4) Myocardium
    h. COMPLICATIONS
            i. Aortic puncture
            ii. Coronary Sinus perforation
            iii. Pericardial Tamponade
            iv. Pericardial Centesis

Pediatric Catheterization Techniques

INDEX: D9 - Pediatric Catheterization Techniques - RCIS removed 2013
1. Equipment . . . . . p. 329 - Review
2. Vascular Access . . . . p. 331 - Review
3. Procedures / Patient Care . . p. 333 - Know
4. Hemodynamics . . . . p. 338 - Review
5. Acyanotic Lesions . . . p. 351 - Review
6. Cyanotic Lesions . . . p. 364 - Review
7. Other Congenital Pathology . . p. 373 - Review
8. Sample Pathology . . . p. 374 - Review
9. Chapter Outline . . . . p. 388

1. Equipment - CCI removed Pediatric Cath category in 2013. Still expect shunt basics.

590. Identify the pediatric catheter labeled #5 on the diagram.
   a. NIH
   b. Berman
   c. Swan-Ganz
   d. Pigtail
   e. Rashkind
   f. Cournand or Lehman
   g. Judkins RCA

Pediatric catheters

ANSWER e. Rashkind atrial septostomy catheter. It is used to enlarge the foramen ovale in certain cyanotic lesions.
CORRECTLY MATCHED ANSWERS ARE:
1. **NIH**: The NIH is a "No End Hole" catheter. It is most commonly used in RV and PA angiography.
2. **COURNAND/ LEHMAN**: A woven Dacron standard wall catheter used for right heart catheterization.
3. **BERMAN**: PVC BALLOON floatation catheter with side holes proximal to the balloon tip. It is the right heart angiographic catheter of choice in infants and children.
4. **SWAN-GANZ**: A whole family of multi-lumen balloon floatation catheters with a rubber balloon at the tip. These catheters have become the standard for right heart cath because they are easy to insert and are safe.
5. **RASHKIND ATRIAL SEPTOSTOMY** catheter. These are sturdy single lumen balloon catheters. They are made to take the abuse of a rapid pullback to tear the atrial septum. This provides increased blood flow to the lungs for oxygenation. Remember

"Rashkind Rips."
6. **JUDKINS RIGHT** coronary catheter: Many coronary catheters & wires may be used on pediatric cases because they are smaller and more readily available.
7. **PIGTAIL**: The pigtail catheter is the most commonly used LV gram and AO-gram catheter. With up to 12 side holes it evenly disperses the dye within the LV. The distal coiled tip prevents spearing, arrhythmia (irritation), recoil, and intra-myocardial injection.

See: Tilkian, CV Procedures, chapter on "Tools for Cardiac Catheterization."
Keywords: Pediatric balloons and angiographic catheters.

591. **In a pediatric heart cath the first ANGIOGRAPHIC flood catheter selected is usually a:**
a. Swan-Ganz
b. Berman
c. Pigtail
d. NIH type

ANSWER b. Berman catheter. In infant or child catheterization the right heart cath is done first because the left side often then becomes accessible through an ASD or other shunt. This makes the flow-directed balloon catheters ideal because they float downstream so easily and are so atraumatic to the soft infant heart.

The Berman is the balloon catheter of choice because of its multiple side holes proximal to a floatation balloon. The only thing it is not good for is wedge pressures- but with a shunt you can get into the LA directly and don't need indirect wedge pressures. Remember "Baby Berman Balloon."

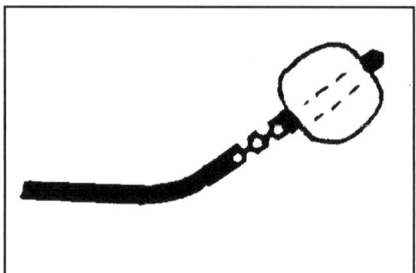

Berman angio cath.

See: Baim and Grossman, Cardiac Cath., Angiog., and Interventions, chapter on "Cardiac Catheterization in Infants and Children." **Keywords**: First pediatric angio. cath chosen usually = Berman

592. **To reduce the amount of contrast and optimize angiographic information retrieved during pediatric caths use _____ .**
a. High concentration low-osmolar or non-ionic contrast media
b. High flow thin-walled catheters with pressure injectors
c. Single plane digital subtraction X-ray equipment
d. Biplane Xray equipment

ANSWER d. Biplane Xray equipment with 2 C arms. Grossman says, "Because of contrast agent constraints and the necessity of acquiring as much anatomic information as possible from each injection, biplane equipment is essential for pediatric catheterization."
See: Grossman, Cardiac Cath., Angiog., and Interventions, chapter on "Cardiac Catheterization in Infants and Children."

593. Pulse oximeters utilize what two light emitting diodes?
a. Red and infrared
b. Red and purple
c. Ultraviolet & green
d. Blue and red

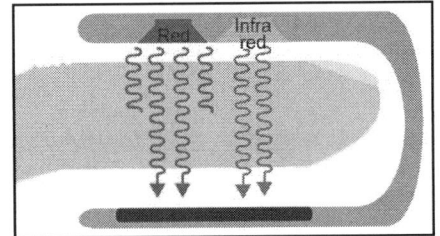

ANSWER a. Red & infrared. Infra-red lies in the invisible heat spectral range. These two colored lights pass through the finger, toes, or ear and the relative intensity of each color determines the % saturation. This is possible because deoxygenated (or reduced) hemoglobin and oxyhemoglobin each has a unique but overlapping absorption spectrum.
See: Daily, chapter on "Hemodynamic Monitoring of Children." **Keywords:** Pulse oximeter wavelengths red & infra-red

594. Pulse oximeters are often inaccurate in the pediatric patient with profound:
a. Anemia and/or hypertension
b. Anemia and/or hypotension
c. Polycythemia and/or hypertension
d. Polycythemia and/or hypotension

ANSWER b. Anemia (<20% Hct.) and/or systemic hypotension. Hypotension is usually associated with peripheral vasoconstriction. Vasoconstricted peripheral capillaries do not move enough arteriolized blood through the finger or toes to give accurate O_2 saturation. Consider how blue your fingers or lips get when cold (peripheral cyanosis). In the low O_2 saturation ranges the O_2 dissociation curve is extremely steep and small changes in PO_2 can dramatically affect the O_2 saturation.
See: Daily, chapter on "Hemodynamic Monitoring of Children." **Keywords:** Pulse oximeters inaccurate in anemia and/or hypotension

2. Vascular Access - Not tested on RCIS

595. An umbilical artery catheter can usually be inserted within the first ___ days of life. When inserted correctly it passes into the _____.
a. 3, IVC & right heart
b. 3, Descending aorta & left heart
c. 10, IVC & right heart
d. 10, Descending aorta & left heart

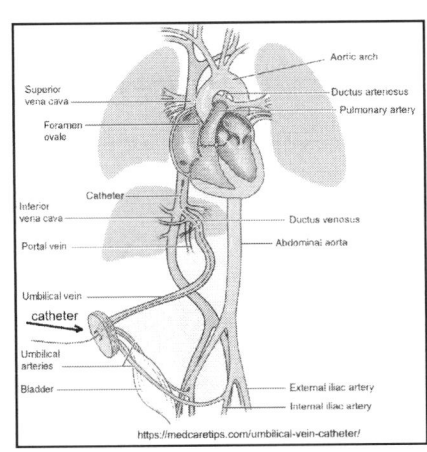

ANSWER d. 10, Descending aorta & left heart. Within the first 10 days of life the umbilical artery can quickly be entered. It passes the internal iliac, the common iliac artery and into the descending aorta & left heart. It is usually a last resort approach - when right heart and femoral arterial cath fail to enter the left heart. Since it may be associated with significant complications it should only be performed by experienced physicians.

The umbilical vein may also be entered within the first 3 days of life. However, Grossman says it is more difficult to enter the RV and PA with this approach than the femoral approach. Clots may block the vein soon after birth.

See: Baim and Grossman, chapter on "Pediatric Interventions" and Daily, chapter on "Hemodynamic Monitoring in Children." **Keywords**: Umbilical artery entry in first 10 days

596. **A pediatric heart cath usually starts with puncture of the _____.**
   a. **Femoral vein**
   b. **Femoral artery**
   c. **Subclavian vein**
   d. **Umbilical artery**

ANSWER a. The femoral vein is the usual first puncture attempted. These are among the largest accessible veins in the body. The left subclavian vein is a second choice. The pediatric cath usually starts with the right heart because the left heart is often accessible through the foramen ovale.

See: Baim and Grossman, chapter on "Pediatric Interventions" and Daily, chapter on "Hemodynamic Monitoring in Children." **Keywords**: First pediatric puncture usually femoral vein

597. **Pediatric transseptal left heart cath may be performed with atrial septal puncture. When advancing the pediatric transseptal heart needle during transseptal puncture Pepine recommends attaching the needle to:**
   a. **A Doppler probe (smart needle)**
   b. **A pressure transducer**
   c. **A syringe of contrast**
   d. **Pressure bag with attached continuous flow device**

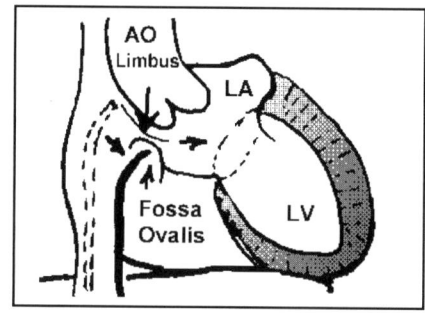

RA-LA, pediatric transeptal

ANSWER c. A syringe of contrast. Although all the authors recommend it, few centers still attach pressure transducers to the transseptal needle. Many make the puncture with fluoroscopy alone. Pediatric transseptal puncture must be done though a much smaller atrial septum.

The advantage of the syringe of contrast is that it makes septal passage easy to detect, when whiffs of dye are seen in the LA. If passage is incomplete a tiny injection stains the atrial septum to mark it on fluoro. This stain then becomes a landmark, should additional sticks be necessary.

See: Pepine, chapter on "The Adult Patient with Known or Suspected Congenital Heart Disease." **Keywords**: Attach transseptal needle to contrast syringe for injection

3. Procedures & Patient Care

598. Compared to an older child or adult, the heart of a fetus or newborn infant has high:
   a. Diastolic reserve (to increase preload)
   b. Inotropic reserve (to increase contractility)
   c. Heart rate reserve ($HR_{max} - HR_{rest}$)
   d. O2 consumption/M^2 (metabolic rate)

ANSWER d. O2 consumption/M^2. Newborns have a high metabolic rate and demand more O2 per M^2 than older individuals. Thus, they have LITTLE RESERVE to either:
   •Increase HR (already near maximum HR)
   •Increase contractility by reducing preload (have weak hearts)
   •Increase diastolic filling (have relatively stiff hearts)
Cardiac output in the neonate can only increase about 25% above resting level. Whereas, by two weeks of age they can double their CO. For all these reasons infants are at high risk with any kind of stress such as cardiac catheterization.
See: Braunwald, chapter on "Congenital Heart Disease." **Keywords:** High O2 consumption/M^2 & diminished cardiac reserve

599. How much heparin should be administered in pediatric left heart catheterization?
   a. None, babies do not clot easily
   b. 10 units/Kg
   c. 100 units/Kg
   d. 5000 units

ANSWER c. 100 units/Kg. In infants, if the left heart cannot be entered via the right heart, arterial left heart cath may be attempted. Then Grossman recommends a bolus of 100 IU/Kg. e.g. in a 22 lb or 10 Kg infant this would equal 1000 units of heparin IV. The heparin anticoagulation dose increases with the child's weight, up to a maximum of 5000 units. Grossman also recommends keeping the ACT over 200 sec.
See: Baim and Grossman, chapter on "Cardiac Cath in Infants and Children." **Keywords:** Heparin in children = 100 IU/Kg

600. What is the age range for a pediatric patient labeled at #3 (neonate)?
   a. Born before "term" or < 5.5 lb.
   b. < 6 months of age
   c. Between 6 months and 1 year of age
   d. Between 1 year and puberty

AGES OF PEDIATRIC PATIENTS:
1. Premature (preemie)
2. Infant
*3. Neonate
4. Child

ANSWER b. Neonate = Less than 6 months of age.
CORRECTLY MATCHED ANSWERS ARE:
AGES OF PEDIATRIC PATIENTS:
1. **Preemie** - born before < 37 weeks of gestation or < 5.5 lb.
2. **Infant** - between 6 months and 1 year
3. **Neonate** - < 6 months of age
4. **Child** - between 1 year and puberty

See: Medical dictionary **keywords:** Pediatric age groups

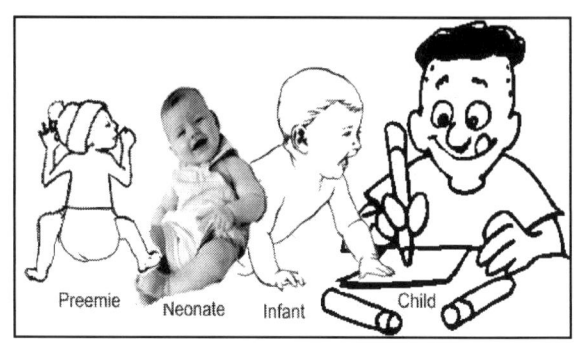
Pediatric age groups

601. In order to reduce the risk of hypovolemia in a 5 Kg neonate, consider blood replacement when the total blood sample size exceeds:
a. 15-25 ml
b. 30-50 ml
c. 60-80 ml
d. 100-150 ml.

ANSWER a. 15-25 ml. Daily says, "Small amounts of blood loss during catheter insertion may represent significant blood loss for the child." For this reason blood sampling bleeding must be minimized in pediatric cath.

Daily recommends that blood transfusion may be necessary when acute blood loss exceeds 3.5-5 ml/Kg of body weight. 3.5 x 5 = 17.5 ml; 5 x 5 = 25 ml. Daily states that this critical blood loss is 2.5-5% of the circulating blood volume of an infant.

Daily says that 8.5-9% of the neonate's body weight is circulating blood volume (less in children and adults). Rounding this to 10% means that in a 5000 gm neonate (11 lb.), 500 ml may be blood. Thus 2.5-5% (12.5-25 ml) of acute blood loss in a neonate may be critical. One way to remember this number might be: *"Never allow pediatric patients to lose more blood in ml. than twice their weight in lb."* E.g. our 5 Kg (11 lb) neonate cannot lose more than 22 ml of blood.

See: Daily, chapter on "Hemodynamic Monitoring in Children." **Keywords:** Minimize infant acute blood loss to fewer ml than 2 x wt. in lb.

602. To take accurate O_2 saturation samples from a catheter during pediatric heart cath, what procedure should be done before withdrawing a blood sample into a heparinized sample syringe?
a. Flush out the catheter with heparinized flush
b. Let 2-3 ml of blood drip out the catheter hub
c. Withdraw 1-2 ml (catheter dead space) into a separate syringe
d. Withdraw 5-6 ml (catheter dead space) into a waste syringe

ANSWER c. Withdraw 1-2 ml (catheter dead space) into a separate syringe. This is necessary to keep saline flush out of the sample. Most pediatric catheters hold around 1.0 ml of dead space. This must be removed before you start to get blood. The sequence is:

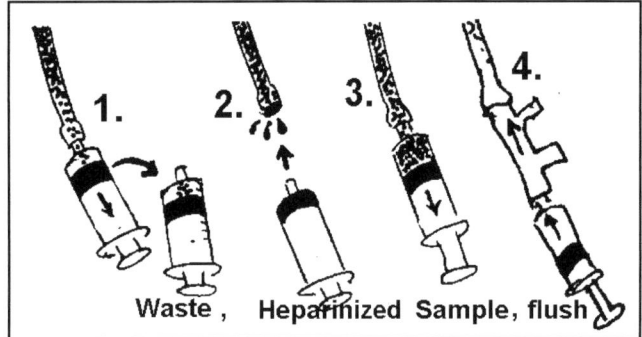

Oximetry sampling - flushing

1. **Withdraw** the catheter dead space in a waste syringe, until blood is seen. (One ml. in pediatric cath.)
2. **Attach** a heparinized sample syringe and draw the 0.5-1 ml necessary for oximetry. Eject air bubbles. RUN on OXIMETER.
3. **The first syringe** (containing dead space flush and blood) should then be reinfused into the catheter. This helps prevent the danger of blood loss described above, using aseptic technique.
4. **Attach manifold,** pullback slightly to eliminate bubbles, and flush catheter with fresh heparinized flush solution.

In addition to the sampling technique described, catheters with multiple side-holes should not be used to sample O_2 saturation because the holes cover such a large area. Use a single end hole Swan-Ganz or other catheter with side holes near the end.
See: Daily, chapter on "Hemodynamic Monitoring in Children." p. 291 **Keywords**: O_2 sampling from catheter = withdraw dead space flush first

603. The simplest way to screen for L-R shunts is to take two blood samples during a right heart cath. A L-R shunt may be suspected if the difference between ____ and ____ samples exceeds a _____ change.
  a. RA - PCW, ≥15-20% O_2 saturation
  b. PA - PCW, ≥15-20% O_2 saturation
  c. SVC - PA, ≥5-8% O_2 saturation
  d. IVC - PA, ≥5-8% O_2 saturation

ANSWER c. SVC - PA, ≥5-8%. Grossman says, "The simplest way to screen for a left-to-right shunt is to sample SVC and PA blood... we routinely obtain blood samples from SVC and PA at the time of right heart catheterization and determine their O_2 saturation by reflectance oximetry. If the ΔO_2 saturation between these samples is ≥8%, a left-to-right shunt may be present at atrial, ventricular, or great vessel level, and a full oximetry run should be done."

Although not as accurate, an alternative screening method is to evaluate the PA blood for elevated O_2 saturation. If it exceeds 85%, a L-R shunt may be stepping-up the right heart saturation. Normal systemic venous (RA-RV-PA) O_2 saturation varies from 67-84% with a mean of 75% O_2.
See: Baim and Grossman, chapter on "Pediatric Interventions."

604. How is the infant usually restrained at cardiac cath for vascular access?
a. Paralyzing agents allow the child to be unrestrained
b. Wrists and ankles are bound with soft gauze strips which are tied at the top and bottom of the X-ray table
c. Arms and legs are bound to an X shaped leg and arm board
d. Legs are bound to a Y shaped board, wrists are also tied with gauze to the top of the X-ray table

ANSWER d. Legs are bound to a Y shaped board, wrists are also tied with gauze to the top of the X-ray table. The legs must be immobilized for percutaneous puncture. They are loosely bound to a Y shaped board. Not too tightly, because good venous pressure is necessary to catheterize the femoral vein. New boards with Velcro straps are available commercially.

The arms, also, may need restraints to prevent flailing and grabbing. They are not usually used for venous access so may be loosely tied above the head. This allows the baby some arm motion and allows the nurse to control the arms.
See: Personal experience

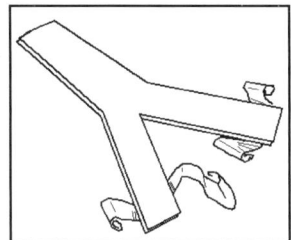

Y board for infants

605. Overhead infrared lamps may be used during a pediatric cath to:
a. Keep the child warm
b. Provide sufficient light for vascular entry
c. Encourage bilirubin photo-oxidation
d. Accelerate vitamin D synthesis

ANSWER a. Keep the child warm. Infra-red over bed warmer lights keep the infant warm. Infants have increased body surface / weight ratio. This makes them lose heat and moisture rapidly, and more prone to hypothermia. In addition infants have no "shiver reflex." Instead, infants must burn fat in a high energy process called "non-shivering thermogenesis." A cool environment forces them to increase their oxygen consumption and cardiac work through this inefficient process. It's very important to keep infants warm.

Infants may be removed from their incubator and placed on a "cold" X-ray table. Methods of body heat preservation are necessary, including heating pads, infra-red lights, and warm blankets.
See: Daily, chapter on "Hemodynamic Monitoring of Children."
Keywords: Thermoregulatory needs of infant = infra-red lights

606. Identify 4 early signs of cardio-respiratory failure in infants. (Select 4.)
a. Skin mottling
b. Peripheral vasoconstriction/cooling
c. Decreased urine output
d. Decreased arterial pulse pressure
e. Arterial hypotension

ANSWERS: a, b, c, & d. Arterial hypotension is NOT correct. Daily says, "The child may maintain a "normal" blood pressure despite the presence of shock or significant hemorrhage. *Hypotension is only a very late sign of cardiorespiratory distress in children and indicates that cardiorespiratory arrest is imminent."*

Signs of poor systemic perfusion in children include nonspecific signs of distress, including:
- tachycardia
- irritability
- tachypnea
- lethargy
- decreased response to pain

Early signs of cardiorespiratory failure include:
- mottling of the skin
- cooling of extremities and peripheral vasoconstriction
- prolonged capillary refill
- decreased urine output (<1-2 ml/Kg/hr)
- decreased intensity of arterial pulses (diminished pulse pressure and damping)

See: Daily, chapter on "Hemodynamic Monitoring in Children." **Keywords:** Children do not show arterial hypotension until too late

607. What is the most common dangerous neonatal and infant arrhythmia?
a. Bradycardia (HR<100)
b. Supraventricular tachycardia (HR>100)
c. Ventricular tachycardia (HR>200)
d. Ventricular fibrillation

ANSWER a. Bradycardia. The average neonatal heart rate is 120-160. This drops to 80-110 for preschool children. Normal adult rate limits of (60-100) do not apply to children. Ventricular arrhythmias are rare in children.

Since children normally have higher heart rates than adults, persistent bradycardia in pediatric patients is usually a sign of hypoxia, vagal stimulation, or catheter manipulation near the tricuspid valve (heart block). Daily says "*Profound or persistent bradycardia in the absence of reversible hypoxia is an ominous finding in the pediatric patient and often indicates impending arrest. In fact, bradycardia (progressing to asystole) is the most common terminal cardiac rhythm in children.*" **See**: Daily, chapter on "Hemodynamic Monitoring in Children."
Keywords: Most dangerous neonatal rhythm = bradycardia

608. Elimination of all bubbles and assuring tight stopcock connections in venous lines is most important in infants and children with:
a. Pulmonary hypertension
b. Systemic hypertension
c. Cyanosis
d. Pulmonary edema

ANSWER c. Cyanotic kids may have a R-L shunt. Bubbles accidentally injected into the right heart may shunt into the left heart leading to stroke.
See: Daily, chapter on "Hemodynamic Monitoring in Children." **Keywords:** Allow no air bubbles in cyanotic kids

609. In most neonates the LA may be entered via a _____.
a. Probe-patent ostium secundum
b. Probe-patent ostium primum
c. Retrograde aortic catheter
d. Pulmonary venous balloon catheter

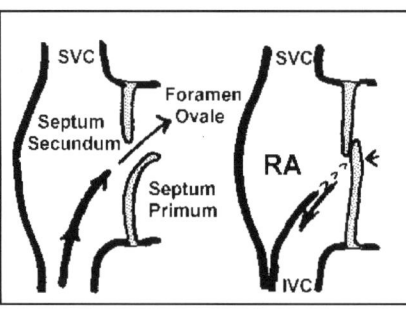
Probe patent fossa ovalis

ANSWER a. Probe-patent ostium secundum. Secundum defects are the most common ASD. And in most neonates the septa have not yet sealed allowing a catheter to "probe" it open.

Remember, the foramen ovale normally closes at the first breath of life. When LA pressures exceed RA pressures, a flap (septum primum) in the LA covers the foramen ovale. It normally grows into and seals to the atrial septum. But most neonates and about 10-25% of normal adults have a "probe patent" foramen ovale which can often be passed with a stiff IVC catheter.

The technique is the same as for a transseptal cath. Start in SVC and pull the tip down the atrial septal wall. When the tip bounces over the limbic ridge and moves to the right - you're in the fossa ovalis. Push the catheter between the septum primum and septum secundum through the foramen ovale into the LA. **See:** Braunwald, chapter on "Congenital Heart Disease." **Keywords:** Most common ASD = ostium secundum

4. Hemodynamics - Tested on RCIS (Not green dye)

610. It is essential to distinguish between reversible and irreversible high pulmonary vascular resistance. The most important diagnostic test for this is:
a. Doppler echocardiography with bubble contrast
b. Two dimensional echocardiography with bubble contrast
c. Right heart cardiac catheterization with inhaled nitric oxide
d. Left heart cardiac catheterization with inhaled nitric oxide

ANSWER c. Right heart cardiac catheterization with nitric oxide (NO) challenge test. Braunwald says "Hemodynamic measurements at cath are the mainstay in assessing the pulmonary vascular bed, especially its reactivity." Right heart cath can evaluate PA and LA pressures (wedge) and CO parameters necessary to calculate pulmonary resistance. If PVR can be reduced with inhaled nitric oxide for 10-30 minutes, then the PA pressures and pulmonary resistance are reversible, and surgery or transplant are likely to be effective. **See:** Braunwald, chapter on "Pathobiology of Pulmonary Arterial Hypertension"

If the pulmonary resistance is NOT reversible it suggests that the lung resistance is fixed and will not adapt to interventions, e.g. if the patient has a longstanding L-R shunt and the perfusion pressure has been so high for so long that even a heart transplant can't effectively pump blood through the stiff lungs. You should know how to calculate pulmonary vascular resistance from hemodynamic data. **See:** Todd, Vol 3, Hemodynamic Calculations, chapter 9.

611. In the cath lab you are testing a pulmonary hypertension patient for vasoreactivity with the nitric oxide inhalation test. Why should you never rely on the hemodynamic computer's calculated mean pressure to make the critical pulmonary vascular resistance (PVR) calculation?
   a. Mean PA pressure varies too much
   b. Mean RA pressure varies too much
   c. You need end expiratory mean
   d. You need end inspiration mean

ANSWER: c. You need end expiratory mean or relaxed breath holding to eliminate the effect of inspiration on the right heart pressures. Inspiration lowers intrathoracic pressure which lowers all right heart pressures - especially deep breathing. You can time these dips with respiration. Accurate mean measurements should be recorded on paper and measured on the plateau before patient inhalation.

Braunwald says, "In addition to confirming the diagnosis and allowing the exclusion of other causes, cardiac catheterization also establishes the severity of disease and allows an assessment of prognosis. By definition, patients with PAH should have a low or normal pulmonary capillary wedge pressure. Because this is a critical measurement in distinguishing a patient with PAH from one with pulmonary venous hypertension, quality measures must be established in the catheterization laboratory to ensure that correct values are obtained. The transducers must be carefully adjusted to reflect the height of the midchest of every patient. Pressures should never be determined by the electronically integrated mean pressure from the laboratory's computer, because these measurements ignore respiratory influences. Instead, measurements of all pressures are properly made at end-expiration to avoid incorporating negative intrathoracic pressures. When a reproducible wedge pressure cannot be obtained, direct measurement of left ventricular end-diastolic pressure is advised. If the wedge pressure is increased, it should be correlated with left ventricular end-diastolic pressure and not attributed to a falsely elevated reading."
See: Braunwald, chapter on "Pulmonary Hypertension"

612. A man with a chronic cyanotic shunt and pulmonary hypertension (PA = 65/30/42) is evaluated for corrective surgery. While breathing 100% O2 (or nitric oxide) his PA pressure falls to 30/15/22 mmHg. This indicates _____ pulmonary resistance, and that surgery _____ considered.
   a. Reversible, WILL NOT BE
   b. Reversible, MAY BE
   a. Irreversible, WILL NOT BE
   b. Irreversible, MAY BE

ANSWER b. Reversible, SURGERY MAY BE CONSIDERED. This is the main reason we test for pulmonary vascular resistance reactivity. Since PVR = (PA-LA)/CO the resistance appears to have dropped in half. Accurate calculations for PVR should be made. But, since it is not likely the CO or LA pressures changed dramatically, the PVR is proportional to PA mean pressure. (PVR ∝ mean PA). This patient's drop in PVR is a good indication that he will be able to adapt to corrective surgery or oral medications

"The nitric oxide study has replaced the oxygen study. Pressure measurements taken

with the patient on room air are compared with measurements while breathing nitric oxide (NO). The pulmonary vascular resistance is calculated for these two conditions. A green light for surgery is when the PVR drops significantly on NO."
See: Braunwald, chapter on "Congenital Heart Disease." **Keywords:** O2 reversibility of high PVR, surgery may now be considered

613. These are GREEN DYE CURVES. Identify the type of shunt detected by the curve labeled #3.
a. Normal
b. L-R shunt
c. R-L shunt

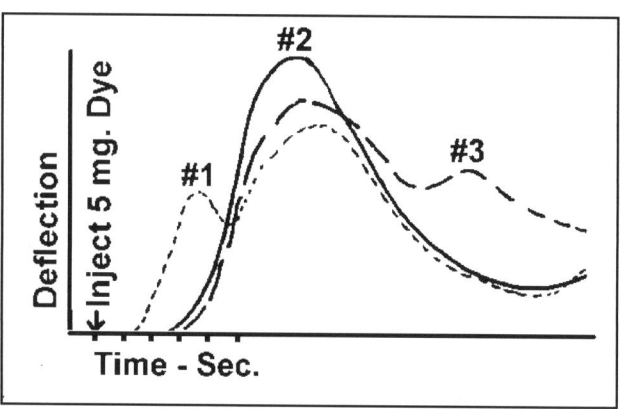
Green dye curves (IVC→AO)

ANSWER b. L-R shunt causes this early bump. Green dye curves have been largely replaced by angiography, echocardiography and thermodilution CO. But the concepts are key to understanding newer techniques like Fast CT shunt detection.

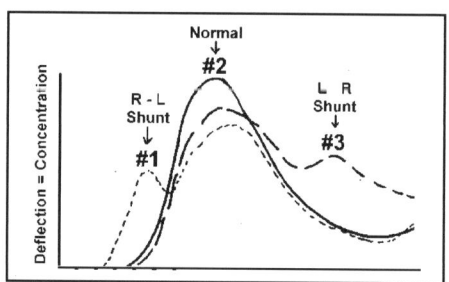
Green dye curves (IVC→AO)

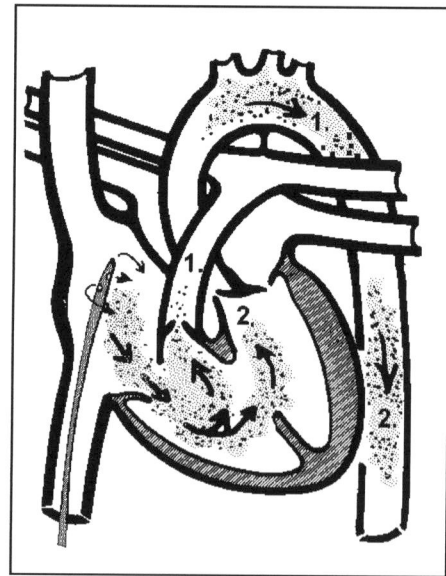
R-L VSD - Shunted Dye (#2) appears early in LV and AO

GREEN DYE CURVES SHOWN ARE:
1. **R-L SHUNT:** The dye divides in the right heart as shunted blood appears early in the left heart - making a distinctive early appearance in the aorta (early bump). Small R-L shunts show the small "early bump" shown while large L-R shunts show large "early bumps." The size of the early bump is proportional to the amount of shunt. At present this sensitive method of R-L shunt detection is the only major application for green dye curves. Note in the diagram that the dye divides (1 & 2) at the VSD shunt. As it passes into the aorta, you see two concentrations of dye (1 & 2 in AO). The amount of the R-L shunt seen at #2 accounts for the curves early hump.
#2. **NORMAL:** The curve rises rapidly to a peak and decays exponentially. As the dye returns through the right and left heart on its second pass it creates the low recirculation curve seen. These were the first indicator dilution curves, before thermodilution. Cardiac output was calculated in a manner similar to TD CO.
#3. **L-R SHUNT:** All the dye circulates through the right heart but as it passes through the left heart some blood is shunted back into the right heart again. This recirculating dye appears as a hump following the primary curve, on the recirculation

curve.

This diagram shows a small R-L shunt with distinct secondary bump. Instead of a "bump" large L-R shunts show reduced peak primary curve concentration and prolong the disappearance of dye at the sampling site (AO).

See: Pepine, chapter on "The Adult Patient with Congenital Disease"

614. You are assisting with a heart cath on a teenager. The girl's skin appears dusky with blue lips, even on O_2. What intra-cardiac pressure would you expect to be most abnormal?
   a. Low AO pressure
   b. High RA (venous) pressure
   c. Low PA pressure
   d. High PA pressure

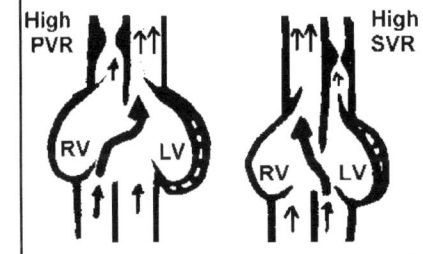

High pulmonary resistance

ANSWER d. High PA pressure. Cyanotic lesions have high right sided heart pressures. Pressure usually builds up over the years to overcome the high pulmonary resistance. When septal shunts are present, blood shunts from high to low pressure areas. Cyanosis implies a R-L shunt. The dark venous blood dilutes the red blood causing an O_2 saturation step-down on the left side and arterial hypoxemia. In R-L shunting 100% O_2 administration will only slightly improve the O_2 saturation and not resolve it.

Shunts are like a river which divides. If the right leg of the river is dammed up (high pulmonary resistance) pressure will build up there and the flow will be diverted into the left side of the river. This is how a R-L shunt usually develops.

Cyanosis like this suggests a R-L shunt. It could be at any level (atrial, ventricular, or PDA). Cyanosis is associated with severe pulmonary disease. But this is unlikely in a normal teenager whois receiving O_2.

The above diagram also shows a L-R shunt which is acyanotic, with a high pulmonary blood flow. This is the most common direction for shunting.

See: Braunwald, chapter on "Congenital Heart Disease."

615. Hemodynamic findings from a heart cath on a child are shown in the box. **CALCULATE THE PULMONARY VASCULAR RESISTANCE (PVR).**
   a. 1 Wood or Hybrid Resistance Unit
   b. 4.2 Wood or Hybrid Resistance Units
   c. 8.0 Wood or Hybrid Resistance Units
   d. 10. Wood or Hybrid Resistance Units

HEMODYNAMICS ON CHILD		
CO	=	2.2 L/min.
RA	=	6/8/(4) mmHg
RV	=	36/4/6 mmHg
PA	=	35/15/(28) mmHg

ANSWER d. 10 Wood or Hybrid Resistance Units.
- PVR = (PA mean pressure - Wedge mean) / CO
- Mean PA pressure is 28 mmHg. Mean LA is mean PA wedge of 6 mmHg.
- PVR = (28-6)/2.2 = 22/2.2 = 10 mmHg/L/min, HRUs or Wood units.
   This is an elevated PVR. Normal PVR is approximately 1.0 HRU. She will be UNABLE

to tolerate and benefit from corrective surgery unless the PVR can be reduced. If it drops too significantly with O_2 or vasodilators - then corrective surgery may be considered and her prognosis improved.
See: Braunwald, chapter on "Congenital Heart Disease." **Keywords:** Calculate PVR

616. In the adult, what is the normal ratio of Systemic Vascular Resistance to Pulmonary Arteriolar Resistance? (SVR/PVR ratio)
  a. 1:7
  b. 2:1
  c. 6:1
  d. 12:1

ANSWER d. 12:1. Since the ratio of pressure gradients across each capillary bed should be the same as the ratio of resistances (assuming the right sided CO equals the left sided CO) it follows that the ratio of resistances is the same as the ratio of pressures (using Kern's normals).
- SVR/PVR = (AO mean pressure - RA mean) /(PA mean pressure - LA or PAW).
- (85-2.8) / (15-7.9) = 12:1

Understand the units of resistance. Wood units = Hybrid Resistance Units (HRU) = mmHg/L/min. CGS units are dyne.cm.sec^{-5} which is 80 x the Wood unit.
See: Kern, chapter on "Hemodynamics." **Keywords:** Ratio SVR/PVR = 12:1

617. After pediatric surgery for a single-ventricle defect, a patient has "Fontan physiology." This means that systemic venous return from the vena cava:
  a. Passes directly into the LV causing cyanosis
  b. Bypass the RV and passes directly into the PA
  c. Is shunted directly into the LA causing cyanosis
  d. Is reversed with the pulmonary venous circulation

ANSWER b. Bypass the RV and passes directly into the PA. Usually the atrial appendage is attached to the PA. This bypasses the RV and corrects the circulation. RA pressures will be elevated but it is tolerated well. Grossman says, "Perhaps the greatest accomplishment in congenital heart disease in the last generation has been the combined surgical/interventional management of patients with functional single ventricles. In these patients, the systemic venous return is rerouted directly to the pulmonary arteries, no longer returning to the heart (RV), leaving only the pulmonary venous return filling the single ventricle and being pumped to the aorta." Since there is no functional RV to increase the right heart pressure, RA pressures must be high enough to push blood through the lungs. So blood flows from vena cava - RA - PA, lungs, LA - LV (common ventricle) - AO. It is amazing that individuals can get along without a functioning RV. These pediatric patients with Fontan surgery have grown up and are now returning to adult cath labs for evaluation and intervention.

Too high a RA pressure may lead to venous pooling and inadequate LV preload. Other problems Fontan patients develop are: atrial arrhythmias, protein-losing enteropathy, pulmonary stenosis, and ventricular dysfunction. **See:** Baim and Grossman, chapter on "Pediatric Interventions." **Keywords:** Fontan physiology

618. A bilateral heart cath was performed with pullback pressures recorded from both sides of the heart. What abnormality is seen on this pullback pressure tracing recorded on X50?
  a. Aortic valve stenosis
  b. Pulmonic valve stenosis
  c. Tricuspid valve stenosis
  d. Tricuspid valve regurgitation

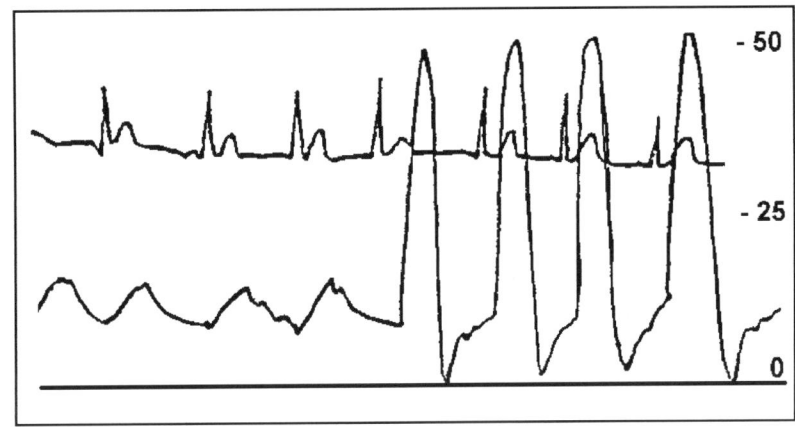

PULLBACK PRESSURES - Recorded X50

ANSWER b. Pulmonic valve stenosis. The first pressure is an arterial pressure (triangular) followed by a ventricular pressure (rapid upstroke and downstroke). The only "pullback" sequence from artery to ventricle is from PA to RV. Also, since the scale is x50 these are most likely right heart pressures. Note the 35 mmHg gradient between systolic PA and systolic RV. This obstruction exists in the pulmonic valve between RV and PA.
See: Kern, chapter on "Hemodynamics." **Keywords:** Pullback through pulmonic stenosis

619. The right heart pullback pressure shown indicates:
  a. Aortic stenosis
  b. Pulmonic valve stenosis
  c. IHSS / HOCM
  d. PA coarctation

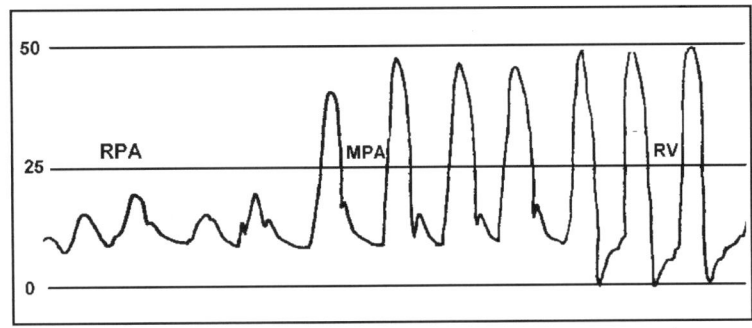

RPA - Main PA - RV pullback recorded 0-50 scale

ANSWER d. PA coarctation. The pullback shows a systolic gradient between RPA and Main PA, indicating a coarctation of the pulmonary artery. There is a 30 mmHg peak-to-peak systolic gradient in the RPA. Often the two diastolic PA pressures are equal. In severe PA coarctation, gradients will increase, and both systolic and diastolic pressures may be reduced, with systole being extremely damped. In this child the left PA may be unobstructed, and will receive the majority of blood flow. Pulmonary hypertension exists. **See:** Criley and Ross "Cardiovascular Physiology."

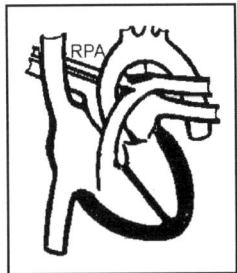

RPA stenosis

Keywords: PA coarctation pullback

620. A right heart catheter was pulled back from the AO. This pullback passes through a/an:
a. PDA
b. ASD
c. VSD
d. Coarctation of AO

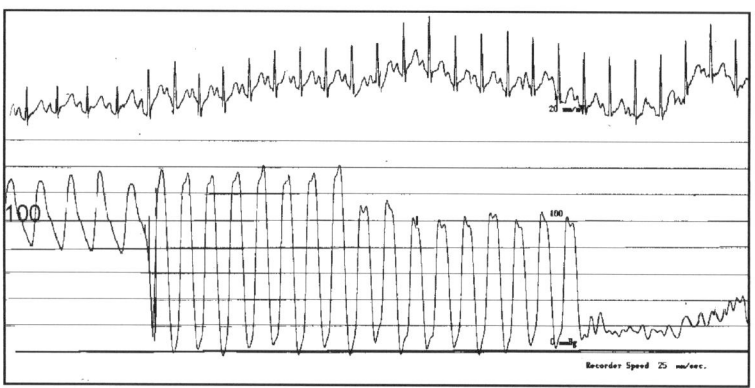
Pullback pressure x200

ANSWER c. VSD. Catheter pressures pass from AO →LV→VSD→RV→RA. Note the 30 mmHg pressure gradient across the ventricular septal defect. This usually indicates a relatively small defect or very high shunt flow. Large VSDs, just like normal valves, show no gradient. Initial catheter position is shown in this drawing. **See:** Kern, Hemodynamic Rounds on "Adult Congenital Anomalies." **Keywords:** VSD

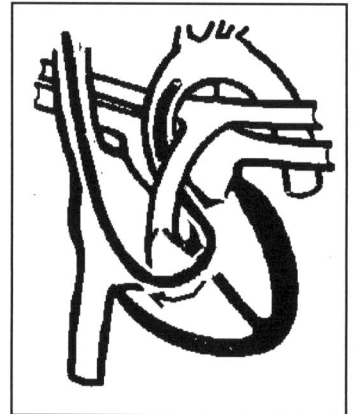
AO →LV→VSD→RV→RA

USE THE TRACING BELOW FOR THE NEXT 2 QUESTIONS. (Same patient as above.)

621. A pediatric Swan Ganz catheter was pulled back from the lungs in the same child shown above. The pressure recording shown suggests a diagnosis of:
a. Aortic stenosis
b. Pulmonic valve stenosis
c. Infundibular stenosis
d. PA coarctation

622. With the above 2 defects, what is the most likely diagnosis for this neonate?
a. Transposition of great vessels
b. Tetralogy of Fallot

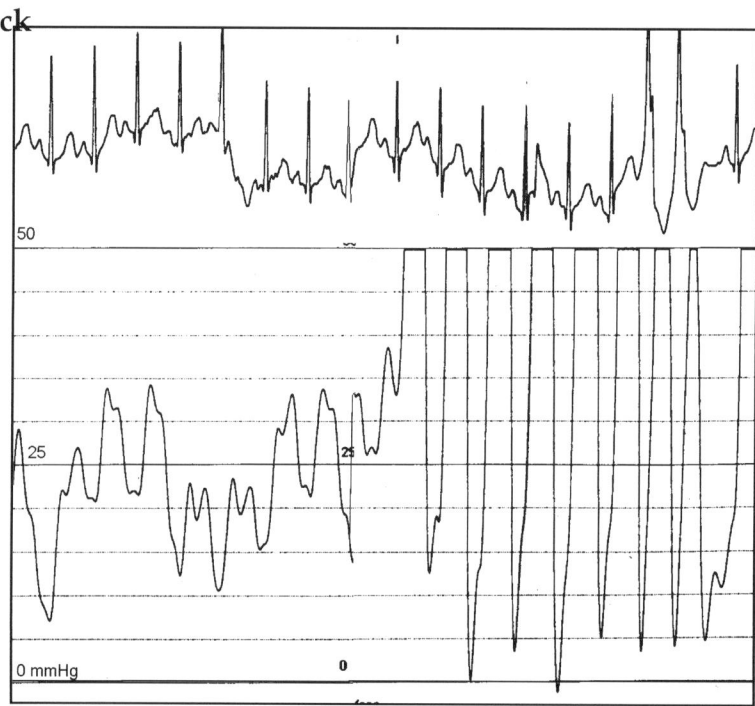
Right heart pullback recorded x50 scale

c. Eisenminger's complex
d. Tricuspid atresia

621. ANSWER b. Pulmonic valve stenosis. This PA→RV pullback shows a large gradient between the PA and RV. The gradient exceeds 25 mmHg. It is impossible to measure the gradient exactly because the RV systolic pressure is "pegged" and "off scale" at the top of the paper. The PA waveform is distorted but does have a dicrotic notch. **See:** Kern, chapter on "Hemodynamics." **Keywords:** Pulmonary valve stenosis (PS)

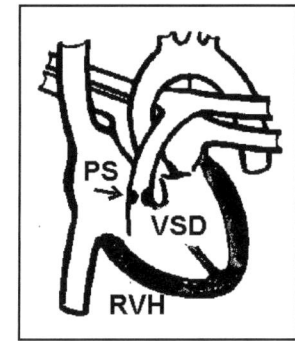
Tetralogy of Fallot

622. ANSWER b. Tetralogy of Fallot. Two of the criteria for TET are shown in the pressure tracings above: VSD and pulmonary stenosis. The other criteria for TET, seen on angio are: RV hypertrophy and overriding aorta.
See: Baim and Grossman, chapter on "Profiles in Congenital Heart Disease." **Keywords:** Tetralogy of Fallot (TET)

623. A child in the cath lab is receiving 100% O_2 by mask. According to Pepine the oximetry data for shunt calculations:
a. Will be inaccurate and should not be done
b. Will be as accurate as room air calculations
c. Should be corrected for dissolved O_2
d. Should be corrected for carboxyhemoglobin

ANSWER c. Should be corrected for dissolved O_2. This involves oximetry as well as running the samples on a blood gas analyzer for PO_2. The high PO_2 levels in arterial blood can make the "physically dissolved" O_2 volume % important.
Usually the small amount of O_2 dissolved in blood plasma at normal room air is insignificant and is neglected in calculations. However, Pepine reports that on 100% O_2, physically dissolved O_2 can make up 14% of the total O_2 content. Physically dissolved O_2 content is calculated by multiplying 0.03 ml O_2/ blood/ mm PO_2 or 0.003 vol%/ mm PO_2. This averages around 1.0 vol% on O_2 and should be **ADDED TO** the hemoglobin O_2 content. For increased accuracy, formulas are:
Hgb O_2 = 1.36 x Hgb x % Sat.
Dissolved O_2 = PO_2 x 0.003 vol%/ mm Hg of PO_2.
For example, if a patient's O_2 content by oximetry is 20 vol% and his PO_2 is 500 mm Hg - calculate the total O_2 content. To the 20 vol% add 0.003 x 500 = 1.5 vol%.
Hgb = 1.36 x Hgb x % Sat = 20 vol%
dis. O_2 = .003 x 500 mmHg = 1.5 vol%
Total O_2= 21.5 vol%
The total O_2 content is significantly increased (Δ7.5%) above the Hgb O_2 calculation. This correction is only made when the patient is breathing O_2 during the oximetry measurements. Fick measurement of O_2 consumption cannot be made because you cannot measure O_2 consumption. It can be estimated from nomograms and BSA but only with considerable error.
See: Pepine, "The Adult Patient with Known or Suspected Congenital Heart Disease."

BOTH QUESTIONS BELOW REFER TO THIS DIAGRAM.

624. Identify the type of pullback pressure and the full scale pressure range for the pullback pressure labeled #1 in the diagram.
  a. LV - AO x 200
  b. LV - $AO_{asc.}$ - $AO_{desc.}$ x 200
  c. PA - RV x 50
  d. PA - RV_{out} - RV_{in} x 50

625. This diagram shows pullback pressure recordings. What congenital defect is diagnosed by the pullback labeled #3.
  a. Coarctation of AO (mild)
  b. Coarctation of AO (severe)
  c. Pulmonic stenosis
  d. Infundibular stenosis
  e. Aortic stenosis

BOTH ANSWERS ARE LISTED BELOW.
624. ANSWER #1 = c. PA-RV x50. By the straight up and down shape of the pressures you should be able to identify ventricular pressure tracings. Likewise the triangular waves with a dicrotic notch are all great vessel pressures. **CORRECTLY MATCHED ANSWERS ARE:**
  1. PA - RV x50
  2. PA - RV_{out} - RV_{in} x50
  3. LV-AO x200
  4. LV-AO_{asc}-AO_{desc} x200
  5. LV - AO_{asc}-AO_{desc} x200

Depending on the systolic pressure level most right heart pressures are recorded on X50, since PA and RV pressure seldom exceeds 35 mmHg. Most left heart pullbacks are recorded on X200, with the top of the paper being 200 mmHg. This keeps systole on the recorder paper.
See: Kern, chapter on "Hemodynamics."
Keywords: ID pullback tracings

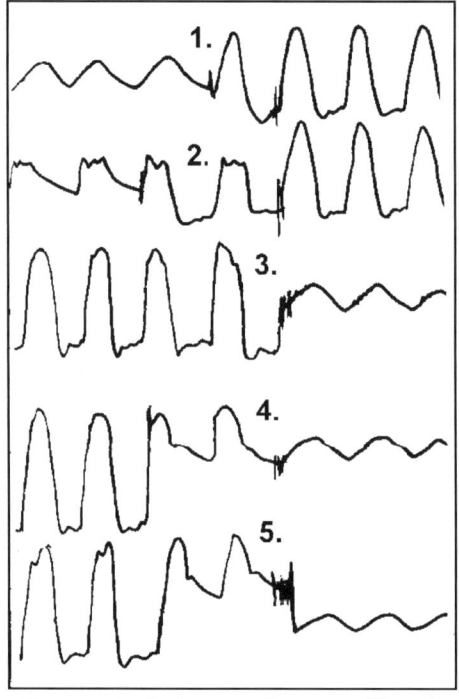
Congenital obstruction - pullback

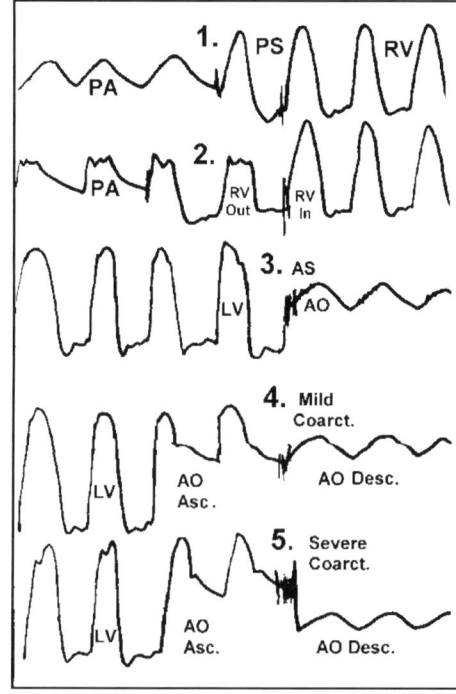
Pullbacks in congenital obstruction

625. ANSWER #3 = e. Aortic Stenosis
1. **PULMONIC STENOSIS:** Pullback from PA to RV on x50. Systolic gradient across the pulmonic valve. Slow upstroke of PA pressure. Simultaneous pressures indicated on diagram at right.
2. **INFUNDIBULAR STENOSIS:** Pullback from PA-RV outflow-RV inflow on x40. It shows subvalvular (infundibular) stenosis. The RV outflow systolic peak appears "chopped off." This is a "dynamic gradient" within the RV outflow tract (infundibulum) similar to IHSS/HOCM on the left side.
3. **AORTIC STENOSIS:** Pullback from LV to AO on x200. Systolic gradient is noted across the aortic valve. Simultaneous pressures indicated on diagram at right.
4. **COARCTATION OF AO (mild):** Pullback from LV-Ascending AO - Descending AO on x200. Systolic gradient within the aorta, across the coarctation. Aortic systolic pressures differ. Diastole is the same. In the early milder stages of coarctation only a systolic gradient is noted. The descending aortic tracing appears damped with a slow upstroke.
5. **COARCTATION of AO (severe):** Pullback from LV-Ascending AO - Descending AO on x200. A severe gradient noted between the two AO tracings both in systole and diastole. This indicates a severe coarctation with a tighter coarctation area.

See: Baim and Grossman, chapter on "Cardiac Catheterization in Infants and Children."

BOTH QUESTIONS BELOW REFER TO THIS DIAGRAM.

626. These diagrams represent the O_2 saturation samples taken at heart cath. Identify the type of shunt labeled #3 on the diagram.
a. L-R, VSD
b. L-R, PDA
c. L-R, ASD
d. R-L, VSD
e. R-L, PDA
f. R-L, ASD

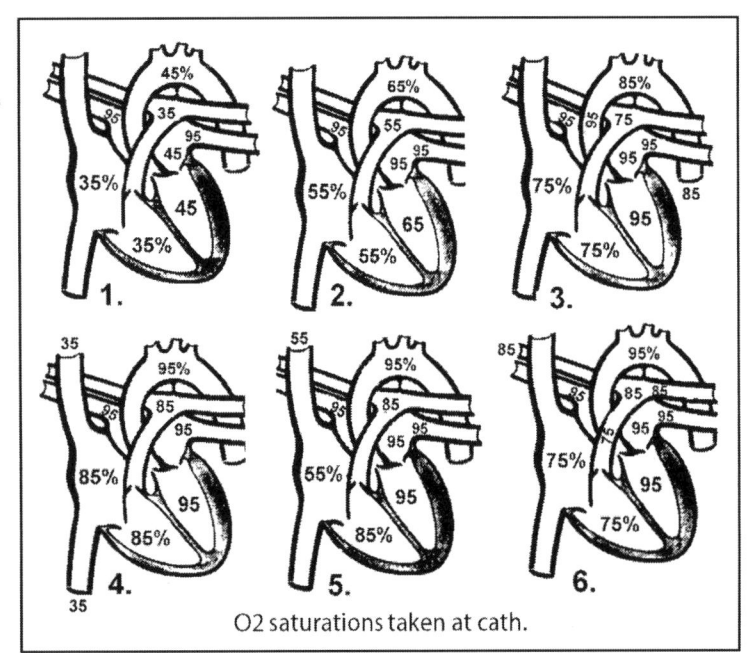

O2 saturations taken at cath.

627. Using the O_2 saturation data in the diagram labeled #4, calculate the ratio of pulmonary blood flow to systemic blood flow (Q_p/Q_s).
   a. 1:2
   b. 1:4
   c. 1:6
   d. 2:1
   e. 4:1
   f. 6:1

BOTH ANSWERS ARE LISTED TOGETHER BELOW.

626. ANSWER e. R-L, PDA = #3
CORRECTLY MATCHED ANSWERS ARE: (Know all these.)
1. **R-L, ASD** step-down in O_2 from 95% to 45% in LA
2. **R-L, VSD** step-down in O_2 from 95% to 65% in LV
3. **R-L, PDA** step-down is O_2 from 95% to 85% in AO. It is usually not this easy to calculate, because of streaming in the AO and the upper extremities receiving saturated blood and the descending receiving desaturated blood.
4. **L-R, ASD** step-up in O_2 from 35% in vena cavae to 85% in RA. Usually not this easy, because IVC sat. does not usually = SVC sat.
5. **L-R, VSD** step-up in O_2 from 55% to 85% in RV.
6. **L-R, PDA** step-up in O_2 from 75% to 85% in PA. Not usually this easy because RPA sat. does not usually equal LPA O_2 sat.
Normally the AO should be constant and fully saturated along its entire course.
   Note the drop in saturation from ascending AO (95%) to descending AO (85%) This is a significant drop in saturation from a R-L PDA shunt. **See:** Baim and Grossman, chapter on "Cardiac Catheterization in Infants and Children." & Braunwald, chapter on "Congenital Heart Disease." **Keywords:** ID direction and location of shunts, L-R, VSD

627. ANSWER f. Diagram #4 is a 6:1 ASD shunt from L-R into the RA. This means that the RV pumps six times as much as the LV.

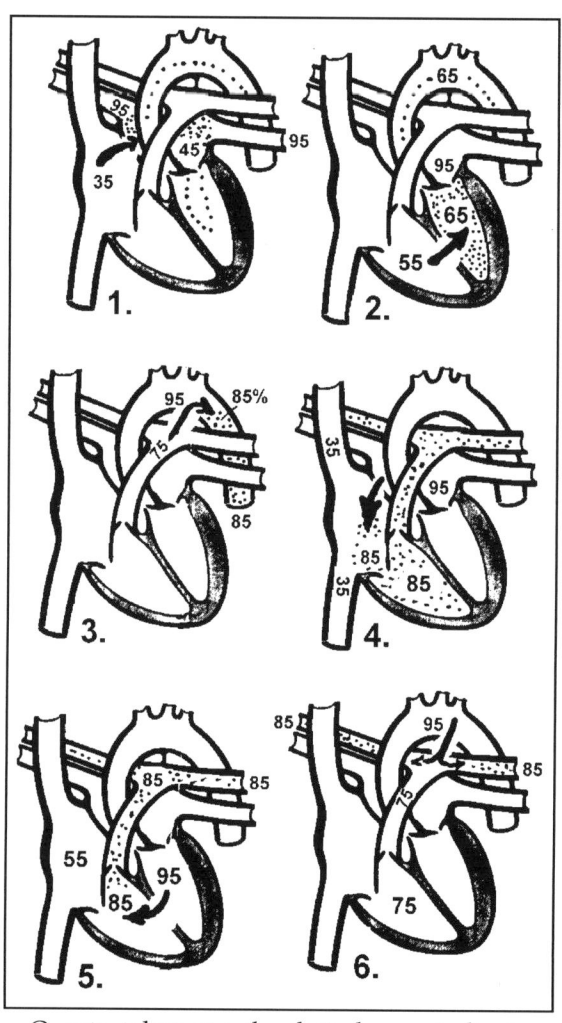

O_2 sats. taken at cath - dotted areas indicate contaminated blood, after the shunt dumps in.

You can tell it is a HUGE shunt because the RA saturation rises from 35% to 85%.

CORRECTLY MATCHED ANSWERS ARE:
1. 1:6 = (45-35)/(95-35) Huge R-L Shunt
2. 1:4 = (65-55)/(95-55) Large R-L
3. 1:2 = (85-75)/95-75) Small R-L
4. 6:1 = (95-35)/(95-85) HUGE L-R Shunt
5. 4:1 = (95-55) /(95-85) Large L-R
6. 2:1 = (95-75)/(95-85) Small L-R

Note how the side of the heart from which the shunt originates always has a constant O_2 saturation, e.g. in all R-L shunts the right heart O_2 sat is essentially the same in RA, RV, & PA. While in all L-R shunts the O_2 sat. is the same in LA, LV, and AO. Also, note that pulmonary venous saturation is 95% regardless of the direction of shunt. This is true if the lungs are oxygenating well. (Baim and Grossman says you can usually estimate PV at 98% sat. even if you can't get in to sample it.)

$$\frac{Q_p}{Q_s} = \frac{(SA - SV)}{(PV - PA)} = \frac{\text{Systemic AV dif.}}{\text{Pulmonary AV dif.}} = \frac{(AO - SVC)}{(PV - PA)}$$

SA = Systemic Arterial (usual distal AO)
SV = Systemic Venous (usually SVC or RA average whichever is lower)
PV = Pulmonary Venous (usually PV average or LA whichever is higher)
PA = Pulmonary Arterial (usually PA or distal PA)

This formula which is easily derived from the Fick formulae, is the ratio of the reciprocal A-V differences of the two systems. Note how Q_p (**pulmonary**) is in numerator on the left. But, Q_p (pulmonary) A-V difference is in the denominator on the right side of equation. This is because of the inverse relation between A-V difference and CO. It looks weird, Q_p looks opposite to pulmonary A-V difference. **But that is the way this formula is always set up.**

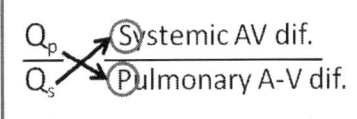

In the 4th diagram: SA = AO = 95% sat.
- SV = SVC= 35%
- PV = LA = 95%
- PA = PA = 85%

Substituting into the Q_p/Q_s formula we get: Q_p/Q_s = (95-35)/(95-85) = 60/10 = 6/1 = 6:1 shunt. That is a BIG ONE. We used SVC or the "Flamm" average, instead of RA for systemic venous because in all shunt calculations we need the O_2 levels just before the shunt dumps in. The RA already has the contaminating red blood in it. So in L-R VSD's we will use an average RA. In L-R PDA's use RV for best mixed systemic venous.

This calculation is tricky when shunts enter atrial or great vessel chambers. This occurs in ASDs and PDAs. Always select the sample which is closest to the capillary system named.

1. **In #1** ask yourself, which sample best represents the pulmonary venous O_2 sat : - 45% or 95%? Well, the 95% PV is closer to the lung capillary system, so 95% is the pulmonary venous O_2 sat. before the shunt dumps in. Thus: Q_p/Q_s = (45-35)/(95-35) = 10/60 = 1:6 . This means six times as much blood goes through the systemic capillary

bed as through the pulmonary system.
2. **In #2** a simple R-L VSD shows a step-down in the LV from 95% to 65%. Since there is no red blood contaminating the right side of the heart, both PA and SV are the same at 55%.
3. **In #3** which sat. represents the best mixed systemic arterial sample 95% or 85%? Since we always select the sample closest to its capillary system, here the AO feeds the systemic capillaries, so the distal AO 85% best represents the systemic arterial O_2 sat.
4. **In #4** since the IVC and SVC are closest to the systemic capillary bed, they best represent the systemic venous blood draining that system. So SV=35%.
5. **In #5**, is a straight-forward Q_p/Q_s = (95-55)/ (95-85) = 4:1 L-R shunt.
6. **In # 6** which sat. best represent PA blood 95% or 85%? The 85% feeds the pulmonary capillary bed, so it best represent pulmonary arterial blood.
Q_p/Q_s= (95-75)/(95-85) = 20/10 = 2:1 shunt.

Note the dotted blood in the diagram represents the mixed arterial and venous blood downstream from the shunt. Also, these shunts are exaggerated and simplified for teaching purposes. **See:** Braunwald, chapter on "Congenital Heart Disease." **Keywords:** Calculate Q_p/Q_s

628. What is a normal cardiac output of a 7 lb. (3 Kg) baby at birth?
a. 60-90 ml/min
b. 100-150 ml/min
c. 200-400 ml/min
d. 600-1000 ml/min

ANSWER d. 600-1000 ml/min. Newborns have extremely high metabolic rates, cardiac index, and heart rates. Normal CO for a newborn is 200 ml/min/Kg (compared to 100 ml/min/Kg for adolescents). So, for a 3-kg baby: 3 x 200 = a CO of 600 ml/min. This is about 1/10 of a normal adult CO of 6.0 L/min.

Hemodynamic values for adults and children are normally referenced to BSA instead of Kg. weight. Normal ADULT and TEENAGER values are:
- V_{O2} index = 125-130 ml O_2/min/ M^2
- CI = 3.5 L/min/M^2

Average infant CI = 4.5 L/min/M^2.
A newborn baby may have a BSA of 0.2 M^2. So: 4.5 x 0.2 = 0.9 L/min = 900 ml/min.

NORMAL RESTING VALUES IN CHILDREN - from Daily				
AGE	CO (L/min)	Ht. Rate	Resp. Rt.	BP
Newborn	0.6-1.0	±145	----	±80/50
Infant (6 mo)	1.0-1.3	±120	30-60	±90/55
Toddler (2 yr)	1.5-2.0	±115	24-40	±100/60
School age (7)	3.0-3.5	±90	18-30	±105/65
Adolescent (15)	±6.0	±70	(± approximates)	±120/70

Note how HR and respiratory rate decrease with age and CO and BP increase with age. **See:** Daily, chapter on "Hemodynamic Monitoring of Children." **Keywords:** Newborn CO = 0.6-1.0 L/min

629. As infants grow the normal PA pressure tends to _____ and the systemic BP tends to _____.
   a. Increase, Increase
   b. Increase, Decrease
   c. Decrease, Decrease
   d. Decrease, Increase

ANSWER d. Decrease, Increase. PA pressure tends to decrease from 90/55 at birth to 25/10 mmHg during teenage, while the systemic BP rises from 85/50 at birth to 120/70 mm Hg during teenage.

Remember that at birth the RV = LV pressure and the RV = LV thickness. During the first few years of life the PA pressure continues to drop and the RV continues to thin. With the first breath the pulmonary resistance drops and the ostium

CARDIOVASCULAR PRESSURES IN CHILDREN			
Age	PVR (u.M^2)	PA(mmHg)	AO(mmHg)
Preemie	8-10	±90/55	±85/50
Neonate	1-3	±50/25	±96/60
Teenage	1-3	±25/10	±120/70

Pulmonary pressures drop and systemic rise with age.

secundum closes. Within 3 days the PDA closes. This separates the right and left heart so that thereafter each side develops to meet its individual needs. The PA resistance is low so it decreases in pressure, while the AO must drive into the high resistant systemic circuit and builds up in pressure.
See: Daily, chapter on "Hemodynamic Monitoring of Children." **Keywords:** As infants grow PA decreases AO increases

5A. Acyanotic Congenital Lesions - General

630. A child with a pulmonary blood flow (PBF) of 3 L/min and a L-R VSD shunt of 1 L/min will have a systemic blood flow (SBF) of ____ L/min.
   a. 2 L/min
   b. 4 L/min
   c. 5 L/min
   d. 6 L/min

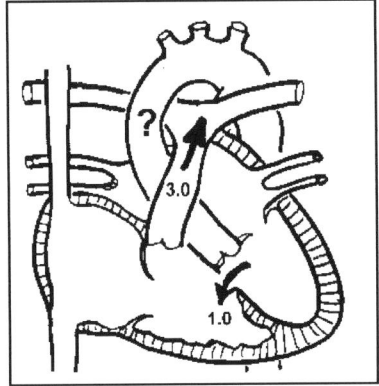

L-R VSD blood flows

ANSWER a. Q_s=2 L/min. Q_p=3 L/min., L-R shunt=1 L/min. The L-R shunt adds to the blood the RV must pump and subtracts from the blood going out the aorta. 3 L/min comes back into the LA, 1 leaks out of the LV into the RV, making aortic flow 2 L/min.
Formulas are:

    L-R shunt flow = PBF - SBF = Q_p - Q_s.

Substituting 3 for PBF and 1 for L-R shunt and then solving gives:

    SBF = PBF - (L-R shunt)
    SBF = 3 - 1 = 2 L/min

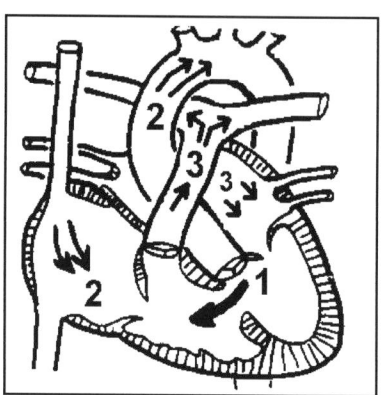
L-R VSD blood flows

Remember, that in common L-R shunts Q_p>Q_s, making the Q_p/Q_s ratio >1. Since this example is a common L-R shunt, Q_p must be greater than Q_s. (If the shunt flow comes out negative then it is a reversed or R-L shunt.)
See: Baim and Grossman, chapter on "Shunt Detection and Measurement." **Keywords**: L-R shunt flow = PBF - SBF.

631. **Many L-R shunts are associated with pulmonary flow murmurs and mild gradients across the pulmonic valve. This gradient is due to:**
  a. **Shunt induced turbulence in RV**
  b. **Increased pulmonary blood flow**
  c. **Associated infundibular stenosis**
  d. **Associated pulmonary stenosis**

ANSWER b. Increased pulmonary blood flow. L-R shunts dramatically increases pulmonary blood flow. This increased flow can cause a gradient and murmur across a normal valve. This is termed a "flow or physiologic murmur." It is normal for the increased flow. These valves do not need repair. The gradient/murmur will disappear once the shunt is corrected and normal flow resumes. Several examples are given in the last section of this chapter.
See: Braunwald, chapter on "Physical Exam."
Keywords: L-R shunts cause flow murmur / gradient due to increased flow

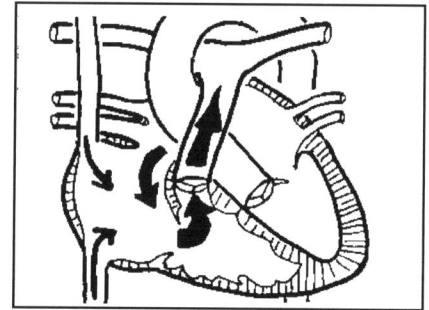
L-R shunt flow murmur

632. Identify the abnormal anatomy shown in the pediatric acyanotic defect labeled #4 in the diagram.
   a. Sinus of Valsalva AV fistula
   b. ASD
   c. VSD
   d. PDA

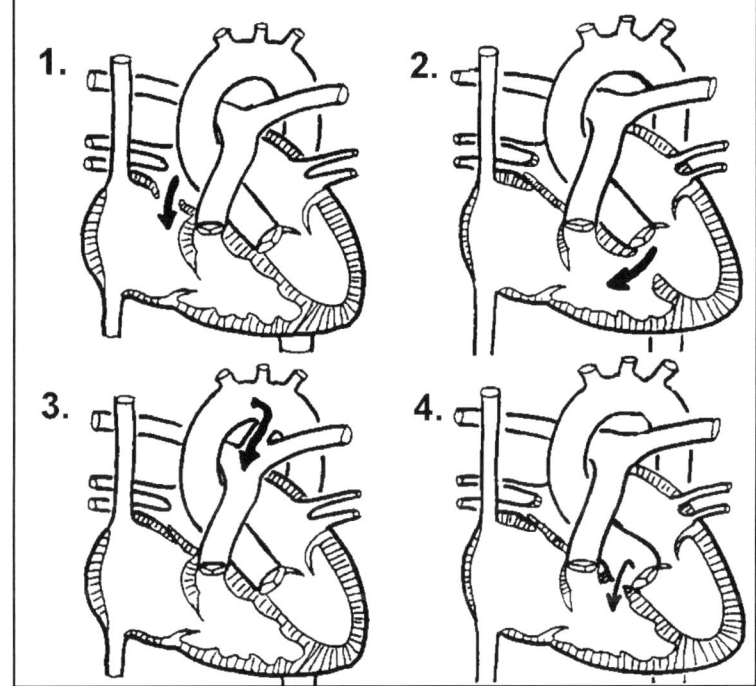

Acyanotic congenital defects

ANSWER a. Sinus of Valsalva AV fistula. These are all L-R shunts. Most shunts go from the high pressure left heart into the low pressure right heart. They are termed "acyanotic" because these children are "pink." This is because with L-R shunts red blood dumps into the blue blood. Central cyanosis only occurs with R-L shunts or lung problems.
CORRECTLY MATCHED ANSWERS ARE:
   1. ASD: L-R shunt through atrial septum (LA-RA)
   2. VSD: L-R shunt through ventricular septum (LV-RV)
   3. PDA: L-R shunt through patent ductus arteriosus (AO-PA)
   4. SINUS OF VALSALVA AV FISTULA: L-R shunt through aortic root into RV or RA. These aneurysms may be imaged during coronary arteriography. They may not rupture until late in life. Then signs of L-R shunt may develop.
See: Braunwald, chapter on "Congenital Heart Disease in Infants and Children."
Keywords: R-L shunts

633. A VSD develops in your adult STEMI patient. This shunt will normally be _____ and the patient will be _____.
   a. L-R, Cyanotic
   b. L-R, Acyanotic
   c. R-L, Cyanotic
   d. R-L, Acyanotic

ANSWER b. L-R, Acyanotic or pink, unless there are related CHF or lung problems. If all cardiac pressures are close to normal, any intracardiac shunts will shunt from left to right. Here the LV pressure is normally much higher than the RV pressure, so the red LV blood will shunt into the blue RV blood. This does not cause cyanosis. The patient will be pink - acyanotic. **See**: Braunwald, chapter on "Congenital Heart Disease in Infants and Children."
Keywords: R-L shunts

634. Chest radiographs with inferior rib margin notching are associated with:
a. Collateral circulation around coarctation of aorta
b. Collateral circulation around thoracic outlet syndrome
c. Mammary artery - Vineberg procedure
d. Mammary artery - coronary bypass surgery

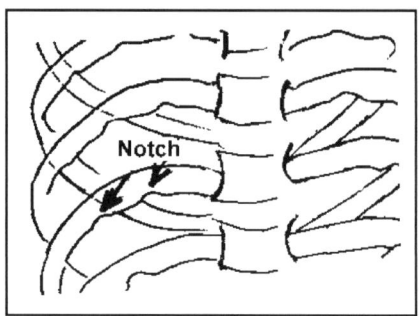
Chest film - rib notching

ANSWER a. Collateral circulation of coarctation of aorta. Coarctation is associated with these notches. The collateral vertebral circulation bypasses the coarctation and becomes so large that these vessels erode the ribs beneath which they pass. **See**: Baim and Grossman, chapter on "Profiles in Congenital Heart Disease." **Keywords**: Rib notching - Coarctation AO

635. From the saturation and pressure samples shown in the diagram, diagnose the direction and location of the shunt (orifice not shown).
a. R-L ASD
b. R-L VSD
c. R-L PDA
d. L-R VSD
e. L-R PDA

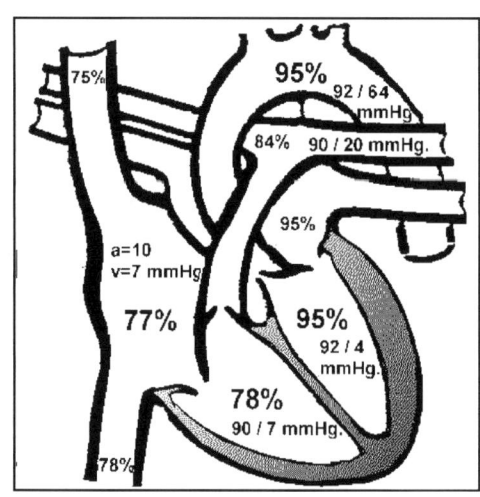
O_2 and pressure data

ANSWER e. L-R PDA. A step-up in saturation of 7% occurs from RV to PA indicating a L-R shunt. No step-down occurs in the left heart. The PDA is a shunt between AO and PA. **See**: Baim and Grossman, chapter on "Shunt detection..."
Keywords: Diagnose PDA from O_2 sat step up.

5B. Acyanotic Lesions - Atrial Septal Defect (ASD)

636. A teenage boy has a small septum secundum defect. His RA receives blood from four different sources. Oximetry samples taken from the part of his RA shown at #3 (IVC) would be expected to be around ± ____ % O_2 sat.
a. 45% O_2 saturation
b. 70% O_2 saturation
c. 80% O_2 saturation
d. 96% O_2 saturation

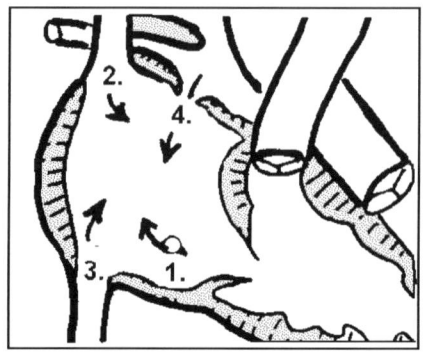
RA blood sampling

ANSWER c. 80% IVC blood is usually several % higher than SVC blood because the kidneys use no O_2 and the brain uses lots. This makes renal vein blood higher and more variable in O_2. Also, the IVC sample mixes with the coronary sinus sample in low RA so that the mixture of the two usually ends up near SVC levels. Pepine gives normal values for SVC as a mean of 78% with a range of 65-87% O_2 sat.

CORRECTLY MATCHED ANSWERS ARE:
1. **Coronary sinus** (low RA) = ± 45% O_2 SATURATION
2. **SVC** = ± 70 O_2 SATURATION
3. **IVC** = ± 80% O_2 SATURATION
4. **LA (ASD shunt)** = ± 95% O_2 SATURATION

Given the disparate saturations coming into the RA it is difficult to get a well mixed sample for shunt calculations. This disparity of O_2 saturations found in the RA makes L-R ASD calculation less accurate than VSD calculations. For more accuracy, the "Flamm" equation may be used to average the two vena cava samples. In ASDs many pediatric cardiologists use SVC as the most representative of the average systemic venous sample. For similar reasons neither are PDA shunt calculations very accurate.

See: Pepine, chapter on "The Adult Patient with Known or Suspected Congenital Heart Disease." **Keywords:** Normal O_2 sats. in IVC = 78%, higher than SVC

637. Depending on what part of the RA or vena cavae is sampled the O_2 saturation may vary considerably. In an adult with an ASD the best mixed systemic venous sample average (Flamm equation) is:
a. The average of 4 RA samples
b. $\dfrac{SVC + IVC}{2}$
c. $\dfrac{(3 \times SVC) + IVC}{4}$
d. $\dfrac{SVC + (2 \times IVC)}{3}$

ANSWER c. {(3x SVC) + IVC}/4. This is the "Flamm" equation. It must be used in the Fick equation for determination of ASD shunt flow. It is an average of SVC and IVC which more heavily weighs the SVC blood sample. This is because the SVC sample is most representative of mixed venous blood. The IVC is higher than SVC O_2 saturation because of the oxygenated renal vein blood. RA blood varies by up to 10% because of streaming from SVC, IVC, coronary sinus and possible ASD shunt blood.

In children the SVC saturation is often used instead of the Flamm equation to estimate systemic venous O_2 sat. It is usually only a few % away from the Flamm average. An ASD is diagnosed with any significant SVC-RA step-up. A significant step-up exceeds ≥5-8% of O_2 saturation on averages of multiple SVC-RA samples.

See: Baim and Grossman, chapter on "Cardiac Catheterization in Infants and Children" & Pepine, chapter on "The Adult Patient with Congenital Disease." **Keywords:** Flamm equation mixed systemic venous O_2 sat. in ASD

638. Depending on where the sample is taken in the RA may show considerable variability within RA O_2 saturations. How large must a L-R ASD be to be detected with a diagnostic O_2 saturation run?
  a. $Q_p/Q_s \geq 0.25\text{-}0.55$
  b. $Q_p/Q_s \geq 0.6\text{-}0.9$
  c. $Q_p/Q_s \geq 1.3\text{-}1.5$
  d. $Q_p/Q_s \geq 1.5\text{-}1.9$

ANSWER d. $Q_p/Q_s \geq 1.5\text{-}1.9$. That's almost a 2:1 shunt. L-R ASD shunts must be quite large to detect them. This is because of the considerable variability in vena caval and RA blood saturation. The "streaming" or black coronary sinus, steady SVC, lower IVC and red LA blood makes for poor blood mixing. SVC is "steady" and usually closest to the systemic venous mixed average O_2. Shunt size must be at least 2:1 before surgery is considered.

Smaller VSD sizes with $Q_p/Q_s \geq 1.3\text{-}1.5$ can be diagnosed with confidence. This is because the LV blood samples are not as scattered. They have had more time and more turbulence to become mixed. PA of course is the BEST MIXED VENOUS blood.
See: Baim and Grossman, chapter on "Shunt Detection and Measurement" and Baim and Grossman, chapter on "Profiles in Congenital Heart Disease." **Keywords:** ASD, minimum shunt diagnosable is $Q_p/Q_s \geq 1.5\text{-}1.9$

639. A large O_2 saturation step-up in the RA can be due to which of the following? (Choose 5 from below.)
  a. Tricuspid Atresia
  b. VSD with Tricuspid Regurgitation
  c. Anomalous Venous Return
  d. Endocardial Cushion Defect
  e. Sinus of Valsalva - AV Fistula
  f. ASD

ANSWERS: b, c, d, e, & f. Tricuspid Atresia is the absence of a tricuspid valve requiring a R-L ASD and a L-R VSD.
CORRECTLY MATCHED ANSWERS ARE:
1. **TRICUSPID ATRESIA:** Here the venous blood is routed R-L through an ASD, then L-R through a VSD into the lungs. The other diagrams all show simple L-R shunts. This heart has 2 shunts going in different directions.
2. **VSD WITH TRICUSPID REGURGITATION:**

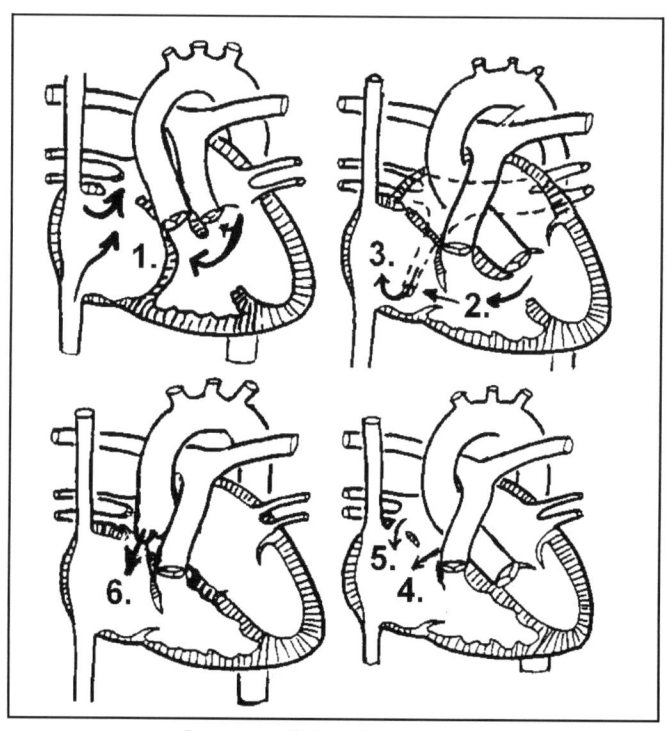

Causes of RA O_2 step-up

Arterialized blood PASSES the VSD into the RV, then backward through the leaking tricuspid valve into the RA.
3. **ANOMALOUS VENOUS RETURN:** Arterialized blood enters the RA through misplaced pulmonary veins. In this diagram the pulmonary veins join behind the LA. This empties into the coronary sinus and RA.
4. **ENDOCARDIAL CUSHION DEFECT**: Septum primum ASD or absent atrial and ventricular septum.
5. **ASD:** Usually L-R shunt because LA pressure is higher.
6. **SINUS OF VALSALVA AV FISTULA**: L-R shunt through aortic root into RA (or RV). These aneurysms may be found at coronary arteriography. They may not rupture until late in life. Then signs of L-R shunt may develop.

See: Baim and Grossman, chapter on "Profiles in Congenital Heart Disease." **Keywords:** Four causes of RA O_2 step-up

640. Most ostium secundum ASDs may be closed via catheter with which 2 of the following devices shown?
   a. Single Clamshell Septal Umbrella
   b. Cardioform Occluder
   c. Single Embolization Coil
   d. Dumbbell Embolization Coil
   e. Amplatzer device

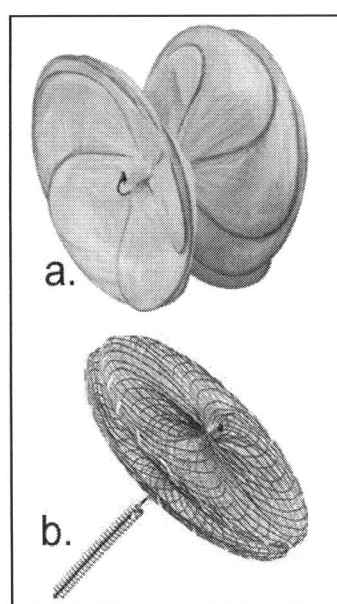

ANSWERS: b & e. Cardioform occluder & Amplatzer device. These are the currently approved ASD occlusion devices. Both devices spring into disc shapes determined by nitinol wires. Each disc supports cloth to encourage tissue ingrowth.

Topol says, "In the United States, two devices are approved for use by the FDA: (1) The Amplatzer Septal Occluder (AGA Medical, Golden Valley MN) and (2) the Helex Septal Occluder (W. L. Gore and Associates, Flagstaff, AZ). [replaced by the Gore Cardioform occluder] While different in design, the principles of function, deployment, and follow-up are similar for the two devices. After deployment, both devices are designed to have two disks connected by a central core or waist. One disk is positioned on the left atrial side of the ASD, with the core or waist straddling the defect, and the other is opposed to the atrial septum from the right atrial side of the defect. The devices have intrinsic recoil that pulls both disks together, holding the devices securely in place on the atrial septum." See: Topol, chapter on "Transcatheter Therapies for Congenital Heart Disease"

641. This diagram shows transcatheter implementation of an occluder device in a congenital defect. From the location of the device, what condition is being treated?
a. PDA
b. Tetralogy of Fallot
c. Pulmonary valve dilation
d. Coronary AV fistula

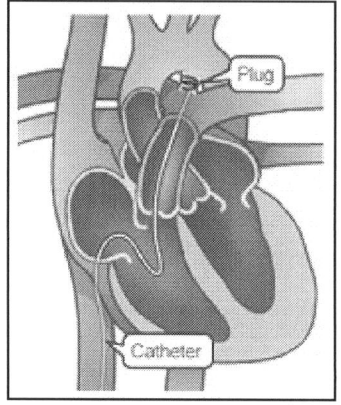

What condition??
After www.aboutkidshealth.ca

ANSWER a. PDA (Patent Ductus Arteriosus). In the picture a long sheath is advanced from the femoral vein into the pulmonary artery and ductus arteriosus. The device is then opened and set in the PDA closing it. The catheter is then detached and removed. Braunwald says: "Although strictly speaking still investigational, substantial experience exists with transcatheter closure of the patent ductus using various approaches, including coils, buttons, plugs, and umbrellas, with each occluder device introduced through a relatively large-diameter sheath from the femoral vein. The approach is especially feasible in patients who weigh more than 10 kg and who have neither a long tubular ductus nor a ductus with a long, narrow aortic end. In experienced hands, initial occlusion is successful in 85 to 90 percent of patients. . . ."

Currently approved devices for PDA closure include the Gianturco coil, Gianturco-Grifka vascular occlusion device and Amplatzer duct occluder.
See: Braunwald, chapter on "Congenital Heart Disease in Infancy and Childhood"

642. Identify the type of atrial septal defect (ASD) shown at #2 on the diagram.
a. Sinus venosus defect
b. Ductus venosus
c. Ostium secundum defect
d. Ostium primum defect

ANSWER c. Ostium secundum defect. **CORRECTLY MATCHED ANSWERS ARE:**
1. **SINUS VENOSUS DEFECT**: These ASDs are high on the atrial septum near the SVC entrance. Remember that the sinus venosus forms the most inferior part of the cardiac tube. When the tube folds these lower veins form the vena cava and pulmonary veins. So sinus venosus defects are often associated with anomalous pulmonary veins.
2. **OSTIUM SECUNDUM DEFECT**: These are located in the mid-atrial septum. They are often large and the most common type of ASD. They are often called "patent foramen ovale" because it is located where the normal fossa ovale occurs. But it is much larger. The foramen ovale normally closes at the first breath. When LA pressures exceed RA pressures, a flap in the LA covers the foramen ovale. It normally seals itself to the atrial septum.
3. **OSTIUM PRIMUM DEFECT**: These are the lowest ASDs. They occur just above the tricuspid

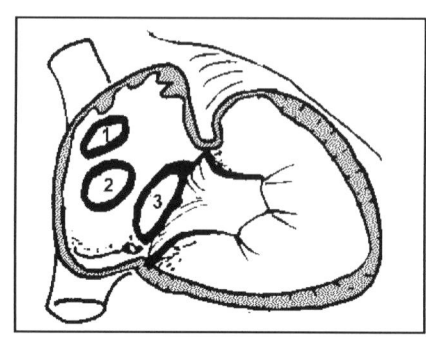

Location of ASDs

valve and are crescent shaped. They are also called "AV canal" or "atrio-ventricularis communis" ASDs. Since they are so low, they are often associated with endocardial cushion defects where part of the mitral valve is absent.

4. **DUCTUS VENOSUS**: (Not shown on the diagram) This is NOT an ASD. It is found in the abdomen. It carries the red blood from the umbilical vein through the liver and into the IVC.

See: Braunwald, chapter on, "Congenital Heart Disease in Infancy/ Childhood."
Keywords: Locations of ASD's

643. A child has a huge L-R ASD shunt seen on echocardiogram. A pulmonary flow murmur is heard. What type of pressures would you expect?

	RA	LA	RV	PA
a.	3	4	38/4	22/10 mmHg.
b.	5	10	30/5	30/10 mmHg.
c.	4	8	25/5	22/10 mmHg.
d.	9	3	30/6	30/10 mmHg.

ANSWER a. RA= 3, LA=4, RV=38/4, PA=22/10 mmHg. Grossman says, "The hallmark of a moderate or large ASD is the equalization of atrial pressures: previous workers have documented that mean atrial pressures are within 1 to 2 mm Hg in a good-sized ASD." Tamponade and other restrictive pathology may also show pressure equalization.

Note also, the systolic gradient between PA and RV. The peak RV and PA should normally be the same. The gradient here is not due to a tight pulmonic valve, but to the huge flow through it. This is termed a "flow" or "functional murmur" not due to pulmonic stenosis. These numbers are from Grossman's example.

See: Baim and Grossman, chapter on "Profiles in Congenital Heart Disease." **Keywords:** Pressures with L-R ASD

644. This oximetry data was taken at infant cath after Rashkind septostomy. What type of shunt has resulted?
a. L-R ASD & R-L PDA
b. R-L ASD & L-R PDA
c. Bi-directional ASD & PA-AO PDA
d. Bi-directional ASD & AO-PA PDA.

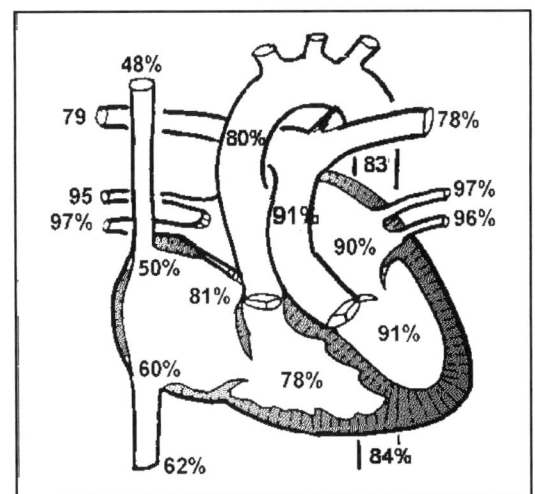

O₂ sats. taken at cath
(shunt orifice not shown)

ANSWER c. Bi-directional ASD & PA-AO PDA. Bidirectional shunts show both step-up in the right heart and step-down in the left heart. The RA shows a large 30% step-up from 50% to 80%. This indicates a large L-R ASD. The LA shows a PV average of 96% which drops to 90% in the LA. This is a 6% step-down, indicating a small R-L ASD. Note both R-L and L-R ASD's (bidirectional). This occurs when pressures alternate across the shunt.

There is also a slight step up in the descending AO from a small PA-AO PDA. It's inaccurate to say it is a R-L PDA because the PA is the left sided great vessel.

In bidirectional shunts, simple calculation of Q_p/Q_s is misleading and low because Q_p/Q_s only measures the net or average flow. E.g., if the amount of R-L shunt = the amount of L-R shunt the Q_p/Q_s would be 1.0. Since 1.0 is normal, this calculation is clearly misleading. The long Armstrong or Q_{eff} formula must be used for calculation of bidirectional shunts.

Infants with compete Transposition of the Great Vessels (TGV) need a large ASD to mix oxygenated blood. Without a large bidirectional shunt TGV patients often die of hypoxemia. The Rashkind balloon septostomy creates this shunt and may be lifesaving.
See: Baim and Grossman, chapter on "Shunt Detection and Measurement." **Keywords**: Bi-directional ASD

5C. Acyanotic Lesions - Ventricular Septal Defect (VSD)

645. What does this transseptal flood ventriculogram show?
  a. Muscular VSD with L-R shunt
  b. Muscular VSD with R-L shunt
  c. Membranous VSD with L-R shunt
  d. Membranous VSD with R-L shunt

ANSWER c. Membranous VSD with L-R shunt. Note the transseptal catheter injecting in the LV. Contrast is seen in the RV shunting across a high VSD in the membranous septum just beneath the aortic valve. Muscular VSDs are lower in the IV septum.
See: Braunwald, chapter on "Congenital Heart Disease."

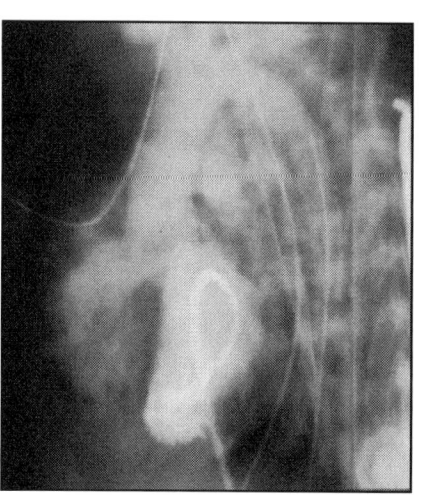
LAO flood ventriculogram

646. Identify the location of the VSD labeled #4 on the diagram.
  a. Muscular - anterior VSD
  b. Muscular - posterior VSD
  c. Membranous - inferior VSD
  d. Membranous - infracristal VSD
  e. Membranous - supracristal VSD

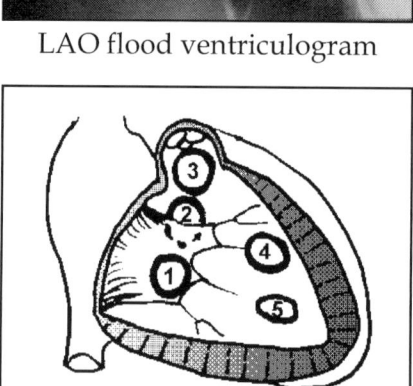
Location of VSDs

ANSWER a. Muscular - anterior VSD.
CORRECTLY MATCHED ANSWERS ARE:
1. **MEMBRANOUS - inferior VSD**: Beneath the septal tricuspid leaflet in the membranous IV septum.
2. **MEMBRANOUS - infracristal VSD**: Beneath aortic valve at the right margin.
3. **MEMBRANOUS - supracristal VSD**: Since it is just above the crista terminalis junction of the RV and PA. These are also called "subpulmonary" or "outlet" VSDs.
4. **MUSCULAR - anterior VSD**: Through the thick anterior aspect of the interventricular

septum. There may be multiple small fenestrations which close with time (it's like Swiss cheese.)
5. **MUSCULAR - posterior VSD:** Through the thick inferior-posterior aspect of the interventricular septum. There may be multiple (Swiss cheese) small fenestrations which close with time. **See**: Braunwald, chapter on "Congenital Heart Disease."
Keywords: VSD locations, membranous supracristal

647. A teenage girl has a large VSD with R-L shunt, pulmonary hypertension and elevated pulmonary vascular resistance. What invasive procedure should be done at heart cath to evaluate whether her hypertension will decrease significantly following corrective surgery?
a. Renal arteriography to evaluate for reno-vascular hypertension
b. Administer NO and measure change in PVR.
c. Measure change in PA pressure after Rashkind septostomy.
d. Measure change in cardiac output with Isuprel drip.

ANSWER b. Administer NO and measure change in PVR. If PVR can be reduced with NO or 100% O_2 for 10-30 minutes, then corrective surgery is likely to reduce the PA pressures and pulmonary resistance. But, if the pulmonary resistance remains fixed, she is NOT a candidate for corrective surgery. In fact, corrective surgery may make her worse. It may act as a kind of pressure release valve that protects from excessive hypertension. A chronic pulmonary hypertensive patient may have been hit with so much PA pressure - for so long, that his pulmonary arterioles will not relax. This increased pulmonary resistance occurs even though the shunt is closed and normal flow resumes. These people are termed "pulmonary vascular hyper-reactors". Another pulmonary vasodilatory drug is tolazoline, which should relax normal pulmonary arterioles in a manner similar to inhaled nitric oxide.
 Therefore, all congenital disease should be carefully followed, with an eye toward pulmonary resistance changes. It takes time for this hypertension to become irreversible, so most patients are operated at a young age. Corrective surgery on infants is becoming more successful. In future years most infants will be operated early to avoid waiting too long, as in this example.
See: Baim and Grossman, chapter on "Cardiac Catheterization in Infants and Children" & Braunwald **Keywords:** Fixed PVR ? => test with O_2 or tolazoline

648. You are assisting with a heart cath on a man with a chronic R-L VSD with pulmonary hypertension (PA = 65/30/42). Even while breathing 100% O_2 or nitric oxide his PA pressures remains high at 60/28/40 mmHg. Neither do vasodilators reduce his PA pressure. This indicates that:
a. Corrective surgery would probably NOT benefit him
b. Corrective surgery would probably benefit him
c. Palliative surgery (PA band) may be considered
d. Interventional angioplasty may be considered

ANSWER a. Corrective surgery would probably NOT benefit him. This is the reason we test for pulmonary vascular resistance reactivity as in the previous question. Since PVR =

(PA-LA)/CO the resistance does not appear to have dropped significantly. Accurate calculations for PVR should be made. But, since it is not likely the CO or LA pressures changed dramatically, the PVR is proportional to PA mean pressure. (PVR ∝ mean PA). This constant PVR is an indication that he is not a good candidate for VSD closure surgery, because his PVR will not adapt to a lower flow rate. The resistance becomes fixed and won't drop.

PA banding surgery is done to protect the lungs against this high pressure. Permanent damage has been done to our patient's lungs. There is nothing here to angioplasty.

See: Braunwald, chapter on "Congenital Heart Disease." **Keywords:** O_2 reversibility of high PVR, surgery may now considered

5D. Acyanotic Lesions - Patent Ductus Arteriosus (PDA)

649. These diagrams show the cardiac silhouette as shown on PA fluoroscopy. With the catheter positioned as seen in PA film #4 the congenital defect most probably is:
a. VSD
b. Left SVC
c. PDA
d. Anomalous venous return

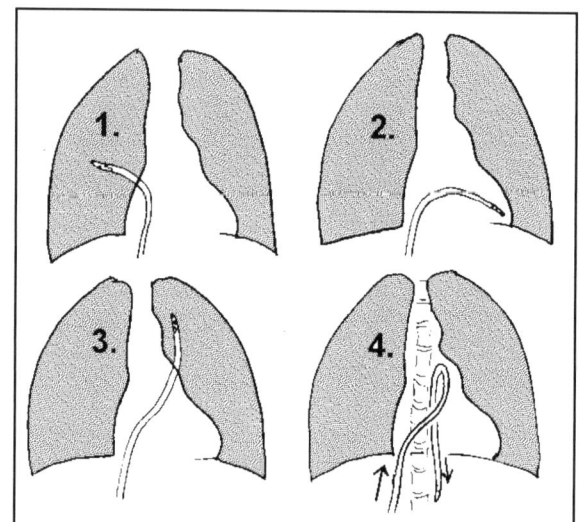

Diagnostic catheter positions

ANSWER c. PDA. Match all below.
CORRECTLY MATCHED ANSWERS ARE:
1. Anomalous venous return (TAPVR) with catheter entering right pulmonary vein.
2. VSD: Catheter enters femoral vein-IVC-RA-RV-LV apex
3. Left SVC: Catheter enters femoral vein-IVC-RA-CS-Left SVC (possible TAPVR)
4. PDA: Catheter enters femoral vein-IVC-RA-RV-PA-PDA-desc. AO

See: Grossman, chapter on "Percutaneous Approaches..." **Keywords:** Catheter positions, PDA, VSD, anomalous PV, anomalous left SVC

650. Identify the use of the PDA or PVR active drug labeled #2.
a. Maintain patency of PDA
b. Closes PDA
c. Pulmonary vasodilator
d. Pulmonary and systemic vasodilator

PDA & PVR ACTIVE DRUGS
1. Indamethacin
2. Prostaglandin E1
3. O_2 administration
4. Tolazoline

ANSWER a. Maintain patency of PDA.
CORRECTLY MATCHED ANSWERS ARE:
1. **INDAMETHACIN**: Closes PDA. It blocks the enzyme that keeps the PDA open (arachidonic acid), thus vasoconstricting the smooth muscle in the PDA.
2. **PROSTAGLANDIN E1**: Maintains patency of PDA. Prostaglandin E1 interferes with the normal vasoconstrictors. Dilating the PDA may be lifesaving in cases where its closure brings on cyanosis and CHF. For example in preductal coarctation of the AO the PDA may be the only way to bring blood to the descending AO. Remember the acronym "din" dilates, "cin" constricts the PDA. (Where din = prostoglanDIN and cin = indomethaCIN.)
3. O_2 **ADMINISTRATION**: Vasodilator. Reduces PVR, unless hypertension has irreversibly damaged the pulmonary arterioles. Nitrous oxide is another pure pulmonary vasodilator.
4. **TOLAZOLINE**: Pulmonary and systemic vasodilator. It reduces PVR and SVR. The drug is infused into the PA for 10 minutes. Its effect is similar to O_2 on the vaso-reactive pulmonary arterioles.

See: Baim and Grossman, chapter on "Cardiac Cath. in Infants and Children." **Keywords:** PDA active drugs = indomethacin

651. In the O_2 saturation diagram shown, where is most of the shunt blood going?
a. LPV
b. RPV
c. LPA
d. RPA

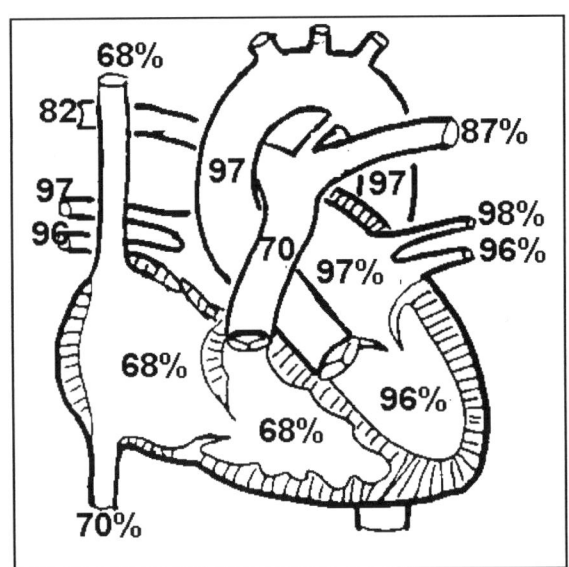

O_2 sat. & pressures

ANSWER c. LPA. This is a L-R PDA which empties into the main PA. Most of the arterial shunt blood empties into the LPA as indicated by the higher O_2 saturation there. This is common. Grossman says, "Because aortic blood crosses into the lungs without passing through a mixing chamber, there is considerable streaming in the PA: the cephalad portion of the MPA is often fully saturated, the left PA usually has a higher saturation than the right PA, and the 'mixed' pulmonary arterial saturation cannot be defined accurately." Therefore when calculating PDA shunt flows, Grossman recommends calculating one using RPA and one using LPA saturations, e.g., calculate PBF as if PA=82, AO=97 % and again as if PA=87, AO=97%. This gives a range with the true average somewhere between the two.
See: Baim and Grossman, chapter on "Profiles in Congenital Heart Disease." **Keywords:** PDA most often selectively shunts into LPA

6A. Cyanotic Lesions - General

652. Peripheral cyanosis is blue skin coloration due to:
a. Desaturated arterial blood
b. Desaturated venous blood
c. Peripheral vasodilation
d. Peripheral vasoconstriction

ANSWER d. Peripheral vasoconstriction. Cyanosis is blue coloration of the skin and mucus membranes brought on by low cardiac output, cold or when our skin becomes vasoconstricted for any reason. Remember how blue your kids' lips looked when they got out of the pool. When this vasoconstriction happens the tissue blood flow is reduced and it extracts more O2 from each ml of blood. This makes the AV difference wider and makes the venous blood a much darker color. It takes 3 gm% of reduced Hgb in the skin capillaries to be detected in Caucasians. Cyanosis is more difficult to diagnose with dark complexion. Any time decreased CO occurs peripheral vasoconstriction and peripheral cyanosis are likely - as in CHF and shock.
See: Braunwald, chapter on "Congenital Heart Disease." **Keywords:** Peripheral cyanosis

653. Cyanosis begins to show in the lips and mouth when arterial blood is desaturated by more than:
a. 10% O2 sat
b. 20% O2 sat
c. 3 gm% O2 content
d. 6 gm% O2 content

ANSWER c. 3 gm% O2 content. This is the serious type of cyanosis and is caused by arterial blood DESATURATION of more than 3 gm%. Remember, a normal Hgb is 15 gm%. Cyanosis is the ABSOLUTE quantity of desaturated Hgb present, NOT the O2 sat. alone. All of the below individuals have 3 gm% desaturated hemoglobin (or 4 vol%). They would all start to show signs of blue skin cyanosis. Note how the saturations vary markedly.

O2 Saturations with 3 gm% DESATURATED HEMOGLOBIN (**CYANOSIS**)

Hematocrit	Hgb.	O2 Cap.	O2 Cont.	O2 Sat.
Polycythemia (60% Hct.)	~± 20 gm.%	28 Vol.%	24 Vol.%	24/28=86%
Normal (45% Hct.)	~± 15 gm.%	21	17 Vol.%	17/21=80%
Anemic (30% Hct)	~± 10 gm.%	14	10 Vol.%	10/14=71%

Cyanosis is more apparent in polycythemic individuals. Since cyanosis becomes apparent when arterial blood has more than 3 gm% of reduced (black) hemoglobin, a normal person with a Hgb of 15 gm% will show cyanosis at saturations of 12/15 gm Hgb (or 17/21 vol.%) <80% O2 sat. For this reason anemic blood does not show the cyanosis until the O2 sat is much lower, e.g. 7/10 (or 10/14 vol.%)= <70% O2 sat. Polycythemic patients will show cyanosis at higher O2 saturations, e.g. 17/20 = 86% sat.

Central cyanosis is usually seen in a shunt patient when a R-L shunt exceeds 25% of the LV CO (Qp/Qs < 1/1.25). Dark skin and blue mucus membrane coloration is evident unless the patient is anemic. **See:** Braunwald, chapter on "Congenital Heart Disease."
Keywords: Central cyanosis → arterial desaturation

654. The fingers in the diagram show ____ which is associated with _____.
  a. Arachnodactyly, Central cyanosis
  b. Arachnodactyly, Peripheral cyanosis
  c. Clubbing, Peripheral cyanosis
  d. Clubbing, Central cyanosis

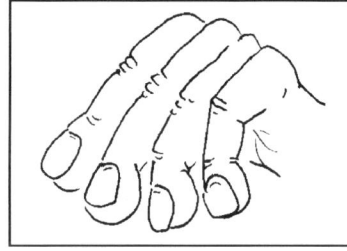
Bulbous fingertips

ANSWER d. Clubbing, central cyanosis. These fingers are dilated at the tips. The earliest forms of cyanosis show glossy fingernails and blue coloration at the root of the nail. As cyanosis progresses the angle the root makes with the finger is over 160 degrees and eventually becomes almost straight. This is associated with chronic hypoxemia from any cause.

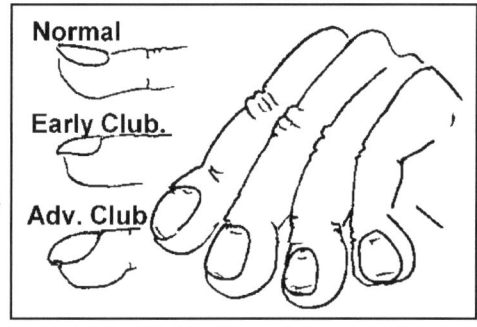
CLUBBING - and nail angle

Arachnodactyly are fingers which are extremely long compared to the torso. They are so long the thumb and little finger can completely encircle the wrist on the other hand. This is seen in Marfan Syndrome, a connective tissue disease associated with dilated AO root and AI. **See:** Braunwald, chapter on "Congenital Heart Disease."
Keywords: Clubbing = Cyanosis

655. In congenital heart disease patients clubbed fingers (as shown in the diagram above) are associated with a _____ shunt and a _____ pulmonary to systemic blood flow ratio (Qp/Qs).
  a. R-L shunt, High Qp/Qs
  b. R-L shunt, Low Qp/Qs
  c. L-R shunt, High Qp/Qs
  d. L-R shunt, Low Qp/Qs

ANSWER b. R-L shunt, Low Qp/Qs. Cyanosis lesions are R-L shunts with dark blood contaminating the red arterial blood. In R-L shunts the systemic blood flow (SBF is Qs) exceeds the pulmonary blood flow (PBF is Qp) by the amount of the shunt. Since Qs exceeds Qp the ratio Qp/Qs is less than one. This ratio can be easily calculated from the O2 saturation data taken during a diagnostic run during cardiac cath, e.g. a child's PBF = 2 L/min. SBF = 3 L/min. (R-L shunt is 1 L/min) Qp/Qs = PBF/SBF = 2/3. This is termed a 2 to 3 or 66% R-L shunt. **See:** Braunwald, chapter on "Congenital Heart Disease."

Keywords: clubbing → L-R shunt, low Qp/Qs

656. R-L shunts may be suspected if the blood O_2 levels show:
   a. $SaO_2 > 95\%$
   b. $SaO_2 < 95\%$
   c. $PvO_2 > 80$ mm Hg.
   d. $PvO_2 < 80$ mm Hg.

ANSWER b. $SaO_2 < 95\%$. R-L shunts will drop the O_2 saturation of arterial blood. You can't tell where the shunt is, or if the desaturation is due to lung disease or hypoventilation - which is usually the case. CHF with pulmonary edema is a common cause of ventilation, perfusion mismatch resulting in arterial hypoxemia/desaturation.

Access to the left side of the heart is necessary to detect the location of any R-L saturation step-down. But if you can't get in, this patient's lungs are normal, and the arterial blood is desaturated, look further for a possible R-L shunt. Perform an RV gram or make another attempt at left heart catheterization (perhaps transseptal).

SYMBOLS USED:
- S = Saturation
- a = Arterial
- SaO_2 = Sat'n. art. O_2
- PvO_2 = PO_2 of venous blood
- v = venous
- P = Partial pressure

Normal O_2 sat should exceed 95%. The PvO_2 is irrelevant (partial pressure of venous O_2 in mmHg). **See**: Baim and Grossman, chapter on "Shunt Detection and Measurement."
Keywords: Suspect R-L shunt if $SaO_2 < 95$ mmHg.

657. During heart catheterization, cyanotic cardiac shunts show a _____ in O_2 saturation on the _____ side of the heart.
   a. Step-up, Left
   b. Step-up, Right
   c. Step-down, Left
   d. Step-down, Right

ANSWER c. Step-down, Left. Cyanotic lesions shunt from right to left (R-L). The dark venous blood is shunted into the red arterial blood lowering its O_2 saturation. This causes the O_2 saturation to drop on the left side of the heart, often so severely that blue cyanosis is seen. Where the O_2 sat. drop occurs is the shunt entry point. The magnitude of the step-down determines the size of the shunt.

Some large shunts which have balanced pressures may show both R-L and L-R shunting. This is termed a "bidirectional shunt." These rare shunts show both saturation step-up on the right side and step-down on the left side.
See: Braunwald, chapter on "Congenital Heart Disease." **Keywords:** Cyanotic = sat. step-down on left side

658. Echocardiography suggests a VSD on a cyanotic child. Although breathing rapidly on nasal oxygen, the child's lips are dusky blue. During a diagnostic heart cath, mixed RA saturation was 70% and mixed arterial blood (AO) sat. was 80%. A diagnostic run through all cardiac chambers would most likely show an O2 saturation: (select only one below)
a. Step down from 97% to 70%, in LV
b. Step down from 97% to 80% in LV
c. Step down from 80% to 70% in RV
d. Step up from 70% to 80% in RV
e. Step up from 70% to 97% in RV
f. Step up from 80% to 97% in LV

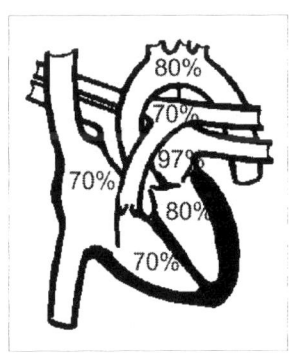

ANSWER: b. Step down from 97% to 80% in the LV. Since the child is cyanotic we know it is a right to left shunt. (All cyanotic shunts are right to left.) Echo tells us the shunt is between the ventricles - VSD. So there should be a drop in blood saturation in the LV. We must assume that the lungs are working correctly and LA saturation is around 97% or higher on O2. If you could get a catheter in the LA, you would use the actual measured O2 sat.

Here, the dark (blue) blood shunts across the ventricular septum from right to left diluting the bright red arteriolized blood. LV saturation drops from 97% to 80%. The larger the R-L shunt the lower the LV & AO sats will be.

It is helpful to write these sats on a heart diagram as shown here. This clearly shows the step down in saturation as blood moves into the LV. Pressures in the right ventricle must be higher than in the LV to cause such a R-L shunt. But, remember the right heart pressures are high at birth, and only go down over several months. With high right heart pressures and pulmonary hypertension a child may develop RVH. This happens in Tetralogy of Fallot with high pulmonary vascular resistance and large VSD.

Simple calculations are the ratio of pulmonary blood flow to systemic blood flow Qp/Qs = (80-70)/(97-70)= 10/27 = 0.37. This means the systemic blood flow (Qs) is much greater than the pulmonary blood flow (Qp), almost 3 times greater. Surgery or patch is indicated. Normal Qp/Qs= 1.
See: Braunwald, chapter on "Congenital Heart Disease"

659. The "Eisenmenger's complex" is characterized by increased pulmonary resistance and reversal of a:
a. L-R shunt into a cyanotic R-L shunt
b. L-R shunt into an acyanotic R-L shunt
c. R-L shunt into a cyanotic L-R shunt
d. R-L shunt into an acyanotic L-R shunt

ANSWER a. L-R shunt into a cyanotic R-L shunt. Eisenmenger has come to represent end stages of a shunt (especially a L-R VSD) in which the pulmonary arterioles have reacted to the high flow and pressure with fixed hypertrophy. When this resistance increases to the point where RV pressure exceeds LV pressure, the shunt will reverse and switch to a R-L shunt. Then cyanosis becomes evident. This diagram shows reversal of the 3 common L-R shunts into cyanotic R-L shunts and RV hypertrophy.

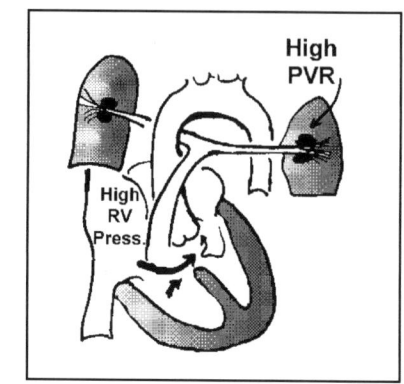
Eisenmenger's

When a high PVR becomes fixed and irreversible like this, it is too late for corrective surgery. The irreversible arteriolar vasoconstriction will not relax and pulmonary hypertension remains despite corrected anatomy. Consequently "Eisenmenger" often refers to the end stage of a congenital L-R shunt which has done permanent damage to the lungs. It is most important to catch these early and prevent Eisenmenger's condition from developing. That is why children with shunts are followed so closely. PA banding surgery may protect the lungs from hypertensive changes.
See: Braunwald, chapter on "Congenital Heart Disease."

660. **An interventional "RASHKIND PROCEDURE" may be performed on cyanotic infants to:**
   a. **Balloon dilate the stenotic pulmonary valve**
   b. **Balloon dilate the coarctation of the aorta**
   c. **Dilate shunts with an umbrella occluder**
   d. **Tear open the atrial septum with a balloon**

ANSWER d. Tear open the atrial septum with a Rashkind balloon catheter. The balloon septostomy procedure was invented by Dr. Rashkind in Philadelphia. A deflated balloon catheter is passed through the ASD or foramen ovale and then inflated with 50-50% contrast/saline mixture. Then it is jerked back hard enough to tear open the atrial septum around the foramen ovale. This provides communication between the two sides of the heart so oxygenated blood can enter the LA, LV and AO. It may make dramatic improvement in cyanotic infants. But this is a temporary palliative (non curative) measure to buy time for the cyanotic child and future corrective surgery. Remember "Rashkind Rips."

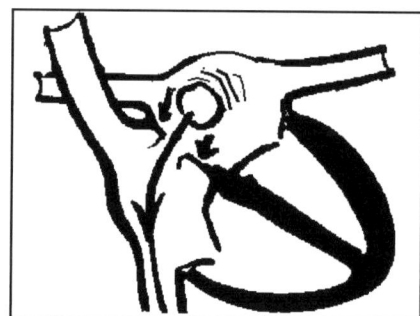
Rashkind Septostomy

See: Braunwald, chapter on "Congenital Heart Disease." **Keywords:** Rashkind balloon procedure → tears atrial septum

661. In the cyanotic neonate "PERSISTENT FETAL CIRCULATION" involves two shunts normal to the fetus. These shunts are a _____ patent foramen ovale and a _____ PDA:
a. L-R, L-R
b. L-R, L-R
c. R-L, R-L
d. R-L, L-R

ANSWER c. R-L Patent Foramen Ovale, R-L PDA.
In the premature infant or neonate these normal shunts do not always close right away. This is usually due to persistent high pulmonary resistance due to hypoxemia, a small PA, or a reduced number of pulmonary vessels. Here right sided pressures continue to exceed left sided pressures and the shunts remain as in uterine R-L.
Normally the foramen ovale closes at birth and the PDA within 3 days after birth.
See: Braunwald, chapter on, "Congenital Heart Disease in Infancy/ Childhood." **Keywords:** "Persistent fetal circulation" = R-L patent foramen ovale, R-L PDA

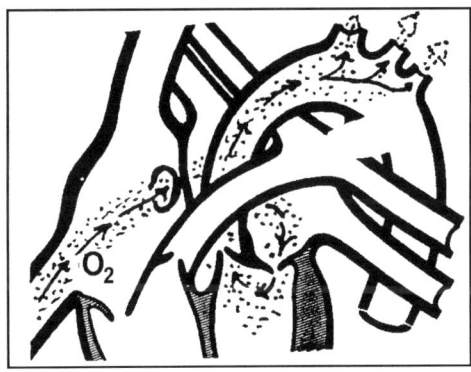
Fetal ASD, PDA

662. Normally the foramen ovale closes _____ and the PDA closes _____.
a. At birth, at birth
b. At birth, within 3 days after birth
c. Within 3 days after birth, within 30 days after birth
d. Within 30 days after birth, within 90 days after birth

ANSWER b. At birth, within 3 days after birth.
At birth, the flap over the foramen ovale closes with the increased pressure in the LA on the first breath. Then as oxygen is sensed at the PDA it begins to slowly close, too. Normally it is totally closed within 3 days.
See: Braunwald, chapter on, "Congenital Heart Disease in Infancy/ Childhood."

663. In this diagram of cyanotic congenital defects, identify the defect labeled #2.
   a. Tricuspid Atresia
   b. Tetralogy of Fallot (TOF)
   c. Truncus Arteriosus
   d. Hypoplastic Left Heart & AO
   e. Total Anomalous Venous Return(TAPVR)
   f. Transposition of Great Vessels (TGV)

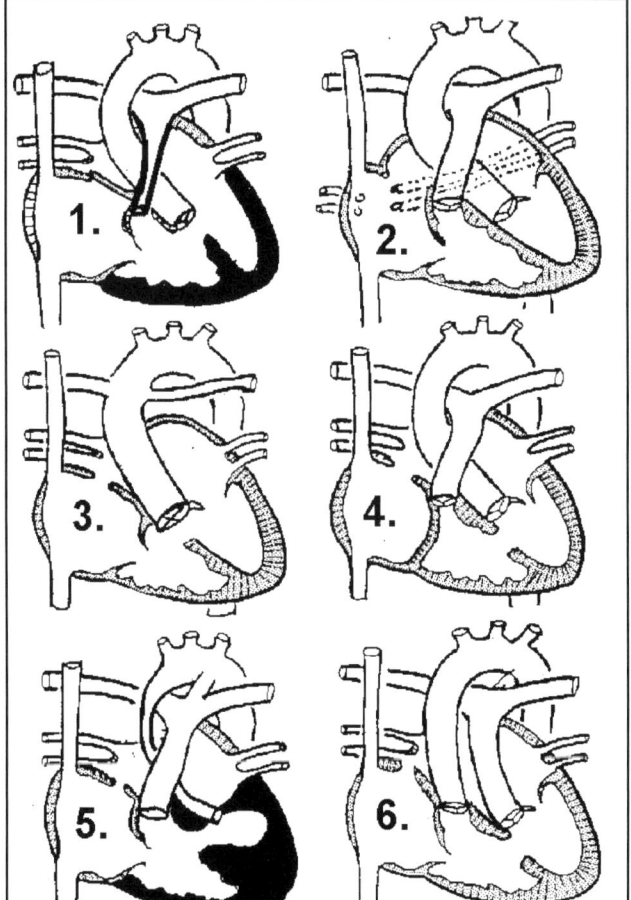

Cyanotic congenital defects

ANSWER e. Total Anomalous Venous Return (TAPVR). **CORRECTLY MATCHED ANSWERS ARE:**
1. **TET FALLOT, SMALL MAIN PA:** Note all 4 components of Tetralogy of Fallot: VSD, overriding AO (over the VSD), RVH from the increased pressures, and some kind of pulmonary obstruction.
2. **TOTAL ANOMALOUS VENOUS RETURN (**TAPVR) - Direct RA connection type: Pulmonary veins drain directly into RA. There is a R-L ASD.
3. **TRUNCUS ARTERIOSUS, TYPE III:** Right and left PA arises from side of ascending AO. This is retention of the embryonogic bulbar trunk. It results from the failure of normal separation and division of this trunk into the AO and PA. This single great vessel overrides the ventricles and receives blood from them through a ventricular septal defect. The entire pulmonary and systemic circulation is supplied from this common arterial trunk.
4. **TRICUSPID ATRESIA,** Large VSD with L-R shunt, and a large ASD with R-L shunt. The tricuspid valve is gone (atretic). All RA blood must pass through the ASD.
5. **HYPOPLASTIC LV** and ascending AO, mitral atresia, L-R ASD shunts arterialized blood into RV, and then LV via VSD. PDA shunts R-L to supply periphery.
6. **TRANSPOSITION OF GREAT VESSELS** (TGV), VSD, PDA. This anomaly is an embryonic defect caused by a straight division of the bulbar trunk without normal spiraling. As a result, the AO originates from the RV, and the PA from the LV.

See: Braunwald, chapter on, "Congenital Heart Disease in Infancy/ Childhood."

6B. Cyanotic Lesions - Tetralogy of Fallot (TET or TOF)

664. In children with Tetralogy of Fallot what catheter position should be avoided because it may lead to a hyper-cyanotic "spell?"
a. RA
b. PA
c. LV
d. AO

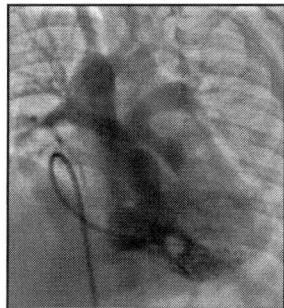

Tetralogy of Fallot

ANSWER b. PA. In children with Tetralogy of Fallot Catheterizing the PA should be avoided if possible because the child may become hypoxemic, cyanotic and begin crying. The crying makes them even more cyanotic. Classically these children "squat" during a "spell" to cut off venous return and reduce R-L shunting. Therapy for these hypertensive and hyper-cyanotic spells involves bagging with 100 % O_2 and narcotics (morphine or fentanyl) to relax the smooth muscle vasculature.

Another position to avoid is passing the catheter from RV through the VSD into the AO. This position is associated with heart block and bradycardia.
See: Braunwald, chapter on, "Congenital Heart Disease in Infancy / Childhood."
Keywords: in TET avoid PA cath. because of cyanotic spells

6C. Cyanotic Lesions - Total Anomalous Venous Return (TAPVR)

665. Besides having anomalous pulmonary veins, patients with total anomalous venous return usually have a _____.
a. R-L shunt through an ASD
b. R-L shunt through a PDA
c. L-R shunt through an ASD
d. L-R shunt through a PDA

ANSWER a. R-L shunt through an ASD. In the TAPVR cyanotic defect, all of the red arterialized blood finds its way into the RA. The pulmonary veins do not enter the LA, but the RA instead. The anomalous venous return is the primary L-R shunt. This shunt causes the cyanosis. Another R-L shunt, usually an ASD, exists to get some oxygenated blood back into the left heart and aorta.

In some pulmonary venous return cases only part of the pulmonary venous blood shunts into the RA - perhaps only one of the 4 pulmonary veins. In this partial-anomalous return the patient's symptoms mimic those of simple ASD.

This diagram shows TAPVR (Total Anomalous

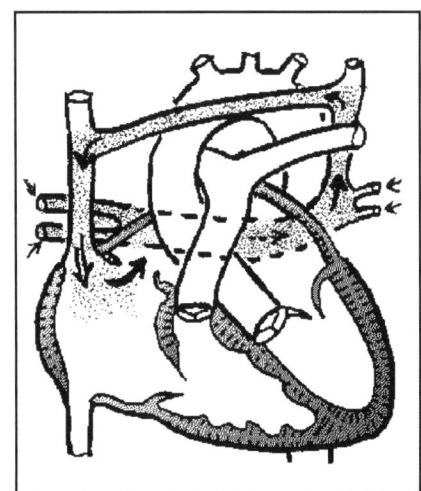

TAPVR

Venous Return) of the "supra-cardiac type." Here the pulmonary veins drain into the cardinal veins and into the SVC.
See: Braunwald, chapter on "Congenital Heart Disease." **Keywords**: TAPVR associated secondary R-L ASD

6D. Cyanotic Lesions - Transposition of Great Vessels (TGV)

666. In the first 10 days of life critical patients with the common form of transposition of the great vessels receive the arterial switch operation. Prior to surgery, what 2 interventions are commonly performed to reduce cyanosis?
 a. Balloon atrial septostomy (BAS) and administration of prostoglandins E_1 (PGE$_1$)
 b. Balloon atrial septostomy (BAS) and administration of indomethacin
 c. Stent enlargement of PDA and administration of prostaglandins E_1
 d. Stent enlargement of PDA and administration of indomethacin

ANSWER a. Balloon atrial septostomy (BAS) and administration of prostaglandins E_1. PGE1 maintains patency of PDA and allows for mixing of oxygenated blood between PA and the aorta. Grossman says: "the most common variety is known as dextro-TGA (DTGA); the ventricle position is normal (i.e. the RV is right-sided and the LV left-sided, with the RV giving rise to a right sided anterior aorta and the LV to a left-sided posterior PA). In the most common form of DTGA...., and in particular, the introduction of the remarkable arterial switch operation in

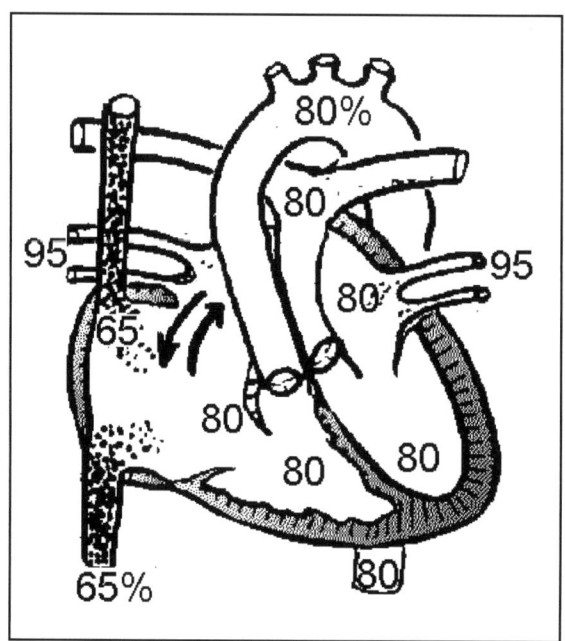

Creating ASD increases mixing in TGV

the first few days of life have made DTGA, with or without VSD, a correctable lesion and no longer a lethal one. . . . Even though an arterial switch operation is performed electively in the first 10 days of life, we continue to perform a BAS in the early neonatal period. Creation of an ASD remains the optimal method for stabilization of these cyanotic infants during the days before surgical repair."
See: Grossman, chapter on "Profiles in Congenital Heart Disease." **Keywords**: TGV needs Rashkind when PA exceeds AO by ≥10% Sat.

7. Other Congenital Pathology - not tested on RCIS

667. Different blood pressures in the upper and lower extremities suggests:
a. Double arch aorta
b. Truncus arteriosus
c. Coarctation of the aorta
d. Patent ductus arteriosus

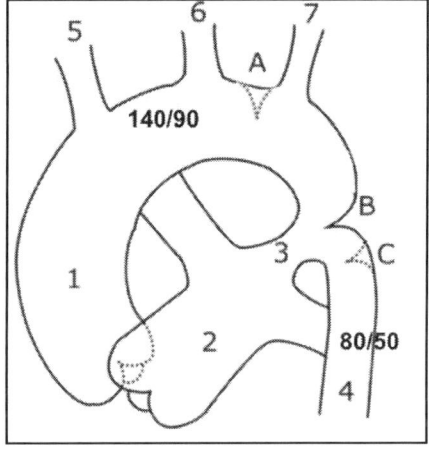

ANSWER: c. Coarctation of the aorta. Coarctation of the aorta is a congenital condition whereby the aorta narrows in the area of the ductus arteriosus #3 (or ligamentum arteriosum). There are 3 types: A. Preductal coarct., B. Ductal coarct., or C. Post ductal coarct. A pressure gradient usually occurs at the level of the coarctation.

Arterial hypertension in the right arm with normal to low blood pressure in the lower extremities is classic (#A is termed the "preductal" type). A coarctation occurring after the left subclavian artery (#B or #C "postductal") will produce synchronous radial pulses but delayed pulses in the legs. If there is a PDA there may be cyanosis below the arms. **See:** https://medlineplus.gov/ency/article/000191.htm **Keywords:** Arm BP > leg BP = coarctation of AO

668. Reversed LA-RA chambers with the LV apex on the patient's left side as shown is termed:
a. Situs Inversus, Levocardia
b. Situs Inversus, Dextrocardia
c. Situs Solitus, Levocardia
b. Situs Solitus, Dextrocardia

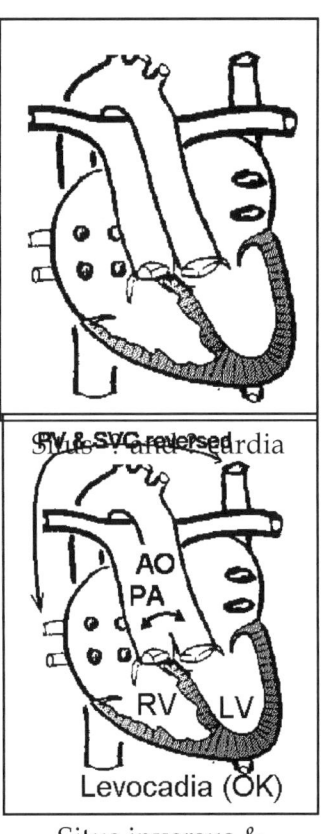

ANSWER c. Situs inversus, levocardia, and right sided aorta. Situs inversus is Latin for inverted visceral position (e.g. liver on the right side). This means the vena caval inflow enters on the left side, PV on the right side. All the viscera are mirror-image reversed in situs inversus. The systemic atrium (RA) and liver is on the left side. The aorta is also reversed because it descends to the right of the patient's backbone.

Levocardia refers to a left sided LV apex (levo means left). If the LV apex points abnormally to the patient's right side it is termed "dextrocardia" (dextro means right).
See: Braunwald, chapter on "Congenital Heart Disease."

Situs inversus & levocardia

8. Sample Pathology

BOTH QUESTIONS BELOW REFER TO THIS DIAGRAM.

4 chamber 2D echo	Right	% Sat.	Press.	Left	% Sat	Press.
	SVC	77%		LPV	%	
	IVC	80%		RPV	97%	
	RA	90%	6/6/3	LA	97%	
	RV	90%	38/4	LV	97%	120/4
	PA	91%	22/8	AO	97%	120/80
	PAW		3	dAO		

669. The angio, O_2 saturation, and pressure data shown in the diagram above is consistent with a diagnosis of:
a. R-L ASD
b. L-R ASD
c. R-L PDA
d. L-R PDA with PS

670. Interventional treatment of the defect above is:
a. Rashkind procedure
b. Rastelli surgery
c. Amplatzer device
d. Dumbbell embolization coil

BOTH ANSWERS LISTED CONSECUTIVELY.

669. ANSWER b. L-R ASD with pulmonary flow gradient. Note the O_2 step-up from SVC (77%) to RA (90%) jumps up 13%. The atrial pressures are equal indicating a huge ASD. The Q_p/Q_s=3.3/1. In pediatrics the SVC O_2 sat. is a good estimate of the mixed venous O_2 average. Gradient across the tricuspid valve is due to high flow not pulmonic stenosis.

The angiogram should be injected in LA and filmed in the LAO cranial view. Angiography is not usually called for, unless a double umbrella occluder is

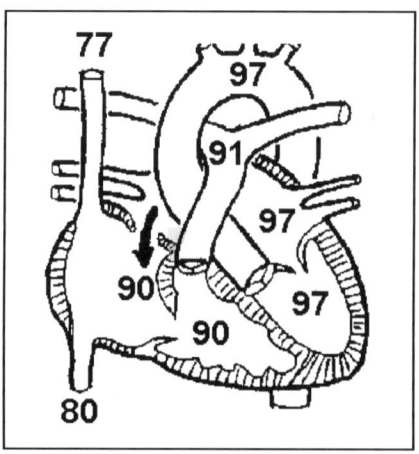

L-R ASD.

going to be placed, or a VSD is suspected.
See: Baim and Grossman, chapter on "Profiles in Congenital Heart Disease." **Keywords:** Large L-R ASD

670. ANSWER c. Amplatzer device or Cardioform devices are nitinol ASD occluders that can be delivered via catheter. Diagram (a) is the Cardioform occluder and diagram (b) is the Amplatzer occluder.
See: Baim and Grossman, chapter on "Pediatric Interventions."

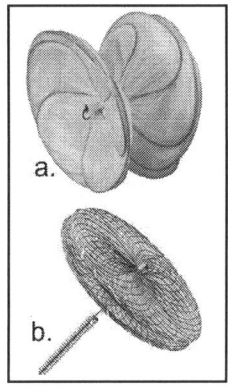

ASD occluders

671. The gold standard and most accurate way to diagnose a patent foramen ovale (PFO) is:
   a. Gated MRI
   b. Transseptal cath & angio
   c. Trans-thoracic echocardiography (TTE)
   d. Trans-esophageal echocardiography (TEE)

ANSWER: d. Trans-esophageal echocardiography (TEE) produces the highest quality LA imaging. Note in echo diagram bubbles passing through the PFO into LA.

Topol says, "Echocardiography plays an important role in the diagnosis of abnormalities of the atrial septum. Traditionally, TEE has been considered the gold standard to diagnose a PFO. The advantage of TEE is that it can identify all portions of the IAS, allowing for the diagnosis of all subtypes of ASDs, a fenestrated atrial septum, and PFOs.... Fundamental imaging trans-thoracic echocardiography (TTE) has been considered inferior for the diagnosis of PFOs. However, the advent of second harmonic imaging has improved the sensitivity of TTE to 90%."

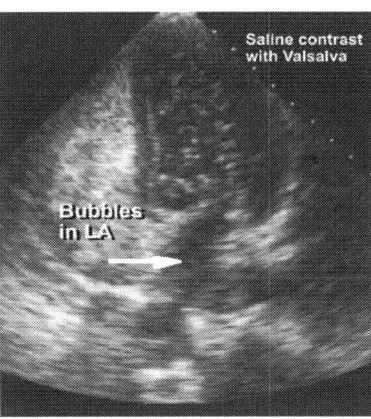

See: Topol, chapter on "Percutaneous Closure of PFO & ASD"

BOTH QUESTIONS BELOW REFER TO THIS DIAGRAM.

672. LV Angio - LAO cran	Right	% Sat.	Press. mmHg	Left	% Sat	Press. mmHg
	SVC	59%		LPV	%	
	IVC	60%		RPV	%	
	RA	58%	8	LA	94%	16
	RV	85%	103/10	LV	94%	110/12
	PA	88%	98/40	AO	94%	110/70
	PAW		16	dAO		

672. The angio, O_2 saturation, and pressure data shown in the diagram above is consistent with a diagnosis of:
a. L-R ASD
b. L-R VSD
c. Pulmonary stenosis with R-L PDA
d. Aortic stenosis with L-R PDA

673. Estimate the Q_p/Q_s in the above shunt.
a. 1:2
b. 1:6
c. 2:1
d. 6:1

BOTH ANSWERS LISTED CONSECUTIVELY.
672. ANSWER b. L-R VSD. The 27% O_2 step-up in RV indicates a large VSD.
   Pulmonary hypertension exists with an RV pressure almost equal to LV pressure. Large shunts often show pressure equalization between chambers. LV filling pressure (wedge of 16) is elevated due to increased pulmonary return.
   Note how the LV angiogram done in a steep LAO cranial view shows the septal surface on edge and nicely delineates the shunt.
See: Baim and Grossman, chapter on "Profiles in

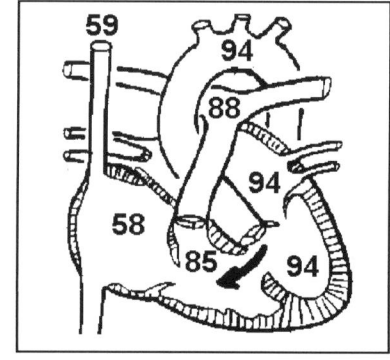

L-R VSD

Congenital Heart Disease." **Keywords:** VSD

673. ANSWER d. 6:1 = Q_p/Q_s = Pulm. Blood Flow/ Systemic Blood Flow

$$\frac{Q_p}{Q_s} = \frac{(SA - SV)}{(PV - PA)} = \frac{94\% - 59\%}{94\% - 88\%} = \frac{35}{6} = 5.8$$

This large 28% step-up in the RV indicates a huge L-R shunt. It is coming into the pulmonary or right side, making it a L-R shunt. This is verified by the Q_p/Q_s > 1.0. The large Q_p/Q_s ratio of 5.8 indicates that almost six times as much blood goes through the pulmonary as through the systemic circuit. That is a BIG shunt.
See: Grossman, chapter on "Shunt Detection and Measurement." **Keywords:** Calculate Q_p/Q_s

BOTH QUESTIONS BELOW REFER TO THIS DIAGRAM.

674. AO Gram 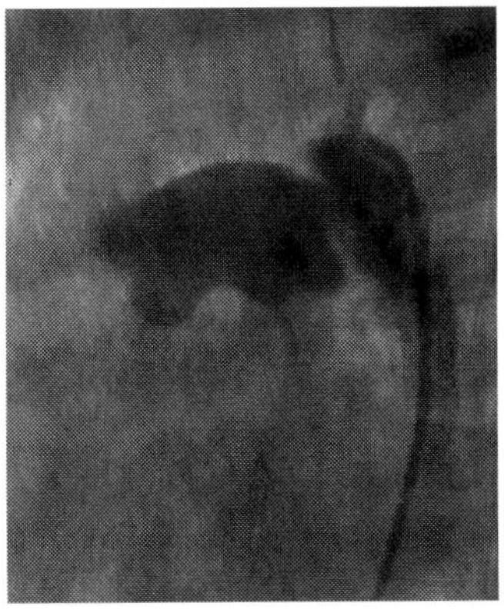	Right	% Sat.	Press. mmHg	Left	% Sat	Press. mmHg
	RA	68%	3	LA	92%	12
	RV	68%	68/5	LV	92%	110/10
	PA	80%	68/28	AO	92%	110/40
	RPA	82%	68/28	dAO	92%	110/40
	LPA	87%	68/28			

674. The angio, O_2 saturation, and pressure data shown in the diagram above is consistent with a diagnosis of:
a. R-L VSD
b. L-R VSD
c. R-L PDA
d. L-R PDA

675. Estimate the ratio of systemic to pulmonary resistance (SVR/PVR).
a. 0.4 : 1
b. 4.2 : 1
c. 2.4 : 1
d. 3.6 : 1

BOTH ANSWERS LISTED CONSECUTIVELY.

674. ANSWER d. L-R PDA. PA shows a 12% O_2 step-up indicating a L-R PDA with 3:1 shunt. Disparate saturations in the right and left PA indicate streaming and incomplete mixing in the PA. Differing PA samples make shunt calculations difficult.

RV pressure indicates moderate pulmonary hypertension due to the large L-R shunt.

With the advent of echocardiography and Doppler diagnosis, angiography is now rarely done in PDA, unless a PDA umbrella occluder is being placed at cath. **See:** Baim and Grossman, chapter on "Profiles in Congenital Heart Disease."

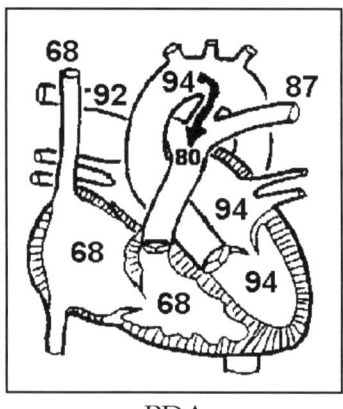
PDA

675. ANSWER c. 2.4 : 1. Calculation is based on the ratio of pressure drops across the two systems. Mean pressures should be used below.
- SVR = (AO - RA) / CO and PVR = (PA-LA) / CO
- SVR/PVR = (AO - RA) / (PA -LA) *note that CO cancels out algebraically.
- SVR / PVR = (70-3) / (40-12) = 67 / 28 = 2.4

Normal ratio SVR/PVR is around 12:1. This low ratio indicates a low resistant pulmonary circuit - necessary to accommodate the L-R large shunt. The ratio may normalize after ligation of the ductus arteriosus. **See:** Baim and Grossman, chapter on "Clinical Measure of Vascular Resistance..." **Keywords:** Calculate SVR/PVR resistance ratio

BOTH QUESTIONS BELOW REFER TO THIS DIAGRAM.

676. RV Angio - Lt. Lat.	Right	% Sat.	Press. mmHg	Left	% Sat	Press. mmHg
	SVC	68%		LPV	95%	
	IVC	%		RPV	95%	
	RA	68%	8	LA	91%	5
	RV	68%	155/10	LV	91%	120/8
	PA	68%	10	AO	91%	120/80
	PAW	68%	5	dAO		

676. The angio, O_2 saturation, and pressure data shown in this diagram is consistent with a diagnosis of:
a. Pulmonic stenosis
b. Infundibular stenosis
c. L-R VSD
d. L-R PDA with AS

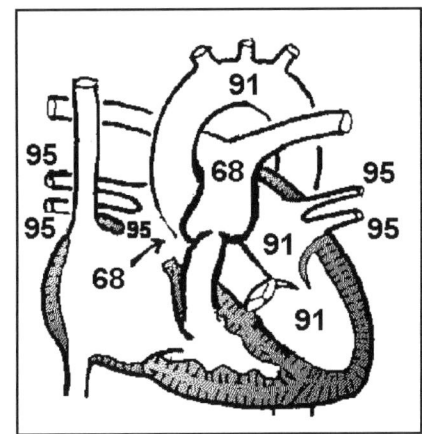
O2 saturation run

677. The interventional treatment of choice for the neonatal defect above is:
a. Pulmonary artery banding
b. PA valve commissurotomy
c. Rashkind procedure
d. Pulmonary valvuloplasty

BOTH ANSWERS LISTED CONSECUTIVELY.

676. ANSWER a. Severe pulmonic valve stenosis. A huge 143 mm Hg gradient exists across the pulmonic valve. A small 4% step-down in O_2 saturation in the LA indicates small R-L shunt through a patent foramen ovale from the increased right sided pressures.
  Extreme RV hypertension exists (systolic of 155 mmHg).
  RV angio in left lateral view shows domed pulmonic valve and post-stenotic dilatation of PA.
See: Baim and Grossman, chapter on "Profiles in Congenital Heart Disease." **Keywords:** Pulmonic stenosis with small R-L ASD

677. ANSWER d. Pulmonary valvuloplasty is replacing valve surgery. In the pediatric groups it is much more successful than in adults. Long term results are excellent. The valves are pliable and heal quickly.
  Neonatal surgery is risky and the infant will soon outgrow an artificial valve.
See: Baim and Grossman, chapter on "Balloon Valvuloplasty." **Keywords:** PS intervention = valvuloplasty

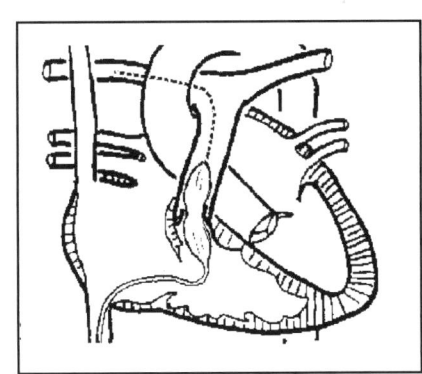
Pulmonary valvuloplasty

BOTH QUESTIONS BELOW REFER TO THIS DIAGRAM.

678. RV Angio - PA cran.	Right	% Sat.	Press. mmHg	Left	% Sat	Press. mmHg
	SVC	75%		LPV	98%	
	IVC	%		RPV	%	
	RA	75%	5	LA	95%	4
	RV	75%	105/5	LV	91%	105/5
	PA	76%	14/6	AO	84%	105/70
				dAO	90%	

678. The angio, O_2 saturation, and pressure data shown in the diagram above is consistent with a diagnosis of:
   a. TOF/TET
   b. L-R VSD
   c. Tricuspid atresia
   d. Truncus arteriosus

679. During the heart cath on the above pediatric patient she becomes cyanotic and begins crying uncontrollably. PA pressure is rising. What therapy is indicated?
   a. Ventilate with 100 % O_2 and IV fentanyl or morphine
   b. Place 5 L/min O_2 nasal cannula and IV epinephrine
   c. Emergency Rashkind procedure
   d. Emergency pericardio-centesis

BOTH ANSWERS LISTED CONSECUTIVELY.
678. ANSWER a. Tetralogy of Fallot (TOF). O_2 data indicate a small R-L ASD and a large R-L VSD. This is about a 1:2 shunt. AO saturation is artificially low (84%) due to streaming. Descending AO shows more thorough mixing at 90%.

Pressures indicate a 91 mmHg systolic gradient across the pulmonic valve. This is severe pulmonic valvular stenosis. Equalization of pressures between the two ventricles (common ventricle) is compatible with a large VSD.

PA cranial angiogram lays out the pulmonic valve and bifurcation. Both PA and AO light up at the same time indicating a large VSD. Besides pulmonic stenosis

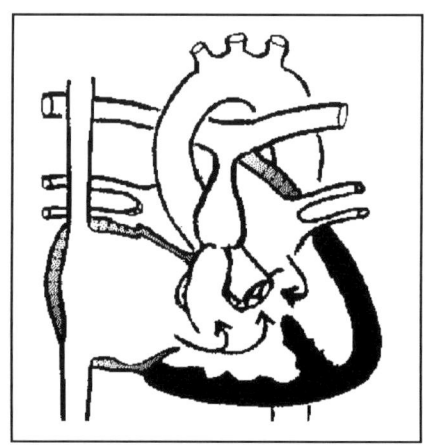

TET/TOF

the pulmonary trunk appears narrowed. The aorta overrides the VSD.
See: Grossman, chapter on "Profiles in Congenital Heart Disease.", p.669 **Keywords:** Tetralogy Fallot (TOF) with R-L VSD and true pulmonary stenotic gradient

679. ANSWER a. Ventilate with 100 % O₂ and IV fentanyl if the child becomes hypoxemic, cyanotic and begins crying. The crying makes them even more cyanotic. Give maximum O₂ - the classic therapy. Administer IV narcotics (morphine or fentanyl) to relax the smooth muscle vasculature and decrease pulmonary vascular resistance.
See: Baim and Grossman, chapter on "Catheterization on Infants and Children."

BOTH QUESTIONS BELOW REFER TO THIS DIAGRAM:

680. RV Angio	Right	% Sat.	Press. mmHg	Left	% Sat	Press. mmHg
	SVC	50%		LPV	99%	
	IVC	55%		RPV	99%	
	RA	70%		LA	95%	4
	RV	72%	90/4	LV	94%	35/5
	AO	72%	90/50	PA	94%	18/10

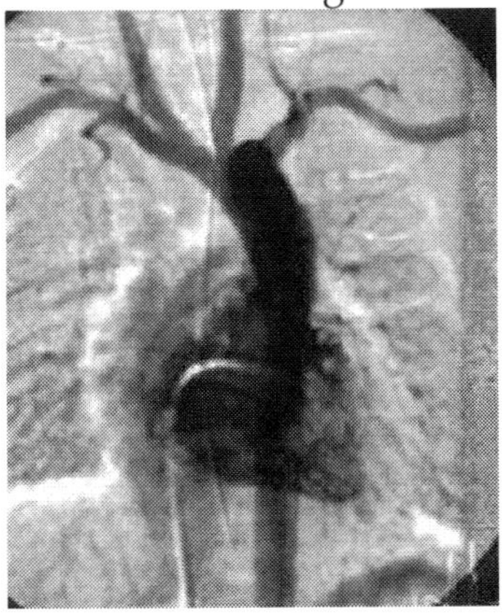

680. The angio, O₂ saturation, and pressure data shown in the diagram above is consistent with a diagnosis of:
   a. TOF/TET
   b. TGV
   c. Tricuspid Atresia
   d. Truncus Arteriosus

681. What palliative interventional procedure is often done on the newborn above?
   a. Blalock-Handlin procedure
   b. Mustard procedure
   c. Rashkind septostomy
   d. Watterston shunt procedure
   e. Angioplasty

BOTH ANSWERS LISTED CONSECUTIVELY.

680. ANSWER b. TGV = Transposition of Great Vessels. On this chart the PA and AO have been switched indicating transposition. A 20% step-up in the RA indicates a large L-R shunt. A small step down in the LA is consistent with a small R-L ASD. Thus, a bidirectional ASD is present. The RA-RV-AO are all desaturated, inadequate systemic oxygen levels. Rashkind septostomy would improve this. Arterial switch surgery is recommended within 10 days.

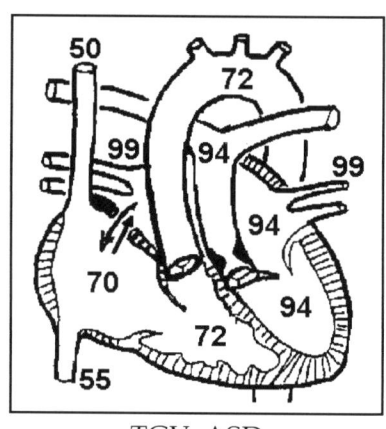
TGV, ASD

Pressures are higher in the RV and AO because of the increased systemic resistance. A systolic pressure gradient of 17 mmHg is present across the pulmonic valve. This is a true gradient because the flow across the LV-pulmonic valve is only 2 L/min compared to 10 L/min across the RV-aortic valve.

The LV angiogram in the RAO view leads to the PA.
See: Baim and Grossman, chapter on "Profiles in Congenital Heart Disease." **Keywords**: TGV with bidirectional ASD and mild PS

681. ANSWER c. Rashkind septostomy. The balloon septostomy procedure was invented by Dr. Rashkind in Philadelphia. A deflated balloon catheter is passed through the ASD or foramen ovale and then inflated. Then it is jerked back hard enough to enlarge the foramen ovale. This provides communication between the two sides of the heart so oxygenated blood can supply the periphery. It may make dramatic improvement in cyanotic infants but it is a temporary non curative (palliative) measure to buy time for the child until the arterial switch surgery can be performed.

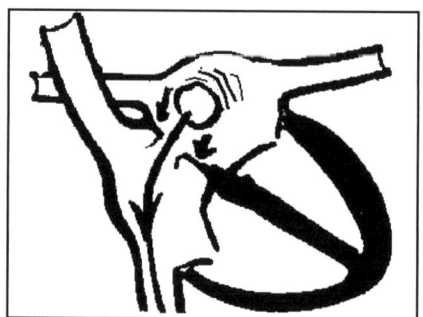
Rashkind Septostomy

Imagine that as you pull back the balloon, you are pulling red blood into the RA, RV, and transposed aorta.
See: Braunwald, chapter on "Congenital Heart Disease." **Keywords**: TGV → Rashkind balloon procedure

THE QUESTION BELOW REFERS TO THIS DIAGRAM.

4 chamber 2D echo	Right	% Sat.	Press. mmHg	Left	% Sat	Press. mmHg
	SVC	65%		LPV	98%	
	IVC	%		RPV	98%	
	RA	65%	5	LA	80%	9
	RV	80%	25/5	LV	80%	100/14
	PA	80%	10/8	AO	80%	100/60
	PAW		8	dAO		

682. The angio, O_2 saturation, and pressure data shown in the diagram above is consistent with a diagnosis of:
a. TOF/TET
b. L-R VSD
c. Tricuspid Atresia
d. Truncus Arteriosus

ANSWER c. Tricuspid Atresia. There is no tricuspid valve, so all blood must route around it. A large O_2 step-down in the LA indicates complete mixing of pulmonary venous and systemic venous blood from the R-L ASD. A small VSD exists. It fills the small RV with mixed blood from the LV. Both PA and AO are desaturated at 80%.

A systolic gradient exists between the RV and PA, indicating some degree of pulmonary outflow obstruction.

The RA angiogram shows LA filling, with nothing crossing the atretic tricuspid valve. The VSD allows rerouted mixed blood to enter the PA and lungs.

See: Baim and Grossman, chapter on "Profiles in Congenital Heart Disease." **Keywords:** Tricuspid Atresia (TA)

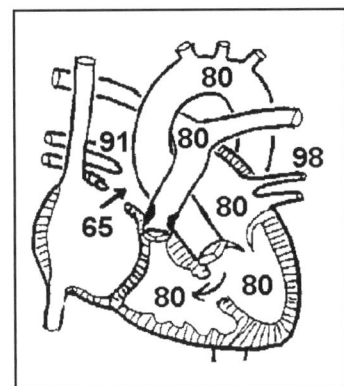

Tricuspid Atresia

BOTH QUESTIONS BELOW REFER TO THIS DIAGRAM.

683. AO gram - LAO view	Right	% Sat.	Press. mmHg	Left	% Sat	Press. mmHg
	SVC	70%		LPV	%	
	IVC	70%		RPV	%	
	RA	70%	5	LA	98%	10
	RV	70%	40/5	LV	98%	110/10
	RPA	82%	40/15	AO	98%	110/70
	LPA	87%	40/15	dAO	98%	30/20
	PAW		10			

683. The angio, O₂ saturation, and pressure data shown in the diagram above is consistent with a diagnosis of:
a. L-R ASD
b. L-R VSD
c. Aortic Stenosis
d. Coarctation AO

684. An interventional therapy for the neonatal defect above is:
a. Aortic banding
b. AO valve commissurotomy
c. Coil embolization of stenosis
d. Coarctation angioplasty

BOTH ANSWERS LISTED CONSECUTIVELY.

683. ANSWER d. Coarctation AO. O₂ sats. show no signs of a shunt. However, an 80-mm Hg systolic and 50 mm Hg diastolic pressure gradient exists between the ascending and descending AO. This is a severe coarctation. Mild coarctation only show a systolic gradient. LAO aorto-gram shows the constriction just below the left subclavian artery. **See:** Braunwald, chapter on, "Congenital Heart Disease in Adults." **Keywords:** Coarctation AO

684. ANSWER d. Coarctation angioplasty may someday replace coarctation corrective surgery. Angioplasty of a

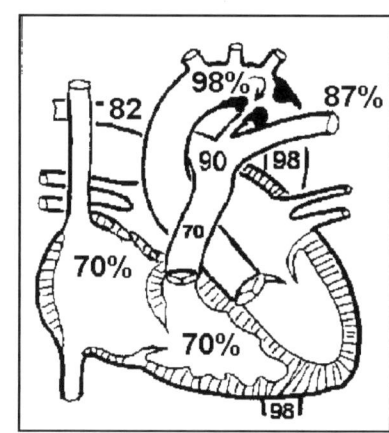
Coarctation AO

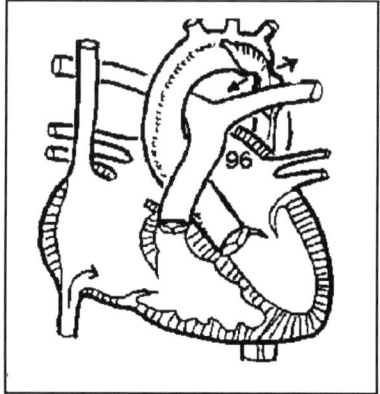
Coarctation angioplasty

coarctation is more likely to be successful if it is discrete or membranous. Large coarct's are difficult to dilate.

Neonatal surgery is risky and the infant will soon outgrow a Dacron graft. That is why "coarct-oplasty" is becoming so popular.

See: Baim and Grossman, chapter on "Pediatric Interventions" **Keywords**: PS intervention = valvuloplasty

THE QUESTION BELOW REFERS TO THIS DIAGRAM.

685. 4 chamber 2D echo	Right	% Sat.	Press. mmHg	Left	% Sat	Press. mmHg
	SVC	60%		LPV	95%	
	IVC	%		RPV	95%	
	RA	60%	12	LA	95%	18
	RV	66%	80/10	LV	89%	80/10
	PA	83%	80/50	AO	83%	80/50
	PAW		18	dAO	83%	80/50

685. The angio, O_2 saturation, and pressure data shown in the diagram above is consistent with a diagnosis of:
   a. TOF/TET
   b. L-R VSD
   c. Truncus Arteriosus
   d. Sinus Valsalva A-V fistula

ANSWER c. Truncus Arteriosus. Oximetry shows an O_2 step-up in the RV and PA, also, a large step-down in the LV and AO. There is bidirectional shunting at the ventricular and great vessel level, consistent with one large common AO-PA called a truncus arteriosus.

Pressures are elevated in the RV and there is no difference between PA and AO because they combine into one trunk.

The right lateral RV gram shows a bidirectional VSD and both chambers filling the large common trunk. A 5-6 cusp semilunar valve can be seen at the base of the large truncus. In this "type 1" truncus arteriosus, a small common PA arises from the back of the truncus and divides into right and left pulmonary arteries. Note the four aortic valve cusps drawn. There may be as many as

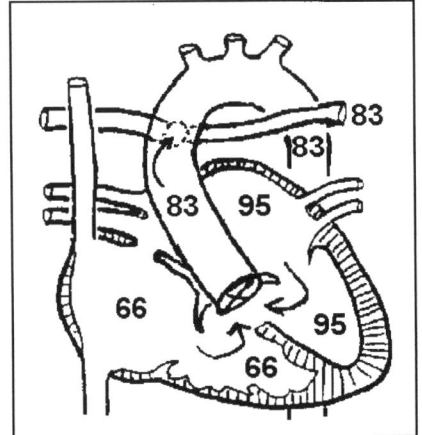

Truncus Arteriosus

6 valve cusps in a large truncus.
See: Braunwald, chapter on, "Congenital Heart Disease in Infancy/ Childhood." **Keywords**: Truncus arteriosus

BOTH QUESTIONS BELOW REFER TO THIS DIAGRAM.

686. AO gram - RAO view	Right	% Sat.	Press. mmHg	Left	% Sat	Press. mmHg
	SVC	70%		LPV	%	
	IVC	75%		RPV	%	
	RA	71%		LA	96%	9
	RV	81%	35/4	LV	96%	90/9
	PA	81%	35/115	AO	96%	90/50
	PAW		9	dAO	96%	

686. The angio, O_2 saturation, and pressure data shown in the diagram above is consistent with a diagnosis of:
a. TOF/TET
b. L-R VSD
c. Truncus Arteriosus
d. Sinus of Valsalva A-V Fistula

687. To quantitate the shunt shown above, estimate the Q_p/Q_s.
a. 0.17 R-L shunt
b. 0.59 R-L shunt
c. 1.7 L-R shunt
d. 5.9 L-R shunt

BOTH ANSWERS LISTED CONSECUTIVELY.

686. ANSWER d. Sinus of Valsalva A-V fistula. Oximetry shows an O_2 step-up in the RV. Pressures step up slightly in the RV and PA.

The aortogram shows a leak from the left coronary sinus of Valsalva into LV. These leaks may enter any right sided chamber and may originate from the aorta or coronary arteries.
See: Braunwald, chapter on "Acquired Heart Disease in

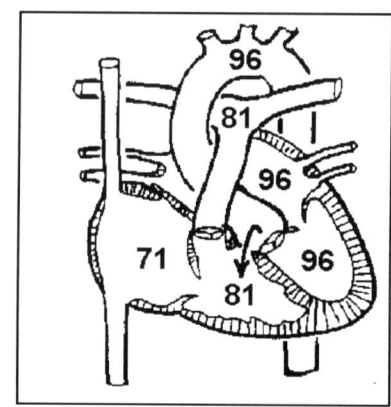

Sinus of Valsalva A-V fistula

Infancy and Childhood." **Keywords:** A-V fistula

687. ANSWER c. 1.7 R-L shunt. This is obviously a L-R shunt because the RV O_2 saturation steps up 10%. The Q_p/Q_s calculation is based on the ratio of A-V differences.

Q_p/Q_s = (AO - RA) / (LA - PA) = (96 - 71) / (96 - 81) = 25/15 = 5/3 = 1.7

See: Grossman, chapter on "Shunt Detection and Measurement." **Keywords:** Calc. Q_p/Q_s

688. What arterial approach provides the safest entry for contrast aortography in an adult with suspected coarctation of the aorta?
a. Femoral artery
b. Femoral vein
c. Brachial artery
d. Axillary artery cutdown

ANSWER c. Brachial or radial artery. If the coarctation is tight, it may be difficult to cross with a catheter. Also, many thin walled collateral intercostal arteries often enter into the post-stenotic segment. These are often fragile and perforate easily with stiff catheter manipulation. An arterial access into the aortic arch, (e.g. as the brachial) avoids having to cross the coarctation. Aortic arch angiography can easily delineate a coarctation.

See: Grossman, chapter on "Aortography." **Keywords:** Enter coarctation from brachial approach

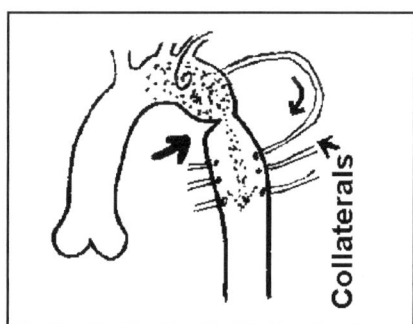

Coarctation of Aorta

REFERENCES

Baim D. S. and Grossman W., *Cardiac Catheterization, Angiography, and Intervention*, 7th Ed., Lea and Febiger, 2006

Braunwald, et. al. Ed., *Heart Disease, a Textbook of CV Medicine*, 9th Ed., Saunders, 2012

Kern, M. J., Ed., *The Cardiac Catheterization Handbook*, 6th Ed., Mosby-Year Book, Inc., 2016

Criley J. M., and Ross, R. S., *CARDIOVASCULAR PHYSIOLOGY*, Tampa Tracings, 1971

Daily, E. K., and Schroeder, J. S., *Techniques in Bedside Hemodynamic Monitoring*, 4th Ed., C. V. Mosby Company, 1989

King & Yeung, Interventional Cardiology, McGraw Hill, Co., 2007

Netter, *CIBA Collection of Medical Illustrations, "The Heart"*, CIBA Pharmaceutical

Pepine, J. C., and Hill, J. A., et. al., *Diagnostic and Therapeutic Cardiac Catheterization*, 2nd Ed., Williams and Wilkins, 1994

Topol, Textbook of Interventional Cardiology Elsevier Saunders, 6th Ed., 2012

Rushmer, R. F., *CARDIOVASCULAR DYNAMICS*, W. B. Saunders Co., 1976

Tilkian, A. G., and Daily, E, J, *Cardiovascular Procedures, Diagnostic Techniques and Therapeutic Procedures*, C. V. Mosby Company, 1986

Watson, Sandy, Ed., Invasive Cardiology, A manual for Cath Lab Personnel, 1st Ed., Physicians Press, 2000

OUTLINE: Pediatric Cath. Techniques

1. EQUIPMENT
    a. Pediatric Catheters
        i. NIH
        ii. Berman
        iii. Swan-Ganz
        iv. Pigtail
        v. Rashkind
        vi. Cournand or Lehman
        vii. Gensini
    b. Other Equipment
        i. biplane filming
        ii. Warmer
        iii. Y-boards (tie down)
        iv. Pulse oximeter
        v. Oximeters
        vi. red-infrared light source
        vii. inaccurate in anemia/hypotension
    c. EVALUATING CARDIAC SHUNTS
        i. Indicator dilution curves
        ii. Early hump = R-L shunt
        iii. Late hump = L-R shunt
        iv. Angiography
        v. Radionuclide
        vi. Oximetry
        vii. H2 curves = I-R shunt
        viii. 2D Echocardiography
        ix. Doppler Ultrasound
2. VASCULAR ACCESS
    a. AGE GROUPS
        i. Preemie born before < 37 weeks gestation or < 5.5 lb.
        ii. Infant between 6 months and 1 year of age
        iii. Neonate < 6 months of age
        iv. Child between 1 year and puberty
    b. INVASIVE MONITORING
        i. Considerations for Pediatric Cath
        ii. small vessels
        iii. small blood volume
        iv. -reduce blood sampling
        v. fluid overload
        vi. -reduce contrast volume
        vii. secure tubing connections
        viii. -small blood loss critical
        ix. lower BP
        x. Risk of infection
    c. VENOUS SITES
        i. umbilical venous cath.
        ii. Subclavian vein cath.
        iii. External Jugular
        iv. Internal Jugular
        v. Femoral venous cath.
            (1) -most common
    d. RIGHT HEART CATH
        i. Insertion Swan-Ganz
        ii. Risks & Complications
        iii. PA and PAW pressures
        iv. CO determinations
        v. Continuous SVO_2 monitoring
        vi. Transseptal pediatric cath
        vii. -attach needle to contrast filled syringe
    e. ARTERIAL SITES
        i. Peripheral Artery Cath.
        ii. Umbilical Artery Cath.
        iii. insertion
        iv. maintenance
        v. Complications
    f. Arterial pressure monitoring
        i. indications
        ii. contraindications
        iii. insertion
        iv. Maintenance
        v. Blood sampling from lines
        vi. Blood sampling from stopcocks
            -Blood sampling
PROCEDURES
    g. GENERAL PROTOCOL
        i. preop-diagnosis
        ii. echo
        iii. ECG
        iv. History and physical Exam
        v. study chart for preop-diagnosis
    h. SPECIAL PEDIATRIC CONSIDERATIONS
        i. umbilical catheter
        ii. strapping down to body board
        iii. Fluid Volume Balance
        iv. entertainment (toys, pacifier)
        v. Limiting the amount of angiographic dye injected
        vi. Reducing blood sampling and bleeding
        vii. Retaining baby's body heat
    i. INVASIVE PROCEDURES
        i. right heart cath.
            (1) -inflate with CO_2 if cyanotic
            (2) -Probe patent Ostium Secundum?
            (3) right heart pressures
            (4) -higher on right than in adult
            (5) right heart saturations
        ii. left heart cath
            (1) heparinization
            (2) cardiac output & O_2 cons.
            (3) EDP pressures (failure)
            (4) SVR, PVR
        iii. angiography
            (1) selective CINE angio.
            (2) focus on suspected pathology
        iv. EP studies as appropriate
        v. renal CINE
        vi. pull catheters
        vii. hold pressure
        viii. SPECIAL PROCEDURES
            (1) Rashkind balloon septostomy
            (2) Rashkind catheter technique
    j. PEDIATRIC MANAGEMENT
        i. Differences from adult physiology:
            (1) CO, CI
            (2) HR
            (3) Resistances
            (4) O_2 consumption
            (5) tachy/brady/arrhythmias

            (6) blood volume
            (7) Maintenance Fluid requirements
            (8) Thermoregulatory
        ii. Signs of poor systemic perfusion
            (1) tachycardia
            (2) irritability
            (3) tachypnea
            (4) lethargy
            (5) decreased response to pain
        iii. Early signs of cardiorespiratory failure
            (1) mottling of the skin
            (2) cooling of extremities and peripheral vasoconstriction
            (3) prolonged capillary refill
            (4) decreased urine output (<1-2 ml/Kg/hr)
            (5) diminished pulse pressure and damping
    k. NONINVASIVE MONITORING
        i. General Assessment
        ii. vital signs
        iii. BP
        iv. Pulse oximetry
        v. O_2 Sat.
        vi. Transcutaneous Blood Gas Mon.
        vii. Automatic BP
    l. PREMEDICATION
        i. Versed
        ii. Ketamine
        iii. Demerol compound (Pediatric cocktail)
        iv. Morphine Sulfate
    m. OTHER MEDICATIONS
        i. Indomethacin: Closes PDA's.
        ii. Prostaglandin E1: Maintains Patency of PDA
        iii. O_2 Administration: Vasodilator.
        iv. Tolazoline: Pulmonary and Systemic Vasodilator
3. HEMODYNAMICS
    a. NORMAL BP
        i. Newborn BP=80/50 mmHg
        ii. Infant (6 mo) BP=90/55
        iii. Toddler (2 yr) BP=100/60
        iv. School age (7) BP=105/65
        v. Adolescent (15) BP=120/70
    b. VASCULAR RESISTANCE
        i. Poiseuille equation
        ii. SVR = (Ao-RA) / SBF(CO)
        iii. PVR = (PA-LA) / PBF(CO)
        iv. Resistance Index = Resistance X BSA
        v. Normal resistance
        vi. Fixed PRV
        vii. dilation test
        viii. Vasodilators/constrictors
        ix. PVR
        x. SVR
        xi. Wood units
        xii. Dyne cm sec-5 (x80)
        xiii. Reversible Pulmonary Hypertension
            (1) -O_2 challenge
            (2) -Tolazoline challenge
            (3) -If significantly lowers SVR surgery considered
    c. Normal O_2 sats in heart (adult)
        i. Coronary sinus (low RA) = ± 45% O_2 SATURATION
        ii. SVC = ± 70 O_2 SAT
        iii. IVC = ± 80% O_2 SAT
        iv. LA (ASD shunt) = ± 95% O_2 SAT
    d. PRESSURES
        i. PULLBACK PRESSURE TRACING
            (1) Aortic valve stenosis
            (2) Pulmonic valve stenosis
            (3) Infundibular Stenosis
            (4) Tricuspid valve stenosis
            (5) Tricuspid valve Regurgitation
            (6) Mild coarctation of AO
            (7) Severe coarctation of AO
    e. SHUNTS
        i. physiology in intracardiac shunting
        ii. normally L-R
        iii. Reversal of shunt to R-L (cyanotic)
        iv. - Eisenminger's complex
        v. Suspect L-R shunts when PA sat. over 80%
        vi. - 5-8% step up significant
        vii. Suspect R-L shunts when AO sat. less than 95%
        viii. volume overloaded ventricles
        ix. Errors in the Fick evaluation of cardiac shunts
            (1) sampling errors (streaming, site, CS..)
            (2) patient movement, crying...
            (3) arrhythmia
            (4) insensitive to small shunts
        x. normal diagnostic saturation run.
        xi. Normal variations
            (1) IVC (Sat higher than RA or SVC
                (a) Renal/Hepatic blood (uses no O_2)
            (2) SVC (Sat closest to RA)
            (3) RA (Flamm equation in ASD)
            (4) RV, PA
            (5) PV (estimate 98% if cannot enter)
            (6) LA, LV, AO
            (7) O_2 sat. step-up and step-down
            (8) Site and direction of shunt
            (9) Significant Step-up in Rt. Ht.=Acyanotic shunt
            (10) Significant Step-down in Lt. Ht.=Cyanotic shunt
            (11) bidirectional shunts
    f. CALCULATION OF SHUNTS
        i. Use the Q_p/Q_s shunt ratio to quantitate shunts.
            (1) SBF
            (2) PBF
            (3) Shunt flow
            (4) direction of shunt
            (5) bidirectional shunt
        ii. select appropriate blood samples
        iii. Best mixed samples
        iv. Site immediately upstream to where shunt dumps in
        v. Estimating mixed systemic venous O_2 content
            (1) -Flamm equation (3xSVC + IVC)/4
        vi. Estimating mixed pulmonary venous

O₂ Sat
- (1) -Estimate PV = 98% if can't enter
vii. L-R shunt flow = PBF - SBF = $Q_p - Q_s$.
viii. Child on O₂ during blood sampling
- (1) -include physically dissolved O₂
g. Types of Intracardiac shunts
  i. Direction, Site
  ii. L-R VSD, PDA, & ASD
  iii. R-L VSD, PDA, & ASD
  iv. Coronary Sinus AV fistula
  v. Endocardial Cushion
4. ACYANOTIC DEFECTS
   a. GENERAL
      i. Sinus of Valsalva AV fistula
      ii. ASD
         (1) -bidirectional
         (2) -Double clamshell umbrella occluder
      iii. VSD
      iv. PDA
         (1) -Ductus active medications
         (2) -Indomethacin (constricts)
         (3) -Prostoglandin E1 (dilates)
      v. VSD
      vi. Valvular Regurgitation
      vii. Infundibular stenosis
      viii. Valvular Stenosis
         (1) -valvuloplasty
      ix. Coarctation of AO
         (1) -Balloon dilation of Coarct
      x. Endocardial Cushion Defect
      xi. Sinus of Valsalva - AV Fistula
   b. ASD
      i. Types ASDs
      ii. Sinus Venosus defect
      iii. Ductus Venosus
      iv. Ostium Secundum defect
      v. Ostium Primum defect
      vi. Single-Bidirectional shunt
   c. TYPES VSDs
      i. Muscular - anterior VSD
      ii. Muscular - posterior VSD
      iii. Membranous - inferior VSD
      iv. Membranous - infracristal VSD
      v. Membranous - supracristal VSD
      vi. Common ventricle
5. CYANOTIC DEFECTS
   a. Tricuspid ATRESIA
   b. Tetralogy of FALLOT (TOF)
   c. Truncus Arteriosus
      i. -Type I, 2, 3
   d. Hypoplastic Left heart
   e. Total Anomalous Venous Return(TAPVR)
   f. Transposition OF GREAT Vessels (TGV)
   g. Eisenminger with ASD, VSD, PDA
   h. Persistent Fetal Circulation
   i. Hypoplastic left heart
6. OTHER
   a. DEFECTS
      i. Endocardial cushion defect
      ii. Ebstein anomaly
         (1) electrode cath pullback diagnosis
      iii. Mitral valve prolapse
      iv. Situs Inversus
      v. Dextrocardia
   b. INTERVENTIONAL PROCEDURES
      i. Double umbrella Closure: ASD, VSD, PDA
      ii. Balloon Valvuloplasty / valvulotomy
      iii. Balloon Angioplasty, Coarctation-oplasty
      iv. Balloon Angioplasty Branch PA Stenosis
      v. Spring Coil Vascular occlusion
   c. SURGICAL PROCEDURES
      i. PA Banding
      ii. Shunt closure / patch
      iii. PDA Ligation
      iv. Fontan procedure
      v. Blalock Taussig procedure
      vi. Rastelli procedure
      vii. Senning/Mustard baffle
      viii. Arterial switch of Jatene
      ix. Watterson-Cooley/Potts procedure

Vascular Angiography

INDEX: D10 - Vascular Angiography
1. General Vascular . . . p. 391 - Know
2. Vascular Procedures . . . p. 394 - Know
3. Aortography . . . . p. 396 - Know
4. Pulmonary Angiography . . p. 401 - Know
5. Abdominal Arteriography . . p. 402 - Review
6. Limb Arteriography . . . p. 406 - Know
7. Cerebral Arteriography . . p. 414 - Know
8. Venography . . . . p. 418 - Review
9. Chapter Outline . . . . p. 420

1A. General Vascular

689. The abbreviation used in vascular procedures labeled at #1 is:
a. BUN
b. CFA
c. DP
d. DSA
e. DVT
f. IVP
g. KUB
h. NG
I. PFA
j. PTA
k. SMA
l. HU

VASCULAR ABBREVIATIONS
* 1. Kidney function test
  2. Artery punctured for AO-gram
  3. Feeding tube to stomach
  4. Artery supplying femur
  5. Computerized digital X-ray imaging
  6. Thrombosis of leg veins
  7. Roentgenogram of the renal pelvis and ureter, abdominal area
  8. Artery to front of foot
  9. Artery of the intestine
  10. Radiodensity measure on CT scan
  11. Vascular angioplasty
  12. X-ray of kidneys excreting contrast

ANSWER. a. BUN = Blood Urea Nitrogen
Along with creatinine evaluates kidney function. **Know all these common abbreviations.**
CORRECTLY MATCHED ANSWERS ARE:
1. **BUN** = Blood Urea Nitrogen = Kidney function test
2. **CFA** = Common Femoral Artery = Artery punctured for AO-gram
3. **NG** = Nasogastric = Feeding tube to stomach
4. **PFA** = Profunda Femoral Artery = Artery supplying femur
5. **DSA** = Digital Subtraction Angiography = Computerized digital X-ray imaging
6. **DVT** = Deep Vein Thrombosis = Thrombosis of leg veins
7. **IVP** = Intravenous Pyelogram = Roentgenography procedure of the renal pelvis and ureter after contrast filling
8. **DP** = Dorsalis Pedis = Artery to front of foot
9. **SMA** = Superior Mesenteric Artery = Artery of the intestine
10. **HU** = Hounsfield Units = Radiodensity measure on CT scan (0 = water)

11. PTA = Percutaneous Transluminal Angioplasty = Vascular Angioplasty
12. KUB = Kidneys, Ureters, and Bladder X-ray film. Immediately after angiography a KUB film shows the kidneys excreting dye. In renal toxicity and shutdown no excretion is seen. **See:** Kandarpa, Handbook of Cardiovascular and Interventional Radiologic Procedures, appendix of "Abbreviations." **Keywords:** Vascular abbreviations

690. During CT angiography the radiologist wants you to set a region of interest in the aorta for a bolus trigger of 270 HU (Hounsfield Units). What is a Hounsfield unit (HU)?
  a. Radiographic density (water = 0)
  b. Radiographic density (air = 0)
  c. Radiation count (1 Gray)
  d. Radiation count (100 Grays)

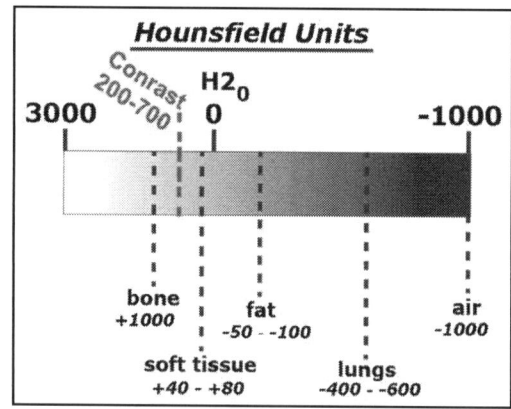

ANSWER: a. Radiographic density (water = 0). Hounsfield units (HU) are a measure of radiographic density (brightness) on CT scanner images calibrated to the brightness of water. The brighter the area on the screen, the higher the HU number. Water is 0 HU, air is -1000 HU, and bone is up to +3000 HU. Thus, positive numbers are more radiodense, like contrast or bone. Negative numbers are less dense, like lung tissue.

Contrast is injected in an arm vein and the radiodensity on the CT image will increase as contrast passes into the area of interest during the arterial phase begins. As the contrast increases in the aorta, the area will brighten until it reaches the trigger point (270 HU). This triggers the start of image acquisition/filming. The scanner will then follow the contrast down the aorta. With an IV contrast injection it usually takes 20-30 seconds for the contrast to pass through the right and left heart into the aorta. Without having to program an estimated time delay to start imaging, bolus triggering is more accurate and reduces radiation exposure. **See:** https://radiopaedia.org/articles/hounsfield-unit

1B. General Vascular - CT & MRI Angiography

691. What type of contrast is used in "contrast-enhanced magnetic resonance imaging" of the vascular system?
  a. Gadolinium
  b. Tc-99m-Sestamibi
  c. Iodine based contrast
  d. Low-osmolar radiographic contrast

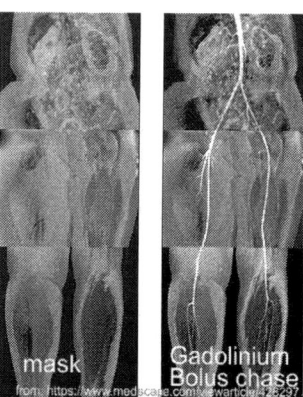
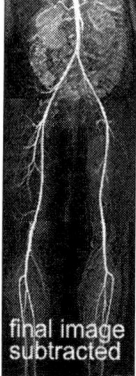

ANSWER a. Gadolinium. Because of its exceptionally high absorption of neutrons, solutions of organic gadolinium compounds are the most popular intravenous MRI contrast agents. In vascular MRI gadolinium is infused IV and makes the vascular system "light up." It is not as good as iodinated contrast for X-ray angiography but is a possible alternative for individuals allergic to iodinated contrast. **See:** Online medical dictionary on gadolineum.

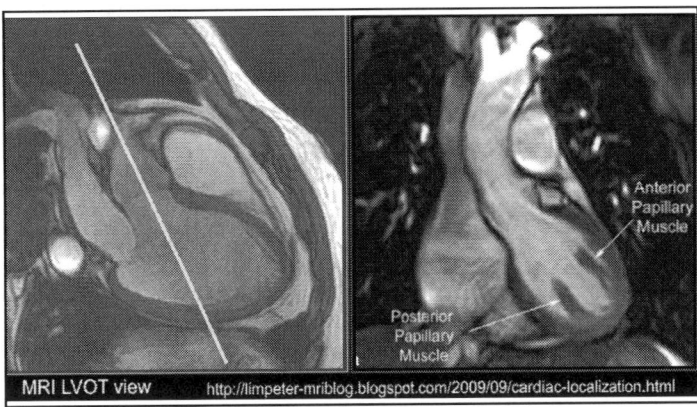
MRI of LV outflow track gadolinium contrast

692. **MRI & CT peripheral artery imaging while moving the patient through the scanner isocenter to image the bolus of contrast as it moves down the legs is termed:**
a. "Bolus chasing"
b. "Time-of-flight"
c. "Table stepping"
d. "Long board runoff"

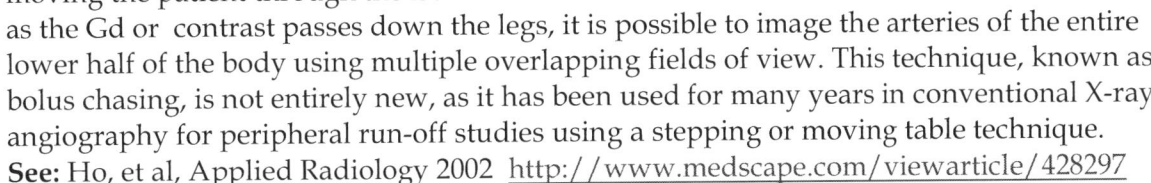

ANSWER a. "Bolus chasing". By imaging rapidly and moving the patient through the isocenter of the scanner as the Gd or contrast passes down the legs, it is possible to image the arteries of the entire lower half of the body using multiple overlapping fields of view. This technique, known as bolus chasing, is not entirely new, as it has been used for many years in conventional X-ray angiography for peripheral run-off studies using a stepping or moving table technique. **See:** Ho, et al, Applied Radiology 2002 http://www.medscape.com/viewarticle/428297

693. **An imaging technique in selective peripheral DSA arteriography that helps visualize the moving catheter uses the initial injected image as a "roadmap"to:**
a. Simplify image post processing
b. Provide a 3D map for catheter manipulation
c. Compare your current catheter position to anatomic landmarks
d. Act as a mask that is subtracted from the fluoro image to give a DSA image

ANSWER d. Act as a mask that is subtracted from the fluoro image to eliminate bones. This simplified image provides a 2D map for your catheter to follow.
   Grossman says, "Another useful technique used in DSA is road mapping. This technique is used for selective catheterization and is a useful aid for visualization of a moving catheter. Prior to moving the catheter, a small amount of contrast is injected. The

image with the filled vessels is stored in memory as a mask (a road map along which the catheter is to be moved). This mask is then subtracted from the following fluoroscopic images, which will display both the vessels and the catheter with its tip. Although it is not used in cardiac work (where cardiac motion precludes acquiring a suitable mask image), DSA is of great value in peripheral angiography as it reduces contrast volume, procedure time, and radiation exposure." **See:** Grossman, chapter on "Angiography of AO & Peripheral Arteries." **Keywords:** Roadmap, DSA

694. **Femoral approach catheters designed for abdominal angiography are usually _____ while those for cerebral angiography are usually _____.**
a. 3-4 French size, 5-7 French size
b. 5-7 French size, 3-4 French size
c. 100-120 cm in length, 60-80 cm in length
d. 60-80 cm in length, 100-120 cm in length

ANSWER d. 60-80 cm in length, 100-120 cm in length. Baim says, "For catheters designed to be positioned in the abdominal aorta, 60-80 cm lengths are sufficient; in the thoracic or carotid areas, 100-120 cm length (similar to those of left heart catheters) may be required. The most common diagnostic catheter sizes are 5 to 7 French, although 3 to 4 French systems have gained popularity when brachial and radial arteries are used for access." **See:** Grossman, chapter on "Angiography of AO & Peripheral Arteries." **Keywords:** short caths for abdominal angio, long for cerebral

2. Vascular Procedures

695. **Bilateral iliofemoral angiograms to image both legs are termed femoral:**
a. **Run-off films**
b. **Levophase films**
c. **Capillary blush films**
d. **DSA films**

ANSWER a. Run-off films. Aorto-iliac-femoral bilateral arteriograms are simply called "run-off films." This is a lot of anatomy and a lot of distance to cover with one injection. You need a wide field of view and multiple images moving down the legs. Because femoral run-off films are so long, adequate imaging requires special equipment, such as a stepping table or moving gantry with bolus chasing ability.
See: Kandarpa, Handbook of Cardiovascular and Interventional Radiologic Procedures, Appendix A, "Anatomy." **Keywords:** Run-off films

696. **Claudication is usually due to _____ in the _____.**
a. **Thrombotic occlusion, Abdominal aorta**
b. **Thrombotic occlusion, Leg arteries**
c. **Atherosclerosis, Abdominal aorta**
d. **Atherosclerosis, Leg arteries**

ANSWER d. Atherosclerosis, Leg arteries. Claudication is a cramping leg pain brought on by walking or running. And like stable angina, it subsides with rest. This pain is typical of atherosclerotic disease of the legs. The ischemic pain results not so much from O2 deficit but more the accumulation of metabolic waste (lactic acid buildup) in the muscles due to inadequate blood flow. The location of the pain is often below the obstruction, usually in the affected thigh or calf.
See: Underhill, chapter on "Vascular Diseases."

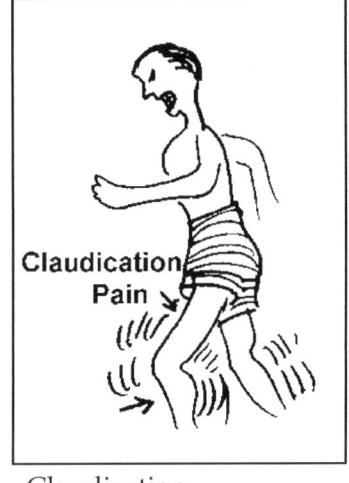

Claudication

697. What 3 types of vascular interventional procedures should be pre-treated with prophylactic antibiotics?
1. Percutaneous gastrostomy
2. Splenic and portal interventions
3. Biliary obstructive jaundice (percutaneous biliary drainage)
4. Urinary obstruction (percutaneous nephrostomy)
5. Tumor devascularization (embolic coil placement)
6. Placement of foreign body in vascular system (stent placement)
   a. 1, 3 & 6
   b. 2, 3 & 5
   c. 2, 5 & 6
   d. 3, 4 & 5

ANSWER d. 3, 4 & 5. Percutaneous biliary drainage, urinary obstruction (percutaneous nephrostomy) and tumor devascularlization (embolic coil placement). Valji says: "Prophylactic antibiotics are NOT indicated in the following cases:
   Most vascular procedures or gastrostomy"
"Bacterial overgrowth is common with biliary obstruction, particularly when caused by malignancy. Infectious complications are one of the common sources of fatal and major nonfatal complications. Biliary colonization with enteric organisms should be assumed in all patients with obstructive jaundice.... Antibiotic prophylaxis is therefore routinely recommended."
   Regarding percutaneous nephrostomy for urinary obstruction Valji says: "Prophylactic antibiotics should be administered intravenously 60 minutes before the procedure. ... The antibiotics should be continued for 24 to 48 hours in patients at low risk of urosepsis and 48 to 72 hours in high-risk patients."
   When the blood supply to a tumor is cut off by embolization therapy, that tissue will deteriorate and may become infected as it is absorbed. See: Valji, chapter on "Patient Evaluation and Care"

3. Aortography

698. Is contrast aortography safe in patients with aortic dissection? It generally:
a. Is contraindicated because the catheter may extend the intimal tear
b. Is contraindicated unless alternate routes of entry allow entry above the dissection (e.g. brachial approach)
c. Should be done by venous injection only using digital subtraction angiography
d. Is safe if contrast is not injected into the false channel

ANSWER d. Aortography is safe if contrast is not injected into the false channel. Usually ultrasound or chest film are the initial lab tests to discover aortic dissections. Follow up studies usually include noninvasive CT and/or MRI. However,
    Braunwald states that "**Aortic angiography is the single most important study in the diagnosis of aortic dissection.** ..The retrograde approach is **now the method of choice.** The hazards of the approach have proved minimal, provided the catheter is carefully inserted and contrast material is **not injected into the false channel.**"
See: Braunwald, chapter on "Diseases of the Aorta."

699. What is the best angiographic X-ray view to show the aortic arch and arch branches with the least foreshortening?
a. 30° to 40° RAO
b. 40° to 60° RAO
c. 30° to 40° LAO
d. 40° to 60° LAO
e. PA & Lateral biplane

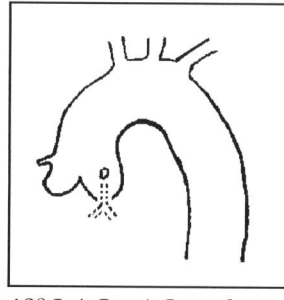

40° LAO, AO arch

ANSWER c. 30° to 40° LAO. The aortic arch "arches" posteriorly to descend to the left and in from of the backbone.
    Kern says, "Standard baseline arch aortography is using a pigtail catheter with power injection (typical volume of 40 cc) in a LAO 30- to 40-degree orientation. There should be limited foreshortening of the catheter. This position permits visualization of the origins and proximal segments of the great vessels and enables determination of arch type, which may indicate any potential technical challenges related to performing selective carotid angiography." **See:** Kern, chapter on "Peripheral Artery Disease and Angiography"

700. How does aortography in the shallow RAO projections show the ascending and descending aortic arch?
a. Ascending to left, descending to right
b. Ascending to right, descending to left
c. Superimposed
d. Anastomosed

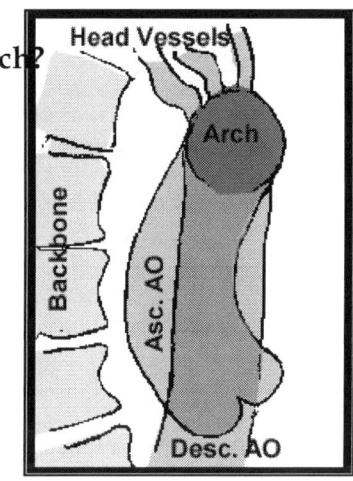
30° RAO view of AO arch

ANSWER c. Superimposed. In the RAO view the arch vessels overlap each other and are often superimposed. The aortic arch is foreshortened. Thus an RAO aortogram does not usually show as many takeoff vessels, and is rarely used. In this view you often see the top of the arch as a circle, termed the "aortic knob." **See:** Grossman, chapter on "Aortography."
Keywords: RAO AO-gram is rarely used. Arch foreshortened.

THE NEXT TWO QUESTIONS REFER TO THIS DIAGRAM.

701. Identify the stenosed artery in the aortogram shown.
a. Right subclavian
b. Right internal mammary (int. thoracic)
c. Right common carotid
d. Innominate (brachio-cephalic)
e. Left common carotid

702. In this type of stenosis, the right subclavian artery may receive collateral flow by "stealing" blood flow from the:
a. Bronchial artery
b. Internal mammary artery
c. Carotid artery
d. Vertebral artery

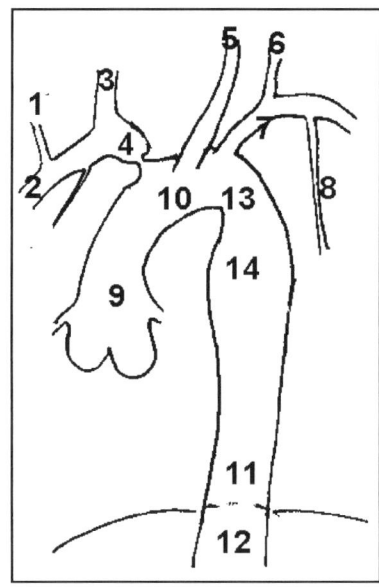
Aortic arch vessels

BOTH ANSWERS TOGETHER BELOW.

701. ANSWER d. Innominate or brachio-cephalic artery. Know all these vessels.
CORRECTLY MATCHED ANSWERS ARE:
   1. Right Vertebral
   2. Right Subclavian
   3. Right Common Carotid
   4. Innominate (Brachio-cephalic)
   5. Left Common Carotid
   6. Left Vertebral

7. Left Subclavian
8. Left Internal Mammary (int. thoracic)
9. Ascending AO.
10. Aortic Arch
11. Descending AO (thoracic AO)
12. Abdominal AO (below diaphragm)
13. Aortic Isthmus - Normal notch, at site of ligamentum arteriosus
14. Aortic spindle - Normal fusiform dilatation below isthmus

See: Snopek, chapter on "Aortography." **Keywords:** RIMA

702. ANSWER d. Vertebral artery. A proximal subclavian obstruction may be bypassed naturally by collateral flow from the contralateral vertebral artery. Normally the two vertebral arteries join in the basilar artery, to supply the circle of Willis in the brain. But, in "subclavian steal" flow can pass retrograde down the ipsilateral vertebral artery, into the stenosed subclavian artery, as shown.
See: Johnsrude, chapter on "Aortic Arch..."

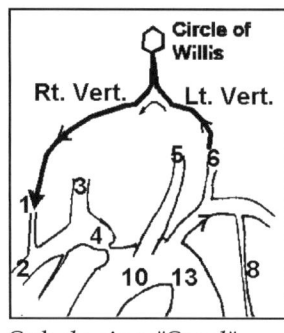
Subclavian "Steal"

703. **Which class of aortic dissection originates in the DESCENDING aorta?**
  a. Type I of Debakey
  b. Type II of Debakey
  c. Type A of Daily
  d. Type B of Daily

ANSWER d. Type B dissection (proposed by Daily et. al.) The simplest aortic classification system of Daily has just two dissection types - A and B. The Debakey and Daily classes include:
  • Debakey class I & II - both originate in the ascending AO
  • Debakey class III (not part of this question) - originate in the descending thoracic aorta
  • Daily Type A = ascending AO origin
  • Daily Type B = descending AO origin

From this one can see that no matter what classification system is used, the first classes originate in the ascending AO. Type A is a medical emergency because they may cut off the carotids, coronaries, and aortic valve. **See:** Braunwald, chapter on "Diseases of the Aorta."

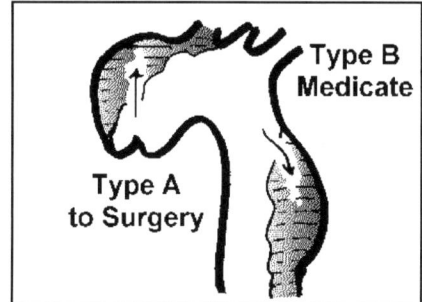
Dissection: Daily types A & B

704. The aortic defect shown is ___ and its most common cause is ___.
   a. AAA, Atherosclerosis
   b. AAA, Marfan syndrome
   c. Aortic dissection, Atherosclerosis
   d. Aortic dissection, Marfan syndrome

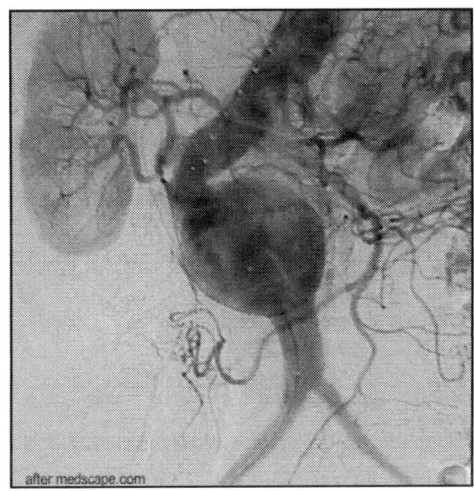

5.5 cm AAA

ANSWER a. AAA, Atherosclerosis. This DSA angiogram shows a large 5.5 cm fusiform (symmetrical) abdominal aortic aneurysm [AAA] which needs repair, because beyond this diameter, they rupture frequently. Note the cm measuring dots on the catheter in the suprarenal aorta.

Lanzer says, "The most common cause of AAA is a dilation type of atherosclerosis (95%). Less common are AAAs of infections or inflammatory origin, or those associated with connective tissue diseases... A common histopathologic element is the inflammatory reaction within the aortic wall that leads to destruction of the entercellular matrix (particularly elastin) and remodeling of collagen, which consequently leads to the loss of aortic wall elasticity and rigidity." See: Lanzer, chapter on "AAA"

705. The greatest risk associated with the large AAA's is:
   a. Kidney failure
   b. Aneurysm rupture
   c. Clot formation and embolization to legs
   d. Dissection of AO with cutoff of vital arteries

ANSWER b. Aneurysm rupture and probable death. Lanzer says, "The prognosis of a patient with AAA is unfavorable. In men older than 55 years, AAA is the 10th most frequent cause of death. The rupture of the aneurysm is the most severe complication and, when untreated, it is usually lethal... The risk of rupture increases with the size of the AAA, with the transverse diameter of the AAA being the most powerful predictor of rupture." Surgery or endovascular stentgrafting is usually done early before the aneurysm gets over 5.5 cm. See: Lanzer, chapter on "AAA"

706. The aortic defect shown at #1 in angio A is ___ and in angio B it is treated with ___.
   a. Large aortic thrombus, Platinum coil embolization
   b. Large aortic thrombus, Stent-graft
   c. Aortic dissection, Stent-graft
   d. Aortic dissection, Platinum coil embolization

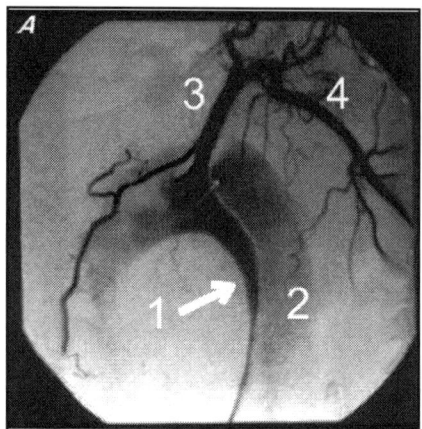

ANSWER c. Aortic dissection, Stent-graft. The true lumen is seen at #1, and the false lumen at #2. The dissected intimal flap is visible as a line between the true and false lumens.

The intimal tear is near the takeoff of the left carotid artery. Intima has been torn (like loose wallpaper) from the descending arch. It obstructs flow to the descending aorta and probably extends into and blocks distal side branch arteries. Some thrombus is often present in the false lumen.

Both angiograms appear to have been injected through a subclavian left arm catheter at #8.

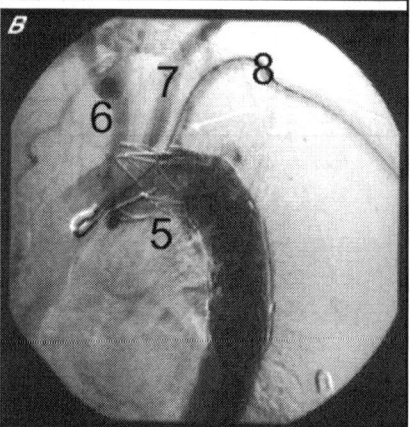

Arch aortogram - from Vasc.Surg.

An aortic arch endograft or cloth covered stent-graft is seen in angio B with the supporting wires at #5. Note the now patent arch vessels in the image at #6, 7 & 8.

The CT shows the various lumens and mural thrombus within the descending aorta. Noninvasive imaging is used extensively to diagnose dissection. **See:** Braunwald, chapter on "Diseases of the Aorta"

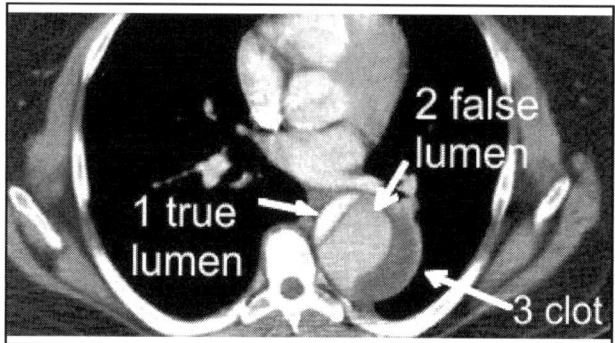

CT cross section of AO dissection

4. Pulmonary Angiography

707. What defect is shown on this CT pulmonary angiogram?
   a. Mitral stenosis
   b. Aortic dissection
   c. Pulmonary valve stenosis
   d. Pulmonary embolism

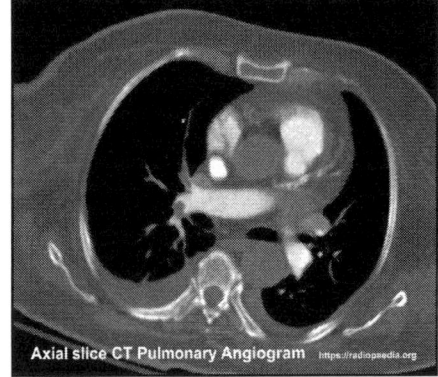

CT pulmonary angiogram

ANSWER d. Pulmonary Embolism due to large thrombus in left pulmonary artery.

Mos et al say, "Computed tomographic pulmonary angiography (CTPA) is the imaging test of choice because of its high sensitivity and specificity. Compression ultrasonography and ventilation perfusion scintigraphy are reserved for patients with concomitant suspicion of deep vein thrombosis or contraindication for CTPA... Several tests are available for the diagnosis of PE. Formerly, the reference standard for the diagnosis of PE was pulmonary angiography. This invasive technique, however, is cumbersome to the patient and is also expensive. It has thus been replaced by computed tomographic pulmonary angiography (CTPA).... Due to the invasive character, including right heart catheterization and injection of contrast material, and the current availability of noninvasive diagnostic imaging modalities like CTPA and V/Q scintigraphy, catheter pulmonary angiography now has an insignificant role."

708. Pulmonary angiography may precede PE intervention. The angiographic features most specific to pulmonary embolism are: (Select 2 below.)
   a. Tortuous PA vessels
   b. Slowed filling from PA into pulmonary veins
   c. Abrupt vessel cut off
   d. An avascular lung area
   e. Intralumen filling defects

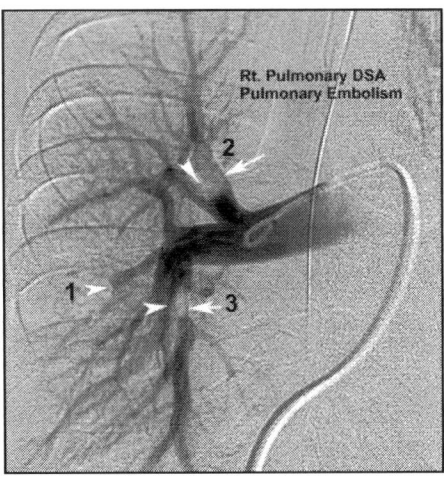

ANSWER c & e. Abrupt vessel cut off and intralumen filling defects. As shown in the diagram, filling defects usually represent an embolus, often with their tail extending downstream (#2 & 3 in this angio image.) It's easy to see why they embolize.

Cut off vessels are completely occluded branches (#1.) They will eventually clot off right up to and appear flush with the main vessel. When that happens it is difficult to tell there was a vessel there in the first place. Balloon occlusion angiography uses smaller amounts of contrast injected distal to an inflated Swan-Ganz type balloon.

The other 3 answers are secondary signs associated with PE, but not in themselves diagnostic. **See:** Grossman, chapter on "Pulmonary Angiography." **Keywords:** PE on PA angiogram ➜ cut off vessels, filling defects

709. An abnormal hemodynamic finding associated with massive pulmonary embolism is:
a. Pulmonary artery hypotension
b. Dilatation and pressure overload of LV
c. IV septum bulges into LV, reducing filling volume and CO
d. Pulmonic valve regurgitation

ANSWER c. IV septum bulges into LV reducing LVEDV
a. **NO, PULMONARY ARTERY HYPOTENSION:** The obstruction of the PA causes the RV to increase its pressure resulting in pulmonary **HYPERTENSION.**
b. **NO, LV DILATATION AND PRESSURE OVERLOAD:** It is the RV which is dilated and pressure overloaded.
c. **YES, IV SEPTUM BULGES INTO LV REDUCING LVedv:** The obstructed PA causes RV pressure overload. As the RV distends maximally it is limited by the pericardium. This causes the RV septum to bulge into the LV, reducing LV preload and CO. This RV pressure overload effect is also seen in cardiac tamponade. Reflexive tachycardia compensates for the decreased LV stroke volume.
d. **NO, PULMONIC VALVE REGURGITATION:** As the RV dilates the tricuspid ring dilates causing tricuspid regurgitation - not pulmonic regurgitation.

See: Braunwald, chapter on "Pulmonary Embolism." **Keywords:** Hemodynamics of PA = IV septal bulging into LV reducing LVEDV.

5. Abdominal Arteriography

710. An otherwise healthy 70 year old man with diabetes is suspected to have secondary hypertension. To diagnose this type of hypertension, what type of angiographic procedure would he most likely be scheduled for?
a. Splanchnic arteriogram
b. Coronary arteriogram
c. Ilio-femoral arteriogram
d. Renal arteriogram

ANSWER d. Renal arteriogram. Reno-vascular obstructive disease involves mostly older men. The stenosis usually occurs near the orifice of the main renal artery. These are usually amenable to

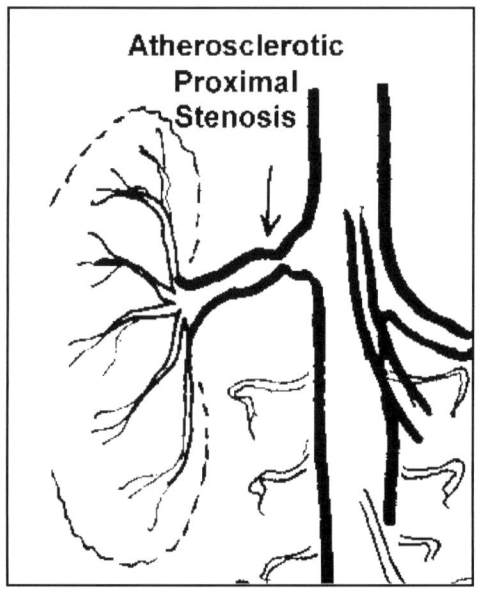

Renal artery stenosis

angioplasty and stenting.

As the kidney becomes more deprived of blood it sends out a hormone call for more blood pressure to increase renal flow. The first hormone produced is renin. It is easily measured in the renal venous blood. Renin triggers angiotensin II release (vasoconstrictor) and aldosterone (a water retainer). All of this leads to a hypertension which can be cured by removal of the obstruction, either by angioplasty or surgery.

Only 1% of hypertensives have renal stenosis. But this is the most common secondary form of hypertension that is correctable with stenting. **See:** Braunwald, chapter on "Systemic Hypertension." **Keywords:** Secondary hypertension → renal artery stenosis

711. **Hemodynamically severe renal artery stenosis occurs when the resting hyperemic peak translesional pressure gradient is _____ or FFR _____.**
a. > 10 mmHg or FFR<0.75
b. > 10 mmHg or FFR<0.80
c. > 20 mmHg or FFR<0.75
d. > 20 mmHg or FFR<0.8

ANSWER d. > 20 mmHg or FFR<0.8
Current guidelines say: "Expert consensus and experimental evidence have determined that a hemodynamically severe renal artery diameter stenosis is present when there exists a resting or hyperemic translesional mean pressure gradient of ≥10 mm Hg, a resting or hyperemic peak systolic translesional pressure gradient of ≥20 mm Hg or renal fractional flow reserve (FFR) ≤0.8. The pressure gradient is best measured with an 0.014" pressure wire and not a catheter." See: http://onlinelibrary.wiley.com/doi/10.1002/ccd.27141/full

712. **What does this arteriogram show on DSA?**
a. **Renal artery occlusion**
b. **Fibromuscular dysplasia**
c. **Left renal artery stenosis**
d. **Right renal artery stenosis**

ANSWER c. Left renal artery stenosis at the origin of the renal artery. Origin-stenosis is the most common location. Severe stenosis like this may lead to secondary arterial hypertension. It is not occluded because we see filling distal to the stenosis. It is not FMD because we do not see a "string of pearls".
See: https://medlineplus.gov/ency/article/000204.htm

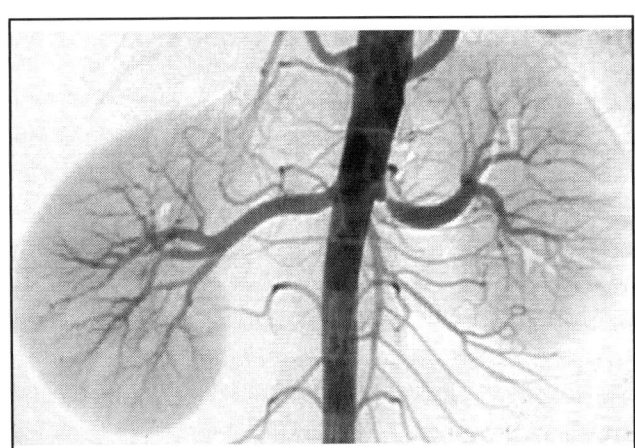

Renal artery stenosis

713. Renal artery pressures were measured through the stenosis shown. This shows a/an:
a. Insignificant mean gradient of 12 mmHg
b. Insignificant mean gradient of 60 mmHg
c. Significant peak to peak gradient of 12 mmHg
d. Significant peak to peak gradient of 60 mmHg

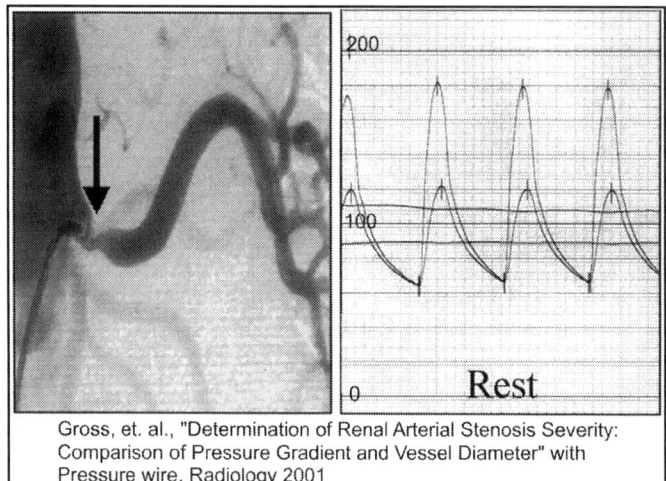
Gross, et. al., "Determination of Renal Arterial Stenosis Severity: Comparison of Pressure Gradient and Vessel Diameter" with Pressure wire, Radiology 2001

Renal artery stenosis

ANSWER d. Significant peak to peak gradient of 60 mmHg. Systolic pressure in the AO is 180 mmHg. Systolic pressure in the renal artery is 120 mmHg. The difference (gradient) between these 2 systolic pressures is 60 mmHg. Renal systolic gradients of 20 mmHg are hemodynamically significant (10 mmHg mean gradient). Hemodynamically significant renal stenosis leads to renin production in the kidneys and often secondary arterial hypertension. **See:** Grossman, chapter on "Angiography of AO & Peripheral Arteries."
Keywords: Significant renal stenotic gradient = 20 mmHg

714. This renal arteriogram on a 31 year old woman with secondary hypertension shows:
a. Renal artery atherosclerosis
b. Fibromuscular dysplasia
c. Renal AV fistula (AVM)
d. Chronic renal parenchymal disease

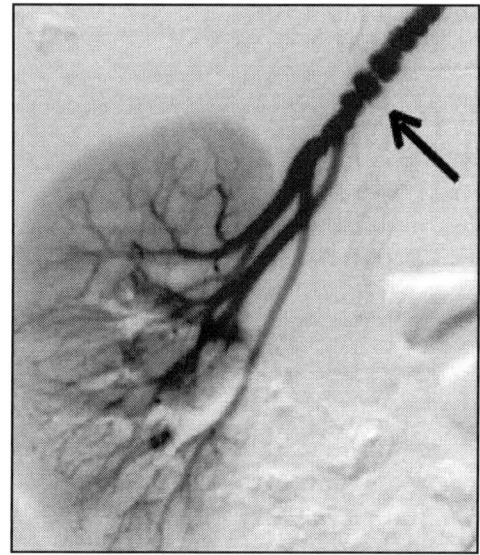
Renal artery - Fibromuscular Dysplasia - "String of pearls"

ANSWER b. Fibromuscular dysplasia. Reno-vascular disease occurs in younger women, and occurs in the distal 2/3 and branches of the renal arteries. This is termed fibro-muscular disease (FMD). These are small aneurysms appearing in the distal renal artery as a "string of pearls" shown at arrow. Other arteries may show similar findings. The cause of FMD is unknown, but it is progressive. Easily treated with angioplasty. **See:** Braunwald, chapter on "Systemic Hypertension." **Keywords:** Fibromuscular Dysplasia

715. In a patient with hypertension due to pheochromocytoma, arteriography may be used to visualize the tumor which is within the:
a. Kidney
b. Liver
c. Adrenal gland
d. Pituitary gland

ANSWER c. Adrenal gland. Pheochromocytoma is a vascular tumor of chromaffin tissue of the adrenal medulla. This is where humoral epinephrine and norepinephrine are liberated into the blood stream. With the tumor, increased epinephrine is released often leading to hypertension. As many as three adrenal arteries may supply different parts of the gland. These may arise from: inferior phrenic artery off the celiac artery, directly from the aorta, or from the renal artery as shown.

Structures shown in the diagram are:
1. Celiac artery
2. Right renal artery
3. Superior mesenteric artery
4. Testicular or ovarian artery
5. Inferior mesenteric artery
6. Right adrenal (suprarenal) gland
7. Right inferior adrenal artery
8. Left adrenal (suprarenal) gland
9. Left middle adrenal artery

See: Johnsrude, chapter on "Adrenal Vascular Studies."

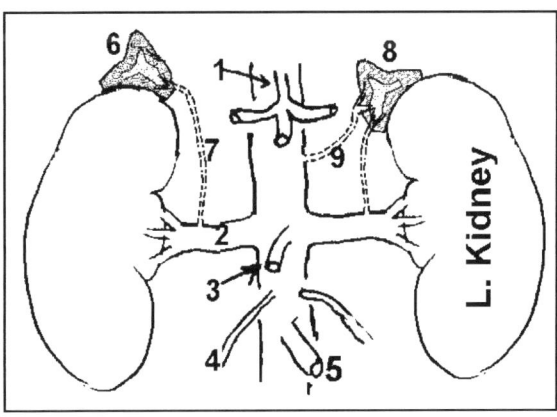

Adrenal (suprarenal) glands

716. Which of the following medications may be used to increase visualization of the portal venous system or during a splenic arteriogram?
a. Pitressin
b. Epinephrine
c. Tolazoline
d. Vasopressin

ANSWER c. Tolazoline and priscoline are vasodilators that may optimize splenic vein filling. Johnsrude says, "Vasodilators may be used when vasospasm detracts from the study..., or more rapid arterial flow or enhanced venous opacification is required." Other vasodilators that may be injected to minimize vascular spasm are nitroclycerin, papaverine, dopamine or nifedipine.
See: Johnsrude, chapter on "Adrenal Vascular Studies."

717. Which angiographic position best delineates the origins of the celiac axis and the superior mesenteric arteries?
  a. PA or AP
  b. 45 degree RPO
  c. 45 degree LAO
  d. Lateral

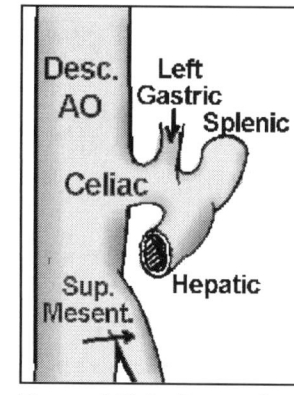

ANSWER d. Lateral. Since the celiac axis and superior mesenteric arise anteriorly off the abdominal aorta, they will be seen in profile in the lateral view. Ballinger says a slight 10° to 15° RPA view may be used to better visualize the superior mesenteric artery. **See:** Grossman, chapter on "Aortography."

Desc. AO in Lateral view

6A. Limb Arteriography - Legs

718. Identify 3 current filming modalities for peripheral arteriograms.
  a. MR Angiogram
  b. CT Angiogram
  c. Stepping table with cut film
  d. Cine angiogram
  e. Digital subtraction angiogram

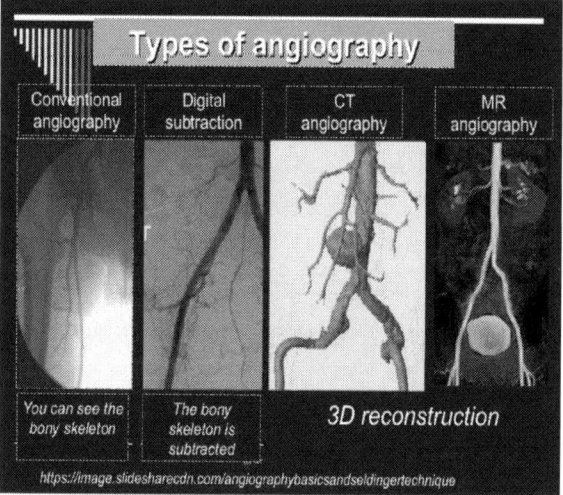

ANSWERS: a, b, & e. Cine and cut film are virtually outmoded with advances in digital imaging. Digital imaging is now state of the art at all major medical centers. It allows postprocessing and computer enhancements of images to improve quality.
  The 2nd diagram shows DSA image after subtraction, #3 shows a CT angiogram reconstruction, and #4 is an MRI angiogram.

719. How does spiral CT Angiography differ from Magnetic Resonance Angiography (MRA) for PAD? CTA uses _____ contrast, and _____ energy detectors.
  a. Gadolinium, X-ray
  b. Gadolinium, radio wave
  c. Iodine based, X-ray
  d. Iodine based, radio wave

ANSWER c. Iodine based, X-ray. Both use a

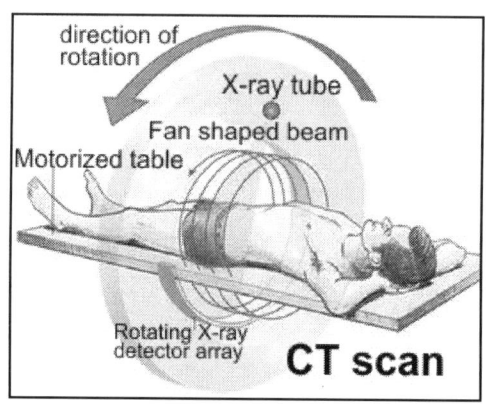

doughnut shaped detector gantry with rotating sensors, where the patient is moved through it's isocenter. CT (Computed Tomography) uses traditional radiographic contrast that absorbs ionizing X-ray radiation; where MRA uses a gadolinium contrast that is pulsed through a strong magnetic field to give off radio waves. Each is less invasive than peripheral arteriography because the contrast is only injected via a vein and must flow through the lungs, left heart and aorta before arriving at the leg arteries. Both use bolus chasing and both make 3-dimensional reconstruction of the anatomic image.

Topol says, "CTA has advantages over magnetic resonance angiography (MRA) in the case of patients with pacemakers and defibrillators and in those with metal clips, stents, or prostheses (no significant artifact is seen in CTA as opposed to MRA) and is significantly faster to perform as compared with MRA. However, CTA requires the use of iodinated contrast and entails exposure to ionizing radiation. Dose-saving algorithms are very effective in reducing radiation exposure and should be used whenever possible."

"The use of spiral CT angiography (CTA) in assessing lower extremity PAD has 93% sensitivity and 96% specificity in detecting >50% stenosis with high accuracy when compared with digital subtraction angiography.... Because CTA reconstructions allow three-dimensional assessment, significant disease may be detected by CTA but not be recognized by angiography,..." See Topol, chapter on Lower Extremity Interventions, 2012

720. When revascularization is expected on a patient's leg arteries, what is the gold standard imaging technique?
   a. CT Angiography (CTA)
   b. Magnetic Resonance Angiography (MRA)
   c. Digital Subtraction Angiography (DSA)
   d. Duplex Ultrasound with Doppler

ANSWER c. Digital Subtraction Angiography (DSA)
Topol says, "Despite recent advances in the noninvasive evaluation of lower extremity PAD, contrast angiography remains the gold standard.... Contrast angiography remains the most easily used and widely available imaging technique in patients with PAD of the lower extremity when revascularization is contemplated. Noninvasive technologies, such as MRA or CTA, may be used prior to contrast angiography to help identify the potential culprit lesion and plan the best approach to study such lesion (access point, catheter selection, etc.) invasively." See Topol, chapter on Lower Extremity Interventions, 2012

721. How long will it take make a contrast injection if the radiologist asks you to program the pressure injector to "12 for 90"?
   a. 6 sec
   b. 7.5 sec
   c. 10 sec
   d. 12 sec

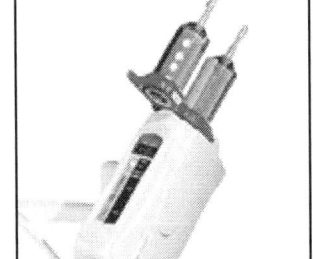

Medrad Injector

ANSWER b. 7.5 sec.
- Injection time = Volume / (flow rate)
- 90 ml / (12 ml/sec) = 7.5 sec.

Note how the ml units cancel out resulting in "seconds." "12 for 90" is a commonly used abbreviation for programming injectors.

The "12" is the flow rate, "90" the total volume. However, when abbreviations like this are unclear you should always respond to the radiologist "That will take 7.5 seconds" to be sure everyone understands. To be precise the injection is for 12 ml/sec for a total of 90 ml over 7.5 sec. **See:** Snopek, chapter of "Aortography."

722. You are running the pressure injector for a DSA on the right carotid artery of an adult patient. The radiologist wants Hexabrix injected 5 for 10 with a film sequence of 3/6. How will the films be exposed?
   a. 2/second for a total of 6 films
   b. 3/ second for a total of 6 films
   c. 3/second for a total of 18 films
   d. 5/second for 2 seconds for a total of 10 films

ANSWER c. 3/second for a total of 18 films with the imaging sequence lasting 6 seconds. So, 3/6 is shorthand for 3 images per second with a 6 second imaging run. So the product of the 2 numbers is the total number of images. Math is (3 images/sec) x 6 sec = 18 images), with the product being 3x6 or 18 total films.
   The first numbers (5 for 10) deal only with the injector settings and has nothing to do with the filming sequence. Only the numerators of the 2 settings are similar with the first number always being a rate/second. **See:** Schneider, chapter on "Arteriography", Table 4

723. With critical limb ischemia, which type of selective arteriogram filming often requires a long time delay of up to 15-20 seconds after aortic contrast injection?
   a. Tibeopedal
   b. Celiac/SMA
   c. Bilateral runoff
   d. Common femoral

ANSWER a. Tibeopedal arteriography (calf & foot) often shows slowed blood flow in the small arteries of the calf and foot, especially with critical limb ischemia. Schneider recommends filming 1/20 with a delay of 3-15 seconds. Most other arterial injection sites allow immediate filming with no delay after selective contrast injection.

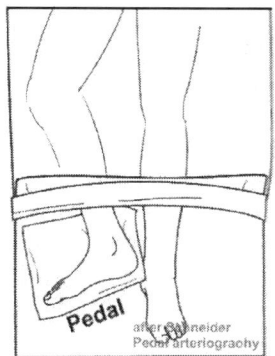

   Schneider says, "Contrast displaces what little blood is flowing to an ischemic foot, so arteriography causes discomfort, which prompts movement. This movement diminishes film quality, but also indicates the timing of the contrast flow to the foot....Once the transit time for contrast to flow from the injection site to the foot has been quantified, the delay can be programmed into the cut film sequence. Patients with very ischemic limbs may require a 20-second delay after administration of contrast into the femoral artery." **See:** Schneider, chapter on "Arteriography", Table 4

724. A patient with a resting a/b ratio of 0.4 has a resting blood pressure of 200/75 mmHg. This means that the systolic BP in the:
a. Lower leg is only 80 mmHg
b. Arm is only 80 mmHg.
c. Lower leg is only 40 mmHg
b. Arm is only 40 mmHg.

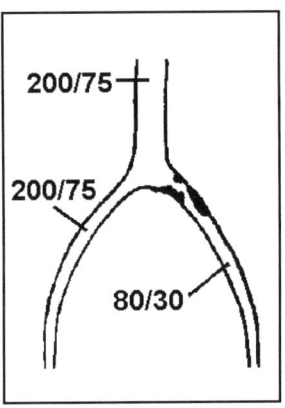

Segmental BP

ANSWER a. Systolic BP in the lower leg is only 80 mmHg. The a/b ratio is the ratio of ankle systolic BP to brachial BP, or 80/200 as shown here. These BP's are taken noninvasively using Doppler sounds and several BP cuffs on the leg. A 40% drop in resting BP is very significant. It usually indicates severe stenosis in the iliac or femoral artery. It will be further reduced on exercise.
See: Johnsrude, chapter on "Arteriography of Extremities."

725. What disease is suggested by the noninvasive segmental pressure recordings shown?
a. Severe right sided stenosis in iliac artery
b. Severe stenosis in right femoral artery
c. Severe stenosis in right peroneal artery
d. Severe left sided stenosis in posterior or anterior tibial artery

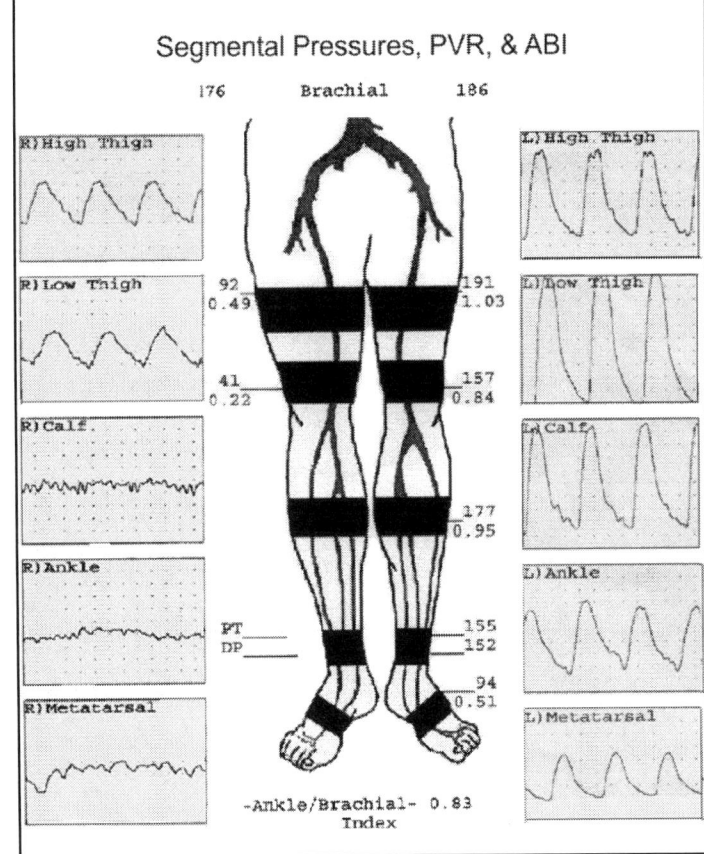

ANSWER: b. Severe stenosis in right femoral artery as the systolic pressure drops from 92 to 41 systolic and the pressure index ratio (ABI) from 0.49 to 0.22. An ankle brachial index of less than 0.40 suggests severe PAD. Segmental pressures in the calf cannot even be measured. Note how the right calf pressure waveform drops dramatically. The lower extremities are the most common location of PVD. Many BP cuffs are placed and many pressures taken after exercise.

Positioning Fem. Angio

See: Lanzer, chapter on "Abdominal AO, Iliac & Lower Extremity Disease" **Keywords:** Segmental pressures & ABI

726. A patient has claudication symptoms in only his left leg. To perform a unilateral left femoral arteriogram the radiologist wants to enter from the right femoral artery, pass the catheter across the iliac bifurcation, and down the left iliac artery. This is termed a/an _____ entry or approach.
   a. Ipsilateral
   b. Contralateral
   c. Retrograde
   d. Antegrade

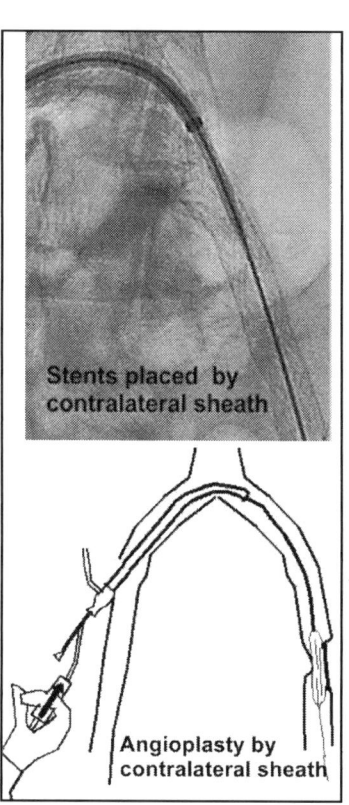

ANSWER b. Contralateral comes from "contra-" meaning "opposite." A contralateral approach is from the opposite side of the body, e.g. a stroke on one side of the brain effects the "contralateral" side of the body.
   Contralateral iliac sheaths like the Balkin sheath are long with a 90 degree bend at the tip specifically for this contralateral bifurcation approach.
   The Balkin sheath is designed to go up-and-over the iliac bifurcation. A standard puncture is made with the wire and placement catheter inserted into the contralateral femoral artery. The standard sheath is then replaced with a Balkin sheath. The Balkin curve then directs the wire and catheter antegrade down the contralateral femoral artery as shown.
   See: Johnsrude, chapter on "Equipment."

727. Noninvasive testing on your obese patient shows severe stenosis in both the right iliac and right common femoral arteries. What initial catheter access site would you recommend for iliofemoral angiography and intervention?
   a. Right common femoral retrograde (distal approach)
   b. Left common femoral antegrade (over aortic bifurcation)
   c. Right brachial (proximal approach)
   d. Translumbar (below 12th rib)

ANSWER b. Left common femoral antegrade (over aortic bifurcation). This is termed the contralateral approach, because it is on the side opposite the stenosis. Several sheath types make this common practice.
   Schneider says, "Infrarenal occlusive disease is usually approached with a retrograde femoral artery puncture on the side opposite the worst disease.... After attempting various maneuvers to cross a lesion, it is sometimes better to approach the lesion from the other end rather than force it and cause a complication. A second puncture is performed in the contralateral femoral artery, a catheter is passed over the aortic bifurcation, and the guidewire is advanced antegrade

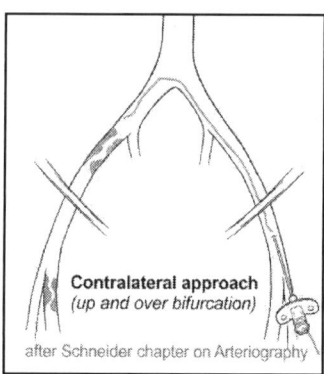

through the iliac lesion."
See: Schneider, chapter on "Arteriography"

728. Noninvasive testing shows severe stenosis in both common femoral arteries and in the right iliac artery. Right ABI is 0.2, left ABI is 0.3. What initial catheter access site would you recommend for iliofemoral angiography and stenting?
   a. Left common femoral retrograde (proximal approach)
   b. Left common femoral antegrade (over iliac bifurcation)
   c. Left brachial (proximal approach)
   d. Translumbar (below 12th rib)

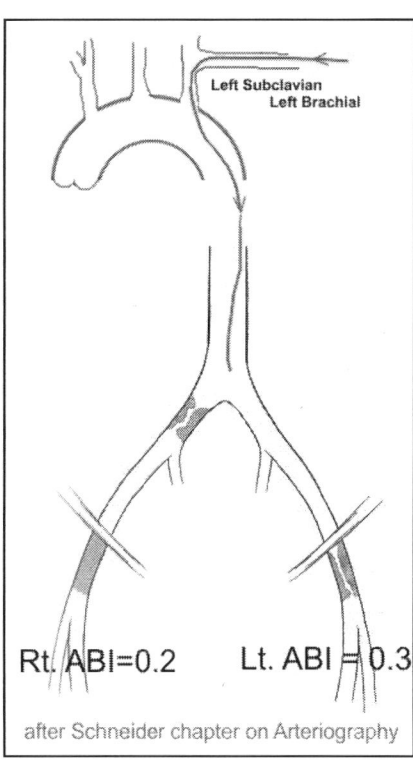

ANSWER c. Left brachial, or radial, is a proximal approach, where you can come down the aorta above the various stenoses. Note the catheter in the descending aorta image. This catheter would initially enter the brachial or radial artery retrograde, pass into the subclavian and aortic arch, and then pass antegrade down the aorta.

With an ABI of 0.2 and 0.3 both femoral stenosis are severe. Even if you accessed the left femoral artery retrograde below the stenosis you still may not be able to pass up through it. If it were possible to pass the left stenosis then up-and-over access might be a possibility. The brachial proximal approach requires very long catheters and may make manipulation difficult. Although the translumbar access is closest to the iliac bifurcation it is risky and would make catheter manipulation and stenting difficult.

Schneider says, "Severe common femoral artery occlusive disease is an indication for a proximal approach....through the brachial or axillary arteries."
See: Schneider, chapter on "Arteriography"

729. Your obese patient with extensive iliofemoral tortuosity has a history of claudication and TIAs. You are assigned to prep the patient for diagnostic runoff angiography. Which arterial access site would you recommend?
   a. Right femoral artery
   b. Left femoral artery
   c. Right radial artery
   d. Left radial artery

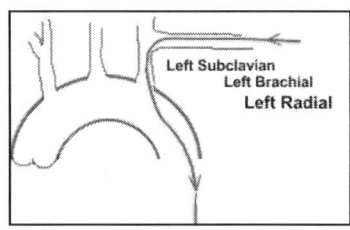

ANSWER: d. The left radial artery avoids the carotid arteries and the fatty groin. Entry into the left radial and left subclavian leads directly down the descending aorta.

Grossman says, "The transradial approach is particularly advantageous for patients with peripheral vascular disease or morbid obesity." **See:** Grossman, chapter on "Percutaneous Approach"

Lanzer says, "In peripheral interventions the left brachial artery is preferred because manipulation across the aortic arch with its attending risk of intracranial embolization is avoided, and the intravascular pathway is shortened." **See:** Lanzer, chapter on "Arteriography"

730. Your patient has severe claudication and has failed exercise and medical therapy. Patient's DSA shows a 60% diameter common iliac artery stenosis. Pressure wire shows a mean gradient of 15 mmHg across the lesion. When do current guidelines recommend <u>stenting</u> for symptomatic common iliac artery stenosis such as this?
   a. > 50% diameter stenosis >20 mmHg mean gradient
   b. > 50% diameter stenosis >10 mmHg mean gradient
   c. > 50% area stenosis >20 mmHg mean gradient
   d. > 50% area stenosis >10 mmHg mean gradient

ANSWER: b. > 50% diameter stenosis >10 mmHg mean gradient. This patient qualifies for stenting. Remember a 50% diameter stenosis is a 75% area stenosis. So a 50% area stenosis is only a small 33% diameter stenosis. These same criteria hold for similar patients with hemodynamically significant stenosis in the abdominal aorta, common iliac and external iliac arteries.

Current guidelines recommend: "Claudication: Provisional or primary stenting for external iliac artery >50% diam. Stenosis and/or resting mean or hyperemic translesional gradient >10 mmHg after having failed pharmacologic and supervised exercise therapy."

ACC/AHA Peripheral Artery Disease guidelines continue to support EVT [EndoVascular Therapy], with primary or provisional stenting, as first-line therapy for symptomatic aorto-iliac occlusive disease. Guidelines state that 'Endovascular procedures are effective as a revascularization option for patients with lifestyle limiting claudication and hemodynamically significant aorto-iliac occlusive disease'. Because of its high success rates and lower morbidity/mortality compared to surgical revascularization, EVT (Endovascular Therapy), with primary or provisional stenting may be considered a first-line treatment strategy for aorto-iliac disease" **See:** SCAI, appropriate use criteria for peripheral arterial interventions: an update 2017 online at:
http://onlinelibrary.wiley.com/doi/10.1002/ccd.27141/full

731. Noninvasive tests suggest that your patient has left bilateral femoral and popliteal stenoses. But the patient is allergic to iodinated contrast and has severely elevated creatinine and BUN blood tests. What contrast agent will be safest to use during the angiography and interventional procedure?
   a. CO2
   b. Gadolinium
   c. Ionic contrast with low iodine content (Hexabrix)
   d. Low osmolar nonionic contrast (Isovue or Visipaque)

ANSWER: a. CO2 gas. Remember elevated creatinine and BUN mean poor renal function and poor excretion of contrast. Neither Hexabrix, Visipaque nor Isovue have a low iodine content. Gadolinium may be considered for iodine allergy, but only if kidney function is normal.

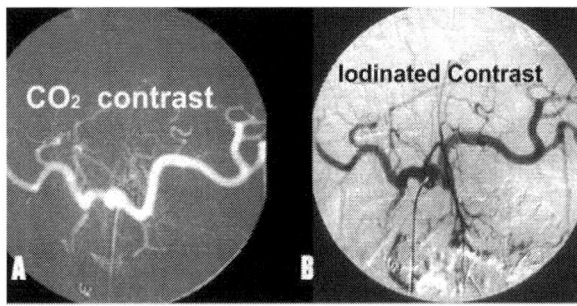

Schneider says, "CO2 is the only proven safe contrast agent in patients with iodinated contrast allergy and renal failure.... CO2 is useful for most interventional procedures of the iliac and lower-extremity arteries in patients with contrast allergy and renal failure. The advantages of the gas are the lack of allergy and renal toxicity, injection of unlimited volumes of CO2, and the low viscosity that permits the injection of CO2 between the needle or catheter and the guidewire.... CO2 can also be used during CT angiography.... Carbon dioxide has also been employed but has some distinct disadvantages. When CO2 encounters occlusive disease, it tends to break up into bubbles, making images difficult to interpret. Since it is a gas, it will rise. The patient must be positioned so that the CO2 will flow and not form an airlock. Brachiocephalic arteriography using CO2 is contraindicated since bubbles may cause stroke." **See:** Schneider, chapter on "Imaging."

Thomsen says, "Nephrotoxicity of gadolinium-based contrast agents when used for radiographic studies, CT and MRI has now been described in both man and animals with renal impairment. Nephrogenic systemic fibrosis is another important adverse reaction after some gadolinium-based contrast media in patients with renal impairment. Gadolinium-based contrast media should not be used as contrast agents for radiography, including CT, in patients with reduced renal function. Gadolinium-based contrast media may be helpful for radiography in patients with normal renal function who have had multiple severe adverse reactions to iodine-based contrast media." **See:** Radiography with Gadolinium-Based Contrast Media, Contrast Media, in Medial Radiology, Thomsen & Leander, https://link.springer.com/bookseries/174

6B. Limb Arteriography - Arms

732. Identify the major arm arteries labeled # 3 in the box (in the forearm - thumb side).
   a. Brachial
   b. Axillary
   c. Radial
   d. Ulnar
   e. Subclavian

LOCATION OF ARM ARTERIES
 1. Shoulder area
 2. Humorous area
*3. Forearm - thumb side
 4. Forearm - little finger side
 5. Thorax - beneath clavicle

ANSWER c. Radial artery. The major **subclavian** arteries become **axillary** vessels after exiting the thorax at the shoulder. Then in the arm the **axillary** becomes the **brachial** artery, and in the forearm becomes the **radial or ulnar** artery. The radial is the one you normally palpate when taking a pulse nearest the thumb. The axillary and brachial arteries are alternate arterial catheterization sites. Be able to ID all these vessels.

LOCATION	ARTERY
1. Shoulder area	Axillary artery
2. Humorous area	Brachial artery
3. Forearm - thumb side	Radial artery
4. Forearm - little finger	Ulnar artery
5. Beneath clavicle	Subclavian art.

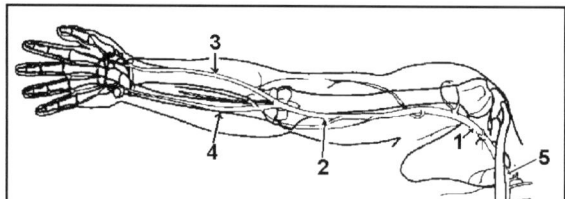
Arm arteries

See: *Grays Anatomy.* **Keywords:** Axillary artery > subclavian artery

733. A young woman has attacks of intermittent vasospasm in both of her hands when exposed to cold or if she becomes emotional. Her fingers become white, numb and painful. These signs and symptoms are most likely due to:
   a. Thromboangiitis Obliterans
   b. Atherosclerosis Obliterans
   c. Raynaud's Disease
   d. Takayasu's Arteritis

ANSWER c. Raynaud's disease is the cold finger disease of young women (feet may also become involved). The cooled fingers become pale then cyanotic. But immediately following the attack they turn red (rubor). This vasospastic action is of undetermined origin, although the defect is probably due to a defect in the sympathetic nervous system supplying the extremities. Sympathetic ganglion-ectomy usually cures the symptoms, especially if the feet are involved. Vasodilatory drugs such as alpha blockers, nifedipine, and/or nitroglycerin ointment may improve the vasoconstriction. Reduction in smoking also reduces vasoconstriction. **See:** Underhill, chapter on "Vascular Diseases." **Keywords:** Raynaud's disease - signs and symptoms

7. Cerebral Arteriography

734. A patient with an occluded right internal common carotid artery may not have signs of a stroke or TIA because of a:
   a. Circle of Willis arterial anastomosis
   b. Carotid sinus arterial anastomosis
   c. Venous plexus at the base of the brain
   d. Collateral circulation from the azygous system

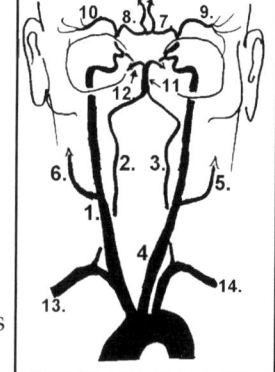
Circle Willis

ANSWER a. Circle of Willis arterial anastomosis. At the base of the brain the internal carotid artery and vertebral arteries form this remarkable circular anastomosis. It helps protect the brain against stroke. If any one of the major arteries feeding the brain occludes, this circle provides an automatic collateral pathway for redirection of blood. This diagram shows the circle of Willis where all arteries supplying the brain join. Note the circle made by #7 & 8 (Anterior cerebral arteries), on the side of the circle (#12 Right posterior communicating artery). **See:** Snopek, chapter on "Cerebral Angiography." **Keywords:** Circle of Willis

735. In this right lateral view of the major neck arteries, what artery appears stenosed?
a. Subclavian artery
b. Common carotid
c. External carotid artery
d. Internal carotid artery
e. Vertebral artery

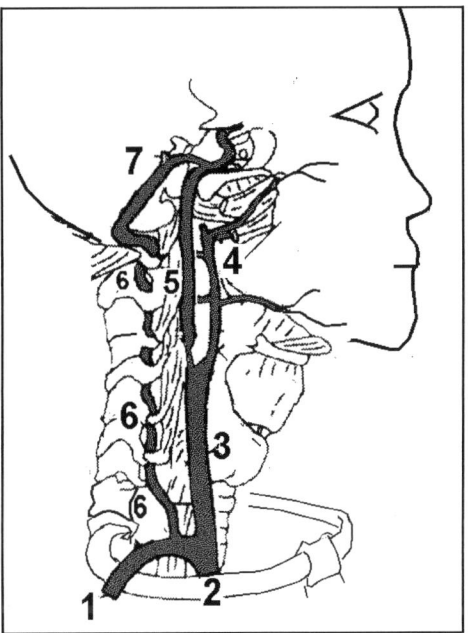
Rt. Sided neck arteries

ANSWER d. Internal carotid artery. This is a 70-80% stenosis in the carotid bulb area of the internal carotid artery, labeled #5.
LABELED ARTERIES ARE:
1. Subclavian artery
2. Innominate or brachio-cephalic artery
3. Common carotid artery
4. External carotid artery
5. Internal carotid artery
6. Right vertebral artery
7. Basilar artery

See: Snopek, chapter on "Cerebral Angiography." **Keywords:** Carotid, vertebral artery

736. Distal to a severe internal carotid stenosis you may see delayed flow through a long thin vessel. This skinny (but normal) vessel is termed:
a. Fibromuscular dysplasia
b. Atherosclerosis obliterans
c. String sign
d. Leriche sign

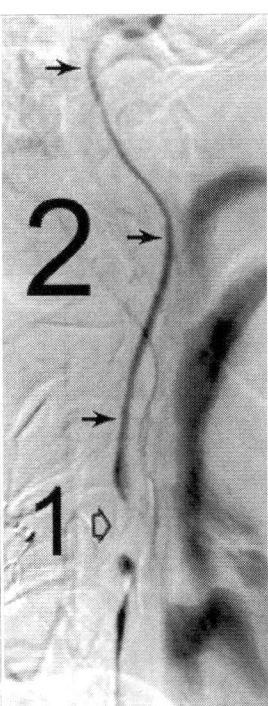
#2 string sign

ANSWER c. String sign. Pappus says, "Perfusion pressures distal to the [internal carotid] stenosis are reduced, which leads to subsequent collapse of the distal ICA vessel lumen and production of the string sign. This collapse is often a result of decreased flow and reduced arterial pressure rather than atherosclerotic disease. Despite the misleading arteriographic appearance of the distal collapsed ICA, the artery is typically not diseased, and there is usually opportunity for successful revascularization once the proximal lesion is repaired..." Not the severe ICA stenosis at the carotid bifurcation at #1. The long skinny ICA vessel distal is at #2.

A "Leriche" is a total occlusion in an aorto-iliac artery, leading to claudication of the buttocks or thighs and impotence in the male.
See: Johnsrude, chapter on "Equipment" and Wojtowycz, chapter on "Basic Principles..."

737. Contrast injections may be painful. In brachio-cephalic arteriography which of the following can be used to reduce pain? (Select 4.)
a. Use reduced strength contrast (<60%)
b. Use non-ionic contrast
c. Use low osmolar contrast
d. Mix local anesthetic (lidocaine) into the contrast
e. IV fentanyl and versed

ANSWERS: a, b, c, & e. Do not mix local anesthetic (lidocaine) into the contrast. Wojtowycz says, "...lidocaine is not combined with the newer media. Lidocaine should never be injected into the brachiocephalic vessels!" This is due to its cerebral effects.

Although some centers use lidocaine in the contrast to reduce pain during other types of peripheral injections, it is relatively ineffective compared to the other alternatives listed. If it is used, the lidocaine **must not have any epinephrine** in it - as local anesthetic often does. The pain is directly proportional to the strength and osmolarity of the contrast agent. Low-osmolar and non-ionic dyes are better tolerated, as are injections with lower concentration contrast medium. **See:** Johnsrude, chapter on "Equipment" and Wojtowycz, chapter on "Basic Principles..."

738. When evaluating a patient for suspected left internal carotid artery stenosis, the first arteriogram should be:
a. Aortic arch aortography
b. Selective left carotid arteriography
c. Selective right carotid arteriography
d. Selective bilateral vertebral arteriography

ANSWER a. Aortic arch aortography. Baim says, "To completely evaluate the cerebral circulation, carotid angiography should be performed in conjunction with arch aortography and selective vertebral angiography. Arch aortography is a crucial first step because it allows characterization of the arch configuration and optimal catheter selection." **See:** Grossman, chapter on "Angiography of AO & Peripheral Arteries."

Kern say, "...given the potential variability in arch configuration and the marked impact that anomalous configurations have on procedural technique, arch aortography is a critical first step." **See:** Kern, chapter on "Peripheral Arterial Disease and Angiography."

739. In which 2 types of cerebral catheterization studies are patients usually sedated with general anesthesia? (Select 2 below.)
a. Children under age of 10
b. Basilar artery stent procedures
c. Cerebral embolectomy procedures
d. Adults with recent history of stroke
e. Patients with tortuous aorto-iliac anatomy

ANSWERS: a & c. Children under age of 10 and cerebral embolectomy procedures. These may be painful procedures, especially for kids. **See:** Howard Riina, MD, Angiography and

Endovascular
Access, video at: https://www.youtube.com/watch?v=ycGKCQ0mUj8

740. **Carotid interventional procedures require careful and frequent catheter flushing and back-bleeding to prevent:**
a. Air embolism
b. Blood clotting in catheter
c. Cerebral aneurysm rupture
d. Dislodging atherosclerotic plaque

ANSWER a. Air embolism is even more critical in cerebral procedures than other types of studies because air or thrombus emboli to the brain may cause TIA or stroke. Catheter clotting is a problem if the thrombus is injected. Clotted catheters should be removed and discarded and certainly not flushed in the patient. Some physicians use a pressure bag for continuous infusion of saline through cerebral catheters and sheaths. Heparin is not added to the flush in embolization procedures because you want the embolized aneurysm to clot.
See: https://www.youtube.com/watch?v=ycGKCQ0mUj8

Kern says, "Meticulous procedural technique must be used during carotid and cerebral angiography. It is recommended that anticoagulation with heparin be achieved to prevent catheter- and/or wire-related thrombosis and embolism. Careful flushing and back-bleeding of every catheter must be performed to prevent air or thromboembolism."

Kessel says one of the "Key steps for safe embolization: Use non-heparinized saline to flush catheters and dilute contrast."
See: Kern, chapter on "Peripheral Arterial Disease and Angiography."

741. **Your cerebral angiography patient is being studied for a right internal carotid artery stenosis with aortogram as shown. Your physician has been unable to selectively cannulate from the arch with multipurpose and headhunter H1 catheters. He asks for a catheter with an "active" or "complex" bend. What catheter do you recommend?**
a. Double curve RDC
b. Judkins LCA or Amplatz Left
c. Simmons or Sidewinder
d. Berenstein or Multipurpose

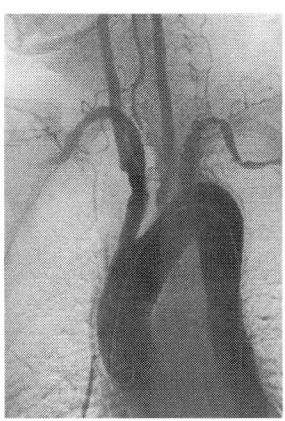

ANSWER c. Simmons or Sidewinder. This catheter uses the hooking maneuver by doubling it over and pulling it back into the brachiocephalic artery as shown. Type 1 arch is normal with the great vessels arising at right angles from the top of the arch. The type 3 arch like this one is hardest to cannulate, because the great vessels arise low and at a sharp angle to the aortic arch.

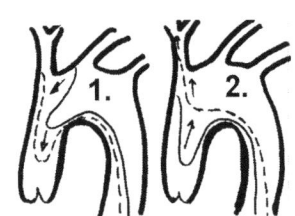

Kern says: "Various-shaped catheters are available for selective carotid and vertebral artery angiography. The catheters can be divided into three groups: passive, intermediate, and active shape designs. Use of a particular category of catheter will depend on the type of aortic arch and the geometry of the origins of the great vessels.

Passive catheters, such as headhunter, multipurpose, vertebral, and Berenstein, are used to access the great vessels in patients with a type-I aortic arch. Intermediate catheters, including the Vitek.. and Bentson..., require more manipulation than passive catheters and are ideal for type-II aortic arches. Active catheters including the Simmons, Sidewinder and Newton catheter are useful for type-II or -III arches but must be shaped in the ascending aorta and therefore may introduce the opportunity for release of atheroemboli." See: Kern, chapter on "Peripheral Arterial Disease and Angiography."

742. You are attempting to selectively catheterize the left subclavian with an H3 catheter. Further advancing the catheter pulls the tip and wire out of the vessel as shown. From the first position shown you should:
a. Pull out and rewire the vessel
b. Pull back the catheter to hook the vessel
c. Exchange catheter for a sidewinder bend
d. Advance the wire to straighten the catheter

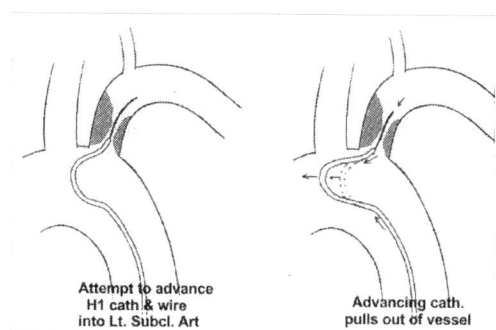

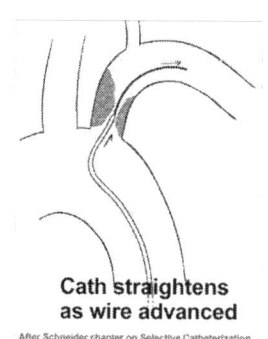

ANSWER d. Advance the wire to straighten the catheter. Guidewire tips are very soft and flexible. As the stiffer wire body is advanced into a catheter it straightens the bend as shown. This makes the catheter pushable and better directs the forward catheter pressure into the subclavian and past the stenosis as shown.

Schneider says, "Selective catheterization of the subclavian artery using a complex-curve catheter. The catheter, in this example an H3 Headhunter, is placed in the aortic arch proximal to the subclavian artery. The catheter is simultaneously withdrawn and selective guidewire is passed into the artery. The guidewire must be advanced gently because if forward pressure is applied too vigorously the catheter will pop out of the artery. As the guidewire passes into the artery, the catheter head straightens and the catheter may be advance." See: Schneider, chapter on "Arteriography"

8. Venography

743. The "Gold Standard" now used to diagnose deep vein thrombosis (DVT) is:
a. Clinical evaluation (leg tenderness, discoloration...)
b. Venography and pulmonary angiography (filling defect in vein)
c. B-mode ultrasound (compressing veins while imaging them)
d. Impedance plethysmography (changes in electrical "impedance" of the legs)

ANSWER c. B-mode ultrasound venous scan. Braunwald says "The introduction of B-mode ultrasonography has revolutionized the diagnosis of DVT... The inability to compress these veins is highly accurate indication of DVT proximal to the calf... B-mode ultrasound ...is so reliable, inexpensive, safe, and nontraumautic that it is rapidly supplanting leg phlebography as the Gold Standard." Phlebography (venography) is seldom done now.

AN EXPLANATION OF ALL ANSWERS FOLLOWS:

a. **CLINICAL EVALUATION** (leg tenderness, discoloration...): helpful but too variable.

b. **VENOGRAPHY AND PULMONARY ANGIOGRAPHY** (filling defect in vein): many deep veins are missed because the entry site bypasses them.

c. **B-MODE ULTRASOUND** (compressing veins while imaging them): The femoral and popliteal veins are imaged with a 2-D transducer in cross section. Slight pressure is applied to the transducer and a normal vein should compress easily. Clotted veins remain distended. Color flow Doppler imaging can also visualize blood flow and its absence. Now used extensively and very sensitive.

d. **IMPEDANCE PLETHYSMOGRAPHY** (changes in leg electrical resistance). The patient's legs and abdomen are encircled with metal tapes that conduct low voltage high frequency electricity. The electrical resistance changes in edematous thrombo-phlebitic legs. This test has been superseded by the more sensitive and specific B-mode ultrasound venous scan.

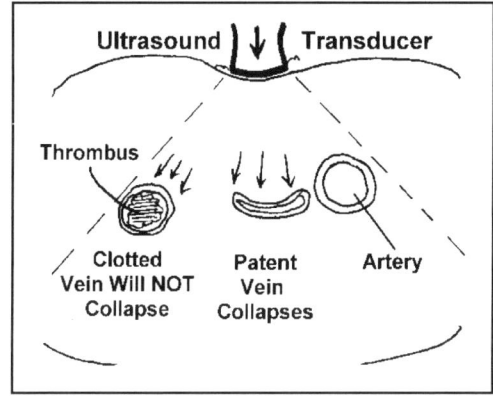

Diagnosis of DVT with ultrasound

See: Braunwald, chapter on "Pulmonary Embolism." **Keywords:** DVT → B mode ultrasound diagnoses

REFERENCES

Baim D. S. and Grossman W., *Cardiac Catheterization, Angiography, and Intervention,* 7th Ed., Lea and Febiger, 2006

Braunwald, et. al. Ed., *Heart Disease, a Textbook of CV Medicine,* 9th Ed., Saunders, 2012

Kern, M. J., Ed., *The Cardiac Catheterization Handbook,* 5th Ed., Mosby-Year Book, Inc., 2016

Hurst, J. W., and Logue, R. B., et. al., *THE HEART Arteries and Veins,* 3rd Ed., McGraw-Hill Book Co., 1995

Johnsrude, I. S., Jackson. D. C., et al., *A Practical Approach to Angiography,* 2nd Ed., Little, Brown and Co., 1987

Kandarpa, K., *Handbook of Cardiovascular and Interventional Radiologic Procedures,* 3rd Ed., Lippincott Williams and Williams, 2002

Lanzer, P., Editor, *Mastering Endovascular Techniques,* Lippincott, 2007

Schneider, Endovascular Skills, Guidewire and Catheter Skills or Endovascular Surgery, 2nd Edition, 1998

Snopek, A. M., *Fundamentals of Special Radiographic Procedures,* 3rd Ed., W.B. Saunders, 1992

Topol, Eric, Textbook of Interventional Cardiology, Elsevier, 6th edition, 2012

Taylor, E. J. Ed., *Dorland's Medical Dictionary,* 27th Eed., W. B. Saunders Co.,1988

Underhill, S. L., Ed., *CARDIAC NURSING,* 2nd Ed., J. B. Lippincott Co., 1989

Valji, Karim, *Vascular and Interventional Radiology,* W.B. Saunders, 1999

Wojtowycz, M., *Handbooks in Radiology, Interventional Radiology and Angiography,* 1st Ed., Year Book Medical Publishers, Inc., 1990

OUTLINE: Peripheral Vascular

2. GENERAL VASCULAR
   a. Abbreviations
      i. CFA
      ii. DSA
      iii. SMA
      iv. PTA
      v. DVT
      vi. IVP
      vii. DP
      viii. HU
      ix. BUN
      x. PFA
      xi. NG
      xii. KUB

3. VASCULAR PROCEDURES
   a. Approaches
      (1) Femoral A.
         (a) contralateral (retrograde)
         (b) distal - proximal approach
      (2) Brachial A.
         (a) L. Brachial avoids carotids
      (3) Axillary A.
      (4) Antegrade (levophase) in right heart
      ii. Anesthesia
         (1) General - ebolization & children
         (2) Local - not if general anesthesia
         (3) Conscious sedation
      iii. Medications
         (1) Priscoline, portal dilator
         (2) Heparin, LMWH
         (3) Thrombolytics
         (4) CO_2 contrast
         (5) Gadolinium contrast

4. AORTOGRAPHY
   a. EQUIPMENT
      i. Catheters, Aortography flood
         (1) Pigtail flood
         (2) Selective
            (a) Active - vs. - passive
            (b) Sidewinder, Simmons
            (c) Headhunters
            (d) Berenstein
         (3) Longer lengths for arch/head
      ii. CTAngiogram
         (1) arm vein injection
         (2) Iodinated contrast
         (3) Bolus chasing
         (4) X-radiation
      iii. MRAngiogram
         (1) arm vein injection
         (2) Gadolinium contrast
         (3) Bolus chasing
         (4) Magnetic pulse - radio waves
      iv. DSA = Dig. Subtraction Angiog.
         (1) Arterial injection
         (2) Iodinated contrast
         (3) Bolus chasing
         (4) X-radiation
   b. VIEWS
      i. Arch 30-40 degree LAO
      ii. Townes & waters cerebral views
   c. AORTOGRAMS
      i. Anatomy of the Aorta and its branches
      ii. Arch: asc, descending (Left sided)
      iii. Arch vessels: innom. subc., vert, mam, carotids
      iv. Abd. Ao.: celiac, hepatic, gastric, splenic, renal,
      v. mesenteric, iliac
   d. AORTIC PATHOLOGY
      i. Ao sinus aneurysm/fistula
      ii. Ao aneurysm
         (1) Fusiform/saccular
         (2) True/false aneurysm
         (3) Debakey Classification (I, II, & III)
         (4) Daily Classification (A & B)
      iii. Dissection
      iv. PDA
      v. Coarctation

5. PULMONARY ANGIOGRAPHY
   a. Risks and contraindications to Pulm. Angiog.
      i. pulmonary hypertension high death rate if RVedp >20
      ii. use balloon occlusion angio. method
      iii. use Lidocaine freely if PVCs
      iv. Identify catheter in PA
   b. Imaging methods used in Pulm. Angiog.
      i. Ultrasound = Gold Standard
         (1) Duplex
         (2) B mode
         (3) DVT
      ii. Large cut film methods -outdated
         (1) Program 3 f/s x 4 sec - 2 f/s x 2 sec - 1 f/s x 4 sec.
            (a) PA phase peaks 2-4 sec after start of injection
            (b) Pulmonary venous phase 5-7 sec
            (c) Systemic arterial phase 7-10 sec
         (2) High resolution
         (3) Large field size (see entire lung)
      iii. Fluoro / cine
         (1) smallest field size
         (2) see 1 lobe only
         (3) flow through motion seen
      iv. DSA
         (1) Roadmap
         (2) subtraction, eliminate bones
      v. MRI
         (1) Gadolinium contrast

c. Discuss interpretation of Pulmonary Angiograms for:
   i. filling defects
   ii. abrupt vessel cutoff
   iii. oligemia
   iv. asymmetry of flow
d. Pulmonary wedge angiography
   i. wedged Swan-Ganz
   ii. hand injection into distal port
   iii. fills segments of PA
   iv. no washout until balloon deflated

6. ABDOMINAL ARTERIOGRAPHY
   a. Abdominal arteries
      i. Branches of Aorta
      ii. gastric
      iii. celiac - use lateral view
      iv. superior mesenteric
      v. posterior mesenteric
      vi. renal arteries
         (1)
      vii. testicular or ovarian
      viii. inferior mesenteric
      ix. common hepatic artery
      x.
   b. Kidney
      i. Minor Calyx
      ii. Major Calyx
      iii. Ureter
      iv. renal artery
   c. Cholangiogram
      i. Ducts
   d. Renal Disease
      i. -Fibromuscular Disease (FMD) = string of pearls
      ii. -Atherosclerotic stenotic disease
         (1) pressure gradient criteria
         (2) stenosis diam. & area criteria
   e. Portal system
      i. -Portal vein
      ii. -Superior Mesenteric vein
      iii. -Inferior Mesenteric vein
      iv. -Hepatic vein
      v. -Splenic vein

7. ARTERIOGRAPHY OF LIMBS
   a. LEG
      i. Equipment
         (1) CTA
         (2) MRA
         (3) DSA
         (4) stepping table
         (5) Injector sequences
         (6) films/sec, number of seconds
      ii. Reducing pain from Fem angio.
         (1) -Use reduced strength contrast (<60%)
         (2) -non-ionic contrast
         (3) -low osmolar contrast
         (4) -local anesthetic (lidocaine) in contrast
         (5) -Fentanyl and versed IV
      iii. Positioning - toes in
      iv. Noninvasive Vascular studies
         (1) Sequential Arterial Pressure
            (a) Reactive Hyperemia
            (b) claudication
      v. Anatomy Leg
         (1) anterior tibial artery
         (2) lateral malleolar branch
         (3) medial malleolar branch
         (4) posterior tibial artery
         (5) peroneal artery
         (6) dorsalis pedis artery of foot
         (7) Popliteal artery
         (8) Pelvic arteries
      vi. Anatomy Alio-femoral
         (1) external iliac artery
         (2) internal iliac artery
         (3) femoral (superficial) artery
         (4) Deep (profundus) femoral
         (5) Superior iliac circumflex artery
         (6) deep iliac circumflex artery
         (7) inguinal ligament
         (8) middle sacral artery
   b. ARM
      i. Anatomy
         (1) Subclavian A
         (2) axillaryA
         (3) radial A
         (4) palmar
         (5) deep brachial
         (6) radial collateral a.
         (7) brachial artery
         (8) Ulnar collateral
         (9) ulnar artery
      ii. Takayau's Arteritis
      iii. Raynaud's Disease

8. CEREBRAL
   a. Anatomy -Neck Arteries
      i. -subclavian artery
      ii. -common carotid
      iii. -external carotid artery
      iv. -internal carotid artery
      v. -vertebral artery
   b. Anatomy - Internal Carotid Arteries
      i. -sylvian artery
      ii. -frontopolar artery
      iii. -Ophthalmic
      iv. -Anterior medial frontal
      v. -Intermediate medial frontal (collosomarginal)
      vi. -Pericollosol
      vii. -Middle cerebral artery group
      viii. -Internal carotid
      ix. -Anterior cerebral
   c. Anatomy Vertebral Arteries
      i. Basilar A.
   d. Anatomy - Circle of Willis
      i. -anterior communicating
      ii. -anterior cerebral
      iii. -Internal Carotid
      iv. -middle cerebral
      v. -posterior communicating
      vi. -posterior cerebral
      vii. -superior cerebral
      viii. -Pontine

ix. -basilar
x. -vertebral arteries
xi. -anterior spinal artery

9. VENOGRAPHY & LYMPHOGRAPHY
    a. Varicose veins
        i. -leaky venous valves
    b. Diagnosis of Deep Vein Thrombosis
        i. B Mode Ultrasound

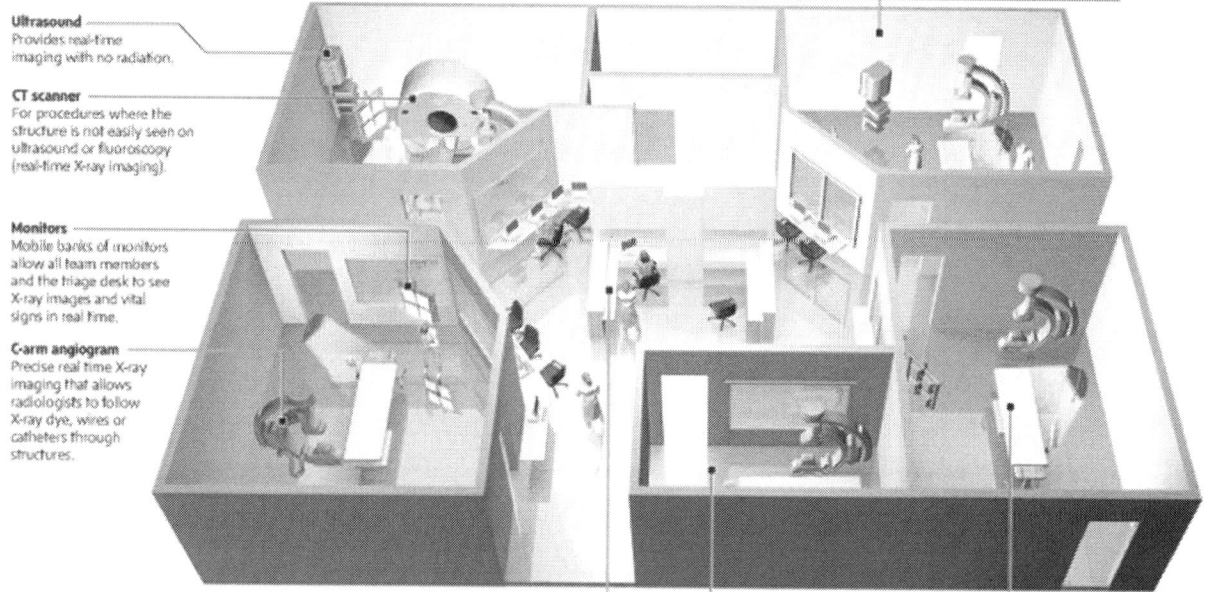

ECG I and ARRHYTHMIAS

INDEX: D11 - ECG1 and Arrhythmias
1. General ECG
   a. General & Terms . . . . p. 423 - Know
   b. Normal Anatomy & Physiology . . p. 426 - Know
   c. Abnormal Anatomy & Physiology . . p. 427 - Know
2. Tracings, Equipment & Measurements
   a. Equipment . . . . . p. 432 - Know
   b. Artifacts . . . . . . p. 434 - Know
   c. Leads & Techniques . . . . p. 436 - Know
   d. Measurements . . . . . p. 437 - Know
   e. Axis & Vectors . . . . . p. 440 - Review
   f. Combined Measurements . . . p. 442 - Know
3. Arrhythmias
   a. Sinus . . . . . . p. 445 - Know
   b. Atrial . . . . . . p. 446 - Know
   c. Junctional . . . . . p. 450 - Know
   d. Ventricular . . . . . p. 450 - Know
   e. Other . . . . . . p. 458 - Know
   f. ACLS Therapy . . . . . p. 459 - Know
4. Chapter Outline . . . . . p. 463

1A. General ECG - General & Terms

744. Match the general class of ECG rhythm labeled #6 (delayed beat, from a lower pacemaker) with its name below.
a. Flutter
b. Fibrillation
c. Arrest
d. Tachycardia
e. Bradycardia
f. Premature
g. Escape
h. Block
I. Paroxysmal

CLASSES OF ARRHYTHMIAS & RHYTHMS	
1.	Slowed or interrupted conduction
2.	Cessation of activity
3.	Chaotic rapid beating (over 300 bpm)
4.	Rapid, but very regular beating (over 200 bpm)
5.	Beat which occurs too soon, early
*6.	**Delayed beat, from lower pacemaker**
7.	Rate over 100 bpm
8.	Rate under 60 bpm
9.	Sudden rhythm or rate change

ANSWER g. Escape. When the normal pacemaker fails to elicit a stimulus for one or more cycles, an impatient ectopic focus fires, this beat is termed an ESCAPE beat. **CORRECTLY MATCHED ANSWERS ARE:**

CLASSES OF ARRHYTHMIAS & RHYTHMS
1. Block = Slowed or interrupted conduction (as in BBB or 3° heart block)
2. Arrest = Cessation of activity (as in SA arrest)
3. Fibrillation = Chaotic rapid beating (over 400 bpm)
4. Flutter = Rapid, but very regular beating (usually over 200 bpm)
5. Premature = Beat which occurs too soon, early (as in PVC)
6. Escape = Delayed beat, from lower pacemaker (as in junctional escape)
7. Tachycardia = Rate over 100 bpm (as in ventricular tachycardia)
8. Bradycardia = Rate less than 60 bpm (or <50 in young athletes)
9. Paroxysmal = Sudden rhythm or rate change (as is paroxysmal atrial tachycardia)

See: Dubin, chapter on "Rhythm."

745. Identify the irregular ECG conduction pattern labeled #3 in the ECG and ladder diagram shown.
  a. Normal sinus rhythm (NSR)
  b. AV junctional beat (PJC)
  c. Ectopic atrial beat (PAC)
  d. Ectopic ventricular beat (PVC)

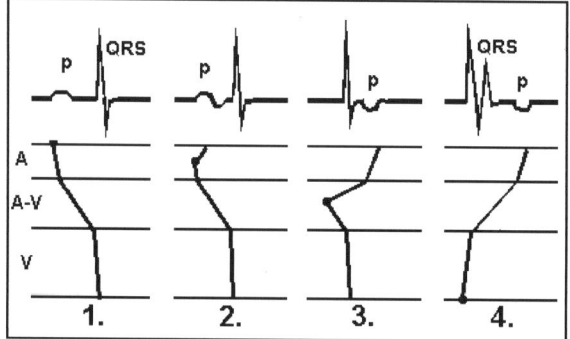

ECG conduction patterns and Ladder diag.

ANSWER b. AV junctional beat (PJC). The ladder diagram depicts depolarization and conduction schematically. Straight or slightly slanting lines drawn on a tiered framework represent electrical events occurring in various cardiac structures (SA or atrium, AV node and junction, and ventricle. The diagram represent electrical activity against a time base. Conduction is indicated by the lines of the ladder diagram sloping in a left-to-right direction. A steep line depicts rapid conduction. This drawing shows the ECG tracing that would be associated with each ladder diagram.

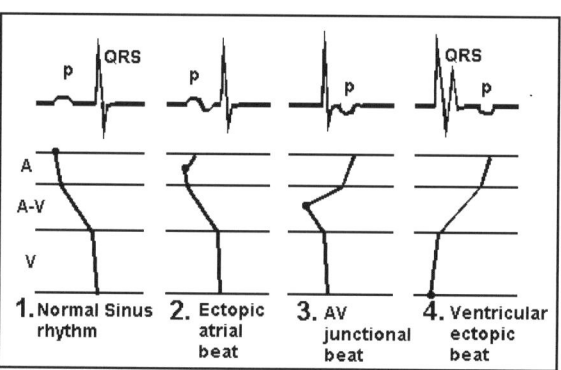

ECG conduction patterns & Ladder diag.

Activity originating in an ectopic site such as the AV junction, is indicated by a dot in that tier of the ladder. Depolarization proceeds rapidly down into the ventricle with a narrow QRS, indicated by the steep line in the V region. Depolarization also proceeds slowly up into the atrium with a delayed and inverted p wave. The T waves are not depicted in a ladder diagram.

See: Braunwald, chapter on "Specific Arrhythmias: Diagnosis and Treatment." **Keywords**: Ladder diagram, ectopic beats

746. If an ideoventricular pacemaker "escapes" it will usually fire at a rate of:
a. 10-20 bpm
b. 30-40 bpm
c. 60-80 bpm
d. 100-200 bpm

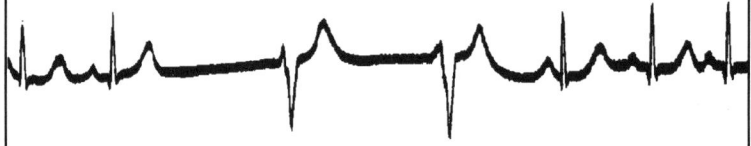

ANSWER b. 30-40 bpm. The ideoventricular pacemaker is the slowest escape rhythm. It is the heart's last resort when all other pacemakers fail. Our hearts have different levels of automatic - "escape" pacemakers to prevent asystole. These "potential" escape pacemakers and their usual rates are:
•Junctional (nodal)   = 40-50 bpm
•Ventricular   = 30-40

The SA node is like a teacher in control of the class. Myocardial cells are like students, they only pay attention to the fastest leader. When the teacher speaks at a normal rate (SA node rate around 60 bpm) everyone follows. But if a fast jazz band were to prance through the hall it would take the students' attention, like an ectopic focus. The teacher then loses control.

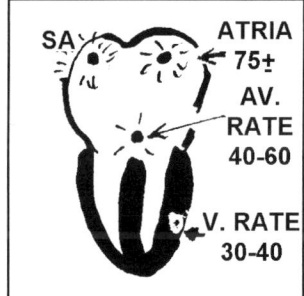

Latent Pacer Rates

Also, if the teacher is too slow, he loses the class' attention - as in sinus bradycardia. A quicker student may stand up and take over. This is analogous to a lower pacemaker that "escapes" at a rate faster than the SA node. A junctional rate of 50 can take over when the sinus node rate falls below 50 bpm.
See: Dubin, chapter on "Rate" **Keywords:** Automaticity, escape pacemakers

747. An impulse may be conducted into part of the conduction system and then dissipate. Since it is not conducted completely through that tissue it may cause refractoriness or distort impulse formation of that tissue. This is termed:
a. Reentry
b. Parasystole
c. Concealed conduction
d. AV block

ANSWER c. Concealed conduction. Since the original impulse dissipates within the tissue, the ECG shows NO impulse, except for its influence on tissue conduction or impulse formation. For example, in ventricular bigeminy, the sinus beat following the PVC is not conducted down the AV node. This is because the AV node and His bundle are still refractory from the concealed retrograde conduction of the PVC into the AV node. Thus, the compensatory pause. **See:** Underhill, chapter on "Arrhythmias." **Keywords:** Concealed conduction

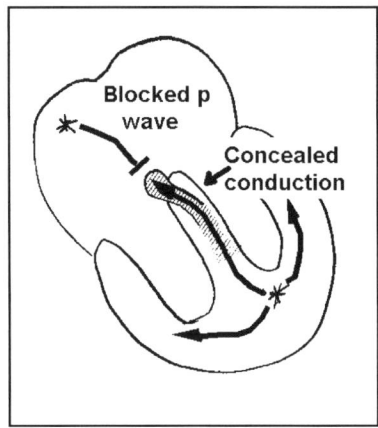

Concealed conduction makes AV node refractory

748. A junctional (nodal) premature contraction may send its impulse upward as well as downward. This may cause a depolarization wave to travel up the atrium in a reverse direction. These inverted "P" waves in lead II are termed:

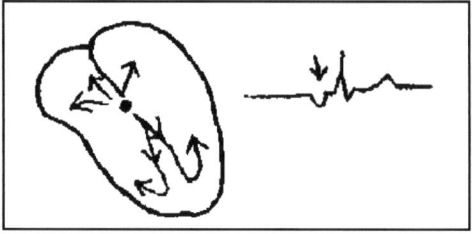

a. Aberrant
b. Antegrade
c. Refractory
d. Retrograde

ANSWER d. Retrograde. Depolarization waves traveling in the wrong direction are termed "retrograde." AV nodal or junctional beats typically conduct into the atria retrograde. These inverted "P" waves may occur with a short P-R interval, in the QRS, or in the ST segment. Ventricular complexes may also conduct retrograde through the AV node into the atria.
See: Braunwald, chapter on "Electrocardiography." **Keywords:** Retrograde conduction

1B. General ECG - Normal Anatomy & Physiology

749. On this ECG identify the segment, wave or interval labeled at #5 in the diagram.
a. "P" wave
b. ST segment
c. PR interval
d. "R" wave
e. RS (QRS)
f. QT interval
g. "T" wave
h. "S" wave

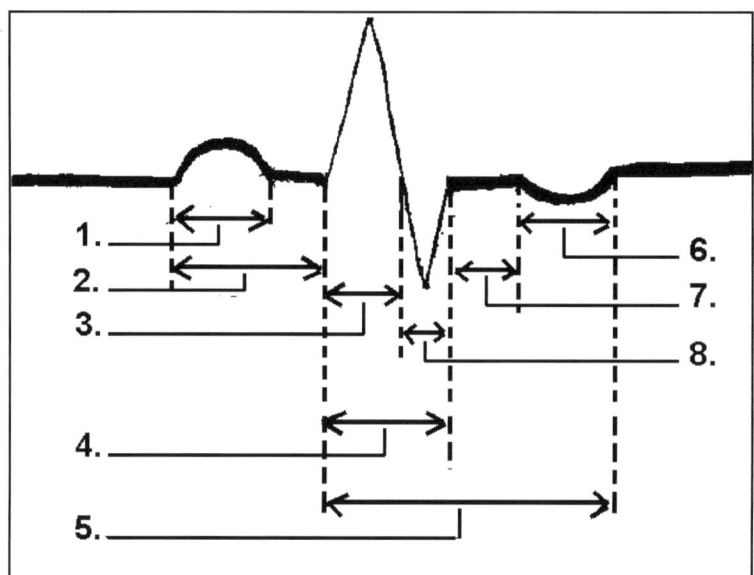

ANSWER f. QT interval. Note that ECG "intervals" are combinations of "waves" plus "segments", e.g. QT interval = QRS waves + ST segment + "T" wave.
  1. "P" wave
  2. PR interval
  3. "R" wave (is always above the baseline)
  4. RS (QRS) is always above then below the baseline
  5. QT interval
  6. "T" wave

7. ST segment
8. "S" wave (is always below the baseline)

See: Davis, chapter on "IV Determination of HR and Normal Heart Rhythms." **Keywords:** ECG intervals, segments & waves

1C. General ECG - Abnormal Anatomy & Physiology

750. The impulse's principal delay in the passage from the SA node to the ventricular myocardial cells occurs in the:
a. Atrial muscle
b. Specialized atrial conduction fibers
c. AV node (upper regions AN-N)
d. AV node (lower region -NH)

ANSWER c. The AV node (upper region) is where the principal AV delay occurs. The slowed conduction occurs in the upper ("AN" and "N") regions of the node. The conduction velocity here is 10 times slower than in the ventricular Purkinje cells. The proper AV delay (PR interval) allows the atrial kick to pack the ventricle with just enough blood (preload) before contraction to optimize systole.

With increased sympathetic tone (e.g., exercise) the AV conduction speeds and the PR interval shortens (dromotropism = increased AV conduction).
See: Underhill, chapter on "ECG" **Keywords:** AV node delay

751. Which of the following is the normal conduction sequence after an electrical impulse has traveled through the AV node?
a. Bundle branches, Bachmann's bundle, Purkinje fibers
b. Bundle branches, bundle of His, Purkinje fibers
c. Bundle of His, bundle branches, Purkinje fibers
d. Purkinje fibers, His bundle, AV junction

ANSWER c. Bundle of His, bundle branches, Purkinje fibers. The sequence is:
- SA node
- Inter-atrial tracts (including *Bachmann's bundle)
- AV Node
  AN = Transitional tissue between atria and AV node
  N = Mid AV nodal tissue (most of the AV time delay occurs in these upper 2 regions of the AV node)
  NH = region where nodal fibers gradually merge with bundle of His tissue
  His = the upper portion of ventricular conduction tissue
- Bundle of HIS
- Right and left bundle branches (Left has 2 fascicles, anterior & posterior)
- Purkinje system - to myocardium

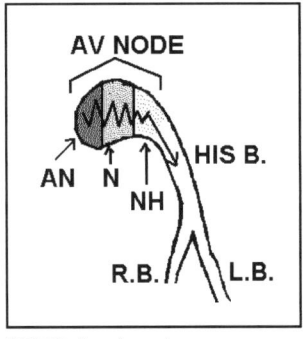

ECG Activation

See: Underhill, chapter on "Cardiac Electrophysiology." **Keywords:** Electrical activation sequence AV, HIS, BB, Purkinje

752. Normal interventricular conduction proceeds from the bundle of His through three major fascicles. Identify these 3 major interventricular fascicles from below.
   a. Right bundle branch
   b. Right posterior fascicle
   c. Left anterior fascicle
   d. Left posterior fascicle
   e. Left lateral fascicle

ANSWERS: a, c, & d. The 3 branches of the conduction system are the: right bundle branch, left anterior fascicle, and left posterior fascicle. The 2 branches of the left bundle go to the 2 papillary muscles attached to the anterior and posterior mitral valve leaflets. This division of the left bundle into 2 is analogous to the way the main left coronary divides into 2 major branches to supply the LV. There is also a common main left bundle between the His and left fascicle division analogous to the main left coronary artery. As with the right coronary, the right bundle branch supplies the RV.
See: Davis, chapter on "IV Conduction Abnormalities." **Keywords:** 3 fascicles

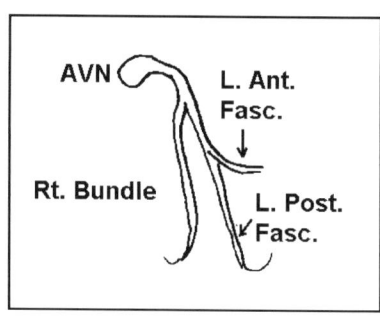
Vent. Conduction

753. When one of the three conduction fascicles becomes blocked it is termed:
   a. 1st degree block
   b. Unidirectional block
   c. Hemiblock
   d. Bifasicular block

ANSWER c. Hemiblock. If any one of these fascicles is blocked, it is a hemiblock. When any 2 fascicles become blocked, it is termed a bi-fascicular block. Any type of bundle branch block (BBB) prolongs the QRS complex and deviates the QRS axis from normal. This diagram shows a right bundle branch block, which is a hemiblock.
See: Underhill, chapter on "Cardiac Electrophysiology."
Keywords: hemiblock

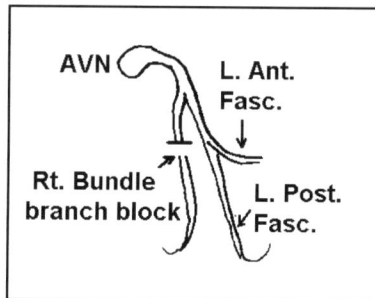
Right bundle branch block

754. The most common dysrhythmia found in SUDDEN DEATH patients is:
   a. Ventricular tachycardia
   b. Ventricular fibrillation
   c. Complete heart block
   d. Asystole

ANSWER b. Ventricular fibrillation. Most sudden deaths are cardiovascular and of these 62% are attributed to ventricular fibrillation (VF) in patients following myocardial infarction. Most of the remainder are due to asystole or severe bradyarrhythmias. Most ventricular tachycardia (VT) is slow enough to sustain a pulse, but it may degenerate into ventricular fibrillation (VF), which, of course, cannot sustain a pulse.
See: ACLS Manual, chapter on "Sudden Death." **Keywords:** Sudden death = ventricular fibrillation

755. Which of the following abnormal accessory pathways may allow a stimulus to bypass the atrio-ventricular node and "pre-excite" the ventricle?
   a. Internodal tracts
   b. Bachmann's bundle
   c. Bundle of Kent
   d. Right or left fascicles

ANSWER c. Bundle of Kent is the common term for any abnormal accessory AV conduction bundle. It is like an extra AV node conducting between atria and ventricle, except it has NO DELAY. It may short circuit and bypass the AV node. This causes pre-excitation (WPW) with a short PR interval. It may create a reentry loop between the normal AV-His-Purkinje network and the accessory bypass tract. This can lead to tachy-arrhythmia. The type shown is the most common type of Kent bundle termed an "atrioventricular" bypass tract. These accessory bundles can be anywhere along the AV groove, on the right or left side. The bypass tracts can also be attached to the AV node, termed, "*nodo-ventricular*" bypass tract or to the His tissue termed a "*atrio-Hisian*" bypass tract. A coronary sinus catheter can usually get close to and record impulses from a left sided accessory pathway.

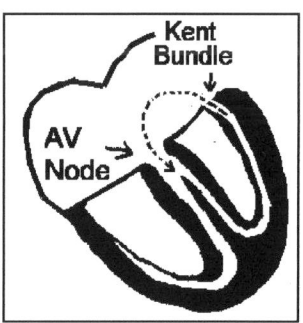

Kent Bundle Accessory pathway

See: Braunwald, chapter on "Electrocardiography." **Keywords:** Bundle of Kent

756. How does a PVC normally affect the blood pressure? The systolic BP associated with the PVC will _____ in pressure, and the following sinus beat will _____ in pressure.
   a. Increase, Decrease
   b. Increase, Increase
   c. Decrease, Decrease
   d. Decrease, Increase

ANSWER d. PVC BP decreases, Post PVC BP increases. The long compensatory pause following the PVC allows for more LV filling and thus a stronger ejection. Patients normally don't feel PVCs - but instead the large surge of blood pumped during the post-PVC beat.
See: Braunwald, chapter on

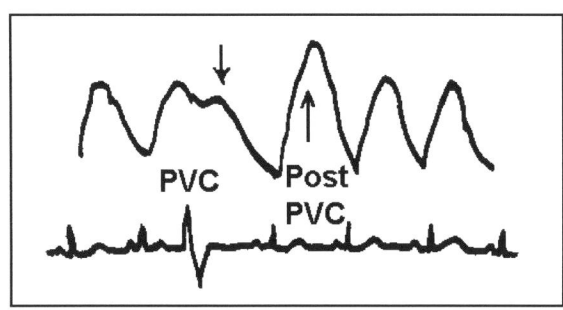

Effect of PVC and post-PVC

"Electrocardiography." **Keywords:** BP increased post PVC

757. Non-compensated pauses are most often seen after a _____ and compensatory pauses are seen after a/an _____.
   a. PAT, PVC
   b. PVC, PAC
   c. PJT, PAT
   d. PAC, PVC

ANSWER d. PAC, PVC. Since PACs (Premature Atrial Complexes) originate in the atria they often penetrate and "reset" the SA node. The SA pacemaker then starts over and resumes firing at the set rate. PVCs (Premature Ventricular Contractions) are not usually conducted retrograde into the atria and may not reset the SA node. The normal "P" wave usually falls in the refractory period of the AV node and is not conducted. This makes the long compensatory pause following most PVCs.
See: Dubin, chapter on "Rhythm." **Keywords:** Compensatory, non-compensatory pauses

758. Extreme bradycardia or asystole frequently leads to syncope or "seizure-like" convulsion. What is this syndrome termed?
   a. Stokes-Adams
   b. Cushing's
   c. Maladie de Roger
   d. Eisenmenger's

ANSWER a. Stokes-Adams (or Adams-Stokes syndrome). When insufficient blood supplies the brain, the patient convulses and goes unconscious. Frequently the eyes roll back and the patient swallows his tongue and gags. The physical convulsion, impact of falling, or recumbent position may be enough to restore consciousness.
See: Medical dictionary **Keywords:** Adams-Stokes/ Stokes-Adams syndrome

759. The imbalance in electrical charge across a cardiac cell membrane is known as:
   a. Polarizing potential
   b. Trans-membrane potential
   c. Ionic channel polarization
   d. Resting membrane potential

ANSWER: b. Trans-membrane potential. These imbalances generate the voltages of the cardiac action potentials. Voltages shown are the voltages inside the cell, relative to the outside of the cell.

760. The cardiac muscle resting interior membrane potential is approximately?
a. +60 mV
b. +90 mV
c. -60 mV
d. -90 mV

ANSWER: d. -90 mV. There are more negative charges inside the muscle cell that average -80 to -100 mV. It is rather like a defibrillator that is charged up. All it takes is for the rapid sodium channels to open and BAM it depolarizes to 0 volts as positive sodium ions rush in. The SA node has a smaller resting voltage around -60 mV.

761. The "ventricular action potential" is comprised of how many phases?
a. 2 Phases
b. 3 Phases
c. 4 Phases
d. 5 Phases

ANSWER: d. 5 Phases. These phases are 0, 1, 2, 3 & 4 You will learn what each phase is and how it relates to the ECG.
- Phase 0: Depolarization upstroke (SA node Ca++ influx, Muscle NA+ influx), P wave or QRS
- Phase 1: Peak, late QRS
- Phase 2: Plateau, time of systole & refractory period
- Phase 3: Repolarization, T wave, vulnerable period
- Phase 4: Resting, restoration of ionic balance, diastole

762. What ion flow across the cardiac muscle cell wall causes it to fire/depolarize?
a. Na+ influx
b. Ca++ influx
c. K+ efflux
d. Cl- efflux

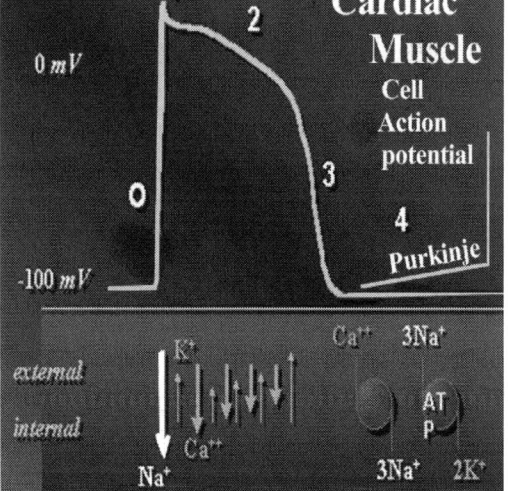

ANSWER: a. Na+ influx. These are termed the FAST channels, because it happens fast. Depending on the muscle cell, it results in the P wave or QRS complex on the ECG. The "firing" is the rapid upstroke of the square wave. There are many ionic channels and exchanges shown in the diagram. See white arrow for rapid depolarization. Purkinje cells have a slowly rising phase 4 which gives them automaticity (20-30 bpm in ventricle). Because of their rapid upstroke, Purkinje cells have the fastest conduction velocity in the heart.

763. What ion flow across the cell wall causes the SA node to fire?
 a. Na+ influx
 b. Ca++ influx
 c. K+ efflux
 d. Cl- efflux

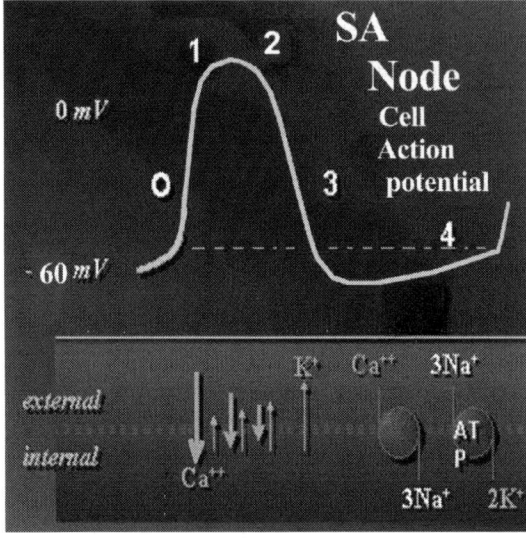

ANSWER: b. Ca++ influx. These are termed the slow calcium channels, because the depolarization is slow and the action potential looks like a sine wave. AV nodal tissue has a similar looking slow action potential. This is the automatic pacemaker of the heart. The slow depolarization in phase 4 determines the intrinsic heart rate. See orange arrows in diagram showing slow Ca influx. The dotted line is the threshold potential, above which it fires and determines the SA rate. The right hand side shows the restoration of ionic balance with the sodium calcium and sodium potassium pumps that require energy.

2A. Tracings, Equipment & Measurements - Equipment

764. This calibration signal on an ECG machine is termed:
 a. Underdamped
 b. Overdamped
 c. Normal
 d. Resonant
 e. Increased high frequency response

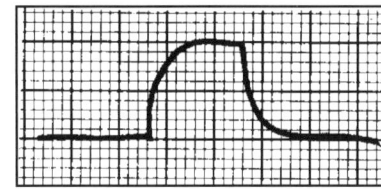
ECG Calibration Signal

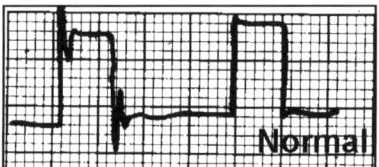
Underdamped Calibration Signal

ANSWER B. Overdamped. This ECG pen responds too SLOW. Damping slows things. This will reduce the recorder's frequency response and impair recording of rapidly occurring waves such as the QRS. Underdamping is the opposite. Underdamping is shown in this diagram. The second diagram shows only slight underdamping (up to 10% overshoot), which is acceptable, since it increases the high frequency response of the recorder.
See: Equipment manuals **Keywords:** ID overdamped stylus

765. If an ECG monitor beeps twice for each heartbeat as shown. Which control of the monitor should be adjusted?
  a. QRS gain
  b. Beeper volume
  c. ECG zero
  d. ECG position

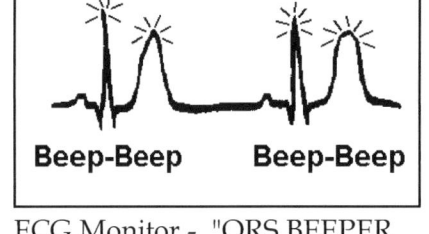
ECG Monitor - "QRS BEEPER ON"

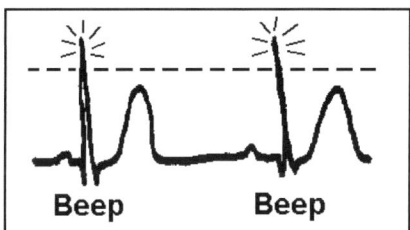
ECG Monitor - "QRS BEEPER ON"

ANSWER a. QRS gain. The high voltage of the "R" and "T" waves exceed the triggering threshold, causing a double beep. Once for each QRS and once for each "T" wave. If the "T" wave cannot be reduced by changing leads, decrease the amplifier gain (or increase threshold level) so the "T" wave is below the threshold level.
See: Equipment manuals Keywords: ECG monitor beeps twice: change QRS gain or threshold.

766. If the 1 mv calibration signal deflects as shown on the ECG paper, what adjustment should be made?
  a. Nothing, it should only go up .5 cm
  b. Turn up the position control
  c. Turn down the position control
  d. Turn down the sensitivity control
  e. Turn up the sensitivity control

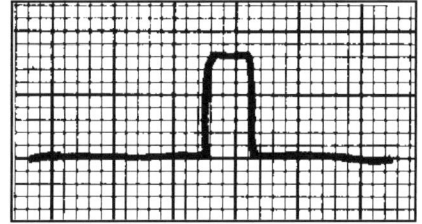
ECG 1 mv Calibration X1

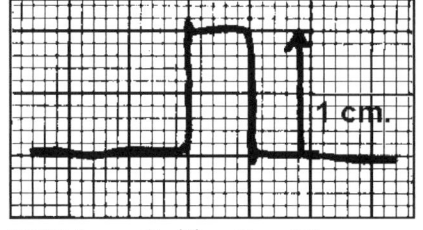
ECG 1 mv Calibration X1

ANSWER e. Turn up the sensitivity (gain) control. The gain sets the relative size of the QRS and other complexes in cm/mv. Standard gain is 1 cm/mv. Gain may be halved if the QRS complex goes off the paper (e.g. in high voltage V leads). Calibration signals (1 mv) should appear on every ECG for accurate voltage measurements.
See: Underhill, chapter on "ECG." Keywords: 1 mv cal = sensitivity (gain) to 1 cm.

767. Calculate the heart rate (HR) if the R-R interval is 920 msec?
  a. 42 bpm
  b. 51 bpm
  c. 65 bpm
  d. 72 bpm

ANSWER c. 65 bpm. Use the basic formula (you should memorize): HR = 60/RR, or HR = (60,000 msec/min)/(r-r interval in msec)
   (60,000 msec/min)/ 920 msec = 65/min.

EP study and pacemaker rates are now calculated not with ECG boxes, or seconds but in milliseconds. Since there are 1000 msec/sec, the standard HR formula uses 60,000 in the numerator. Note how the units cancel to give beats / min.
See: Braunwald, chapter on "Electrocardiography." **Keywords:** Calculate HR using msec.

768. What is the QRS complex shown at #5 termed?
a. QR
b. QRS
c. QRSR'
d. QS
e. RS

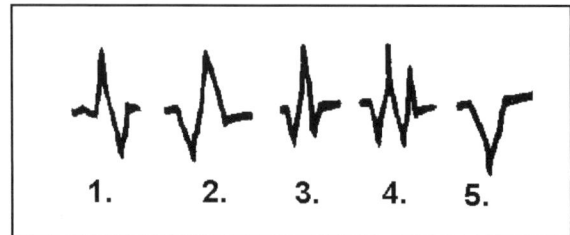
Label the Ventricular Complexes

ANSWER d. QS wave. Being all negative with no "R" wave, it is considered a large "Q" or "S" wave, or together a "QS." The "Q" wave is the first negative deflection, the "S" wave is the second. "R" is the first positive deflection, R' the second, R" the third, etc. In addition some authors use upper and lower case letters to

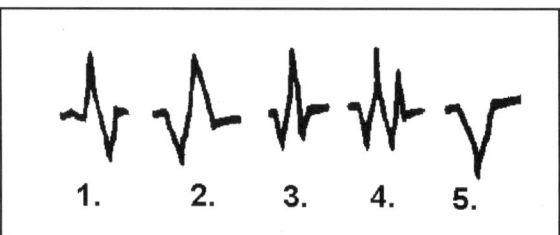
Labeled Ventricular Complexes

indicate the relative size of the complexes. Classic rSR' is termed a "rabbit ears" and is seen in RBBB.
BE ABLE TO MATCH ALL ANSWERS BELOW:
1. RS
2. QR
3. QRS
4. QRSR'
5. QS

See: Davis, chapter on "IV Determination of HR and Normal Heart Rhythms." **Keywords:** Label QRSR' complex

2B. Tracings, Equipment & Measurements - Artifacts

769. You observe a muscle tremor artifact on ECG leads I and II, but NOT on lead III. Which ECG electrode is probably causing this artifact?
a. Left arm
b. Left leg
c. Right arm
d. Right leg

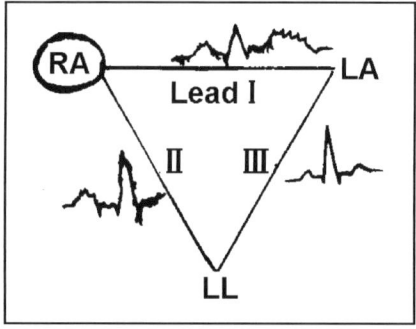
Einthoven's Triangle

ANSWER c. Right arm. The electrode resistance is probably increased on the right arm electrode. The RA is the only electrode common to lead I and II. Draw an Einthoven triangle and note how lead I and II intersect at the right arm. Try re-prepping that electrode to improve the artifact. Poor skin prep is the usual cause of ECG artifacts. With a roughening of the skin, and application of electrode paste, good ECGs can even be obtained during exercise. Also, move the electrodes up to the shoulders, where arm motion will not be sensed.
See: Phillips, The Cardiac Rhythms, chapter on "The Electrocardiogram." **Keywords:** Reducing ECG artifacts, Einthoven

770. How could you reduce the artifacts seen on this ECG?
  a. Relax and quiet the patient
  b. Check for electric motors & improper ground
  c. Increase the damping on the machine
  d. Reapply the ECG limb electrodes more distally

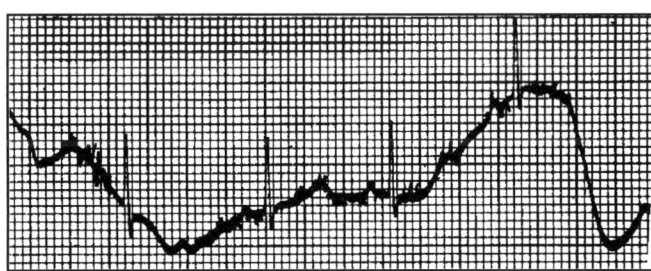
Monitoring Lead II ECG

ANSWER a. Relax and quiet the patient. This artifact is a somatic muscle tremor with wandering baseline due to motion. Make the patient comfortable and ask him to relax all over. If this fails to eliminate the noise, the electrodes should be moved more proximally, onto the shoulders and hips after thoroughly prepping the skin. This kind of noisy ECG signal can interfere with ECG interpretation.
See: Davis, chapter on "12 Lead ECG Interpretation." **Keywords:** Muscle tremors

771. A patient's monitor alarm has just sounded. You come running and see this ECG. What do you do?
  a. Defibrillate
  b. Call for help and begin CPR
  c. Awake the patient by shaking and shouting
  d. Check ECG electrodes and leads

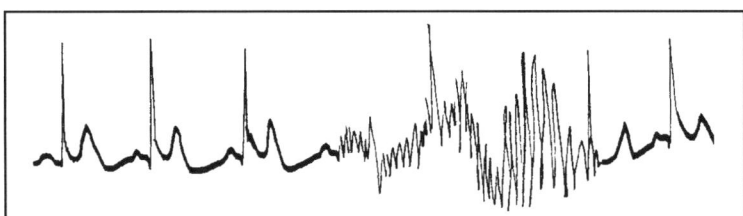
Monitoring Lead II ECG

ANSWER d. Check ECG electrodes and leads. This is a normal sinus rhythm disturbed by motion artifact. Noisy ECG artifacts may occur due to patient motion or a loose electrode. Although this artifact resembles ventricular fibrillation it returns to sinus rhythm at the end of the strip. No patient should be resuscitated or treated based on the ECG alone. *Treat the patient, not the monitor.*
See: ACLS Manual **Keywords:** ECG artifact, check patient first

772. The irregularity seen in the baseline of the ECG tracing below is:
a. DC interference
b. AC (60 Hz) interference
c. Muscle tremors
d. Wandering baseline

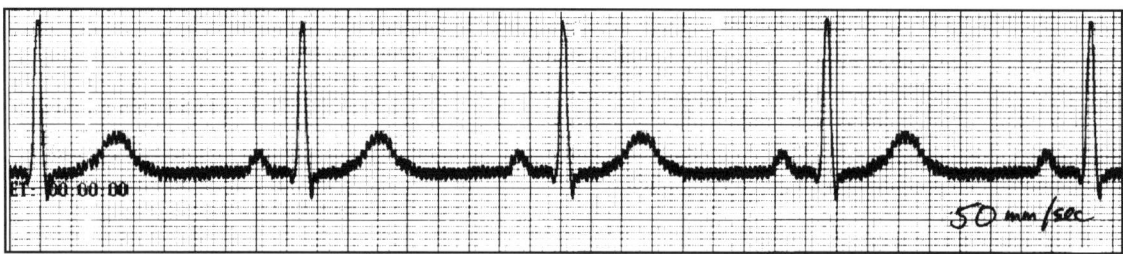

Baseline ECG artifact - recorded at 50 mm/sec

ANSWER b. AC (60 Hz) interference. This is due to 60 cycle interference from such appliances as electric motors(beds), transformers (fluorescent lights), or improper electrical ground. Turn off all electrical appliances close to the patient and check all machine grounding. On slower paper speeds this may appear as a very wide regular baseline. But if you look closely there are tiny sine wave vibrations within the baseline.
See: Davis, chapter on "12-Lead ECG Interpretation. **Keywords:** 60 cycle artifact

2C. Tracings, Equipment & Measurements - Leads & Techniques

773. Which monitoring lead would record the normal ECG shown here?
a. Bipolar lead II
b. Bipolar lead I
c. Marriott MCL1
d. Modified V6

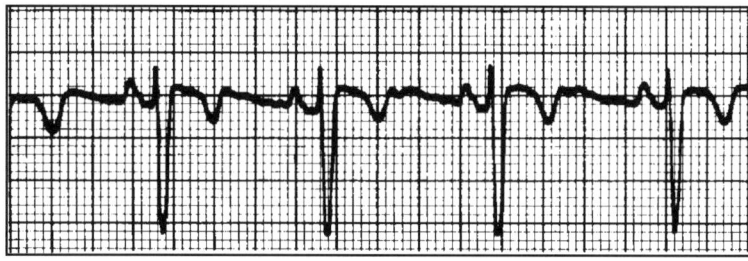

What monitoring lead is shown?

ANSWER c. Marriott MCL1 or monitoring chest lead V1. This common monitoring lead has a large easily monitored negative QS complex and clear biphasic "P" wave. It is similar in configuration to a lead V1. It is useful because it distinguishes well between RV and LV PVCs (LV-PVCs deflect UP).
See: Underhill, chapter on "ECG." **Keywords:** Marriott MCL1 ECG monitoring lead

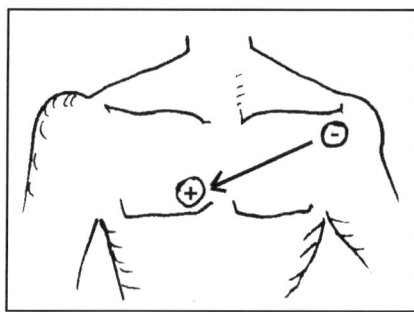

Marriott monitor Lead MCL1

2D. Tracings, Equipment & Measurements - Measurements

774. Determine the heart rate. HR= ?/min
- a. 40-50
- b. 50-65
- c. 65-75
- d. 75-85

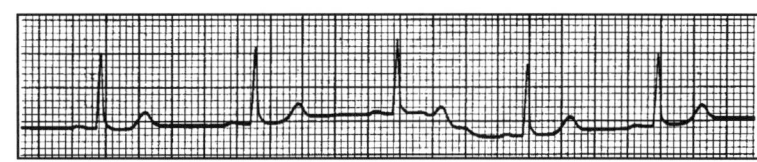
Measure Heart Rate variation on this ECG

ANSWER c. 65-75 beats/min. Remember the quick "box counter" method: 300-150-100-75-60-50 beats/min. The first beat R-R interval measures 5 large boxes = just over 60/min. The last R-R interval is 4 large boxes = 75/min.
   Another method is to calculate the RR interval by counting the number of small boxes between QRS complexes. Remember the normal ECG paper speed is 25 mm/sec., so each small box is .04 sec. Count the number of boxes, multiply times .04 sec/box and then divide that time into 60 sec/min, for beats/min where HR = 60/RR int.
See: Dubin, chapter on "Rate." **Keywords:** Measure HR

USE THE ECG COMPLEX BELOW FOR THE NEXT 3 QUESTIONS.

775. On this magnified ECG, measure the PR interval.
- a. 0.06 sec
- b. 0.10 sec
- c. 0.14 sec
- d. 0.18 sec

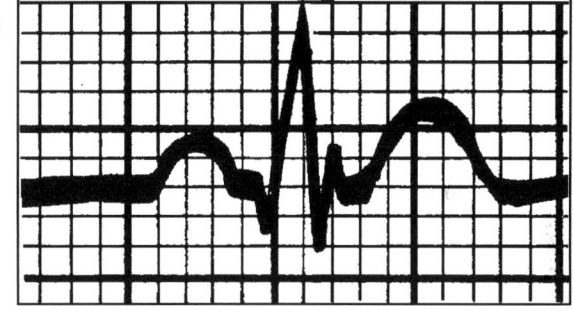
Magnified ECG 25 speed, X1 cal

776. On this magnified ECG measure the QRS duration.
- a. .08 sec
- b. .12 sec
- c. .16 sec
- d. .24 sec

777. On this magnified ECG measure the "R" wave voltage.
- a. 0.6 mV
- b. 1.0 mV
- c. 1.6 mV
- d. 3.2 mV

ALL THREE ANSWERS LISTED CONSECUTIVELY BELOW.

775. ANSWER c. 0.14 sec. Measure from the beginning of the "P" wave to the beginning of the QRS and find 3.5 boxes. Each box is .04 sec. Interval = 3.5 x .04 = .14 sec. PR interval is key to evaluating AV node conduction. Normal adult PR interval = .12 - 2.0 sec.
See: Davis, chapter on "IV Determination of HR and Normal Heart Rhythms." **Keywords:** Measure PR interval

776. ANSWER b. 0.12 sec. From the beginning of the "q" wave to the end of the r' wave it is 3 boxes (leading edge to leading edge). Interval = # boxes x .04 sec/box = 3 x .04 = .12 sec. QRS duration is key to evaluating abnormally conducted ventricular complexes. Normal range for QRS duration in the limb leads is 0.04 - .10 sec.
See: Davis, chapter on "ECG Graph Paper and Measurements." **Keywords:** Measure QRS duration

777. ANSWER a. 0.6 mV. Voltage is measured vertically. Remember the calibration signal is 1 mV = 1 cm. Each small box is 0.1 mV. The "R" wave deflects 6 boxes above the baseline or 0.6 mV. R wave voltage is key to evaluating hypertrophy of a chamber. **See:** Davis, chapter on "ECG Graph Paper and Measurements." **Keywords:** Measure "R" wave voltage

778. Identify the name for the abnormal ECG measurement labeled #2 (short PR interval) in the box.
   a. BBB or PVC
   b. Hypocalcemia
   c. Hypercalcemia
   d. 1° Heart Block
   e. WPW or LGL Syndrome

ECG Measurements
1. Long PR Interval
*2. Short PR Interval
3. Long QRS Duration
4. Long QT Interval
5. Short QT. Interval

ANSWER e. WPW or LGL Syndrome. This is pre-excitation or premature excitation of the ventricles. The sinus impulse is conducted into the ventricle through an AV bypass tract. Delta waves are seen in WPW sinus beats with a short PR interval.
CORRECTLY MATCHED ANSWERS ARE:
   1. Long PR Interval   =   1° Heart Block
   2. Short PR Interval   =   WPW or LGL Syndrome*
   3. Long QRS Duration   =   BBB or PVC
   4. Long QT Interval   =   Hypocalcemia**
   5. Short QT Interval   =   Hypercalcemia
*WPW = Wolf Parkinson White. LGL = Lown-Ganong-Levine. Both are pre-excitation syndromes. **See related question in electrolyte section of this chapter.
See: Davis, chapter on "IV Conduction Disturbances." **Keywords:** Significance of abnormal ECG measurements

779. From this ECG recorded with 0.1 second time lines, determine the heart rate.
   a. 30 bpm
   b. 45 bpm
   c. 50 bpm
   d. 56 bpm

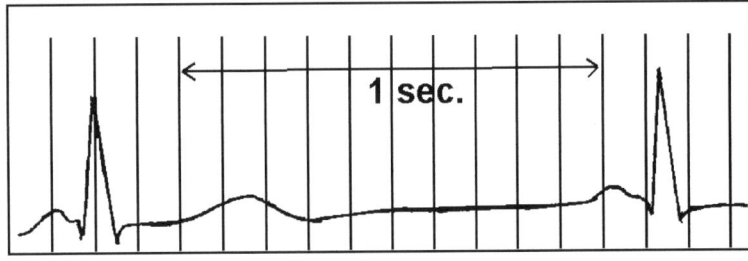
ECG recorded at time lines 0.1 sec

ANSWER b. 45 bpm. RR interval is 1.33 sec. If the paper speed is 100 mm/sec or the time lines are 0.1 as shown, it is EASY to calculate the rr interval and heart rate. Just use the time lines to count up the rr time interval, as shown. Note how easily the 1.33 sec (1,330 msec) is measured on the graph.

Know the formula: HR = 60/ r-r interval
HR (Bts/min) = 60 (sec/min) / r-r interval in (sec)
HR = 60 sec/min / 1.33 sec = 45 bpm
Note the unit cancellation resulting in beats/min.

You may include a paper speed factor in the numerator to convert the r-r interval

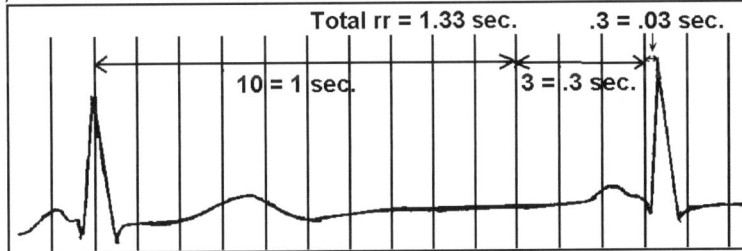
ECG recorded at time lines 0.1 sec

measurement from mm to seconds. Then you can use a mm ruler to measure the paper speed and rr interval.
   HR (Bts/min) = 60 (sec/min) x Paper speed (mm/sec)/ r-r (mm)
See: Grossman, chapter on "Assessing Valvular Stenosis." **Keywords:** Calculate HR

780. **Calculate the heart rate of an ECG when the RR interval averages 20 mm running on 25 mm/sec paper speed as shown.**
   a. 60
   b. 75
   c. 85
   d. 100

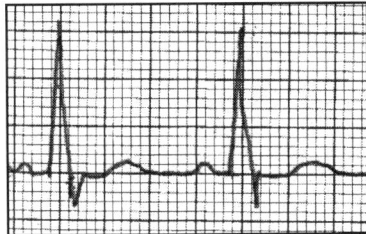

ANSWER: b. 75 beats/min. To measure heart rate easily remember the numbers "300-150-100-75-60-50". Each of those numbers estimates the HR when you measure one RR interval by counting the 5 mm time lines on the ECG paper. Each time you jump 5 mm you recite these numbers. Here there are four 5 mm intervals (20 cm) between R waves, so recite 300-150-100-75, and stop at the 4th number. Here there are 4 boxes between R waves, so the HR = 75 bpm. It is most accurate to start with an R wave on one of the dark ECG paper lines, then count dark lines as you recite these numbers. If the next R wave is exactly on a dark line, the HR is exactly that number.

Or, if you are good at math, you can use the formula HR =60 / RR int. = (60 sec/min)

/ .8 sec = 75 b/min. **See:** Dubin, Rapid Interpretation of EKGs **Keywords:** Measure HR

2E. Tracings, Equipment & Measurements - Axis & Vectors

781. A mean QRS axis of the angle labeled #2 (+130°) in the frontal plane is indicative of:
a. Normal axis
b. Right axis deviation
c. Left axis deviation
d. Extreme or indeterminate axis

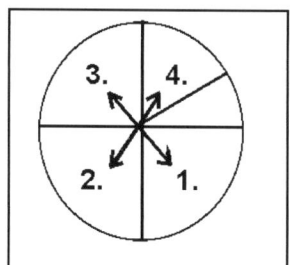

ANSWER b. Right axis deviation (RAD). Mean QRS axis plotted in the lower right quadrant have Right Axis Deviation (RAD). RAD is between +90 and +180 degrees in the lower right quadrant. RAD may be found in hearts with Right Ventricular Hypertrophy (RVH) and RBBB. The mean QRS axis is always close to the frontal lead with the most positive deflection e.g. lead 2 is usually the largest QRS, so the normal mean QRS is at +60°.

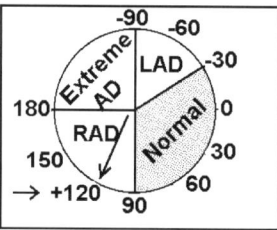

CORRECTLY MATCHED ANSWERS ARE:
1. NORMAL AXIS: =   -30 to 90 degrees
2. RIGHT AXIS DEVIATION: +90 to +180°
3. EXTREME AXIS: =   +180 to -90° (also termed indeterminate or extreme right axis deviation)
4. LEFT AXIS DEVIATION: =   -90° to -30°

See: Davis, chapter on "QRS AXIS." **Keywords:** 120 degree axis = RVH.

782. The mean QRS axis shows left axis deviation when the largest frontal plane QRS complex is a large:
a. Upright R wave in lead III
b. Negative QS wave in lead III
c. Upright R wave in lead II
d. Negative QS wave in lead II

ANSWER b. Large negative "QS" wave in lead III. Since the greatest QRS deflection is measured along a lead parallel to it. A simple way to find the axis is to find the biggest QRS in the frontal plane (limb leads). A negative or downward "QS" wave in lead III means depolarization is AWAY from the lead III positive electrode - which is at the right leg. So the depolarization is away from the right leg or upwards to the patient's left (-60°). This axis is within the left axis deviation quadrant. See mean QRS measurement later in this chapter. **See:** Davis, chapter on "QRS AXIS."
Keywords: Axis quadrants

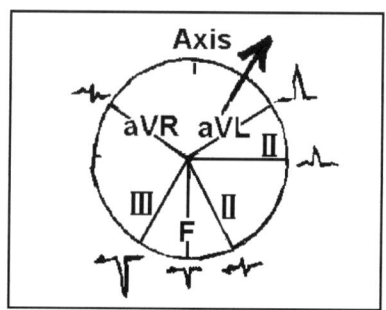

Mean QRS Axis

783. The ECG rhythm shown demonstrates an R wave height abnormality. This is termed ___, which is associated with___.
a. Bigeminy, CHF
b. Bigeminy, Cardiac tamponade
c. Electrical Alternans, CHF
d. Electrical Alternans, Cardiac tamponade

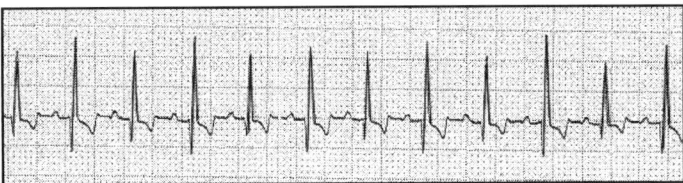

ANSWER: d. "Electrical alternans is an alternating QRS complex amplitude between beats.... It is seen in cardiac tamponade and is thought to be related to changes in the ventricular electrical axis due to fluid in the pericardium." The heart is swinging back and forth in the fluid-filled pericardial space, so the QRS voltage varies, beat-to-beat depending on the heart's orientation.
"Pulsus Alternans" (not seen here) is when this happens to the arterial pulse -high systolic, low systolic, hi, lo, hi, lo... This is associated with CHF.
See: http://emedicine.medscape.com/article/154706-overview#showall Keywords: Electrical alternans = cardiac tamponade

784. This ECG shows:
a. Mobitz II with 2:1 AV block
b. Mobitz II with 3:1 AV block
c. Atrial flutter with 2:1 response
d. Atrial flutter with 3:1 response

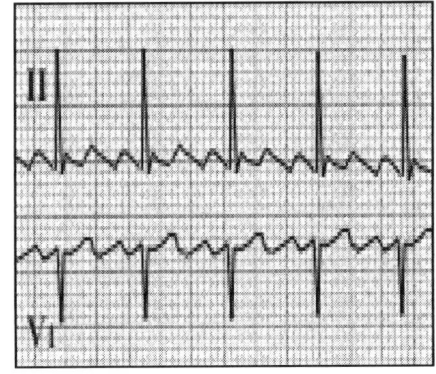

ANSWER: d. Atrial flutter with 3:1 response. Note the two triangular flutter waves between QRS complexes. The third flutter wave is buried in the QRS complex. Here the atria beat 3 times faster than ventricles.
"Atrial flutter is caused by a reentrant rhythm in either the right or left atrium. Typically initiated by a premature electrical impulse arising in the atria, atrial flutter is propagated due to differences in refractory periods of atrial tissue. This creates electrical activity that moves in a localized self-perpetuating loop. Each cycle around the loop results a flutter wave.
See: http://emedicine.medscape.com/article/151210-overview#showall Keywords: AF

785. This lead II ECG shows___.
a. Sinus tachycardia
b. Atrial fibrillation
c. Wandering atrial pacemaker
d. Accelerated junctional rhythm

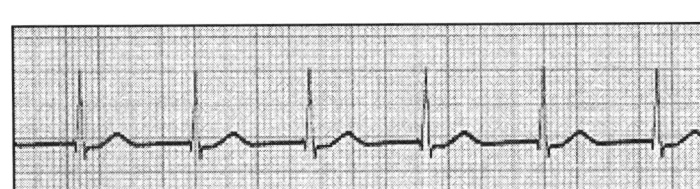

ANSWER: d. Accelerated junctional rhythm. P waves are not seen or are buried in these narrow QRS complex. In junctional rhythms P waves may be upside down or late, because they conduct superiorly from the AV junction. Here the heart's atrioventricular node (junction) takes over as the pacemaker. The atria will still contract by retrograde conduction, but since they arrive too late they may not aid in ventricular filling. The junctional rate is normally slow - 40-50 bpm. This rate is 85, much faster than expected for the junction. Thus, it is accelerated. This is a supraventricular arrhythmia with narrow QRS complexes. **See:** http://emedicine.medscape.com/article/155146-overview#showall
Keywords: Accelerated junctional rhythm

2F. Tracings, Equip. & Measurements - Combined Measurements

Use "Mr. Jones" FULL PAGE 12 lead ECG below for the following 7 questions.

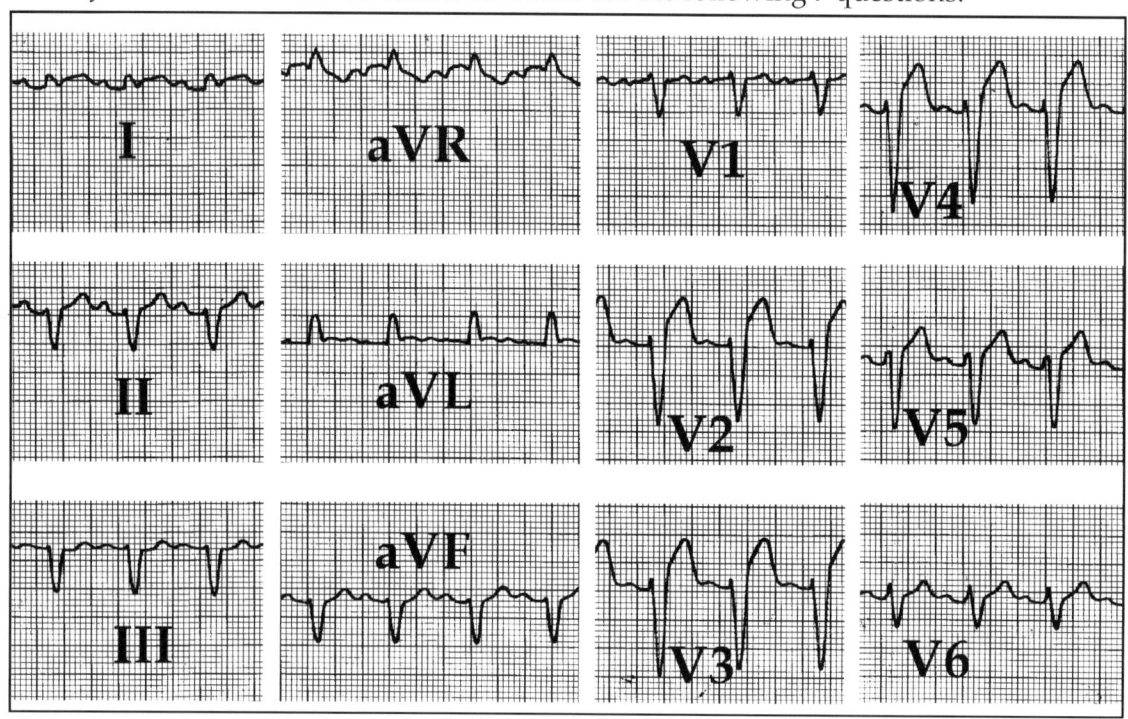

"Mr. Jones" - 12 lead ECG

786.   Measure "Mr. Jones" mean QRS axis.
   a. -90°
   b. -45°
   c. +60°
   d. +90°

Diagnostic Techniques: D11 - ECG 1 and Arrhythmias

787. Evaluate "Mr. Jones" mean QRS axis.
   a. Normal
   b. Left axis deviation
   c. Right axis deviation
   d. Extreme right axis deviation

788. Determine the average heart rate on the "Mr. Jones" 12 lead ECG.
   a. 80
   b. 100
   c. 120
   d. 140

789. What arrhythmia does "Mr. Jones" have?
   a. Sinus tachycardia (with first degree block)
   b. Atrial flutter (2:1 block)
   c. Slow ventricular tachycardia
   d. VVI pacing

790. Determine the QRS duration of "Mr. Jones" ECG above.
   a. .08 sec
   b. .10 sec
   c. .14 sec
   d. .20 sec

791. What does the QRS duration of "Mr. Jones" ECG suggest?
   a. Pacemaker rhythm
   b. Ventricular tachycardia
   c. PVCs
   d. Bundle branch block (LBBB)

792. Measure the PR interval on "Mr. Jones" ECG.
   a. .08 sec
   b. .12 sec
   c. .18 sec
   d. .22 sec

ALL SEVEN ANSWERS FOR "MR JONES" ECG ARE BELOW.

786. ANSWER a. -90°. Look for the largest positive QRS or "R" wave. It is in lead aVL. This tells you that the mean QRS axis is upward and to the patient's left. The most negative is either II or III. To fine tune the axis, look for the isoelectric or equiphasic (= up and =down) lead - with smallest or most equiphasic QRS. The smallest QRS is in lead I. This lead is perpendicular to the mean QRS axis. Lead aVF is perpendicular to lead I. Lead aVF is

strongly negative, indicating the axis away from the foot or straight upward at -90°. Use Davis' three ways to find the axis:
1. Tallest ECG points toward the axis.
2. Most negative points away from the axis.
3. The equiphasic QRS is at right angles (perpendicular) to the QRS.

See: Davis, chapter on "QRS AXIS." **Keywords:** Measure axis

787. ANSWER b. Left axis deviation. Since the LV receives the conduction impulse last, LV depolarization proceeds slowly from the septum posterior and leftward. This shifts the axis leftward. Note the negative rS complex in aVF.
See: Davis, chapter on "Interventricular Conduction defects." **Keywords:** Measure QRS axis in LBBB

788. ANSWER b. 100 beats/min. The R-R interval is 3 large boxes or 100 beats/min. **See:** Davis, chapter on "IV Determination of HR and Normal Heart Rhythms." **Keywords:** Measure rate

789. ANSWER a. Sinus tachycardia. Heart rate just slight over 100. "P" waves precede each QRS (positive in lead II), indicating sinus rhythm. First degree heart block is present as indicated by long PR interval >.20 sec.
See: Davis, chapter on "IV Determination of HR and Normal Heart Rhythms." **Keywords:** Sinus rhythm

790. ANSWER c. 0.14 sec. Look at lead II. the rS complex is 3.5 boxes wide. 3.5 x .04 = .14 sec. The QRS even looks broad. Normal QRS complex is less than .12 seconds wide.
See: Davis, chapter on "IV Determination of HR and Normal Heart Rhythms." **Keywords:** Measure QRS duration

791. ANSWER d. Bundle branch block. The very broad QRS (0.14 sec) is primarily negative in V1. The RV depolarizes first (small "R" wave in lead V1). The LV depolarizes last, with strong leftward forces (rS or RR' in V6). This LBBB pattern is similar to that seen with an RV pacemaker.
See: Davis, chapter on "IV Conduction disturbances." **Keywords:** LBBB

792. ANSWER d. .22 sec. In lead II the distance from beginning of "P" wave to beginning of QRS is 5.5 boxes. 5.5 x .04 = .22 sec. Normal is less than .20 sec. So, first degree AV block is present.
See: Davis, chapter on "IV Conduction disturbances." **Keywords:** Measure PR interval, long = 1st degree block

3A. Arrhythmias - Sinus

793. Slight sinus node arrhythmia occurs normally and is due to:
a. Erratic pacemakers
b. Occasional PVCs
c. Occasional PACs
d. Respiration
e. Sinus node anoxia

ANSWER d. Respiration. Respiratory receptors effect the tone of autonomic nerves supplying the SA node. Inspiration usually causes the HR to increase - expiration causes it to slow. Wide variation in the rate occurs normally in young people. When the sinus heart rate varies by more than 10% it is termed "sinus arrhythmia." **See:** Davis, chapter on "IV Determination of HR and Normal Heart Rhythms." **Keywords:** Sinus node arrhythmia

794. "Sick Sinus Node Syndrome" is associated with ____.
a. Sinus bradycardia
b. Sinus tachycardia
c. A nodal (junctional) pacemaker escaping
d. A ventricular pacemaker escaping

ANSWER a. Sinus bradycardia. The term "Sick Sinus Syndrome" is loosely used to describe any severe bradycardia at rest that does not speed appropriately with exercise. Sick Sinus Syndrome (SSS) also has an absence of escape rhythms, so the rate may drop very low. This SA node disease is often treated with an atrial (AAI or DDD) pacemaker.
See: Marriott, chapter on "Decreased Automaticity." **Keywords:** Sick Sinus Syndrome

795. The long pause in this ECG is probably:
a. A compensatory pause
b. A non-compensatory pause
c. Mobitz type I heart block
d. Sinus pause

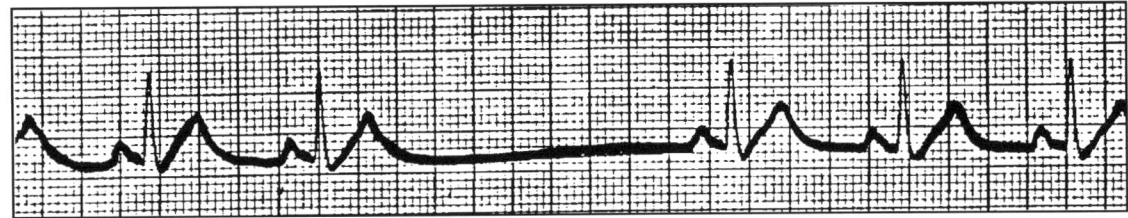

ANSWER d. Sinus pause. There are no "p" waves during the 2 ½ sec. period of asystole. Since the asystolic period is not an even multiple of the normal R-R interval this is called a sinus pause. If the asystolic period had been exactly 2 or 3 times the R-R interval this would be called "SA block." No escape pacemaker takes over if there is failure of all pacemaker cells. When these pauses are brief, no treatment is usually needed.
See: Marriott, chapter on "Decreased Automaticity." **Keywords:** Sinus pause

3B. Arrhythmias - Atrial

796. Identify the atrial heart rate range for the narrow complex supraventricular tachy-arrhythmia labeled #1 in the box (atrial fibrillation.)

a. 100-180 /min
b. 150-250 /min
c. 250-350 /min
d. 300-600 /min

<u>ATRIAL TACHY-ARRHYTHMIAS</u>
*1. atrial fibrillation
2. atrial flutter
3. atrial tachycardia with block
4. sinus tachycardia

ANSWER d. 300-600 / min. Of all supraventricular tachycardias, the atrial rate is most rapid in atrial fibrillation. It may be so fast that it only shows on the ECG as a small irregular baseline undulations of variable amplitude, called "f" or flutter waves. No effective atrial contraction is present.
TACHY-ARRHYTHMIA RATE RANGES SHOWN ARE:
  1. Atrial fibrillation . . 300-600 / min
  2. Atrial flutter . . . 250-350 / min
  3. Atrial tachycardia with block . 150-250 / min
  4. Sinus tachycardia . . 100-180 / min
See: Braunwald, chapter on "Specific Arrhythmias: Diagnosis and Treatment." **Keywords:** Atrial rate range in atrial tachyarrhythmias

797. What is the irregular heart rhythm shown?

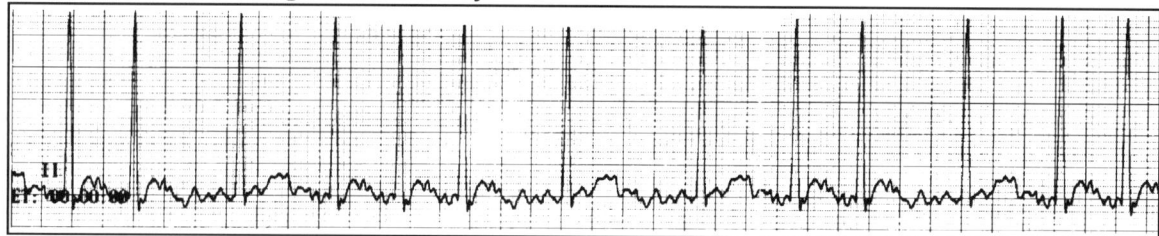

Lead II ECG

a. **Atrial fibrillation**
b. **Atrial flutter**
c. **Sinus tachycardia**
d. **Junctional tachycardia**

ANSWER a. Atrial fibrillation. Atrial fib. is an irregular undulation of the baseline with an "irregularly irregular" ventricular rhythm. Atrial fib. ("f" waves) occurs at atrial rates between 300-600/min. The undulations may be distinct or barely perceptible (coarse or fine fib.). Atrial Fib. is best diagnosed by noting the irregular RR intervals, because sometimes you cannot see the atrial fib. waves. If the ECG switches back and forth between atrial flutter and fibrillation it is termed flutter/fib.

Only when a large enough "f" wave enters the AV node is a beat conducted. As shown in this ladder diagram, most "f" waves are blocked. Although it may look musical, it is not. There is no meter or "beat" to atrial fibrillation. Ventricular response varies irregularly between 100-160/min. Many supraventricular tachycardias can be terminated by DC cardioversion.

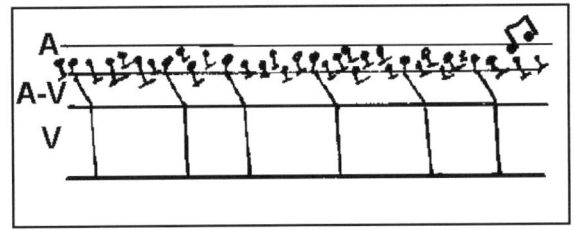

See: Marriott, chapter on "Atrial Fib/Flutter." **Keywords:** Atrial fib.

798. This ECG shows:

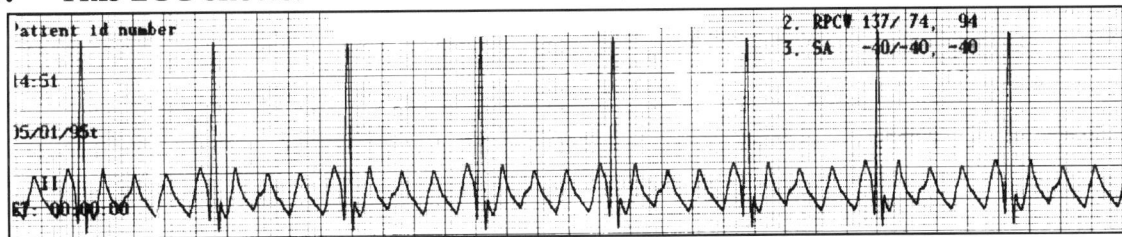

Lead II ECG showing?

a. Atrial fibrillation
b. Atrial flutter
c. Atrial tachycardia
d. Sinus tachycardia

ANSWER b. Atrial flutter. The regular shaped flutter (F waves) appear as a "sawtooth" baseline. Here 4 "F" waves are blocked at the AV node for every one conducted through to the ventricle. This indicates 4:1 AV block. Atrial rate is 280 while ventricular rate is 1/4 of that 70/min. The origin of the "F" waves is a single macro reentry circuit in the atria. Often the atria are enlarged. It may be terminated by DC cardioversion.
See: Marriott, chapter on "Atrial Fib/Flutter." **Keywords:** Atrial flutter

799. The tachycardia shown on the last ½ of this ECG is:

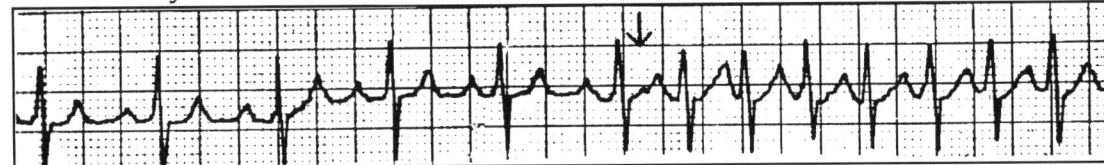

ECG - Lead II

a. Ventricular tachycardia
b. Accelerated junctional escape rhythm
c. Paroxysmal supraventricular tachycardia
d. Torsade de pointes

ANSWER c. Paroxysmal Supraventricular Tachycardia. The tachycardia develops suddenly at the arrow so it is termed "paroxysmal." Since the QRS complexes appear narrow and

normal, the rhythm comes from above the ventricles (supraventricular). This is probably an atrial tachycardia as opposed to a junctional tachycardia because in the end of the strip, the "T" waves appear to contain P' waves.
See: ACLS Manual, chapter on "Arrhythmias." **Keywords:** Paroxysmal supraventricular tachycardia, PSVT

800. The early 3rd beat seen on this ECG is a/an:

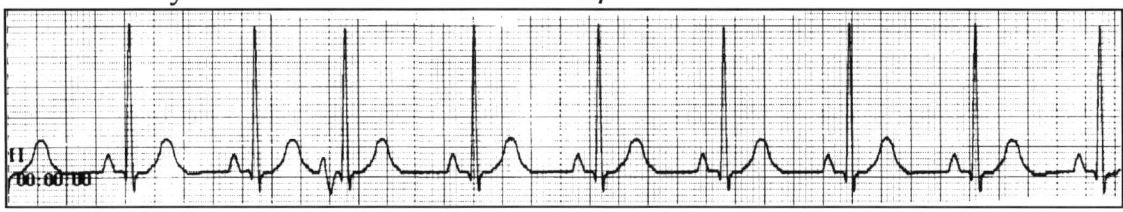

Early beat on ECG lead II

a. Atrial Premature Complex (APC/PAC)
b. Ventricular Premature Complex (VPC/PVC)
c. Premature Sinus Beat (PSB)
d. Junctional Escape Beat (JEB)

ANSWER a. Atrial Premature Complex (APC/PAC). APCs are recognized by these criteria:
- Premature abnormal looking P' wave. Here the P' wave appears biphasic.
- QRS is similar to the sinus beats - not broad.
- No compensatory pause.

Note the same R-R interval after the PAC. These beats commonly occur while manipulating a catheter in the atria.
See: Marriott, chapter on "Atrial Fib/Flutter." **Keywords:** APC/PACs

801. This ECG shows :
a. Frequent PACs
b. Atrial flutter
c. Atrial fibrillation
d. AV nodal reentrant tach.
e. Accelerated junctional rhythm

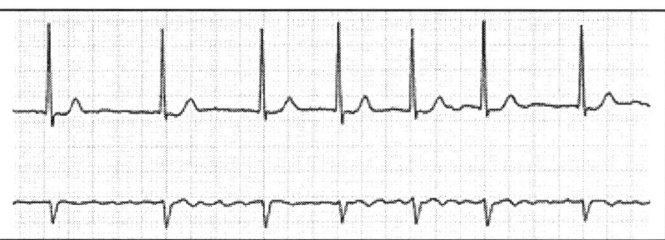

Early beat on ECG lead II

ANSWER c. Atrial fibrillation is characterized by an irregularly irregular ventricular response, and the absence of discrete P waves. The atrial activity seen in the lower lead resembles old saw-teeth (as opposed to the new, sharp saw-teeth of atrial flutter).
See: Marriott, chapter on "Atrial Fib." **Keywords:** AF

THE NEXT 2 QUESTIONS REFER TO THIS ECG.

802. This arrhythmia is an example of:

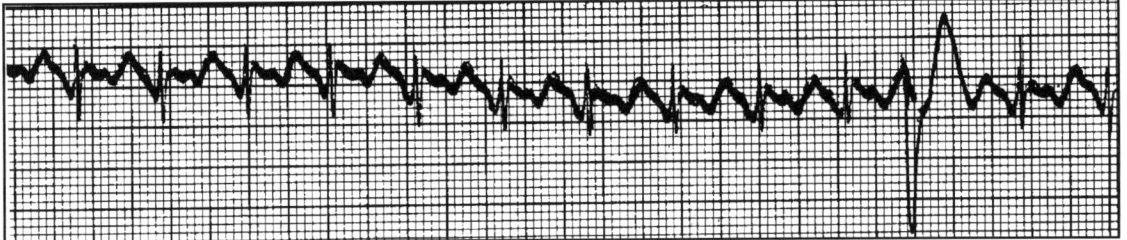

a. Atrial flutter with 2:1 conduction
b. Atrial flutter with 4:1 AV conduction
c. Second degree AV block, Mobitz I
d. Second degree AV block, Mobitz II

ANSWER a. Atrial flutter with 2:1 AV conduction. The regular shaped flutter (F waves) appear as a "sawtooth" baseline. Here 2 "F" waves are seen for every QRS. One is buried in the QRS complex. This indicates 2:1 AV block. Atrial rate is 280, ventricular response is ½ of this or 140/min. What appears to be a down-sloping ST segment is really the end of a flutter wave.
See: Dubin, chapter on "Rhythms." **Keywords:** Atrial flutter

803. In a patient with the tachycardia shown above, increased AV block and slowing of the ventricular rate may occur with:
a. Mild aerobic exercise
b. Mild anaerobic exercise
c. Neck vein massage
d. Valsalva maneuver

ANSWER d. Valsalva maneuver. Patients often learn to Valsalva with these arrhythmias because they feel more comfortable with a lower heart rate. The Valsalva maneuver increases the vagal tone and the amount of AV block. So instead of 2:1 block, the AV node may block 3:1 or 4:1. This lets fewer "F" waves pass into the ventricle, and lowers the ventricular rate. Carotid sinus massage is another maneuver that may increase vagal tone and reduce the ventricular rate. The carotid sinus is at the bifurcation of each common carotid artery. It is not in a vein.
See: Marriot, chapter on "Accelerated Automaticity." **Keywords:** Carotid sinus massage

3C. Arrhythmias - Junctional

804. This ECG strip show sinus slowing. What type of rhythm takes over during the end of the ECG strip?

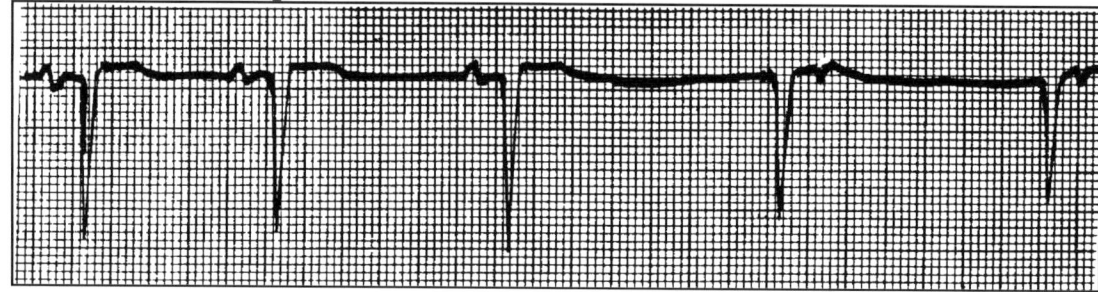

a. Ventricular escape rhythm
b. Junctional escape rhythm
c. Sinus bradycardia
d. Electro-mechanical dissociation

ANSWER b. Junctional escape rhythm. As the sinus rhythm slows from 60 to 50, the 4th beat loses its "P" wave. This is a junctional or nodal escape beat. The QRS configuration remains narrow and normal, so the rhythm is supraventricular. Junctional rhythms may have an inverted "P" wave in lead II (retrograde) that may be buried within the QRS or behind it - as seen in the last 2 beats.
See: Marriott, chapter on "Decreased Automaticity." **Keywords:** Junctional escape

3D. Arrhythmias - Ventricular

805. PVC complexes are distinguished from simple supraventricular QRS complexes in that in PVCs the QRS complexes are _____ and the T waves are _____.

a. Narrow and inverted, Large and in an opposite direction
b. Narrow and negative in polarity, Asymmetrical and positive in polarity
c. Broad and bizarre in shape, Large and in an opposite direction
d. Broad and bizarre in shape, Asymmetrical and positive in polarity

ANSWER c. Broad and bizarre in shape and the T waves are large and in an opposite direction. Braunwald says of PVCs, "A premature ventricular complex is characterized by the premature occurrence of a QRS complex that is

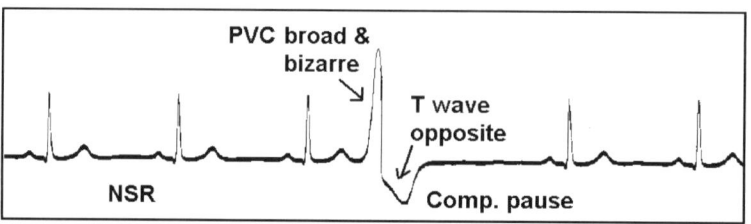

Premature Ventricular Contraction

bizarre in shape and has a duration usually exceeding the dominant QRS complex, generally greater than 120 mSec. The T wave is commonly large and **opposite in direction** to the major deflection of the QRS. The QRS is not preceded by a premature P wave..."
See: Marriot, chapter on "Accelerated Automaticity." **Keywords:** Carotid sinus massage

806. Identify the ventricular heart rate range for the ventricular arrhythmia labeled #1 in the box (ventricular tachycardias.)
   a. <40 min
   b. 50-110
   c. 110-250
   d. 150-300
   e. 400-600

> **VENTRICULAR ARRHYTHMIA**
> 1. Ventricular tachycardia
> 2. Ventricular flutter
> 3. Ventricular fibrillation
> 4. Accelerated idioventricular rhythm
> 5. Idioventricular rhythm with AV block

ANSWER c. 110-250. Braunwald says, "The electrocardiographic diagnosis of ventricular tachycardia is suggested by the occurrence of a mature ventricular complexes whose duration exceeds 120 mSec, with the ST-T vector pointing opposite to the major QRS deflection"Ventricular rates range from 110 to 250 beats/min,..."

RATE RANGES SHOWN VENTRICULAR ARRHYTHMIAS:
   1. Ventricular tachycardia   .   .   110-250 /min
   2. Ventricular flutter   .   .   .   150-300
   3. Ventricular fibrillation   .   .   400-600
   4. Accelerated ideoventricular rhythm   50-110
   5. Ideoventricular rhythm with AV block   <40 min

See: Braunwald, chapter on "Specific Arrhythmias: Diagnosis and Treatment."
Keywords: Ventricular rate range in ventricular arrhythmias

807. Ventricular tachycardia may be mimicked by:
   a. **Disconnected leads**
   b. **Paroxysmal atrial tachycardia**
   c. **Supraventricular tachycardia with aberrancy**
   d. **Mobitz II block with rapid ventricular response**

ANSWER c. Supraventricular tachycardia with aberrancy. An ongoing problem for CCU nurses is to distinguish SVT with aberrancy from VT. Both are wide complex tachycardias, but with totally different implications and treatments.

This diagram compares ventricular tachycardia and supraventricular tachycardia with aberrant conduction. Although they look similar on ECG, the ladder diagram below clearly shows the different origins of the rhythms. Marriott suggests using lead V1 or MCL1 to distinguish the QRS morphology. Supraventricular aberrant beats

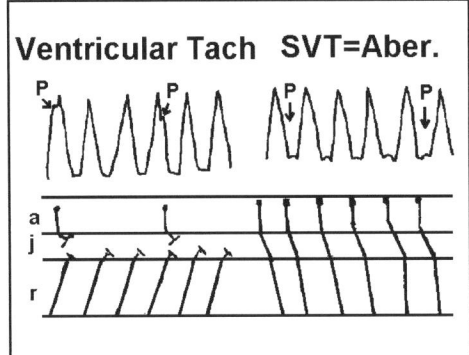

V. Tach. mimicked by SVT with aberrancy

resemble triphasic (rabbit ears rsR') RBBB pattern. Ventricular ectopic beats are more likely to be monophasic (R) or a biphasic (qR). **See:** Marriot, chapter on "Ventricular Tachyarrhythmias" **Keywords:** Aberrancy simulates VT

808. The arrhythmias shown on this ECG (consecutively) are:

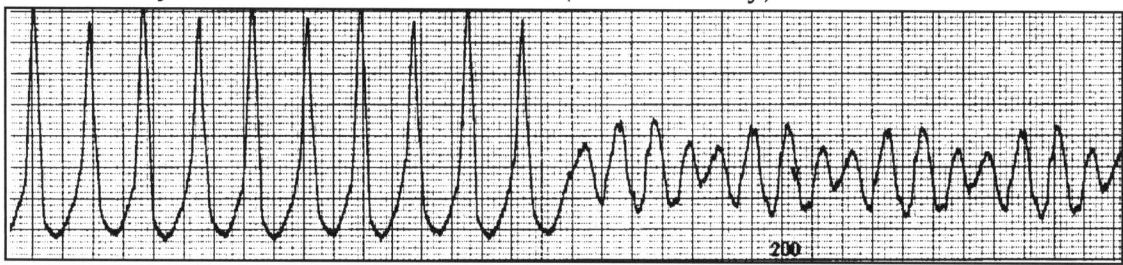

ECG Monitoring Lead II

a. Ventricular fibrillation & ventricular tachycardia
b. Ventricular tachycardia & ventricular fibrillation
c. PVCs & ventricular flutter
d. Ventricular flutter & ventricular tachycardia

ANSWER b. Ventricular tachycardia & ventricular fibrillation. The ventricular tachycardia (VT) may deteriorate to ventricular fibrillation (VF) as it does here. That is the problem with VT, it may lead to lethal VF.
See: ACLS manual, chapter on "Arrhythmias." **Keywords:** VT leading to VF

809. Patients with this arrhythmia will be:

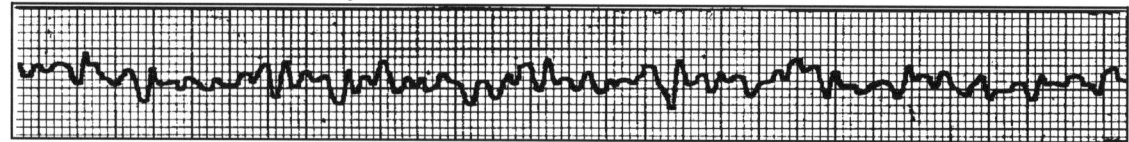

ECG Monitoring lead II

a. Lethargic with a weak pulse
b. Unconsciousness with a pulse
c. Clinically dead
d. Biologically dead

ANSWER c. Clinically dead. Ventricular fibrillation provides NO pulse or cardiac output. The patient is clinically dead, with no vital signs. Within 4-10 minutes brain damage begins, leading to brain death (also termed biological death). Clinical death requires immediate defibrillation and resuscitation for survival. However, be sure to *treat the patient, not the monitor.* Loose electrodes may mimic ventricular fibrillation.
See: ACLS manual, chapter on "Arrhythmias." **Keywords:** V. Fib = clinical death

810. An 80 year old man comes to your lab in NSR with a prolonged QT interval. Before the cath starts he develops the tachy-arrhythmia shown. He is conscious but complains that his heart is pounding. His BP drops from 120/80 to 100/70. What is the rhythm?

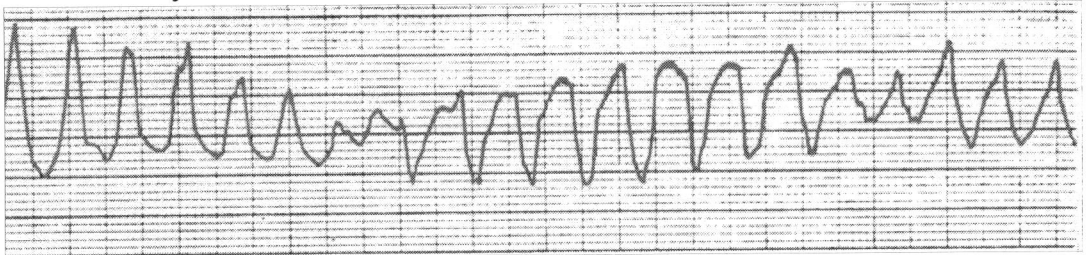
ECG Lead II

a. Ventricular fibrillation (VF)
b. Ventricular flutter
c. Monomorphic VT
d. Torsade des pointes

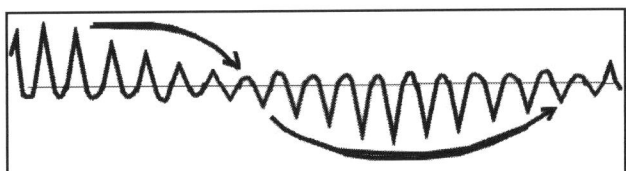
Torsade des pointes - twisting around center

ANSWER d. This is torsade des pointes, a type of VT which tends to increase then decrease in amplitude in an envelope as shown. The QRS complexes point up, then down. In this tracing, note how the first 6 beats point up; the next 8 beats point down. When the patient is in NSR they may have long QT intervals and electrolyte disorders. Commonly treated with IV magnesium or overdrive pacing in 10 second bursts at a rate slightly faster than the tachycardia. Cardioversion may be necessary if the patient becomes unstable. Braunwald says: "The term torsades de pointes refers to a VT characterized by QRS complexes of changing amplitude that appear to twist around the isoelectric line and occur at rates of 200 to 250/min. . . . Torsades de pointes can terminate with progressive prolongation in cycle length and larger and more distinctly formed QRS complexes and culminate in a return to the basal rhythm, a period of ventricular standstill, and a new attack of torsade des pointes or ventricular fibrillation."
See: Braunwald, chapter on "Specific Arrhythmias: Diagnosis and Treatment"

811. The extra ECG beat recorded on lead V1 as shown is an:
a. RV-PVC
b. LV-PVC
c. RA-PAC
d. LA-PAC

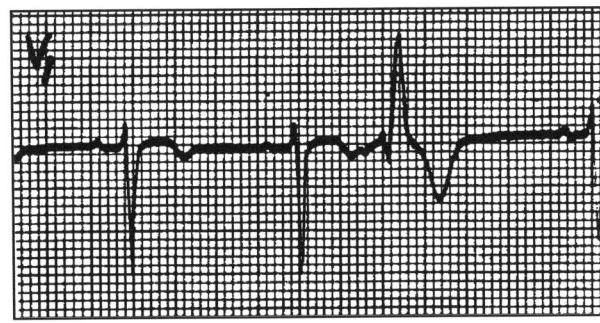
ECG lead V1

ANSWER b. LV-PVC (Left Ventricular Premature Contraction). PVCs are broad and bizarre with a compensatory pause. If PVCs originate in the LV the impulse travels anteriorly making a large positive "R" wave on lead V1. RV PVCs show largely negative (rS) waves on lead V1. Left sided PVCs are more likely to precipitate ventricular fib. and more often associated with heart disease. LV-PVCs are also termed LVPCs. The MCL1 monitoring lead is especially helpful in distinguishing RVPCs from LVPCs. Note in the diagram how the RV-PVCs form a broad QS pattern in lead V1, while LV-PVCs are in the opposite direction, and resemble a RBBB pattern.
See: Marriot, chapter on "Premature Beats"
Keywords: PVC

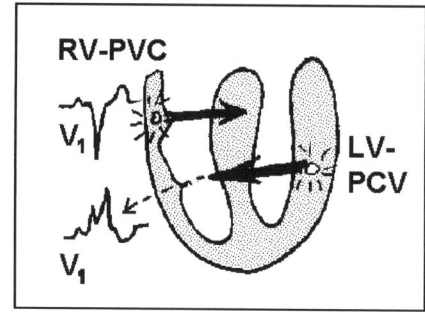
V1 distinguishes RVPCs/LVPCs

812. This arrhythmia shows:

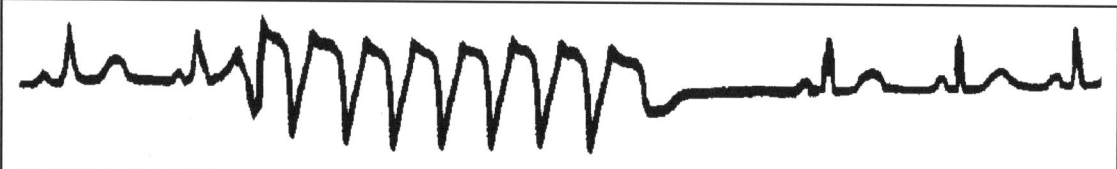

ECG Lead II, 25 mm/sec speed

a. Nonsustained ventricular fibrillation
b. Nonsustained ventricular tachycardia
c. A run of ventricular flutter
d. A run of ventricular fibrillation

ANSWER b. Nonsustained ventricular tachycardia. A short run of PVCs becomes VT after 3 consecutive beats. If the run lasts less than 30 seconds, as this one does, it is termed "nonsustained VT", longer and it is termed "sustained VT." If the ventricular complexes are identical in shape (morphology), as these are, it is termed a monomorphic or uniform VT. If the VT complexes vary they are termed polymorphic or multiformed. **See:** Marriot, chapter on "Ventricular Tachycardia." **Keywords:** Nonsustained VT = tun of PVCs

813. A run of PVCs lasts for 1 minute and then reverts to sinus rhythm, it is termed:
a. Sustained VT
b. Nonsustained VT
c. Monomorphic VT
d. Polymorphic VT

ANSWER a. Sustained VT. If the run lasts more than 30 seconds, it is termed "sustained VT", shorter than 30 seconds is nonsustained VT. **See:** Marriot, chapter on "Ventricular Tachycardia." **Keywords:** Nonsustained VT = run of PVCs

THE NEXT 2 QUESTIONS REFER TO THE ECG AND PRESSURE BELOW.

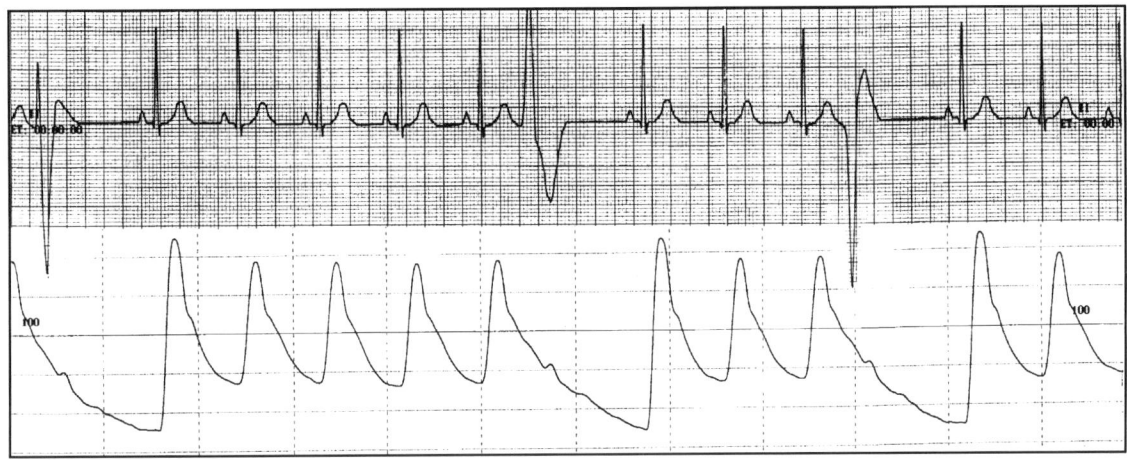

Lead II ECG and arterial pressure

814. The extrasystoles recorded above with an arterial blood pressure are:
a. PAC (Premature Atrial Contraction)
b. PJC (Premature Junctional Contraction)
c. Unifocal Premature Ventricular Contractions (PVCs)
d. Multifocal Premature Ventricular Contractions (PVCs)

815. The premature beats above are followed by a _____ pause.
a. Interpolated
b. Non-compensatory
c. Compensatory
d. Aberrant

ANSWERS TO ABOVE 2 QUESTIONS LISTED BELOW.

814. ANSWER d. Multifocal PVCs. The 2 premature beats are broad and different in shape. This indicates each comes from a different focus in the ventricle, and that ventricular conduction is slow since it must go through the ventricular muscle, not the faster Purkinje system.
   If this were lead V1, the first PVC would be an "LV-PVC" and the second an "RV-PVC." Note that these PVCs occurred too early to generate any significant blood pressure.
See: Marriot, chapter on "Premature Beats." **Keywords:** Multifocal PVCs

815. ANSWER c. Compensatory. The PVCs are not usually conducted retrograde into the atria and do not reset the SA node. The normal sinus "P" wave usually falls in the refractory period of the AV node and is not conducted. This makes the long compensatory pause following most PVCs. These beats can occur while manipulating a catheter in either ventricle.
See: Marriot, chapter on "Premature Beats." **Keywords:** Compensatory pause

816. This ECG trace shows a/an _____ leading to _____.

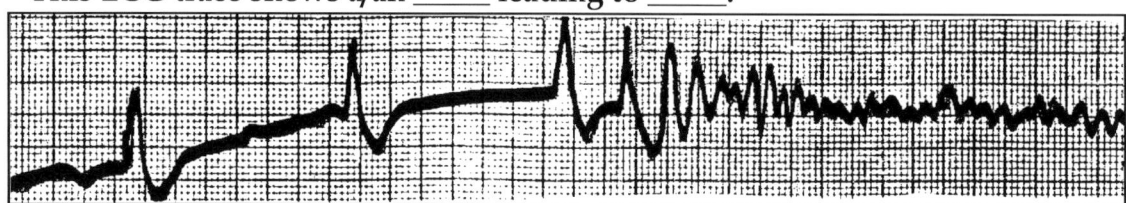

a. PVC on a "T" wave, Ventricular fibrillation
b. PAC on a "T" wave, Ventricular flutter
c. PVC on a "T" wave, Vventricular tachycardia
d. PAC on a "T" wave, Vventricular flutter

ANSWER a. PVC on a "T" wave, ventricular fibrillation. PVCs can be dangerous, when they interrupt the preceding "T" wave's vulnerable period. Premature beats falling on "T" waves may trigger a tachycardia such as VT or VF. Such premature beats may be ominous in patients following MI, with hypokalemia, or with long QT intervals. Treatment is cardiopulmonary resuscitation and emergency defibrillation.
See: Marriot, chapter on "Premature Beats." **Keywords:** PVC on "T" leading to VF

THE NEXT 2 QUESTIONS REFER TO THE ECG AND PRESSURE BELOW.

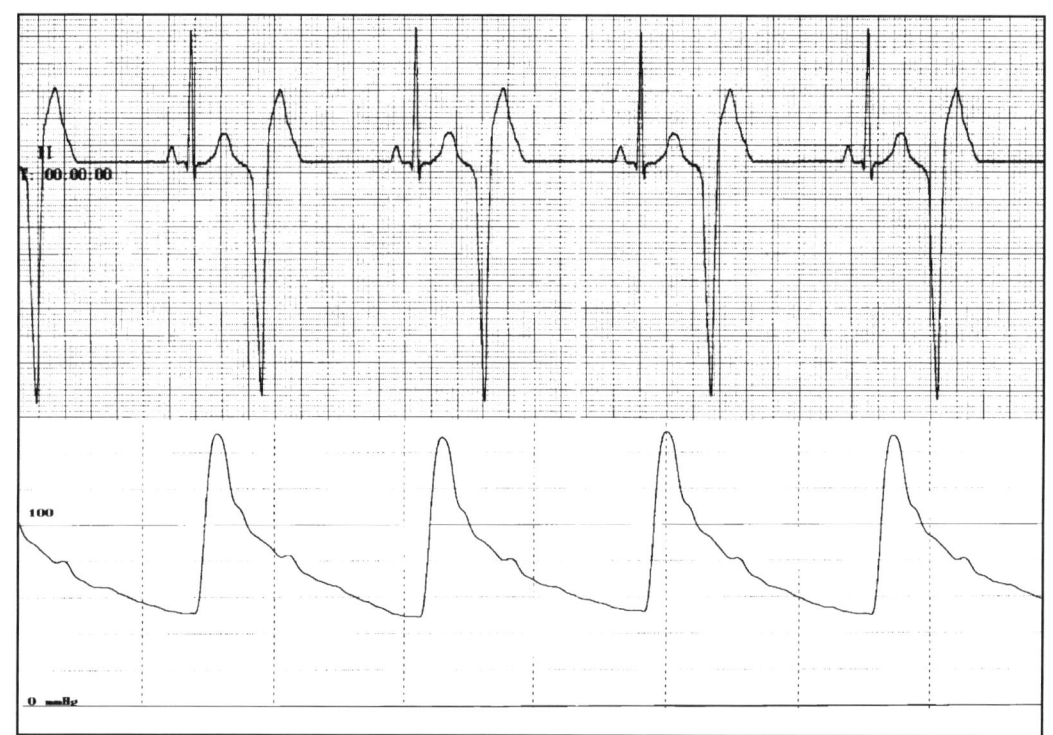

817. The arrhythmia recorded above with an arterial pressure shows:
a. Couplets (pairs of PVCs)
b. Interpolated PVCs
c. Multifocal PVCs
d. Ventricular bigeminy

818. In the ECG and pressure above, why is the pulse rate half the ECG heart rate?
a. Electromechanical dissociation occurs
b. Pulsus alternans occurs due to CHF
c. PVCs too early to allow filling
d. PVCs do not contract the heart

TWO ANSWERS LISTED TOGETHER BELOW.

817. ANSWER d. Ventricular Bigeminy. Each sinus beat is followed by a PVC. Constant coupling intervals occur between each pair of normal sinus and premature beats. Note that the PVCs are too early to generate any significant blood pressure.
See: Marriot, chapter on "Premature Beats." Keywords: Ventricular bigeminy

818. ANSWER c. PVCs too early to allow filling. The ECG shows ventricular bigeminy with a rate of 70/min. The pulse rate is only 35/min. Note. The PVCs do cause a small contraction, seen near the dicrotic notch. These premature beats have just barely enough pressure to open the aortic valve.
   Premature beats have less diastolic filling time than slower beats. Depending on how early the beat is, there may not be enough blood in the ventricle to pump effectively. The reduced preload diminishes their contractile force and resulting blood pressure. With premature beats an apical pulse rate is more accurate than a radial pulse rate. See: Marriot, chapter on "Premature Beats." Keywords: Ventricular bigeminy hemodynamics

819. The arrhythmia labeled at #1 in the diagram is:
a. Sustained polymorphic VT
b. Sustained monomorphic VT
c. Nonsustained polymorphic VT
d. Nonsustained monomorphic VT
e. Ventricular flutter

ANSWER b. Sustained monomorphic ventricular tachycardia (VT). If the VT complexes are all NOT identical, they appear to be multifocal (most dangerous type). And if the run of

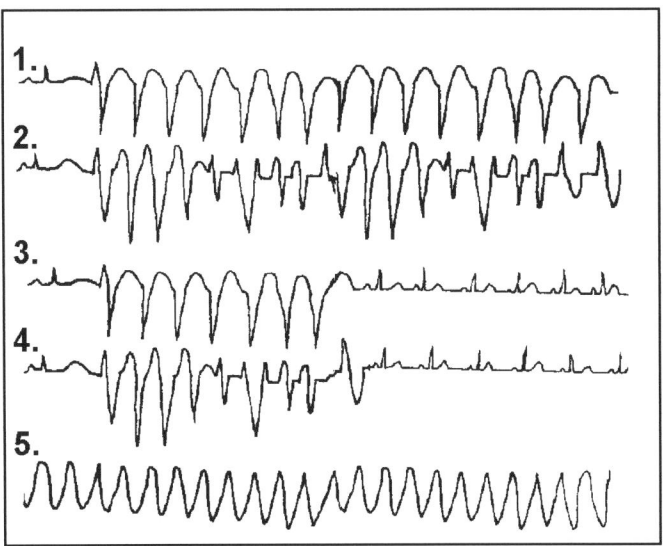

Types of Ventricular Tachycardia/flutter

VT lasts over 30 seconds is termed "sustained."
CORRECTLY MATCHED ANSWERS ARE:
   1. Sustained monomorphic VT
   2. Sustained polymorphic VT
   3. Nonsustained monomorphic VT
   4. Nonsustained polymorphic VT
   5. Ventricular flutter

See: Marriot, chapter on "Ventricular Tachycardia." **Keywords:** Identify nonsustained polymorphic VT run over 30 seconds in duration

3E. Arrhythmias - Other

820. Electro-mechanical dissociation (PEA) is defined as:
   a. Asystole
   b. Ventricular fibrillation
   c. Complete heart block (3°)
   d. Visible ECG but no detectable pulse

ANSWER d. Visible ECG but no detectable pulse. PEA is pulseless electrical activity. It is a state in which organized cardiac electrical depolarization but mechanical contractions are absent or undetectable. The ECG may look like any rhythm (usually bradycardia), but no pulse is detectable. The most common cause of PEA is hypovolemia, which can usually be corrected with fluid administration. Pulseless Electrical Activity or PEA was previously called electro-mechanical dissociation (EMD).
See: ACLS manual, chapter on "Essential of ACLS." **Keywords:** EMD, PEA

821. What arrhythmia may mimic asystole on the ECG monitor?
   a. Ventricular tachycardia - with no pulse
   b. Complete heart block
   c. Fine ventricular fibrillation
   d. Electro-mechanical dissociation

ANSWER c. Fine ventricular fibrillation may appear as a flat line unless the gain is increased. The monitoring lead should to be switched to the one that shows the largest QRS. This is because if your lead is perpendicular to the mean QRS axis, the QRS will be very small. Lead II is usually best. See: ACLS manual, chapter on "Arrhythmias." **Keywords:** Fine VF mimics asystole, isoelectric lead

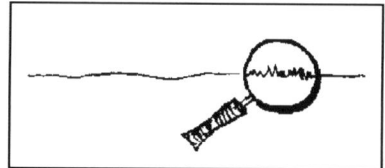
Asystole? NO! fine V. Fib.

822. What rhythm is most often seen in a patient with an acute MI?
a. PSVT
b. PVCs
c. Atrial fibrillation
d. Sinus bradycardia

ANSWER: b. PVCs are very common when the ventricle is irritable due to ischemic myocardium. PVCs in STEMI do not necessarily precede ventricular arrhythmias, so are no longer commonly treated with antiarrhythmics. Early treatment when PVCs are seen during acute MI, is directed at treating electrolyte deficits and sympathetic tone.
See: Braunwald, chapter on MI Keywords: in MI, PVCs common

3F. Arrhythmias - ACLS Therapy

823. Which patients have a narrow complex tachycardia with heart rate over 150, are not in cardiac arrest, yet should be cardioverted starting at the lowest energy (50 J)?
  1. Ventricular fibrillation
  2. Ventricular tachycardia (polymorphic)
  3. Atrial flutter
  4. Supraventricular tachycardia
  5. Atrial fibrillation
   a. 1, 3
   b. 2, 3
   c. 3, 4
   d. 3, 5

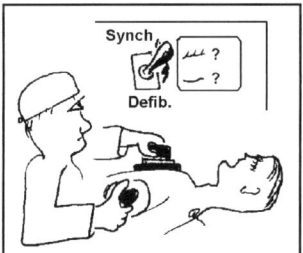

DC Cardioversion

ANSWER c. 3 & 4 (Atrial flutter and supraventricular tachycardia.) These rhythms have a strong narrow QRS complex necessary to trigger the cardioverter. Many of these rhythms can be converted with smaller amounts of energy. These rhythms are not usually emergencies so you have time to optimize the ECG leads and the patient's condition.

Ventricular fib and pulseless ventricular tachycardia should receive emergency defibrillation. Asystole cannot be converted with high voltage shock (unless it is really fine ventricular fib.).

Current guidelines say, "Synchronized cardioversion is recommended to treat supraventricular tachycardia due to reentry, atrial fibrillation, atrial flutter, and atrial tachycardia. Synchronized cardioversion is also recommended to treat monomorphic VT with pulses. Cardioversion is not effective for treatment of junctional tachycardia or multifocal atrial tachycardia."

"Synchronized cardioversion must not be used for treatment of VF as the device may not sense a QRS wave and thus a shock may not be delivered. Synchronized cardioversion should also not be used for pulseless VT or polymorphic (irregular VT). These rhythms require delivery of high-energy unsynchronized shocks (i.e., defibrillation doses)."

The recommended initial biphasic energy dose for cardioversion of adult atrial fibrillation is 120 to 200 J (Class IIa, LOE A). If the initial shock fails, providers should increase the dose in a stepwise fashion. Cardioversion of adult atrial flutter and other supraventricular tachycardias generally requires less energy; an initial energy of 50 J to 100 J is often sufficient. If the initial shock fails, providers should increase the dose in a stepwise fashion." See: ACLS manual, chapter on "Defibrillation."

824. This ECG rhythm should be treated with: (Select 2 below)
a. Defibrillation
b. Cardioversion
c. Pacemaker
d. CPR

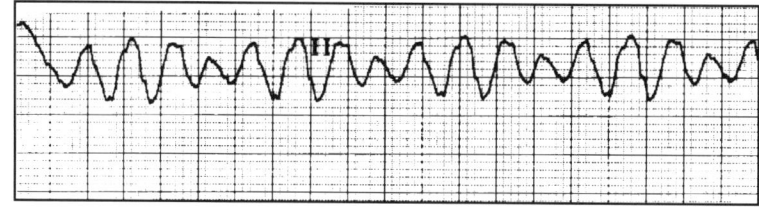

ANSWER a & d. Defibrillation and CPR. This is ventricular fibrillation. This is a resuscitation emergency and should be treated as follows:
- Check ABCs
- Perform CPR until defibrillator attached
- Defibrillate at 200 J, 200-300 J, and 360 Joules

Ventricular Fib should not be cardioverted because there is no clear QRS to trigger from. Since pacemakers are usually used to treat bradycardia, they are not usually used for rapid chaotic rhythms. VF is chaotic and rapid enough. You don't need anything to speed it.
See: ACLS manual, "VF Algorithm" **Keywords:** Treat ventricular fibrillation

THE NEXT TWO QUESTIONS REFER TO THIS ECG AND PRESSURE.

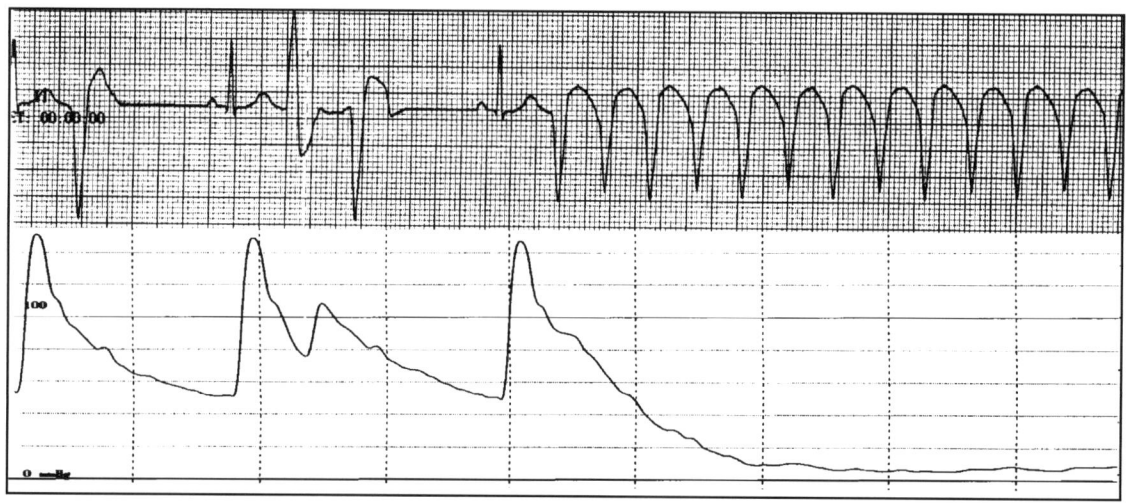

ECG with arterial pressure x 200

Diagnostic Techniques: D11 - ECG 1 and Arrhythmias   461

825. The ECG and arterial pressure ABOVE show PVCs leading to:
   a. Electro mechanical dissociation
   b. Pulseless ventricular fibrillation
   c. Polymorphic ventricular tachycardia
   d. Pulseless ventricular tachycardia

826. You are alone in the cath lab with a patient post coronary angiography. You are ready to remove the arterial line when you hear a snoring sound. Then the patient's eyes roll back. You look at the monitor and see the ECG and arterial tracing above. After calling for help you should:
   a. Administer a precordial thump
   b. Administer 0.5 mg epinephrine IV
   c. Apply oxygen by nasal cannula 5 L/min
   d. Begin endotracheal intubation
   e. Apply an external transthoracic pacemaker

BOTH ANSWERS TOGETHER BELOW.

825. ANSWER d. Pulseless ventricular tachycardia. The multifocal PVCs trigger VT and the blood pressure falls to zero. The patient will be unconscious within 10 seconds. Defibrillation and basic life support resuscitation are needed. VT patients often have a pulse and may not need emergency treatment.
See: Marriott, chapter on "Ventricular Tachyarrhythmias." **Keywords:** Pulseless VT

826. ANSWER a. Precordial thump. Only recommended for witnessed VT by health professionals. This rhythm shows multifocal PVCs leading to a lethal arrhythmia - pulseless VT. After checking the pulse, a forceful precordial thump is administered by "hammering" your fist from 1 foot above the patient's sternum. It generates 10-20 joules of energy and may convert VT into a perfusing arrhythmia in (successful in 11%-25% of cases). It is recommended only immediately in monitored VT when a defibrillator is not available. If the precordial thump proves ineffective, the patient will require CPR and defibrillation. Beware, that a precordial thump may make VT deteriorate into VF. The precordial thump is NOT likely to convert ventricular fib.

   The definitive treatment is defibrillation. Your lab will have a defibrillator, but as here, it may not be readily available. Other options to consider are: begin airway management, begin CPR, to ready the defibrillator, and to record the ECG so it will be documented. **See:** ACLS manual, chapter on "VF/VT Algorithm" and "Defibrillation" **Keywords:** Precordial thump

827. During a heart cath, your patient goes into sustained VT at a rate of 175/min. He is still wide awake. Expect to:
a. Administer amiodarone IV
b. Defibrillate (sync mode is off)
c. Cardiovert (sync mode is on)
d. Let the patient continue in asymptomatic VT

ANSWER: c. Cardiovert (sync mode is on). As long as the QRS complex can trigger the defibrillator, it is safer to shock in synchronized mode. This avoids shocking on the vulnerable period on the T wave which could result in VF. However, the awake patient will not appreciate this shock, and the patient should be sedated, unless he becomes unconscious first. "It is usually possible to terminate a VT episode with a direct current shock across the heart. This is ideally synchronized to the patient's heartbeat. As this is quite uncomfortable, shocks should be delivered only to an unconscious or sedated patient. A patient with pulseless VT or a ventricular fibrillation will be unconscious and treated as an emergency on an ACLS protocol, given high energy (360J with a monophasic defibrillator, or 200J with a biphasic defibrillator) unsynchronised cardioversion. Patients with a stable VT are given cardioversion if the tachycardia exceeds 150 bpm." See: https://medlineplus.gov/ency/article/007110.htm **Keywords:** Cardiovert sustained VT

REFERENCES

Baim, D. S. and Grossman W., *Cardiac Catheterization, Angiography, and Intervention*, 6th Ed., Lea and Febiger, 2006

Braunwald, Eugene, Ed., *HEART DISEASE A Textbook of Cardiovascular Medicine*, 9th Ed., W. B. Saunders Co., 2012

Conover, M. H., *Cardiac arrhythmias, Exercises in Pattern Interpretation*, 2nd Ed., C.V. Mosby Co., 1978

Davis, Dale, *How to Quickly and Accurately Master ECG Interpretation*, 2nd Ed., J. B. Lippincott Co., 1985

Dubin, Dale, *RAPID INTERPRETATION of EKG's*, 3rd Ed., Cover Publishing Co., 1982

Fogoros, R.N., *MD, Practical Cardiac Diagnosis, ELECTROPHYSIOLOGIC TESTING*, 4th Ed., 2006

Hurst, J.W., and Logue, R.B., et. al., *THE HEART Arteries and Veins*, 3rd Ed., McGraw-Hill Book Co., 1974

Kern, M. J., Ed., *The Cardiac Catheterization Handbook*, 6th Ed., Mosby-Year Book, Inc., 2016

Thaler, M. S., *The Only EKG Book You'll Ever Need*, , J. B. Lippincott Co., 1988

Underhill, S. L., Ed., *CARDIAC NURSING*, 2nd Ed., J. B. Lippincott Co., 1989

Textbook of ADVANCED CARDIAC LIFE SUPPORT, American Heart Association, 2017

Wagner, G. S., *MARRIOTT'S Practical Electrocardiography*, 9th Ed., Williams & Wilkins, 1994

OUTLINE: ECG 1 and Arrhythmias

1. GENERAL ECG
   a. General & Terms
      i. Block = Slowed or interrupted Conduction
      ii. Arrest = Cessation of activity
      iii. fibrillation = Chaotic rapid beating (over 300)
      iv. Flutter = Rapid, but very regular beating
      v. (over 200 bpm)
      vi. Premature = Beat which occurs too soon, early
      vii. Escape = Delayed beat, from lower pacemaker
      viii. Tachycardia = Rate over 100 bpm
      ix. Bradycardia = Rate less than 60 bpm
      x. Paroxysmal = Sudden rhythm or rate change
      xi. aberrant
      xii. antegrade
      xiii. refractory
      xiv. retrograde
   b. Normal anatomy & Physiology
      i. Waves of ECG
         (1) "P" wave
         (2) PR interval
         (3) "R" wave
         (4) RS (QRS)
         (5) QT interval
         (6) "T" wave
         (7) ST segment
         (8) "S" wave
      ii. Segments & Intervals
      iii. Normal values for:
         (1) PR int.
         (2) QRS duration
         (3) QT interval
      iv. Anatomy
         (1) SA node
         (2) Inter-atrial tracts (including *Bachmann's bundle)
         (3) AV Node
         (4) AN = Transitional tissue between Atria and AV ode.
         (5) N = Mid AV nodal tissue
         (6) NH = region where nodal fibers gradually merge with bundle of His tissue.
         (7) His = the upper portion of ventricular conduction tissue
         (8) Bundle of HIS
         (9) Right and Left Bundle branches (Left has 2 fascicles, ant. & Post.)
         (10) Purkinje System - to myocardium
         (11) internodal tracts
      v. Bachmann's bundle
      vi. Right or Left fascicles
   c. Abnormal anatomy and Physiology
      i. Bundle of Kent, James, Mayheim
      ii. Intrinsic rates
         (1) SA Node = 60-100 bpm
         (2) Junctional (nodal) = 40-50 bpm
         (3) Ventricular = 30-40 bpm
      iii. Sudden death usually VF
      iv. Effect of PVC
         (1) compensatory pause
         (2) interpolated PVC
2. ECG TRACINGS
   a. EQUIPMENT
      i. Gain: 1 Mv= 1 cm
      ii. Damping: Over & under
   b. Artifacts
      i. 60 cycle
      ii. Wandering baseline
      iii. muscle tremor
      iv. monitor settings
         (1) MCL1 lead position
         (2) sensitivity/gain
         (3) position, threshold
      v. Correcting artifacts
   c. leads & Techniques
      i. Frontal
         (1) Unipolar, bipolar
         (2) Einthoven triangle
         (3) Positive negative poles
      ii. Chest/precordial leads
         (1) position
   d. Axis, Vectors
      i. NORMAL AXIS: -30-90 degrees
      ii. RIGHT AXIS DEVIATION: +90 to +180°
      iii. EXTREME AXIS: +180 to -90° (also Termed Indeterminate or Extreme Rt. Axis deviation)
      iv. LEFT AXIS DEVIATION: -90° to -30°
   e. Combined measurements of all above
3. ARRHYTHMIAS
   a. causes: reentry, automaticity
   b. Sinus
      i. Sinus arrhythmia
      ii. SSS
      iii. Sinus pause/block
   c. Atrial
      i. PAC
      ii. Atrial tach, PAT, SVT
      iii. A. Fib/flutter
      iv. Carotid Sinus Massage
      v. Wandering Pacemaker
      vi. Noncompensatory pause
   d. Junctional
      i. JPC
      ii. Junctional escape beats/rhythm
   e. Ventricular
      i. PVC, RV-pvc, LVpvc
      ii. PVC on T

- iii. Bigeminy, effect on BP
- iv. Ventricular Tachycardia
  - (1) Sustained >30 sec
  - (2) Mono-poly-morphic
  - (3) Unifocal - multifocal
  - (4) Compensatory pauses
  - (5) Torsade De Pointes
- v. Ventricular Fibrillation
  - (1) Fine V. fib. - Asystole
    - (2) Resuscitation, defib.
    - (3) Clinical - biological death
- f. Other
  - i. EMD - PEA
  - ii. Asystole
- g. ACLS Therapy
  - i. Defibrillation
  - ii. Cardioversion
  - iii. Precordial thump

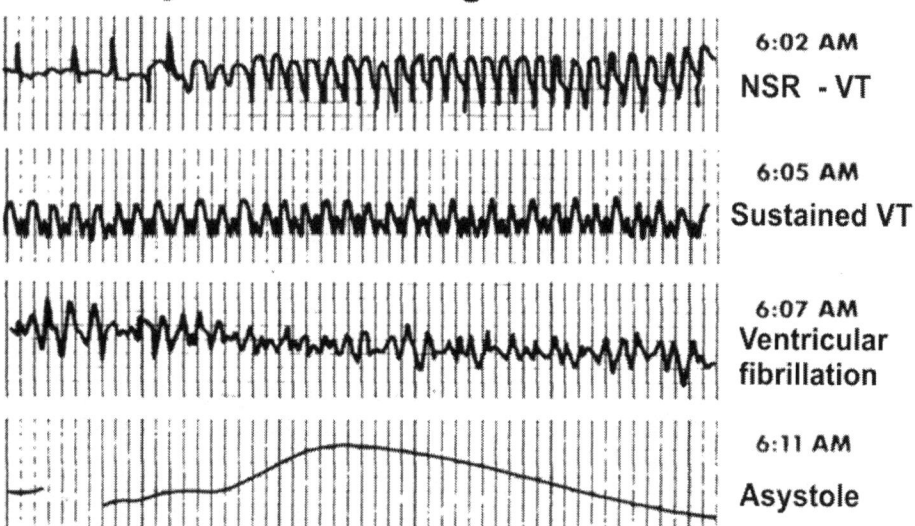

Arrhythmias leading to death

- 6:02 AM NSR - VT
- 6:05 AM Sustained VT
- 6:07 AM Ventricular fibrillation
- 6:11 AM Asystole

ECG II: Blocks, 12 Leads & Pacers

INDEX: D12 - ECG II: Blocks, 12 Leads and Pacers
1. Blocks
   - a. AV Block (1°, 2°, & 3° Block) . . p. 465 - Know
   - b. BBB . . . . . p. 471 - Know
   - c. ACLS Therapy . . . p. 474 - Know
2. Twelve Lead ECGs & Infarct Patterns . p. 475 - Know
3. Hypertrophy & Electrolytes. . . p. 484 - Review
4. Pacemaker Modes . . . p. 485 - Know
5. Chapter Outline . . . . p. 492

1A. Blocks - AV Blocks

827. Match the level of AV block labeled at #3 in the box with its name below (Two out of every 3 "P" waves are not conducted.)
a. Complete heart block
b. Second degree block (type 2)
c. Second degree block (Wenckebach)
d. First degree AV block

LEVELS OF AV BLOCK
1. Prolonged PR interval
2. Gradual lengthening of PR interval until a QRS is dropped
3. **Every third "P" wave is conducted**
4. Unrelated "P" & QRS rhythms

ANSWER b. Second degree block (Mobitz type 2). This is a fixed ratio AV block (e.g. 2:1, 3:1, 4:1 etc.). In the 3:1 AV block shown, three "P" waves occur for every one that is conducted down the AV node. The other two "P" waves are blocked by the AV node. There is no

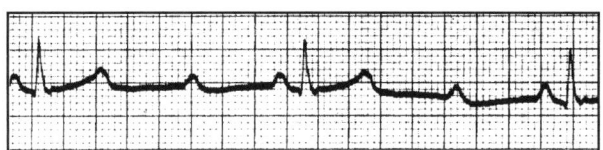

3:1 AB block

gradual lengthening of the PR interval before the dropped beat, as in Wenckebach. The degree of block may vary e.g. in 2:1 AV block, every other "P" wave is blocked by the AV node. **BE ABLE TO MATCH ALL ANSWERS BELOW.**
<u>ECG Finding</u> <u>Levels of AV Block</u>
1. PROLONGED PR INTERVAL = first degree Block
2. LENGTHENING OF PR INTERVAL - UNTIL QRS IS DROPPED = second degree Block (type I Wenckebach)
3. THREE "P" WAVES FOR EACH QRS (Only every 3rd "P" wave conducted) = second degree Block (type II)
4. INDEPENDENT "P" & QRS RHYTHMS = complete heart block
See: Hurst and Logue, The Heart, chapter on "Disturbance of Cardiac Rhythm."
Keywords: EP, Heart Block

828. Lev's disease and Lenegre's disease in aged patients causes calcification or degeneration around the superior interventricular septum. These diseases often result in _____ that is best treated with a/an _____.
   a. V. Tach. or Fib., Antiarrhythmic drugs
   b. Valvular stenosis, Artificial valve replacement
   c. Wolf-Parkinson-White syndrome, Ablation
   d. Heart block, Pacemaker

ANSWER d. Heart block, Pacemaker. These two diseases involve the conduction fascicles. Both lead to AV and intraventricular blocks, such as complete heart block that may require a pacemaker.
See: Hurst and Logue, The Heart, chapter on "Disturbance of Cardiac Rhythm."
Keywords: EP, heart block, Lev, Lenegre

829. What type of heart block is this?

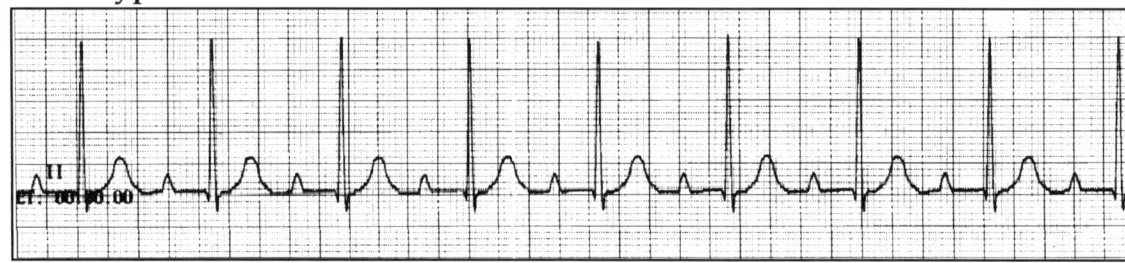

Lead II ECG

   a. First degree
   b. Second degree (Mobitz I)
   c. Second degree (Mobitz II)
   d. Third degree

ANSWER a. First degree. The PR interval measures 7 boxes or .28 sec. PR intervals longer than 0.20 sec indicate 1° heart block in the AV node. This is not usually a serious abnormality, but may progress to higher degrees of block.
See: Marriott, chapter on "AV Block." **Keywords:** First degree block

830. This ladder diagram is an example of what type of heart block?

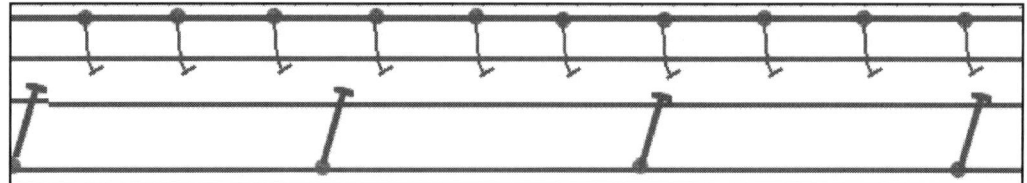

   a. First degree AV block
   b. Second degree AV block - Type I
   c. Second degree AV block - Type II
   d. Third degree AV block

ANSWER c. Second degree AV block - Type II. This is a 3:1 fixed ratio block. Note the 3 "P" waves for each QRS complex. This is a high degree of AV block. Each QRS complex is preceded by a P wave arising from the SA node (marked with a ● at top diagram) with a constant PR interval. QRS complexes arise from the ventricle (marked with a ● at bottom of the diagram) with a broad complex, not conducted by Purkinje system, as indicated by the

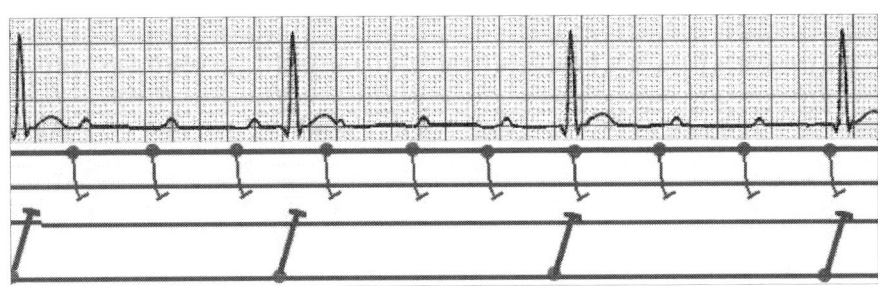

ECG with associated Ladder diagram

sloping line. Here is what the ECG and ladder diagram look like together. **See:** ACLS Manual, chapter on "Arrhythmias." **Keywords:** ID complete or 3rd degree AV block

831. **Mobitz I type heart block is another name for:**
   a. First degree heart block
   b. Sick sinus syndrome
   c. Wolf Parkinson White syndrome
   d. Wenckebach phenomenon

ANSWER d. Wenckebach Phenomenon = Second degree AV block type I or Mobitz I. Progressive lengthening of PR interval until one beat is dropped.
See: ACLS manual, chapter on "Arrhythmias." **Keywords:** Wenckebach

832. **This ladder diagram is an example of what arrhythmia?**

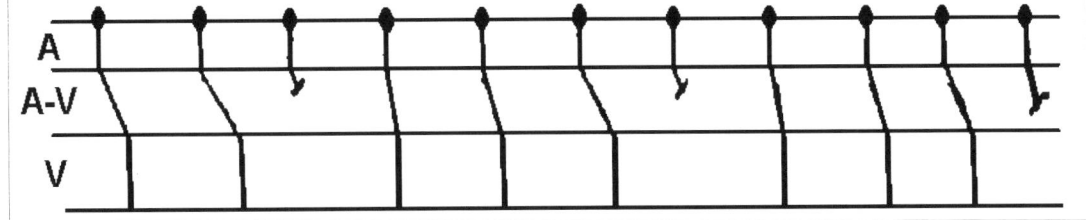

Ladder diagram

   a. First degree AV block
   b. Second degree AV block - Type I
   c. Second degree AV block - Type II
   d. Third degree AV block

ANSWER b. Second degree AV block - Type I - Wenckebach. Shows progressive lengthening of the PR interval until one "P" wave is not conducted though the AV node. Note the 2 "P" waves following each group of 3 QRS complexes. This is 4:3 block. Four "P" waves occur for each three QRS complexes. The dots at the top of the ladder represent SA ode firing. Then atrial conduction occurs, drawn as a straight line down to the AV node.

The slope within the AV band decreases as AV conduction lengthens. The 4th "P" wave is blocked, as shown within the AV band, by ending the conduction with a perpendicular line. These ladder diagrams help to understand complex arrhythmias. A good example of this ECG is seen in the next question.
See: ACLS manual, chapter on "Arrhythmias." **Keywords:** ID Wenckebach or second degree type I

833. This ECG is an example of what type of arrhythmia?

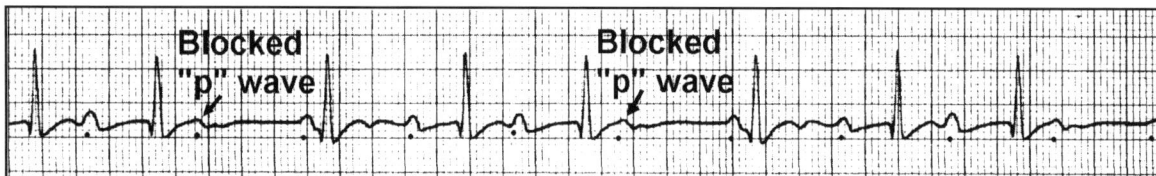
Heart block ECG

a. Mobitz I, with 2:1 conduction
b. Mobitz I, with 4:3 conduction
c. Mobitz II, with 2:1 conduction
d. Mobitz II, with 4:3 conduction

ANSWER b. Mobitz I or Wenckebach with 4:3 conduction. Note that there are 4 P waves for every 3 QRS complexes. Thus, every fourth P wave is dropped (non-conducted). Note the regularity of P waves indicated with "dots." Note also that a P wave is buried within every third T wave. This P wave is not conducted through the AV node, and is not followed with a QRS complex. Note also, the grouping of 3 QRS complexes together.
See: ACLS manual, chapter on "Arrhythmias." **Keywords:** Ladder diagram of Wenckebach

834. This ECG ladder diagram is an example of what type of arrhythmia?

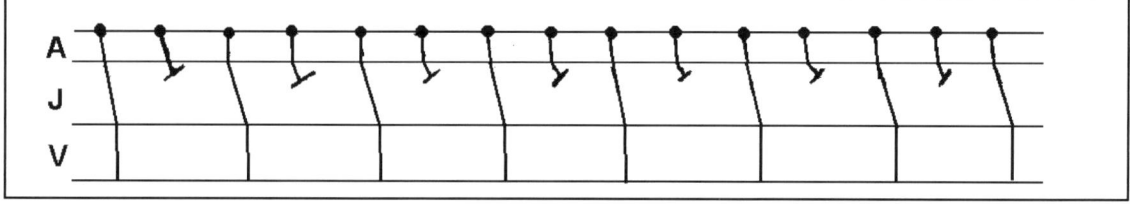
Ladder diagram

a. First degree HB
b. Second degree HB, Mobitz I
c. Second degree HB, Mobitz II
d. Third degree HB

ANSWER c. Second degree HB, Mobitz II. Every second "P" wave is blocked within the AV band. Normal conduction occurs every other beat.
See: ACLS manual, chapter on "Arrhythmias." **Keywords:** Ladder diagram second degree block type II with 2:1 conduction

835. **A patient comes to the cath lab with a left bundle branch block (LBBB) ECG pattern. While passing a right heart catheter through the RV he develops an additional right bundle branch block. The ECG would show:**
   a. Right fascicular block pattern
   b. Bifasicular block with PVCs
   c. Second degree heart block
   d. Complete heart block

ANSWER d. Complete heart block occurs when both left-sided fascicles and the right fascicle are blocked. The heart's normal sinus pacemaker impulse cannot get through the bundle branches into the ventricle. Complete heart block results with junctional or ventricular escape bradycardia taking over. Patients coming to right heart cath with LBBB are at risk of going to complete heart block. Therefore a pacing Swan-Ganz or Baim-Turi catheter should be used and the temporary pacemaker readily available.
See: Kern, chapter on "Electrophysiology." Keywords: RBBB + LBBB = complete heart block.

836. **What type of ECG is shown on this rhythm strip?**

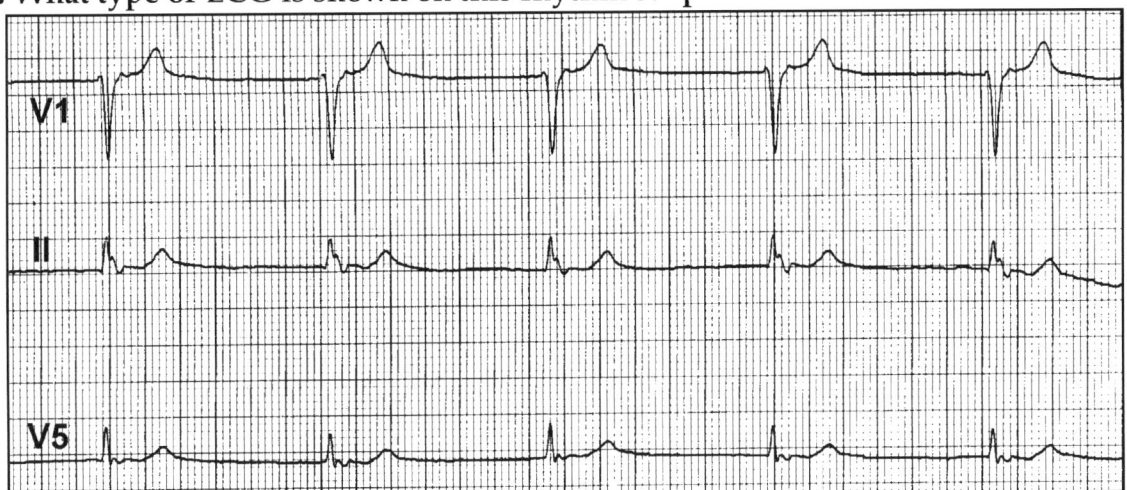

   a. Junctional escape rhythm
   b. Ventricular escape rhythm
   c. 2rd degree block
   d. 3rd degree block

ANSWER a. Junctional escape rhythm. When the SA node is inactive (no P waves are seen here) the junctional pacemaker may "escape" with its slow rhythm (40-50/min). QRS complexes will be narrow (here 0.10 sec) and the same shape as this patient's sinus QRS. This cannot be classed as 3rd degree block because there are no P waves to block. This is a "sick sinus node" or "sinus node arrest."
See: ACLS manual, chapter on "Arrhythmias." Keywords: Junctional escape rhythm

837. What type of heart block is this?

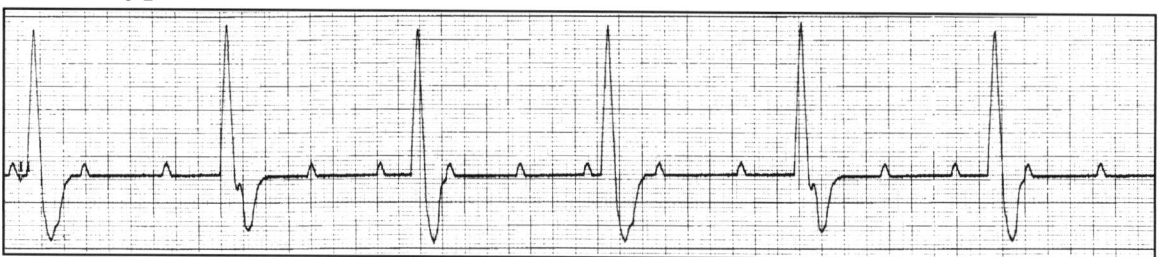

a. First degree
b. Second degree (Wenckebach)
c. Second degree (2:1) fixed ratio
d. Third degree

ANSWER d. Third degree or complete heart block with ventricular escape rhythm. The QRS complexes are broad and bizarre with T waves opposite in direction to the RS waves. The ventricular rate is a "ventricular escape" or "ideoventricular" rhythm. Note how the "P" waves have no relation to the QRS complexes. (This was generated by a machine so some relation may exist). Although the atrial rate is 100, ventricular rate is 35 / min (normal ventricular escape rate is 30-40/min). Use a calipers to "walk" out the nonconducted "P" waves. Some "P" waves are buried in the QRS-T complexes.
See: ACLS manual, chapter on "Arrhythmias." **Keywords:** Third degree block

838. Which of the following would present the greatest risk of leading to a Stokes-Adams attack?
a. LBBB
b. Mobitz I
c. Mobitz II
d. Mobitz III
e. Atrial fibrillation

ANSWER: c. Mobitz II occurs when some P waves are not conducted to the ventricle. It may progress to complete heart block. Stokes-Adams attack is a sudden loss of consciousness due to heart block and bradycardia. The ECG for type 2 second-degree AV block, also known as Mobitz II, shows intermittently nonconducted P waves.

The significance of Mobitz II heart block is that it may progress rapidly to complete heart block, where no escape rhythm may emerge. In this case, the person may experience a Stokes-Adams attack, cardiac arrest, or sudden cardiac death. The definitive treatment for this form of AV block is an implanted pacemaker. In the alternatives, Mobitz I is Wenckebach. There is no Mobitz III - perhaps they meant 3rd degree or complete heart block. **See:** Dubin, Rapid Interpretation of EKGs and http://emedicine.medscape.com/article/161919-overview. **Keywords:** Mobitz II - Stokes-Adams

1B. Blocks - Bundle Branch Block (BBB)

839. Supraventricular beats may have a broad QRS (>0.12 sec) if conducted with:
a. Aberrant conduction
b. Concealed conduction
c. Retrograde conduction
d. Second degree AV block

ANSWER a. Aberrant conduction. Aberrant beats are conducted slowly with a broad QRS. The AV node is still partially refractory. It is a supraventricular impulse with abnormal, bizarre interventricular conduction. If the "P" waves are not evident, these beats may be confused with ventricular beats because of their PVC shape.
See: ACLS manual, chapter on "Arrhythmias." Keywords: Aberrancy

840. This ECG shows what abnormality?

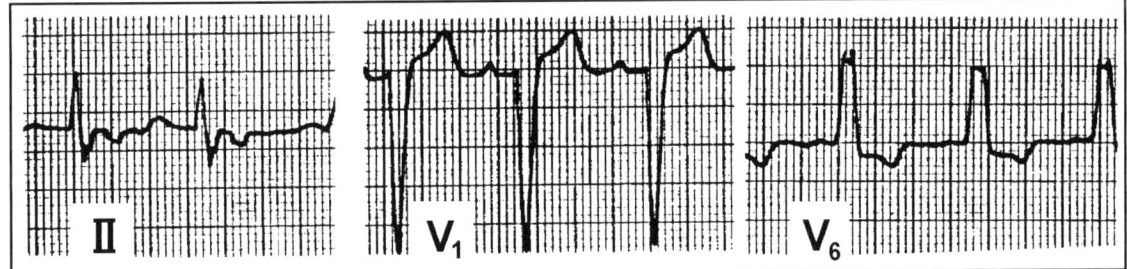

a. Atrial hypertrophy
b. Ventricular hypertrophy of LV
c. Ventricular hypertrophy of RV
d. RBBB
e. LBBB

ANSWER e. LBBB. When the main left bundle branch becomes blocked (or both left fascicles) the RV depolarizes first. The depolarization wave slowly travels across the septum and depolarizes the LV last. This makes a posterior traveling depolarization wave. Since the QRS complex is distorted in BBB it is difficult to diagnose infarction or hypertrophy. The following signs are seen in the QRS with LBBB:
- broad distorted QRS (>0.12sec)
- monophasic QS complex in V1 (V1 negative)
- rR' wave in V6

An easy way to remember the V1 in LBBB is relate it to your car turn signal. V1 QS wave is down in LBBB just like the direction you push your turn signal - down to turn left.
See: Davis, chapter on "Interventricular Conduction Disturbances." Keywords: LBBB

841. In LBBB the ____ ventricle fires first, causing a characteristic V1 ____ pattern.
a. Left, Broad QS
b. Left, Narrow QR
c. Right, Broad QS
d. Right, Broad Rr'

ANSWER c. Right, Broad QS. Since the left bundle is blocked the conduction proceeds down the His bundle into the right bundle branch. Since the RV depolarizes first the depolarization wave must travel across the septum to depolarize the LV. This makes a slow posterior traveling wave of depolarization. Note the broad QS pattern in V1, and the broad Rr' in V6.
See: Davis, chapter on "Interventricular Conduction Disturbances." **Keywords:** LBBB

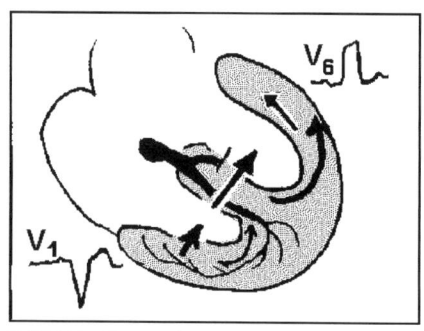
LBBB, Depol. away from V1

842. This ECG shows what abnormality?

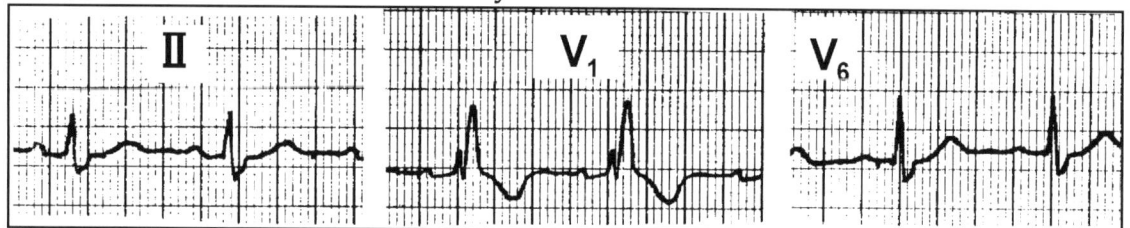

a. Atrial hypertrophy
b. Left ventricular hypertrophy
c. Right ventricular hypertrophy
d. RBBB
e. BBB

ANSWER d. RBBB = Right Bundle Branch Block. When the right bundle branch becomes blocked the depolarization wave is rapid in the LV. The impulse must travel slowly through IVS, and into the RV last. This makes an anterior traveling wave of depolarization. The following signs are seen in the QRS with RBBB:
• Broad distorted QRS (>0.12sec)
• Biphasic rsR' complex in V1
• Negative "S" wave in V6

RBBB moving toward V1

See: Davis, chapter on "Interventricular Conduction Disturbances." **Keywords:** RBBB

843. This precordial lead ECG pattern (rSR' "rabbit ears" in lead V1) is associated with:
a. Acute anterolateral MI
b. Right bundle branch block
c. Left ventricular hypertrophy
d. Sinus bradycardia; left bundle branch block

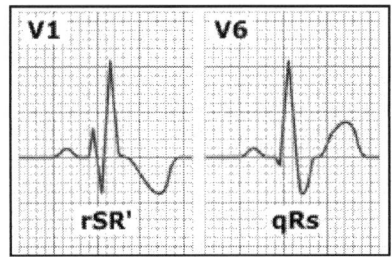

ANSWER: b. Right bundle branch block. Precordial lead V1 and V6 are all that are needed for RBBB. Dubin uses the shortcut method of looking for broad QRS and a "Rabbit Ear" pattern. If the rabbit ears are in V1 it is RBBB. If the rabbit ears are in V6 it is
LBBB. Remember the "turn signal" mnemonic for BB patterns in V1. A car's turn signal is pulled up to turn right - RBBB = R wave up; and pushed down QS for LBBB in V1.

In RBBB there is a wide QRS complexes and T wave inversion in lead V1. Note the typical wide and deep S wave in V6. The small Q wave in V6 may not always be present. Below each QRS complex is its designation (rSR' and qRs) according to standard nomenclature. **See:** Braunwald, chapter on, "Electrocardiography" **Keywords:** RBBB

844. The ECG pattern resulting from a standard right ventricular pacemaker, shows a pacer spike followed by an:
a. RVH pattern
b. LVH pattern
c. RBBB pattern
d. LBBB pattern

ANSWER: d. LBBB. "Each QRS complex is preceded by a pacemaker stimulus - not shown in this diagram. The QRS complex is abnormal, wide, and bizarre, resembling a ventricular beat. The QRS complexes usually have a left bundle branch block configuration since the ventricular lead is most commonly located in the right ventricle."

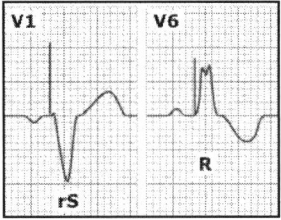

The RV lead stimulates the RV first, then the impulse is conducted slowly to the LV, just like it would in LBBB. This diagram shows LBBB with the wide negative RS pattern in V1, and does not show the pacemaker spike. Note the small "rabbit ears in V6".

845. This ECG shows:
a. Mobitz I
b. Mobitz II
c. Mobitz III
d. 3rd degree HB

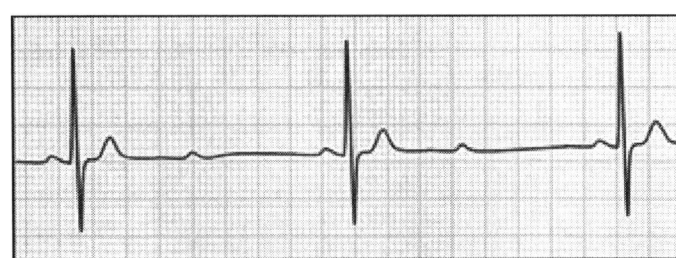

ANSWER: b. Mobitz II or 2nd degree block-type II. "In type II AV block, most beats are conducted with a constant PR interval, but occasionally atrial

depolarization is not followed by ventricular depolarization. Type II is pathological and indicates disease of the conduction system distal to the AV node. It can frequently lead to complete AV block, causing Stokes–Adams attacks. Therefore, temporary and then permanent pacing (DDD) is indicated in most patients, even those who initially present without symptoms."

Second degree heart block has 2 types: Mobitz I and Mobitz II. Mobitz I is Wenckebach which has a longer and longer PR interval until one P is not conducted. This example is type II, with two non-conducted P waves. Other beats have fixed PR intervals.
See: https://www.ncbi.nlm.nih.gov/books/NBK2219/ **Keywords:** Mobitz II = some P waves not conducted down AVN

1C. Blocks - ACLS Therapy

846. This patient's BP is 60/40 mmHg. His arrhythmia is ____ with a definitive treatment of ____.

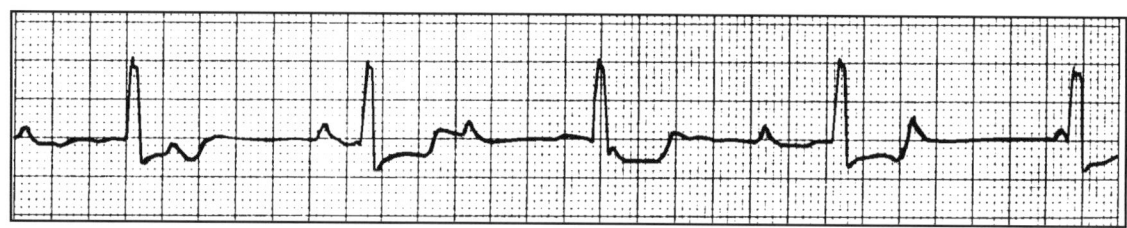

ECG lead II
a. Complete heart block, Defibrillation
b. Complete heart block, Pacemaker
c. Wandering pacemaker, Defibrillation
d. Wandering pacemaker, Pacemaker
e. Second degree AV block, Antiarrhythmic drugs

ANSWER b. Complete heart block (3rd degree), Ventricular pacemaker. This shows an ideoventricular bradycardia with a ventricular rate of 45. "P" waves are seen with a rate of 75 and no relation to the QRS complexes. Blood pressure is 60/40 mmHg. A patient with such a low BP would probably be in a decreased state of consciousness. Stimulant drugs and a ventricular pacemaker may be needed to increase the heart rate and cardiac output.
See: Davis, chapter on "Interventricular Conduction Disturbances."

847. The recommended therapy for first degree heart block is:
a. Lidocaine 1 mg/Kg
b. Atropine .5-1 mg
c. Pacemaker
d. None

ANSWER d. None. Treatment is not usually needed unless the patient exhibits symptoms.
See: ACLS, chapter on "Arrhythmias." **Keywords:** 1st degree block requires no treatment

848. The initial recommended therapy for bradycardia with hypotension is:
a. Dopamine 5-10 mcg/kg/min
b. Atropine .5-1 mg
c. Transcutaneous pacing
d. Cardioversion 50-100 J

ANSWER b. Atropine .5-1 mg. ACLS says, "If bradycardia produces signs and symptoms of instability, the initial treatment is atropine. If bradycardia is unresponsive to atropine, intravenous (IV) infusion of ß-adrenergic agonists with rate-accelerating effects (**dopamine,** epinephrine) or transcutaneous pacing (TCP) can be effective while the patient is prepared for emergent transvenous temporary pacing if required." See: ACLS manual

2. 12 Lead ECGs and Myocardial Infarction Patterns

849. In the progression of a myocardial infarction, as seen on an ECG, an early sign of acute injury to the myocardial cells is seen as:
a. Inverted "T" waves
b. An inverted QRS
c. ST segment elevation
d. "Q" waves of significant size

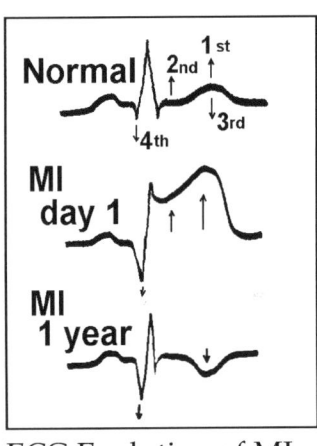

ECG Evolution of MI

ANSWER c. ST segment elevation is the first sign of acute injury to the myocardium. Sometimes called a "current of injury" the ECG begins to resemble an action potential. Electrodes facing the injury register ST elevation. Those on the opposite side of the heart may register ST depression, termed reciprocal ST changes.
   Some authors say that hyperacute "T" wave elevation is an even earlier sign than ST elevation. These hyperacute "T" waves are often tall and narrow, and are termed "peaked." The "T" waves flip and invert soon after the acute injury begins, showing signs of continued ischemia in the area around the injury. See: Dubin, chapter on "Infarction."

850. When a positive ECG electrode is placed over an area of myocardium experiencing myocardial infarction, four basic patterns can be seen. The ECG pattern labeled at #3 on the diagram is indicative of an area of myocardial:
a. Infarction
b. Injury
c. Ischemia
d. Hyperacute ischemia

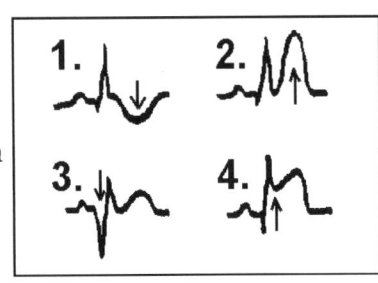

ECG signs seen in MI

ANSWER a. Infarction or dead tissue. "Q" waves must be deep and wide to be significant for MI (>1/3 the height of the QRS and > .04 sec wide). Significant "Q" waves indicate a transmural infarction and remain on the ECG even after it scars over. No ECG lead normally displays large Q waves unless infarct of BBB is present.

BE ABLE TO MATCH ALL ANSWERS BELOW:
1. Inverted "T" wave = Ischemia
2. "T" wave elevation/broadening = Hyperacute ischemia
3. "Q" waves = Infarction
4. ST elevation = Injury

See: Kern, chapter on "Electrophysiology." **Keywords:** ECG signs of MI, ischemia, injury

851. What are the three I's for the different stages of a heart attack (STEMI) in order of occurrence?
a. **Ischemia, Injury, Infarction**
b. **Injury, Ischemia, Infarction**
c. **Infarction, Intense chest pain, Intervention**
d. **Ischemia, Inverted T waves, Indicative ST elevation**

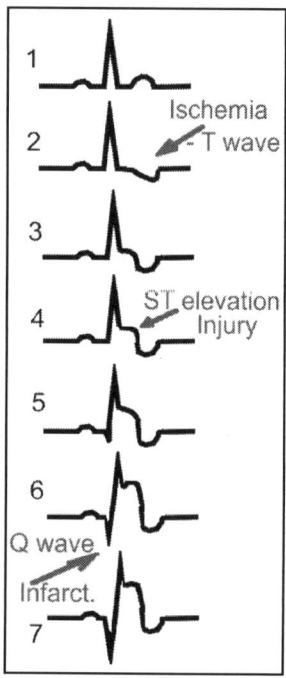

ANSWER: a. Ischemia, Injury, Infarction for ECG, T wave changes, ST elevation, and large Q waves. With STEMI first the tissue gets reduced blood flow (**Ischemia**) then it becomes **Injured** (ST elevation) and finally dies or **Infarcts** (Q waves). Typical stages of MI progression are:
1. Initially T waves peak (often early, transient and may not be seen).
2. ST segments elevate within hours.
3. Q waves (or loss of R wave) develop within 1-2 days.
4. ST segment elevation gradually resolve over several days. Inverted T waves may then develop.
5. Q waves or loss or R wave remain permanently.
6. Inverted T waves may or may not resolve.

Braunwald say, "Ischemic ST-segment elevation and hyperacute T wave changes may occur as the earliest sign of acute infarction (STEMI) and are typically followed within a period ranging from hours to days by evolving T wave inversion and sometimes Q waves in the same lead distribution." **See:** Braunwald, chapter on "MI"

852. In STEMI, what are "reciprocal" ECG changes when viewing the ECG?
a. **When the ST segments flip from negative to positive**
b. **When the T waves flip over from positive to negative**
c. **When viewing the same MI at a 90 degree orthogonal angle**
d. **When viewing the same MI from opposite 180 degree angle**

ANSWER d. When viewing the same MI from opposite 180 degree angle. It is a mirror image recording made by the ECG lead recorded from the opposite wall. Note in inferior

STEMI how the "reciprocal" leads are flipped/inverted.

Kern says, "The ECG findings of acute infarction occur in a stepwise temporal fashion. The earliest phase of infarction is associated with tall upright T waves that are referred to as hyperacute T waves. These T wave changes are usually followed shortly by the development of ST segment elevation in the region where myocardial damage is occurring. ...Within hours of the onset of myocardial infarction, Q waves appear as a result of damage that occurs throughout all layers of the myocardium, resulting in a transmural or Q wave myocardial infarction....Conversely, reciprocal ST segment depression can be noted in the ECG leads recording from the opposing surface of the heart. In an acute inferior myocardial infarction, ST segment elevation is present in the inferior leads (II, III, and aVF), whereas ST segment depression is recorded simultaneously in the anterior leads (I, aVL, V, and V2). **See:** Braunwald, chapter on "MI"

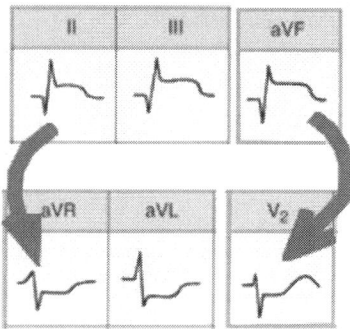

853. Identify the 4 ECG changes associated with myocardial infarction (STEMI). (Select 4 below.)
   a. Q waves
   b. Heart blocks
   c. Preexcitation
   d. ST depression
   e. T wave inversion
   f. Long QT interval

ANSWERS: a, b, d, & e.

The most common coronary ischemic patterns associated with MI include Q, ST, and T wave changes as follows:
1. Inverted "T" wave = ischemia
2. "T" wave elevation/broadening = hyperacute ischemia
3. ST elevation = injury. Right coronary infarction commonly affects the AV node and causes heart blocks.
4. "Q" waves = infarction

Preexcitation comes only through accessory pathways that bypass the AV node and excite the ventricle early. Accessory pathways are normally congenital and not associated with MI.

See: Braunwald, chapter on, "Electrocardiography" **Keywords:** ECG changes of MI

854. What coronary lesion would cause this ECG pattern?

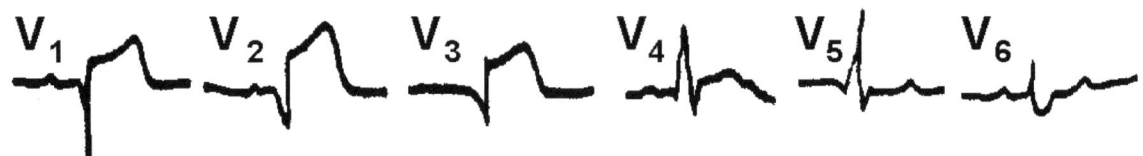

Precordial ECG leads

a. LAD, Infarction
b. LAD, Ischemia
c. RCA, Infarction
d. RCA, Ischemia

ANSWER a. LAD, Infarction. Note elevated ST segments in leads V1-V3. These are the anterior leads. Remember that ST elevation indicates acute injury. Large "Q" waves are seen in V1-V3 indicating infarction. Combining these findings, we can diagnose a fresh anterior septal myocardial infarction and acute injury pattern. The LAD coronary artery normally supplies the anterior LV wall.
See: Dubin, chapter on "Infarction." **Keywords:** Acute anterior MI

855. What coronary lesion would cause this ECG pattern?

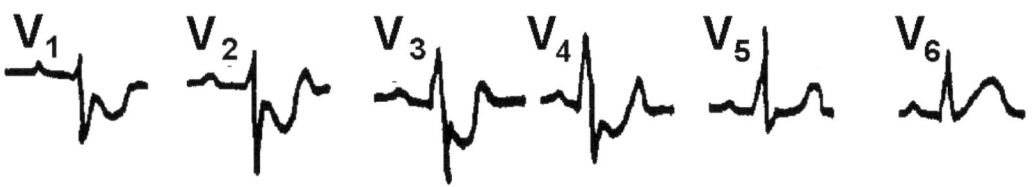

Precordial ECG leads

a. LAD, Infarction
b. LAD, Ischemia
c. Posterior, Infarction
d. Posterior, Ischemia

ANSWER c. Posterior, Infarction. Note the ST depression seen in V1-V4. This pattern is a mirror image of acute anterior septal infarction. The opposite of anterior is posterior, so this is an acute posterior infarction. If we had ECG leads around the back of the patient, they would show the ST elevation. But since electrodes are hard to place there, we rely on the opposite leads to show "reciprocal" changes.
See: Dubin, chapter on "Infarction." **Keywords:** Acute posterior MI

856. An acute myocardial infarction in the LV, labeled #2 on the drawing, is best seen on ECG leads:
a. I, aVL
b. V1, V2, V3, V4
c. II, III, aVF
d. V1, V2

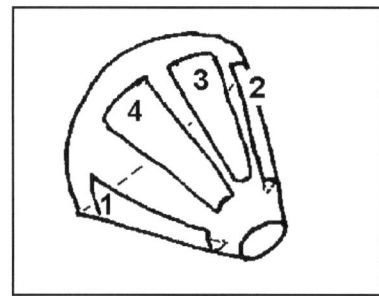
LV areas best seen on ECG

ANSWER a. I, aVL looks at the lateral LV wall. The ECG leads closest to the LV wall injured see it the best.
1. Inferior wall   = II, III, aVF
2. Anterior wall   = V3, V4
3. Lateral wall   = I, aVL
4. Septal wall   = V1, V2

See: Kern, chapter on "Electrophysiology." **Keywords:** LV areas seen on ECG, localizing MI

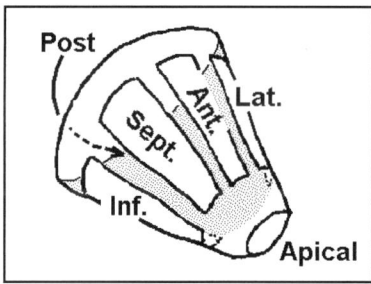
LV areas best seen on ECG

857. This 12 lead ECG was record during PTCA balloon inflation. Which coronary artery is being angioplastied?

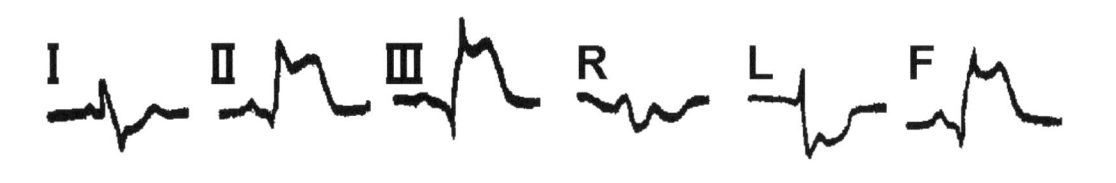
Precordial ECG leads

a. LAD
b. RAD
c. Right (RCA)
d. Circumflex (LCX)

ANSWER c. Right Coronary Artery. The inferior leads II, I II, aVF show ST elevation as sign of myocardial injury. The inflated balloon in an RCA temporarily cuts off blood to the inferior wall. The inferior leads II, III, and aVF show an ST elevation pattern similar to that seen in early myocardial infarction. When monitoring for PTCA, the best monitoring leads are the same ones that best reflect MI changes in that area of the heart.
See: Dubin, chapter on "Infarction." **Keywords:** Monitor II, III, aVF in RCA-PTCA

858. This ECG shows:

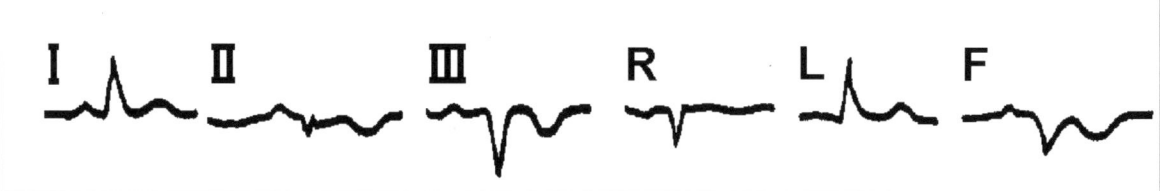

Precordial ECG leads

a. Acute lateral infarct
b. Acute anterior-septal infarct
c. Old lateral infarct
d. Old anterior-septal infarct

ANSWER d. Old anterior-septal infarct. Leads V1-V3 shows significant "Q" waves. These are the anterior and septal leads. So this is an old anterior-septal infarction of undetermined age. ("Undetermined" age because the infarct may have been weeks or years ago.)
See: Dubin, chapter on "Infarction." Keywords: Old anterior MI

859. This ECG shows:

Precordial ECG leads

a. Fresh lateral infarct
b. Fresh anterior infarct
c. Evolving inferior infarct
d. Evolving anterior infarct

ANSWER c. Evolving inferior infarct. Leads III and aVF show significant "Q" waves (infarction). Leads II, III, and aVF show inverted "T" waves indicative of ischemia. II, III and aVF are the inferior leads. So this is an old inferior infarction which still shows signs of ischemia of undetermined age. There are no signs of acute injury (ST elevation).
See: Dubin, chapter on "Infarction." Keywords: Old inferior MI

860. To be significant for myocardial infarction "Q" waves must be more than _____ wide or _____.
   a. .02 sec, 1/6 ht. of QRS
   b. .04 sec, 1/3 ht. of QRS
   c. .06 sec, ½ ht. of the QRS
   d. .08 sec, As deep as the QRS

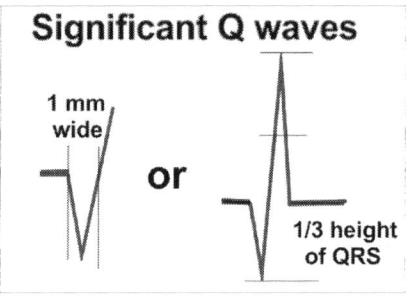

ANSWER b. .04 sec, 1/3 ht. of QRS. To be significant for MI, "Q" waves must be deep and wide. Many leads have small normal "Q" waves. But they are always less than .04 seconds wide. Deep and wide "Q" waves indicate dead infarcted tissue. **See:** Dubin, chapter on "Infarction."

861. After a myocardial infarction has healed and the patient has recovered, what sign usually remains on the ECG for the rest of that patient's life?
   a. Frequent PVCs
   b. Larger than normal "Q" waves
   c. ST elevation in some leads
   d. "T" wave inversion in some leads

ANSWER b. Larger than normal "Q" waves. The necrotic or dead tissue leaves an electrically silent area. ECG leads over this area look through the silent area at the remainder of the myocardium depolarizing away from it (Q waves). The "Q" waves develop within 1 day and over the area of dead (infarcted) tissue. They seldom resolve, but remain as telltale signs of the old transmural infarction. **See:** Dubin, chapter on "Infarction."

862. An acute anterior MI is best seen in leads:
   a. I & V1
   b. II, III, AVF
   c. V2, V3, V4
   d. V4, V5, V6

ANSWER: c. V2, V3, V4. The best leads for simple anterior MI are V2, V3 & V4 as they lie directly over the LV. But, acute changes may extend all across the left chest leads, and in the leftward directed limb leads (aVL & I). V1 & V2 evaluate the septal wall. II, III & aVF evaluate the inferior wall. V5, V6, I & AVL evaluate the lateral wall. **See:** Braunwald, chapter on "Electrocardiography"

863. ECG leads V3 and V4 best evaluate the:
   a. LV lateral wall
   b. LV anterior wall
   c. LV inferior wall
   d. LV anteroseptal wall

ANSWER: b. LV anterior wall. The best leads for simple anterior MI are V2, V3 & V4 as they lie directly over the LV. V1 & V2 evaluate the septal wall. II, III & aVF evaluate the inferior wall. V5, V6, I & AVL evaluate the lateral wall. This table summarizes the leads that show different MI ECG patterns. It has the same pattern as a 12 lead ECG strip, and can be laid over a 12 lead ECG to visually find the area of infarct, e.g. If you see ST elevation in leads V3 & V4 (diagonal line boxes) it is an anterior MI.
See: Braunwald, chapter on, "Electrocardiography" **Keywords:** 12 lead, MI location

I Lateral MI	aVR don't use	V1 Septal MI	V4 Anterior MI
II Inferior MI	aVL Lateral MI	V2 Septal MI	V5 Lateral MI
III Inferior MI	aVF Inferior MI	V3 Anterior MI	V6 Lateral MI

864. These precordial ECG leads show an:
 a. Old anterior MI
 b. Old lateral MI
 c. Acute anterior MI
 d. Acute lateral infarct

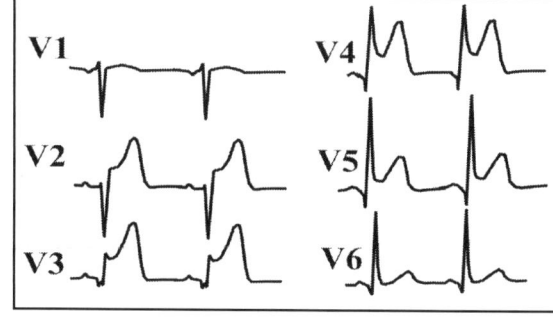

ANSWER: c. Acute anterior MI. Large ST elevation in V2-V4 indicates acute anterior MI. If it were an old MI, there would be large Q waves. If it were a lateral MI, the ECG changes would occur in leads V5 & V6. **See:** Braunwald, chapter on, "Electrocardiography"

865. What ECG leads best diagnose an acute posterior myocardial infarction?
 a. V1-V4 as ST elevation
 b. V1-V4 as ST depression
 c. Lead I and V5 -V6 as ST elevation
 d. Lead I and V5 - V6 as ST depression

ANSWER: b. V1-V4 as ST depression. Occlusion of the right coronary artery produces posterior infarction and/or inferior infarction. Anterior infarct shows best on the leads nearest the infarct V1, V2 & V3. A posterior infarction is difficult to diagnose because there are no ECG leads on the patient's back, nearest the infarct. Instead the posterior infarct is seen as a mirror image of an anterior infarct in anterior leads. These are termed "reciprocal" changes.

"True posterior infarction may produce changes only in lead V1 and V2. The ECG changes of posterior infarction are "reciprocal" changes, that is, they are seen "backwards" on the front of the heart in lead V1. Q waves become big R's, ST elevation is seen as depression, T inversion is seen as an upright T. Lead V1 and V2 have large R waves, which are "reflected Q waves" from the back of the heart. The ST segment depression is seen as "reciprocal" or "reflected" ST elevation from the back of the heart..... posterior infarction is usually accompanied by infarction of another area, such as the inferior wall."
See: www.madsci.com **Keywords:** "reciprocal" changes

866. This ECG is from a 65 YOM with crushing chest pain. What does it show?
   a. LBBB block ECG pattern with NSTEMI of the LM
   b. LBBB block ECG pattern with STEMI of the LAD
   c. Tombstone ECG pattern with NSTEMI of the LM
   d. Tombstone ECG pattern with STEMI of the LAD

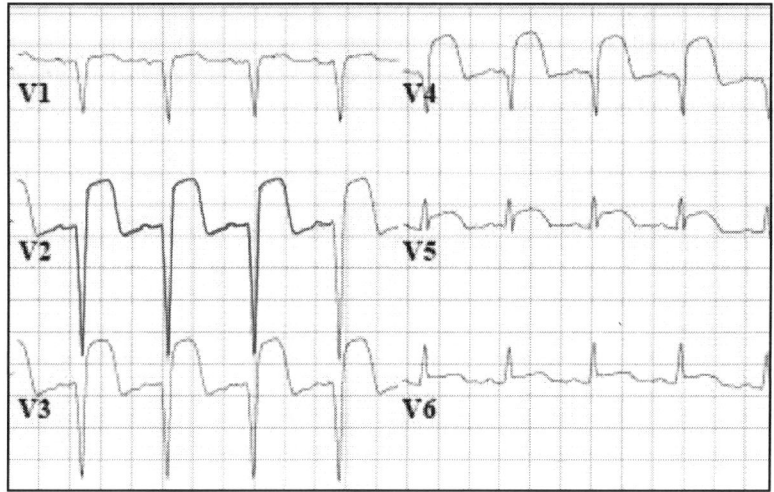

ANSWER: d. Tombstone ECG pattern with STEMI of the LAD.

Steven Lome's blog says, "Identifying an acute MI on the 12-lead ECG is the most important thing that you can learn in ECG interpretation! Time is muscle when treating heart attacks.... This is the big one that carries a high mortality if not treated rapidly. An anterior STEMI is usually from acute thrombotic occlusion of the left anterior descending coronary artery a.k.a. the LAD or the "widow maker".... Recall as well that a STEMI is a STEMI is a STEMI...treatment for ALL of them is the same regardless of what pattern it takes...quick coronary revascularization."

See: http://www.healio.com/cardiology/learn-the-heart/blogs/stemi-mi-ecg-pattern

Urgent revascularization can be with thrombolytic drugs, emergency CABG surgery, or stenting in the cath lab. The term "Widowmaker" can be applied to severe left anterior descending (LAD) lesions or the left main (LM) coronary artery lesions, which is even worse as it would affect the circumflex artery and lateral areas of the heart as well as the anterior LV. NSTEMI is a form of unstable angina. Non-ST-elevation Myocardial Infarction is an MI without ST elevation on ECG, suggesting the artery is not completely blocked as in STEMI. Only measuring cardiac enzymes will tell you whether the NSTEMI patient is stable or having an MI that needs intervention. Although the large Q waves are deep, they are not wide enough to be LBBB.

3. Hypertrophy and Electrolytes

867. Match the "hypertrophy" pattern labeled at #3 in the box, with its name below.
  a. Right Atrial Enlargement (RAE)
  b. Left Atrial Enlargement (LAE)
  c. Right Ventricular Hypertrophy (RVH)
  d. Left Ventricular Hypertrophy (LVH)

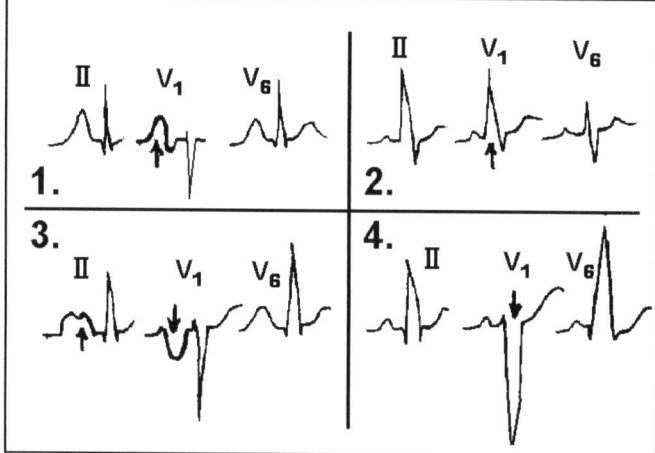

Hypertrophy patterns- leads II, V1, & V6

ANSWER b. Left Atrial Enlargement (LAE). The RA is closer to the SA node and depolarizes before the LA. The terminal "P" wave is LA depolarization. If the "P" wave is enlarged and/or notched in lead II (P mitrale pattern), and/or strongly negative in V1, the LA is enlarged or hypertrophied.

HYPERTROPHY PATTERNS SHOWN ARE:
1. **Right Atrial Enlargement (RAE):** Initial large positive "P" wave in lead II
2. **Right Ventricular Hypertrophy (RVH):** Elevated "R wave " in V1
3. **Left Atrial Enlargement (LAE):** Notched P in II, biphasic late negative "P" in V1
4. **Left Ventricular Hypertrophy (LVH):** Large "S" in V1 and "R" in V6 totaling >35 mm.

See: Marriott, chapter on "Hypertrophy."

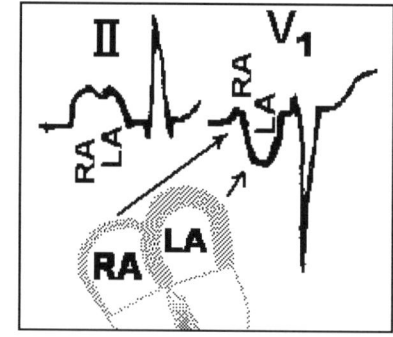

RA fires 1st, LA 2nd in LAE

868. These precordial ECG leads show:
  a. LV hypertrophy with strain
  b. LV myopathy with ischemia
  c. LA hypertrophy
  d. RA hypertrophy

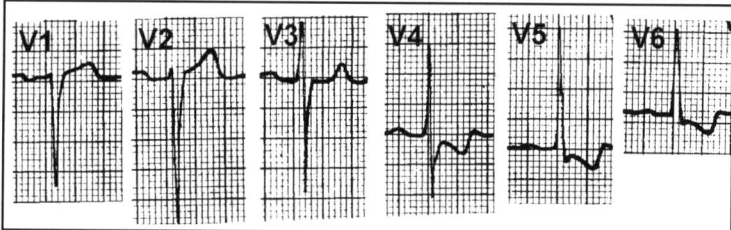

Precordial ECG leads

ANSWER a. LV hypertrophy with strain. Note the high negative voltage in V2 and the high positive voltage of V5. When added these deflections exceed 35 mm - Dubin's criteria for LVH. If V2(S wave) + V5(R wave) > 35 then voltage criteria for LVH exists. The ST depression and "T" wave inversion seen on leads V4-V6 indicates strain or ischemia, due to insufficient coronary supply. **See:** Dubin, chapter on "Hypertrophy." **Keywords:** LVH with strain

869. The ECG labeled #1 in the diagram shows what electrolyte imbalance?
a. Moderate hyperkalemia
b. Moderate hypokalemia
c. Hypercalcemia
d. Hypocalcemia

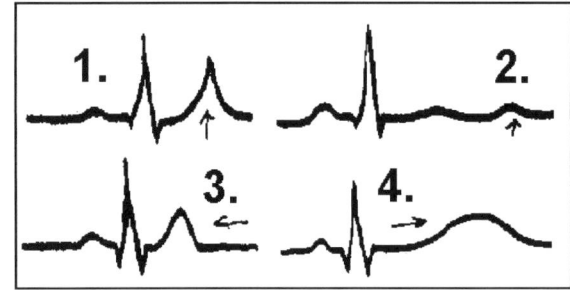
Electrolyte imbalance patterns

ANSWER a. Moderate hyperkalemia shows peaked or tent shaped "T" waves during repolarization. Remember hyperkalemia exists whenever the serum K^+ exceeds 5.0 mEq/L. In extreme hyper K^+ the "P" waves flatten and the QRS broadens. (Too many bananas and you too will live in a "tent" in South America.) **BE ABLE TO MATCH ALL ANSWERS BELOW.**
    1. Moderate hyperkalemia   = peaked/tented "T" wave
    2. Moderate hypokalemia   = prominent u wave
    3. Hypercalcemia   = short Q-T interval
    4. Hypocalcemia   = prolonged Q-T interval
See: Marriott, chapter on "Hypertrophy." **Keywords:** ECG in hyperkalemia

4. Pacemaker Modes

870. Identify the NASPE/BPEG pacemaker mode letter labeled at #4 in the box.
a. Chamber sensed
b. Chamber paced
c. Programmable functions
d. Mode of response
e. Tachy-arrhythmia functions

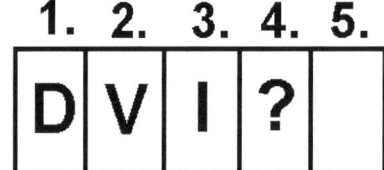
FIVE letter Pacer Code

ANSWER c. Programmable functions include: Simple programmability, multi-programmable, telemetry, or rate responsive. This five letter code was adopted by the NASPE/BPEG as the "generic pacemaker code." In this example, the letters, DVIR signify is a very common pacing mode with: Dual chamber pacing, Ventricular sensing, in Inhibition mode. If the 4th letter is R, this would indicate a Rate responsive pacemaker (responsive to exercise). **BE ABLE TO MATCH ALL ANSWERS BELOW.**
1. **Chamber paced:** "D" indicates Dual chamber pacing (AV sequential)
2. **Chamber sensed:** "V" indicates Ventricular sensing (Senses R waves)
3. **Mode of Response:** "I" indicates Inhibited mode (Inhibits pacing output when it senses an intrinsic R)
4. **Programmable functions:** "R" indicates that the pacing rate is responsiveness to exercise. Most pacemakers already have "P" programmability, "M" Multi-programmable, and "T" Telemetry.
5. **Tachy-arrhythmia functions:** "S" shock or "P" for antitachy-Pacing (None in this example)

See: Braunwald, chapter on "Cardiac Pacemakers and Antiarrhythmic Devices."

871. The most common sensor in Medtronic VVIR pacemakers is:
   a. PR interval
   b. QRS duration
   c. Motion
   d. Venous PO2
   e. Temperature

ANSWER c. Motion/acceleration. VVIR pacemakers sense and pace in the ventricle. The pacing rate is set to a minimum level, but can increase with exercise. "R" means Rate responsive. Medtronic pacemakers are designed to detect patient exercise through a motion sensor - usually a piezoelectric crystal in the battery pack. The more the patient exercises and shakes the sensor, the faster the pacemaker beats. One problem with motion sensors is they may increase in rate during a bumpy train ride. Pacemakers with motion sensors are sometimes called "shaker cans."
   Other sensors are possible (QT interval, PO2, temperature) but rarely used as indicators of exercise level. Another common rate responsive pacemaker responds to minute ventilation, by measuring the changes in resistance across the chest wall.
See: Underhill, chapter on "Pacemakers." **Keywords:** VVIR senses motion

872. Identify the MODE of the schematic pacemaker labeled #2 on the diagram.
   a. VVI
   b. AAI
   c. VDD
   d. DVI

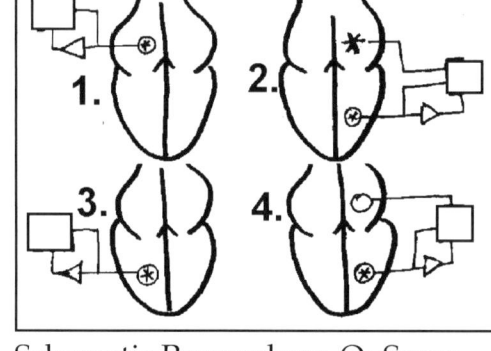
Schematic Pacemakers O=Sense, *=Pace ▼=amplifier

Note that the triangle in the diagrams ▼ represent a sensing amplifier and a square □ indicates stimulation & processing circuitry in the pacer can.

ANSWER d. DVI (or AV sequential) paces in the atrium and ventricle. When it fires, two sequential spikes are always seen, an "A" and a "V." It only senses the ventricle, so it cannot track normal sinus beats in a physiologic mode. It inhibits firing when an intrinsic (normally conducted) QRS is sensed, thus saving power and allowing sinus beats to provide atrial kick. DVI pacer mode may be used in sick sinus syndrome with AV block. This diagram shows how the inhibition mode works in a VVI pacemaker. **BE ABLE TO MATCH ALL ANSWERS.**

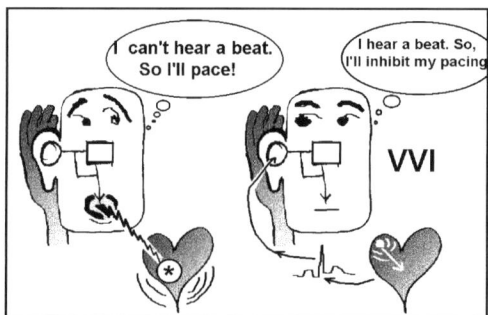
VVI pacemaker - Inhibited Mode

   1. **AAI** = Atrial demand pacemaker
   2. **DVI** = AV sequential
   3. **VVI** = Ventricular demand pacemaker. (See diagram above.)
   4. **VDD** = Atrial synchronous, ventricular demand pacemaker

See: Underhill, chapter on "Pacemakers." **Keywords:** Modes of pacing

873. **In the following types of paced beats, match the mean QRS direction of each to its expected morphology in leads I and aVF. Note: + indicates positive R wave, - indicates negative QRS wave, 0 indicates isoelectric (equal up and down)**

1. (Lead I=0, F=+) conducts mostly downward
2. (Lead I=+, F= 0) conducts mostly leftward
3. (Lead I=0, F=-) conducts mostly upward
4. (Lead I=-, F= 0) conducts mostly rightward

a. LV pacing
b. RV pacing
c. BiV pacing
d. Sinus conducted beat

Correctly matched answers are:
1. d, Sinus (Lead I=0, F=+) conducts mostly downward
2. b. RV pacing (Lead I=+, F= 0) conducts mostly leftward
3. c. BiV pacing (Lead I=0, F=-) conducts mostly upward
4. a. LV pacing (Lead I=-, F= 0) conducts mostly rightward

See circular diagram, showing the 4 orthogonal directions. Of course this is an oversimplification, because you never see perpendicular cardiac vectors like this at 0, 90, 180 and 270 degrees. The heart is more aligned along a 60 degree axis; and the paced vectors vary depending on the location of the pacing electrode. But, in general these are the main QRS axes in pacing. Lead I and V1 tell whether the ventricular vector is RV or LV. The lead aVF and III tell whether the depolarization is starting in the atrium and conducts down (+ in aVF) or whether the depolarization starts in the ventricle (BiV) and conducts upward (- in aVF). If the vector is perpendicular to a lead, that lead will be isoelectric with either a small deflection or a biphasic deflection. Note lead I is perpendicular to the LV paced QRS with a small biphasic RS wave.

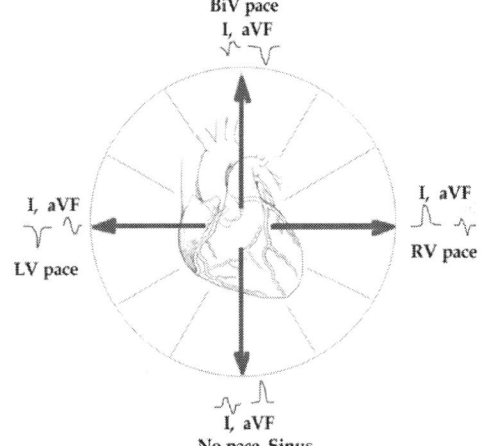

You must know your hexiaxial reference system and where each lead is positive. Start with Einthoven's triangle (I, II, & III), then add the augmented leads (aVR, aVF, aVL). One way to remember this is that in normal sinus beats the mean QRS is upright in all limb leads except aVR (the upside down lead). This is the same reasoning you use to localize the site of a VT. **See:** www.sjm.com, PPT download, Cardiac Rhythm Management CRT EGMs

874. Which physiologic pacemaker mode is rate responsive? (A sensed "P" wave precedes each ventricular artifact.)
   a. AAI
   b. VDD
   c. VVT
   d. DVI

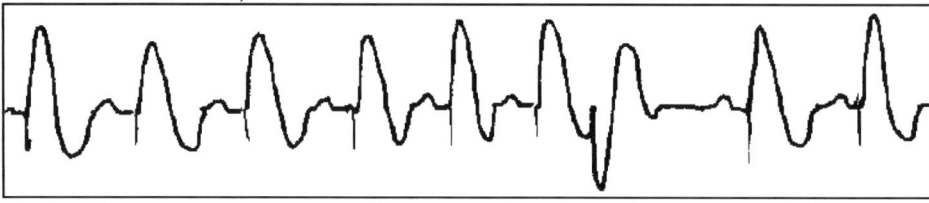
Rate responsive pacemaker

ANSWER b. VDD or VAT are atrial triggered ventricular pacers. It replaces the AV node and provides a physiologic rate responsive pacing. This pacer requires 2 leads, one sensor in the atrium and another pacing lead in the ventricle. The VDD pacer can also act in VOO, VAT or VVI modes.

This pacer requires 2 leads, one sensor in the atrium and another pacing lead in the ventricle. A sensed P wave triggers an AV delay and QRS sensor. If no intrinsic QRS is sensed within the programmed AV delay the ventricular pacer fires at its low rate interval. The upper rate interval shown is the maximum rate the pacer will track the P waves. Above that URL the pacer Wenckebachs and refuses to pace the ventricles any faster. For rate-responsive pacing, the NBG pacer code must be either T or D to indicate that triggering is present. The sensed or paced atrial wave must trigger the ventricular pacer to fire after an appropriate AV delay. **See:** Underhill, chapter on "Pacemakers."

875. This ECG shows:
   a. Atrial bigeminy
   b. Ventricular bigeminy
   c. AAI pacing
   d. VVI pacing

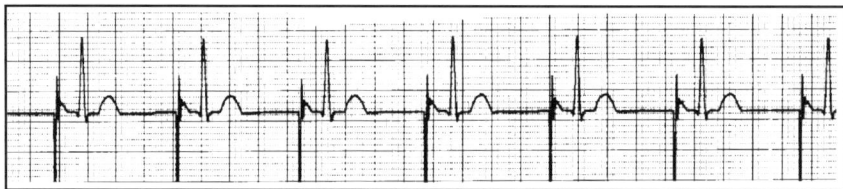

ANSWER c. AAI pacing. Since pacemaker artifacts (negative spikes) precede each "P" wave atrial pacing. In this example we do not see any normal "P" waves. This could also be AOO mode, since, atrial pacing occurs with every beat. We can only be sure that the sensing mode in AAI mode is operational when we see this second diagram. The first complex has a pacemaker spike preceding the atrial complex (a). The second

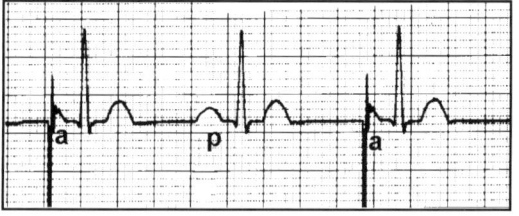
AAI Mode - showing inhibition

complex is a sinus beat with a normal P wave. It was sensed by the pacemaker which inhibits its output. Then no spike would be seen in the second beat. In the third beat, no P waves was sensed so the pacemaker sent a pacemaker spike into the atrium. It is followed by an "A" wave.
See: Underhill, chapter on "Pacemakers."

876. Prior to an RCA intervention, your physician orders that a temporary VOO pacemaker be set up. This will require:
  a. One pacing lead and measuring capture threshold
  b. One pacing lead and measuring sensing threshold
  c. One pacing lead and measuring both capture and sensing thresholds
  d. Two pacing leads and measuring both capture and sensing thresholds

ANSWER a. One lead and measuring capture threshold. Only a ventricular lead is placed. No sensing threshold is possible in VOO mode. This mode has no sensing, since there is a 0 in the 2nd position. Capture threshold should be measured to be sure your electrode is in a good RV position and that you have enough current to stimulate the ventricle. Once the threshold is determined, you should double the output current for a 2:1 safety margin. The pacer will remain turned off unless it is needed. **See:** Underhill, chapter on "Pacemakers."

877. This ECG shows:
  a. Atrial bigeminy
  b. Ventricular bigeminy
  c. AAI pacing
  d. VVI pacing

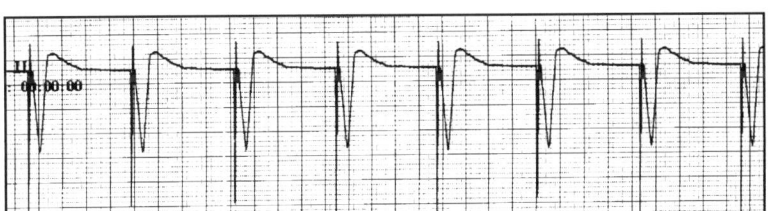

ANSWER d. VVI pacing.
This is ventricular pacing since pacemaker artifacts (negative spikes) precede each QRS complex. This could however, be VOO, or fixed rate ventricular pacing mode. However, VOO is seldom used. It is a primitive mode, and may lead to dangerous pacing on the "T" wave of intrinsic beats. The second tracing shows an intrinsic sinus beat during which the pacemaker output (spike) was inhibited. **See:** Underhill, chapter on "Pacemakers." **Keywords:** VVI pacing

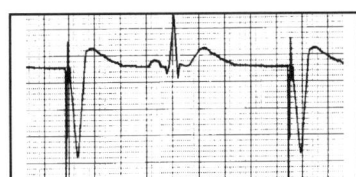

VVI pacemaker showing inhibition

878. A patient with a DDD pacer develops SVT. The physician decides to reprogram the pacer to DDI/R mode, because this mode:
  a. Slows the atrial rate
  b. Only speeds up on exercise
  c. Will switch to Wenchebach mode
  d. Excludes physiological VAT pacing

ANSWER d. Excludes physiological VAT pacing. Without a T or D in the 3rd position this pacer cannot trigger from the atrium into the ventricle. Fast supraventricular rates will not be tracked and triggered. VVI pacing will remain the dominant mode when needed. **See:** http://www.ncbi.nlm.nih.gov/pubmed/15807297 **Keywords:** DDI/R mode

879. This ECG and arterial pressure shows:

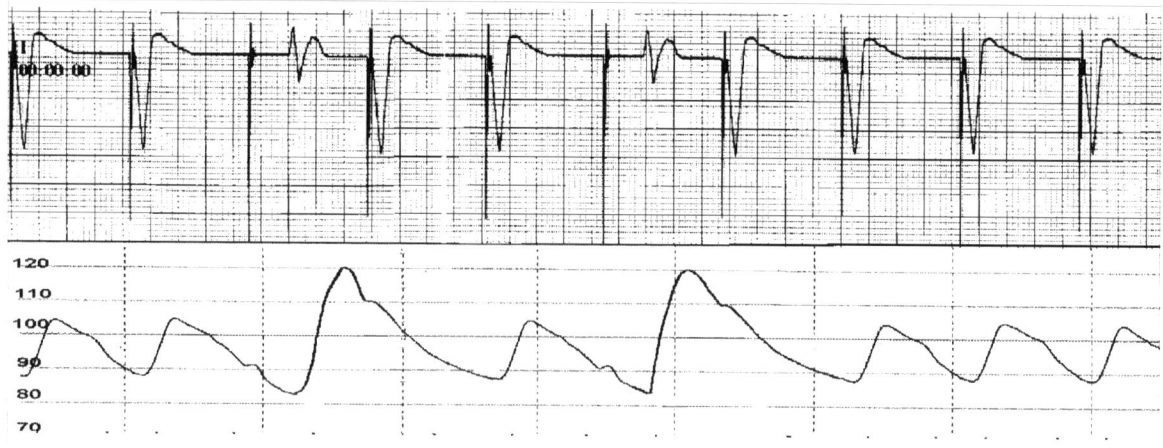

Paced rhythm - Recorded with arterial pressure

a. Atrial bigeminy
b. Ventricular bigeminy
c. AAI pacing with occasional loss of capture
d. VOO pacing with occasional loss of capture

ANSWER d. VOO or VVI pacing with occasional loss of capture. The pacemaker artifacts (negative spikes) precede most QRS complexes indicating ventricular pacing. But the 3rd and 6th pacer artifacts do not capture the ventricle (No QRS immediately follows). The heart responds to the pause with a broad complex ventricular escape beat. Note the large blood pressure with this escape beat. This increase is due to longer filling time following the ineffective pacer spike. It is analogous to the large arterial pressure seen in post-PVC beats.

The solution is to increase the pacer voltage or reposition the electrode to get better contact in the RV.

See: Underhill, chapter on "Pacemakers." **Keywords:** VVI pacing with loss of capture

880. In this ECG what does the notched "T" waves (shown at the "?") indicate?

a. Hyperkalemia
b. Hypocalcemia
c. Bigeminal PVCs with "R" on "T"
d. Retrograde "P" waves

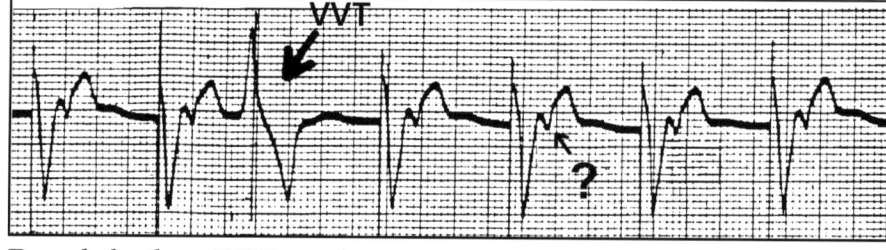

Paced rhythm, VVT mode

ANSWER d. Retrograde "P" waves. The negative "T" waves in lead 2 indicate VA conduction backwards into the atrium. If a DDD pacer were in place, this could lead to a disastrous pacemaker mediated tachycardia (PMT), where the pacer might trigger from the retrograde/re-entrant "P" waves.

The beat marked with an arrow shows VVT mode. In VVT mode a sensed QRS triggers the pacer. The pacer spike falls directly on the QRS complex. This wastes battery energy, but it may be useful in faster intrinsic rates as a marker to indicate that the pacemaker is sensing properly. **See:** Underhill, chapter on "Pacemakers." **Keywords:** Re-entrant P-waves.

881. This ventricular pacemaker ECG shows what problem?

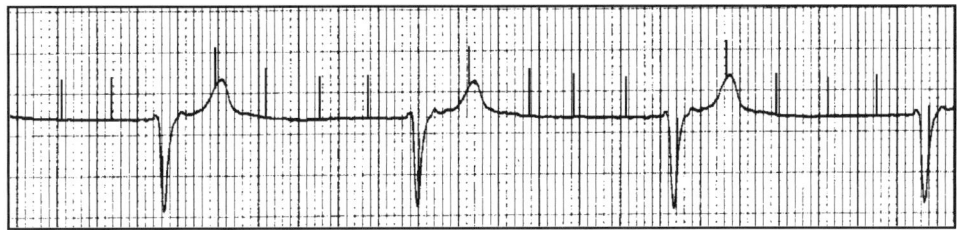

a. 3rd degree block with rapid atrial response
b. Second degree block with 5:1 conduction
c. Anti-tachy pacemaker with severe over sensing
d. Runaway pacemaker with non-capture

ANSWER d. Runaway pacemaker and non-capture. This pacer is firing at over 200/minute. This rate is not physiologic and may trigger a ventricular arrhythmia. Neither are the pacer spikes capturing the ventricle. This pacemaker had a system failure and was dangerously out of control. **See:** Underhill, chapter on "Pacemakers." **Keywords:** Runaway pacer

REFERENCES

Baim, D. S. and Grossman W., Cardiac Catheterization, Angiography and Intervention, 6th Ed., Lea and Febiger, 2006
Braunwald, Eugene, Ed., HEART DISEASE A Textbook of Cardiovascular Medicine, 7th Ed., W. B. Saunders Co., 2008
Braunwald, Eugene, Ed., *HEART DISEASE A Textbook of Cardiovascular Medicine*, 9th Ed., W. B. Saunders Co., 2012
Conover, M. H., *Cardiac arrhythmias, Exercises in Pattern Interpretation*, 2nd Ed., C. V. Mosby Co., 1978
Cummins, R. O., Ed., *Textbook of ADVANCED CARDIAC LIFE SUPPORT*, American Heart Association, 1994
Davis, Dale, *How to Quickly and Accurately Master ECG Interpretation*, 2nd Ed., J. B. Lippincott Co., 1985
Dubin, Dale, *RAPID INTERPRETATION of EKG's*, 3rd Ed., Cover Publishing Co., 1982
Fogoros, R.N., MD,*Practical Cardiac Diagnosis, ELECTROPHYSIOLOGIC TESTING*, Blackwell Scientific Pub., 2006
Hurst, J. W., and Logue, R. B., et. al., *THE HEART Arteries and Veins*, 3rd Ed., McGraw-Hill Book Co., 1974
Kern, M. J., Ed., *The Cardiac Catheterization Handbook*, 6th Ed., Mosby-Year Book, Inc., 2016
Thaler, M. S., *The Only EKG Book You'll Ever Need*, , J. B. Lippincott Co., 1988
Underhill, S. L., Ed., *CARDIAC NURSING*, 2nd Ed., J. B. Lippincott Co., 1989
Wagner, *MARRIOTT'S Practical Electrocardiography*, 9th Ed., Williams & Wilkins, 1994

OUTLINE: Electrocardiography II

1. BLOCKS
   a. Conduction, ladder diagrams
   b. 1st degree (1°)
      i. PR int. > 0.20 sec
   c. Second degree (2°)
      i. Type I (Mobitz I = Wenckebach
      ii. Type II (Mobitz II)
   d. Third degree (3°)
      i. with junctional Escape
      ii. with ventricular Escape
   e. BBB
      i. aberrancy
      ii. RBBB
      iii. LBBB
   f. ACLS Therapy
      i. Brady-arrhythmias, pacemaker
      ii. Defib./Cardioversion
      iii. Lethal - Innocent rhythms
2. 12 lead ECGs, Ischemia
   a. Coronary disease
   b. General areas LV effected
      i. Inferior wall   = II, III, aVF
      ii. Anterior wall   = V3, V4
      iii. Lateral wall   = I, aVL
      iv. Septal wall   = V1, V2
   c. Ischemia
      i. inverted "T" wave   = ischemia
      ii. "T" wave elevation/broadening =Hyperacute ischemia
   d. Injury
      i. ST elevation = injury
      ii. ST depression, reciprocal changes
   e. Infarct
      i. Significant "Q" waves = infarction
      ii. Age of MI
      iii. Evolution of MI
3. HYPERTROPHY, ELECTROLYTES
   a. Atrial (RA- LA)
   b. Ventricular LV - RV)
   c. Electrolytes
      i. moderate Hyperkalemia = peaked/tented "T" wave
      ii. moderate hypokalemia = prominent u wave
      iii. Hypercalcemia = short Q-T interval
      iv. hypocalcemia = prolonged Q-T interval
4. PACERS
   a. Modes
   b. Pacemaker Code
      i. Chamber paced
      ii. Chamber sensed
      iii. Mode of Response
      iv. Programmable functions
      v. Tachy-arrhythmia functions
   c. Pacer names
      i. AAI = Atrial Demand pacemaker
      ii. DVI = AV sequential
      iii. VOO = asynchronous
      iv. VVI = Ventricular Demand pacemaker. (1 lead)
      v. VDD = Atrial Synchronous, Ventricular Demand pacemaker
      vi. DDI/T - no triggered mode, for SVT
   d. Rate Responsive
      i. motion sensor
   e. Problem Solving
      i. Sensing, capture, run-away
      ii. Retrograde P wave

X-Ray

INDEX: D13

1. Introduction to X-ray . . page 493 Review
2. X-Ray Equipment . . . page 494 Know
3. Interaction with Matter. . . page 512 Review
4. Image Production . . . page 515 Review
5. Radiation Safety . . . page 522 Know
6. Digital Radiography . . page 531 Know

Introduction to X-ray

882. The person who discovered X-rays in 1895 was:
a. Whitehead
b. Coolidge
c. Roentgen
d. Curie
e. Crook

ANSWER c. Roentgen. Bushong describes Roentgen's accidental discovery as follows"
"On November 8, 1985, Roentgen was working in his laboratory at Wurzburg University in Germany. He had darkened his laboratory and completely enclosed his Crookes tube with black photographic paper so that he could better visualize the effects of the cathode rays in the tube. A plate coated with barium platinocyanide, a fluorescent material, happened to be lying on a bench top several feet away from the Crookes tube... Roentgen noted that the barium platinocyanide fluoresced regardless of its distance from the Crookes tube.... For this work he received the first Nobel price in physics. Finally, Roentgen recognized the value of his discovery to medicine. He produced and published the first medical x-ray, one of his wife's hand."
See: Bushong, chapter on "Concepts of Radiation." **Keywords**: Roentgen, discoverer of x-rays

883. The person who developed the fluoroscope in 1898 was:
a. Crooke
b. Coolidge
c. Edison
d. Snook
e. Dally

ANSWER c. Edison. Bushong relates this sad tale:

> "The fluoroscope was developed by the American inventor Thomas A. Edison. . . . There is no telling what further inventions Edison might have developed had he continued his x-ray research, but he abandoned it when his assistant and long-time friend, Clarence Dally, suffered a severe x-ray burn that eventually required amputation of both his arms. Dally died in 1904 and is counted as the first x-ray fatality in the United States."

This emphasizes the health risks involved in handling x-radiation. There is no completely SAFE dose of x-rays. **See**: Bushong, chapter on "Concepts of Radiation." **Keywords**: Developed the Fluoroscope, Thomas Edison

884. Materials that emit light when stimulated by X-radiation are termed:
a. Photoelectric
b. Phosphors
c. Irradiators
d. Radiolucent

ANSWER b. Phosphors emit visible light when exposed to x-rays. Bushong says:

> "Any material that emits light in response to some outside stimulation is called a luminescent material, or a phosphor, and the visible light so emitted is called luminescence."

Fluoroscopes and intensifying screens contain phosphorescent material. This phosphor, usually cesium iodide, is similar to Roentgen's original fluoroscope screen. When an X-ray photon hits it, the X-ray's energy is converted into a burst of light.
See: Bushong, chapter on "Intensifying Screens." **Keywords**: Phosphorescent screens luminesce when hit by radiation

X-RAY EQUIPMENT
X-ray Tube

885. Label the component of the X-ray tube labeled #1 in the diagram.
a. Anode (rotating)
b. Focusing cup
c. Target
d. Filament

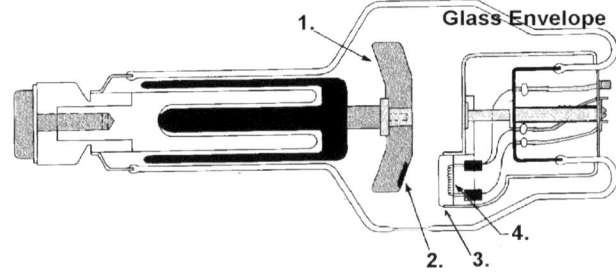

ANSWER a. Anode (rotating). The large rotating disc has one spot on it where the electron beam is focused. This is the target where x-rays are generated. The Cathode is the right-hand negative side, with a heated filament. Thermionic emission generates a cloud of electrons which are focused with the focusing cup toward the target on the anode.

BE ABLE TO MATCH ALL ANSWERS BELOW:
   1. Anode
   2. Target
   3. Focusing cup
   4. Filament

See: Bushong, chapter on "The X-ray Machine." **Keywords**: parts of x-ray tube: anode, cathode, focusing cup, filament, target

886. Identify the function of the X-ray tube component labeled #1 (Anode) in the box.
   a. Area of the anode struck by the electron beam
   b. Negative side of tube containing focusing cup
   c. Heater that "boils" off electrons
   d. Positively charged metal wheel that dissipates heat
   e. Metal shroud around filament that condenses electron beam

*1. Anode (rotating)
 2. Cathode
 3. Target
 4. Filament
 5. Focusing cup

ANSWER d. Positively charged metal wheel that dissipates heat.
BE ABLE TO CORRECTLY MATCH ALL ANSWERS BELOW:
   1. **Rotating Anode** - Positively charged metal side of tube that attracts the electron beam
   2. **Cathode** - Negative side of tube containing focusing cup - generates electrons
   3. **Target** - Area of the anode struck by the electron beam
   4. **Filament** - Heater that "boils" off electrons
   5. **Focusing cup** - Metal cup around filament that directs the electrons into a beam

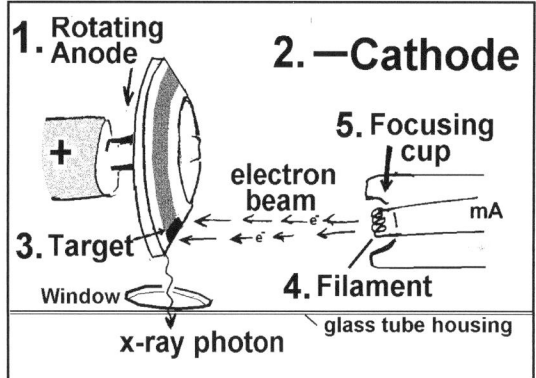

X-ray tube cross section

There are two primary parts of the x-ray tube: anode and cathode. Like in any vacuum tube, electrons are given off by the cathode, and attracted to the anode, to form an electron beam. How does it do this?

   The cathode contains a focusing cup that contains a heater coil (filament). When current (mA) passes though this heater it gets red hot and gives off electrons (thermionic emission). These electrons are focused by the cup and accelerated towards the positively charged anode by the kV. The spot on the anode where the electron beam hits, is termed the target. In the diagram the stippled area the shows typical heat damage burned onto the rotating anode by the electron beam. When the electron beam hits this focal spot or target, most of the electrons are converted into heat. But, some of the electrons interact with the tungsten target to give off x-rays. Some of these x-rays pass downward though an unshielded window in the glass housing to become the primary x-ray beam. **See**: Bushong, chapter on "The X-ray Machine." **Keywords**: Functions of parts of x-ray tube: anode, cathode, focusing cup, filament, target

887. Which of the following tubes can theoretically take X-rays with the greatest detail and finest resolution?
   a. 0.6 mm focal spot, long focal film distance (source image distance)
   b. 0.6 mm focal spot, short focal film distance (source image distance)
   c. 1.0 mm focal spot, long focal film distance (source image distance)
   d. 1.0 mm focal spot, short focal film distance (source image distance)

ANSWER a. 0.6 mm focal spot, long focal film distance (source image distance). Ideally for best resolution you want a point source. The smaller the focal spot the more of a point source or focused the beam will appear be. And the further the focal spot is from the film the smaller a source it will appear to be.

For example, consider the sun as a light source. Because it is so large a light source, a shadow cast by the sun is rather blurred at the edges. However, if the sun were smaller (God forbid) or further away (even worse) the resulting shadow would be less fuzzy. Bushong says,

> "The focal spot is the area of the target from which x rays are emitted. It is the source of radiation. Radiology requires small focal spots because the smaller the focal spot, the sharper the radiographic image."

See: Bushong, chapter on "The X-ray Machine." **Keywords**: greatest detail = small focal spot or long focal film distance

888. When you increase the X-ray tube mA, you are increasing the:
   a. Anode rotation speed
   b. Cathode to anode voltage
   c. Electron acceleration to anode
   d. Filament temperature

ANSWER d. Filament temperature. The more current passing through the filament the hotter it gets and the more electrons are boiled off. This tube current is the mA. When mA is multiplied by the emission time (seconds) you get milli-Amp-seconds (mAs), the best indicator of X-ray quantity. Bushong says,

> "The x-ray tube current is adjusted by controlling the filament current. . . .X-ray quantity is directly proportional to the mAs. When the mAs is doubled, the number of electrons striking the tube target is doubled, therefore the number of x rays emitted is doubled."

Although tube current (mA) is linearly related to X-ray quantity, a small percentage rise in filament current (A) results in higher filament temperatures and a large percentage rise in tube current (mA). **See**: Bushong, chapter on "The X-ray Machine." **Keywords**: increased filament current (A) causes increased tube current (mA) that in turn generates increased quantities of x-rays (Roentgens)

D13: DIAGNOSTIC TECHNIQUES: X-Ray

889. Which part of an X-ray tube produces the X-ray photons?
  a. Flat plate selenium detector
  b. Filament passing mA current
  c. Focusing cup on the cathode
  d. Target on the rotating anode

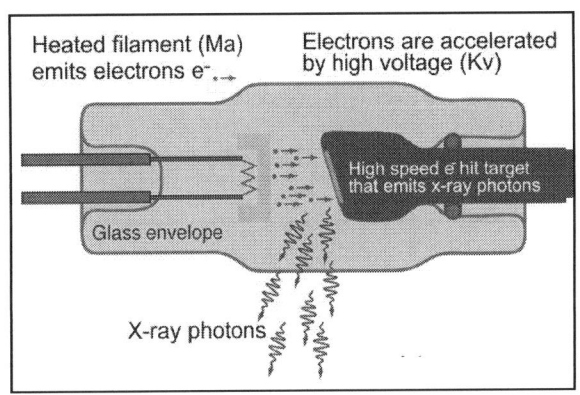

Answer: d. The target is a spot on the rotating anode where the x rays are generated. As the target on the anode is hit by accelerated electrons, some of the anode metal atoms change their energy state and generate X-rays. It is called "characteristic radiation" because it is characteristic of the metallic element in the anode. Anodes made from different elements produce different characteristic radiation. Tungsten is the best element for diagnostic radiology because of its high melting point.

The diameter of this target where the electrons hit is the "focal spot." The smaller the focal spot the more the resolution - just like a candle shadow has poor resolution, unless it passes a small hole or lens to focus it to a small spot. Image intensifiers and flat plate detectors then convert the Xrays into electrons for display. See: Bushong, chapter on "Radiographic Technique" Keywords: Target =focal spot on anode

890. The source of electrons within an X-ray tube is the:
  a. Focal spot
  b. Collimator
  c. Anode
  d. Filament

ANSWER d. Filament. Bushong says:
  "The filament is a coil of wire similar to that in a kitchen toaster except much smaller. The coil is usually about 2 mm in diameter and 1 to 2 cm long. In the kitchen toaster an electric current is conducted through the coil, causing it to glow and emit a large quantity of heat. The filament emits electrons. . . . the outer-shell electrons of the filament atoms are literally boiled off and ejected from the filament."
A vacuum tube is another analogy. The hotter the filament, the more electrons are boiled off the cathode, and more tube current can be generated.
See: Bushong, chapter on "The X-ray Machine." **Keywords**: filament = source of electrons

891. Tungsten is frequently utilized for both the filament and target of an X-ray tube chiefly because of its high:
  a. Melting point
  b. Mass and radiopacity
  c. Number of outer shell electrons
  d. Electrical conductivity

ANSWER a. Melting point. Temperature overload is a major limiting factor to increasing radiation. The anode may reach 2000° C. It must rotate fast enough to prevent its melting (around 3410° C). Heat must be conducted away rapidly into the surrounding oil bath (thermal conductivity). **See**: Bushong, chapter on "The X-ray Machine." **Keywords**: Tungsten anode = high melting point, thermal conductivity, atomic number

892. What component of an X-ray tube is negatively charged?
a. Anode
b. Cathode
c. Target
d. Output phosphor

ANSWER b. Cathode. Cathodes are always negatively charged. Anodes are positive. As the filament boils off electrons (negative charge) they are attracted and accelerated to the positive rotating anode. This electric charge between the anode and cathode is the important kV factor that determines the energy level of the resulting x-ray photons.

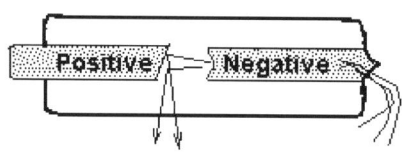

See: Bushong, chapter on "The X-ray Machine." **Keywords**: cathode = negative charge

GENERATION

893. One X-ray photon is generated in the X-ray tube when a high velocity:
a. Electron is suddenly slowed
b. Electron bounces off the target
c. Tungsten atom is thrown off the rotating anode
d. Photon is emitted by radioactive decay

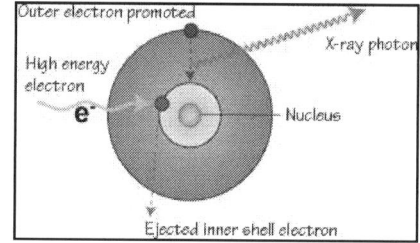

ANSWER a. Electron is suddenly slowed (or stopped). When a high energy electron beam hits the tungsten target some electrons slam into the target and either slow down or stop. In the process they convert some of their energy into X-radiation. This dramatic collision produces x-radiation. Bushong says,

> "When these projectile electrons impinge on the heavy metal atoms of the target, they interact with these atoms and transfer their kinetic energy to the target. . . . The projectile electrons slow down and finally come nearly to rest, . . . The projectile electrons interact with either the orbital electrons or the nuclei of target atoms. The interactions result in the conversion of kinetic energy into thermal energy and electromagnetic energy in the form of x rays."

See: Bushong, chapter on "X-ray Production." **Keywords**: X-ray Production due to slowing of electrons when they hit the metal target

IMAGE INTENSIFIER

894. In an image intensifier what is the function of #1 (input phosphor)?
a. Light stimulates it to emit electrons
b. X-rays stimulate it to emit light
c. Converts electrons to light
d. Accelerates electrons
e. Focus electron beam

* 1. Input Phosphor
2. Photocathode
3. Electrostatic lenses
4. Anode
5. Output Phosphor

ANSWER b. X-rays stimulate it to emit light. The input phosphor is cesium iodide. This phosphor is similar to Roentgen's original fluoroscope screen. When an X-ray photon hits it, its energy is converted into a burst of light.

The image intensifier increases the brightness of the original fluoroscopic image up to 1000 times. It does this in 3 stages. First the remnant beam x-rays hit the input phosphor which gives off light. Second, this light hits the photocathode layer which gives off electrons. These are accelerated by the anode and focused onto the output phosphor which is a small but very bright image. This is then picked up by the cine or TV camera. **BE ABLE TO CORRECTLY MATCH ALL ANSWERS BELOW:**
1. **Input Phosphor** - X-rays stimulate it to emit light
2. **Photocathode** - Light stimulates it to emit electrons
3. **Electrostatic lenses** - Focus electron beam to form image on the output phosphor
4. **Anode** - Accelerates electrons toward the output phosphor
5. **Output Phosphor** - Converts electrons to light and visible image

See: Bushong, chapter on "Special X-ray Equipment and procedures." **Keywords:** Receives remnant radiation converts it to light

895. Identify the part of an image intensifier tube labeled #2 (Thin metal layer) shown in the diagram.
a. Output phosphor
b. Anode
c. Photocathode
d. Input phosphor
e. Electrostatic lenses

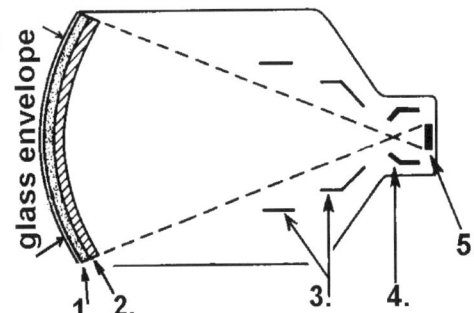

Image intensifier tube cross section

ANSWER c. Photocathode. The photocathode is a layer of thin metallic cesium and antimony compounds bonded to the input phosphor. Light photons from the input phosphor stimulate it to emit electrons by the process of "photoemission." This is similar to the process of "thermionic emission" in the X-ray tube. These electrons are attracted by the anode to the output phosphor where they form a bright image.

The image intensifier tube works rather like a TV tube in reverse, because the electron beam is reversed. When an X-ray image hits the large end of the tube, it generates an electronic image and beam inside. This is transferred to the small viewing screen at the right via an electron beam. A video camera then picks up this image and transfers it to our video monitors.

The image intensifier increases the brightness of the original fluoroscopic image thousands of times. This diagram shows the various stages of amplification. In this example when one X-ray photon hits the input phosphor it releases enough energy to generate 1000 light photons. Each of these can hit the photocathode and generate 50 photoelectrons. In turn, each of these is accelerated to the output phosphor where it may generate 50-75 light photons. The product of each of these 3 stages is the tube's brightness gain, in this diagram, around 3000. (1000 x 50 x 60 = 3000.) This output light becomes our intensified fluoroscopic image.

BE ABLE TO MATCH ALL ANSWERS BELOW:
1. **Input phosphor** (glows when hit with x-ray photons)
2. **Photocathode** (generates electrons)
3. **Electrostatic lenses** (focus electrons)
4. **Anode** (accelerate electrons)
5. **Output phosphor** (converts electron beam back into a light image)

See: Bushong, chapter on "Special X-ray Equipment and procedures."

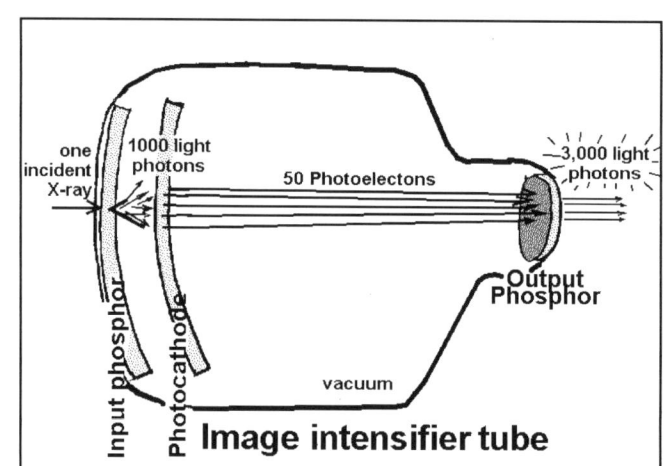

896. Your image intensifier probably has three fields of view: 9", 6" and 4.5". Compared to the 9" mode, the 4.5" mode requires _____ radiation levels and gives ___ magnification.
   a. Increased radiation requirement and Increased magnification
   b. Increased radiation requirement and Decreased magnification
   c. Decreased radiation requirement and Increased magnification
   d. Decreased radiation requirement and Decreased magnification

ANSWER a. Increased radiation requirement and Increased magnification. The 4.5 inch "mag-mode" enlarges the image making it easier to image stents or discrete lesions. However, the mag-modes have drawbacks in that they do not have as good a resolution. Peterson says,

"*As an image is magnified, however, increased radiation is necessary to achieve a high-contrast image that, consequently, leads to increased scatter radiation and a reduction in the signal-to-noise radio.*"

See: Peterson, chapter on "Radiographic Angiocardiography." **Keywords**: 4.5 " mag-mode requires more radiation that increases scatter and noise.

FLAT PLATE FLUOROSCOPY

897. During modern cath lab digital fluoroscopy the image receptor is:
   a. The TV camera
   b. The cassette
   c. The flat plate detector
   d. The Image intensifier

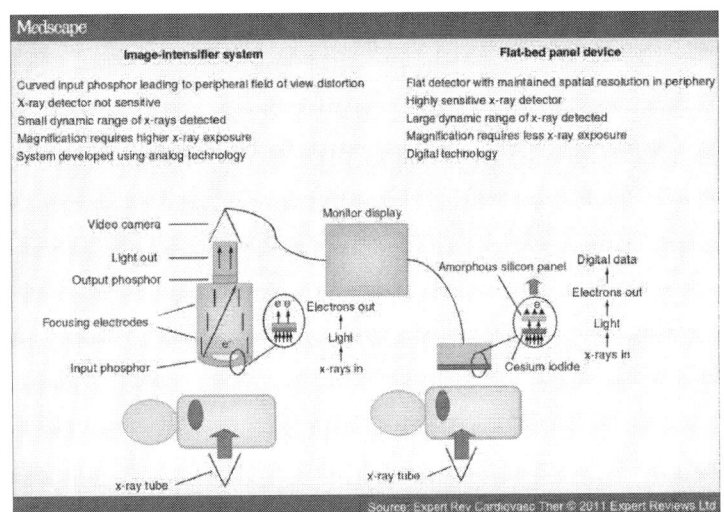

Image intensifier tube cross section

ANSWER The flat plate detector has replaced most image intensifiers because of improved resolution and imaging, such as contrast enhancement. X-ray film is now rarely shot and developed. It is faster and immediately viewable and storable. The electrons go straight to digital sensors (photodiodes) instead of being focused and amplified with electronic lenses.

898. Three differences between image intensifier and digital fluoroscopy systems is that digital systems generally have: (Select 3 answer.)
   a. No optical lenses
   b. Less collimation
   c. No anti-scatter grids
   d. Square images instead of round
   e. A thin film transistor array (TFT)

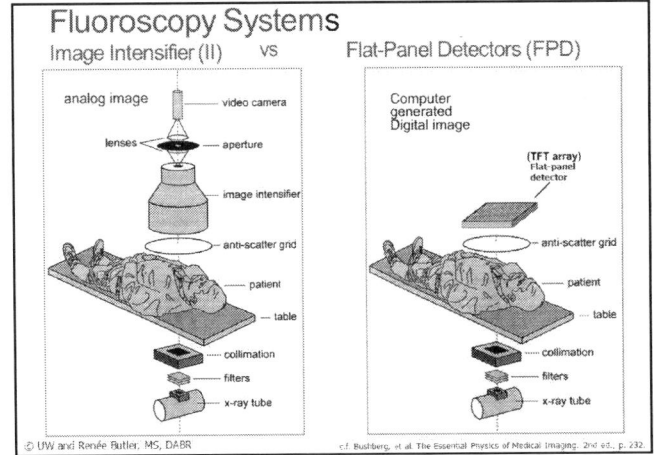

II vs. Flat panel fluoro.

Answer: a, d, & e No lenses, square images, & a Thin film transistor. (TFT) array. The image shows these differences.

Bhatt says, "Digital flat-panel detectors have replaced the older image intensifier technology in virtually all modern CCL equipment. The vast majority of these detectors uses an amorphous silicon detector coupled with a two-dimensional thin-film transistor (TFT) array. The physical size of detector elements (pixels) ranges from 80 to 200 microns, or one twelfth to one fifth of a millimeter." See Bhatt, chapter on, Radiation safety in the cardiac catheterization laboratory

899. What part of a digital X-ray imaging system converts photons into visible light?
   a. Target/photoanode
   b. Focusing cup/emitter
   c. Input phosphor/sensor
   d. Photocathode/scintillator

Answer: d. Photocathode/scintillator. In the II tube and flat plate detector there is a layer of metallic cesium and antimony attached to the input phosphor that converts the light. In the Flat panel detector uses charge coupled devices, photodiodes or scintillators to convert the phosphor generated light into electrons.
   Scintillators in flat panels work by converting X-ray energy into visible light. Scintillators differ from phosphors, in using crystalline materials such as NaI and CsI, while II's use granular phosphors such as rare earth oxysulphides.

VIDEO

900. Most modern digital X-ray imaging systems use the _____ standard for compressing and storing digital data.
   a. GIF (Graphical Interface Format)
   b. DICOM (Digital Imaging and Communications in Medicine)
   c. JPEG (Joint Photographic Expert Group)
   d. CDRA (CD ROM Archiving)

ANSWER b. DICOM (Digital Imaging and Communications in Medicine). There are many methods of compressing the enormous amount of digital data acquired in a digital angiogram. But, DICOM is the current standard.
   Lifewire says, "DICOM is an acronym for Digital Imaging and Communications in Medicine. Files in this format are most likely saved with either a DCM or DCM30 (DICOM 3.0) file extension, but some may not have an extension at all.
   "DICOM is both a communications protocol and a file format, which means it can store medical information, such as ultrasound and MRI images, along with a patient's information, all in one file. The format ensures that all the data stays together, as well provides the ability to transfer said information between devices that support the DICOM format. See: https://www.lifewire.com/dicom-file-2620657 "

901. The mode of digital fluoroscopy used to acquire angiographic images sufficient for single-frame viewing is _____ that uses _____ radiation.
   a. Pulsed fluoro, low mA dose
   b. Pulsed fluoro, high mA dose
   c. Cinefluorographic imaging, low mA dose
   d. Cinefluorographic imaging, high mA dose

ANSWERS: d. Cinefluorographic imaging, high mA dose. We often use the term "cine" for recording high resolution digital angiograms even though there is no film involved. Cine or fluorographic images are higher resolution because they use a higher mA patient dose.

Anderson says, "You should know the difference between fluoroscopy and fluorography. Fluoroscopy is routine real time imaging, performed at a relatively low dose rate. The noise on fluoroscopic images is not apparent when averaged over moving images. Fluorography is high dose rate imaging with quality equivalent to "plain films." An example of fluorography is cineangiography with or without digital subtraction."
See: An Introduction to Fluoroscopy Safety : Anderson & Leidholdt, An Introduction to Fluoroscope Safety, 2013
https://www.mpcphysics.com/documents/IntroductiontoFluoroscopySafety8-20-13.pdf

Shavelle says, "Two different imaging modes are available using the C-arm; pulsed fluoroscopy ('Fluoro') and cinefluorographic acquisition ('Cine'). 'Fluoro' provides low-resolution real-time X-ray imaging (with resolution measured in pulses/second), allowing observation of the moving coronary tree in the two-dimensional plane. Although image quality can be adjusted by increasing the radiation dose [mA] and the pulse rate (normally 10–15 pulses/second in angiography), the generally low-resolution images mean that 'Fluoro' is normally used for catheter advancement and manipulation. By contrast, 'Cine' (with resolution measured in frames/second) provides images of sufficient quality for single-frame viewing. It is, therefore, used to acquire the angiographic images during contrast media injection. Due to the dynamic nature of the heart and rapid flow down the coronary arteries, frame rates of 10–15 frames/second are generally used for acquisition. 'Fluoro' images are, thus, moving images and are not routinely stored, unless specifically requested or done so retrospectively by the operator after acquisition. Due to the higher resolution of 'Cine' images, however, the radiation dose needed is approximately 10 times that used in 'Fluoro'. Activation of 'Fluoro' or 'Cine' is usually via a foot pedal placed next to the operator or radiographer, with a separate pedal for each." **See**: Shavelle, Basic Coronary Angiography: Take Home Points Cardiovascular Medicine Boards and Clinical Practice, British Journal of Cardiology 2016

RADIATION MEASURES

902. The new Standard International (SI) unit for #1 (REM = Radiation Equivalent in Man) is the:
a. Gray (Gy)
b. Sievert (Sv)
c. R or C/Kg
d. Ci or Bq

*1. REM
2. RAD
3. Roentgen
4. Curie

ANSWER b. Sievert (Sv). BE ABLE TO **CORRECTLY MATCH ALL ANSWERS BELOW:**
 1. **REM** - unit of Sievert (Sv)
 2. **RAD** - unit of Gray (Gy)
 3. **Roentgen** - unit of R or coulombs/kg (C/kg)
 4. **Curie** - unit of Curie (Ci) or becquerel (Bq)

This makes the two newer units essentially equal 1 Gray = 1 Sievert (depending somewhat on the tissue absorbing the radiation). A way to remember what the new units correspond to is with their vowels. Gray is the new unit relating to Rads. Both contain the letter "a." Sievert is the new unit corresponding to Rem. Both contain an "e." **See**: Bushong, chapter on "Concepts of Radiation." **Keywords**: new unit for rem = sievert or Sv

903. What X-ray quantity does the RAD measure:
a. The amount of radiation in air
b. Radiation generated at the anode
c. Radiation scattered from a patient
d. The amount of radiation absorbed by a patient
e. The amount of radiation received by radiation workers

Answer: d. The amount of radiation absorbed by a patient. RAD is the Radiation Absorbed Dose (also known as total ionizing dose, TID) is a measure of the energy deposited in a medium (the patients body) by ionizing radiation. It is equal to the energy deposited per unit mass of tissue, and so has the unit J/kg, which is given the special name Gray (Gy). Biologic effects usually are related to the rad, and therefore the rad is the unit most often used when describing the radiation quantity received by a patient. Roentgen is measured in air, and not related to tissue absorption.
See: Bushong, chapter on 'Concepts of Radiation' Keywords: rad = patient absorbed

904. Which one of the following radiation measurement units is 100 times larger than the others below?
a. Rem
b. Rad
c. Roentgen
d. Gray

ANSWER d. Gray. In diagnostic radiology for practical purposes, REM = RAD = Roentgen. The newer units of Gray and Sievert are 100 times larger than the older terms. So, to calculate the smaller older unit (rad), divide the newer larger number (Grays) by 100. One way to remember this is that "Gray" and "Sievert" are larger words than "RAD" or "REM." Baim says,
> "In newer literature, the RAD has been supplanted by a newer unit termed the Gray (one Gy = 100 Rads). . . . an equivalent dose is often expressed in REM (radiation equivalent in man), or the newer unit the Sievert (1 Sv = 100 REM)."

See: Baim and Grossman, chapter on "Angiography..." Keywords: New unit for RAD = Gray

905. Which 3 of the following units of X-radiation are approximately equal to each other (in soft tissue)? (Check 3 below.)
a. Rem
b. Sievert (Sv)
c. Rad (rad)
d. Roentgen (R)
e. Hounsfield (HU)

ANSWERS: a, c, & d.

a. Rem - YES

b. Sievert (Sv) - NO. Sievert and Gray are larger units - just like meters are larger than cm. 1 Gray= 100 Rads and 1 Sievert =100 Rems.

c. Rad - YES

d. Roentgen ® - YES

e. Hounsfield (HU) - NO

A way to associate the new with the old units is: Gray and RAD both have "a" while REM and Sievert both contain an "e". A way to remember which is larger is: "Gray" and "Sievert" are larger words than "RAD" or "REM." Bushong says,

"In diagnostic radiology we may consider 1 roentgen equal to 1 RAD equal to 1 REM."

Baim says that.

"The distinction between Rads and REMs is largely semantic, since the RAD and the REM are essentially equivalent for diagnostic x-rays."

This makes the two newer units essentially equal 1 Gray = 1 Sievert (depending somewhat on the tissue absorbing the radiation). Hounsfield units are a unit of density or brightness seen on CD scans. See: Bushong, chapter on "Concepts of Radiation" and Baim and Grossman, chapter on "Angiography..."

906. All cath lab staff wear radiation film badges. What alternate units can be used to measure radiation exposure by cath lab personnel?
   a. **Rad or Gray**
   b. **Rad or Sievert**
   c. **Rem or Gray**
   d. **Rem or Sievert**

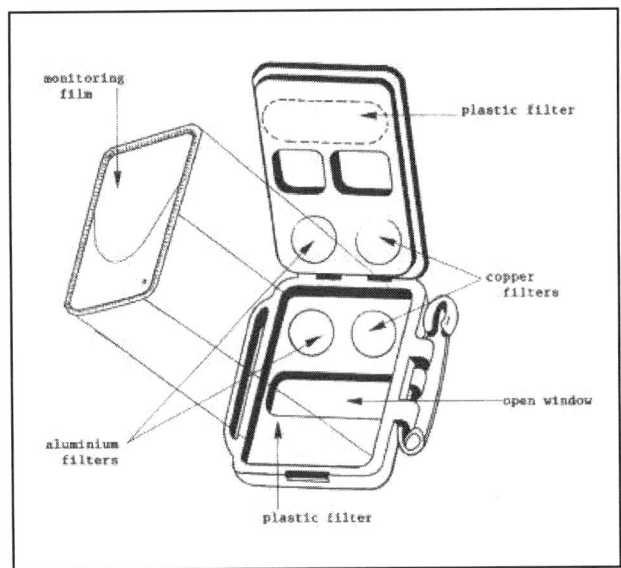

Answer: d. Rem or sievert. Rem is the <u>Roentgen equivalent in man</u> is the traditional unit of radiation <u>dose equivalent</u>. It is the product of the absorbed dose in rads and a weighting factor, which accounts for the effectiveness of the radiation to cause biological damage. A rem is a large amount of radiation, so the millirem (mRem), which is one thousandth of a rem, is used on medical radiation badges. Bushong says, "rem is the unit of dose equivalent to <u>occupation exposure</u>. It is used to express the quantity of radiation received by <u>radiation workers</u>... in the SI system the rem x 0.01 = Sievert (Sv)."

"The rad is the unit of <u>radiation absorbed dose</u>. Biologic effects usually are related to the rad, and therefore the rad is the unit most often used when describing the radiation quantity received by a <u>patient</u>.... Rad x 0.01 = Grays (Gy)" Note that both the new units, Sv and Gy are 100 times larger than the older and smaller units, rem and rad. See, Bushong, chapter on 'Concepts of Radiation' Keywords: Rem & sievert= film badge dose equivalent

907. The milli-REM is related most closely (by a factor of 100) to:
a. The Gray
b. The Joule
c. The Sievert
d. The RAD

Answer: c. The sievert is the unit of occupational exposure like milli-REM (which is reported on your film badge). Say your film badge reads 50 mREM exposure. If this was reported in Seiverts, it would read 5,000 milli-Seiverts. With the modern trend toward smaller and safer exposures these newer units magnify the numbers giving them more significance. Note, 5,000 milli-Seiverts is 5 Seiverts. See: Bushong, chapter on "Concepts of Radiation" Keywords: : occupational exposure measured in mRem

RADIATION PHYSICS

908. Electromagnetic radiation may interact in different ways with matter. Interaction #1 (Attenuation) can be described as:
a. Reduction in beam energy as it passes through tissue
b. When an energy beam completely disappears in tissue
c. Photons emerging from tissue interaction change direction - also termed "refraction"
d. Turning back of a ray that does not penetrate the tissue

*1. Attenuation
2. Absorption
3. Scatter
4. Reflection

ANSWER a. Attenuation. BE ABLE TO MATCH ALL ANSWERS BELOW:
1. Attenuation - Reduction in beam energy as it passes through tissue
2. Absorption - When an energy beam completely disappears (is absorbed) in tissue
3. Scatter - Photons emerging from tissue interaction change direction - also termed "refraction"
4. Reflection - Turning back of a ray that does not penetrate the tissue, like light reflecting from a mirrored surface.

Note that when x-rays are absorbed or scattered by their interaction with matter they remove electrons from that atom. This ionization process is the mechanism of biological damage. See: Bushong, chapter on "X-ray interaction with matter" Keywords: attenuation = reduction

909. The iodine content of angiographic contrast makes it absorb X-radiation. This property is termed:
a. Photo-emission
b. Fluorescence
c. Radiopacity
d. Radiolucence

ANSWER c. Radiopacity. Contrast is radiopaque, to X-rays, just like black glass is opaque to light. Air is radiolucent, just like clear glass is transparent or lucent to light.
See: Bushong, chapter on "Concepts of Radiation" Keywords: contrast is radiopaque

910. X-rays are different from Alpha and Beta rays in that X-rays:
a. Possess an electrical charge
b. Have a very small mass
c. Travel at the speed of light
d. Change direction in presence of a magnetic field
e. Are subatomic particles

ANSWER c. Travel at the speed of light. Alpha and Beta are atomic particles that are big and slow. X-rays have no mass and travel at the speed of electromagnetic radiation - the speed of light. Unlike Alpha and Beta radiation they have no charge, so they cannot be seen, felt, heard, focused, or their direction predicably altered. See: Bushong, chapter on "Concepts of Radiation" Keywords: Properties of x-rays, travel at speed of light

911. Name the smallest quantity of any type of electromagnetic energy. These small energy disturbances (like X-rays) move through space at the speed of light.
a. Atoms
b. Photons
c. Sine waves
d. Electrons

ANSWER b. Photons. Bushong says, "A photon is the smallest quantity of any type of electromagnetic energy, just as an atom is the smallest quantity of an element. A photo may be pictured as a small bundle of energy, sometimes called a quantum, that travels through space at the speed of light. We speak of x-ray photons, light photons, and other types of electomagnetic energy as photon radiation." See: Bushong, chapter on "Electomagnetic Energy" Keywords: photon smallest EM quantum

912. X-rays are a form of:
a. Subatomic particle
b. Supratomic particle
c. Microwave radiation
d. Electromagnetic radiation

ANSWER d. Electromagnetic radiation. X-rays are produced outside the nucleus in the electron cloud. When a rapidly traveling electron slams into metal and suddenly decelerates it produces x-ray photons. They have no mass, no charge and travel at the speed of light. They are considered energy disturbances in space.
See: Bushong, chapter on "Concepts of Radiation"

913. Identify 3 characteristics of X-radiation.
   a. X-rays can be focused with electrostatic lenses
   b. X-rays can penetrate tissue and bone
   c. X-rays travel with the speed of light
   d. X-rays are electromagnetic radiation
   e. X-rays are in the visible light spectrum

ANSWERS: b, c, & d.
a. X-rays can be focused with electrostatic lenses - NO
b. X-rays can penetrate tissue and bone -YES
c. X-rays travel at the speed of light - YES
d. X-rays are electromagnetic radiation - YES
e. X-rays are invisible to the eye

They are electromagnetic radiation that travels with the speed of light. X-rays cannot be focused with any type of lenses. To control their direction, you must restrict the beam size (collimate) or remove non-parallel X-rays (use a grid). Electrostatic lenses are used in image intensifiers to focus an electron beam - not the x-ray beam. X-ray and gamma rays all have no mass and no charge. X-rays themselves are not visible. **See:** Bushong, chapter on "Concepts of radiation" **Keywords:** Properties of x-rays

914. X-rays are "ionizing radiation" capable of injuring human tissue because when they strike an atom of human tissue they can:
   a. Increase the subatomic particles (radioisotope)
   b. Split subatomic particles (release proton)
   c. Add an orbital electron (e⁻)
   d. Remove an orbital electron (e⁻)

ANSWER d. Remove an orbital electron. Ionization has the potential of breaking electron bonds between atoms. If genetic material is ionized it can disrupt the genetic code leading to cancer or mutation. Bushong says,
   "Ionizing radiation is a special type of radiation that includes x rays. Ionizing radiation is any kind of radiation capable of removing an orbital electron from the atom with which it interacts. ...X-rays and gamma rays are the only electromagnetic radiation with sufficient energy to ionize matter. ...Many types of radiation are harmless, but ionizing radiation can severely injure humans." See: Bushong, chapter on "Concepts of radiation"

RADIATION QUALITY/QUANTITY

915. In chest radiography, what is the primary effect of changing the X-ray tube technique factor labeled #1 (Increasing kilovoltage)?

*1. Increasing kilovoltage (kV)
2. Decreasing kilovoltage (kV)
3. Increasing milli- Amp-sec (mAs)
4. Decreasing milli-Amp-sec (mAs)

a. Increasing the quantity of radiation in the primary beam, resulting in increased film blackness
b. Decreasing the quantity of radiation in the primary beam, resulting in decreased film blackness
c. Hardening the quality of the X-ray primary beam to make it more penetrating, resulting in more shades of grey
d. Softening the quality of the X-ray beam to make it more penetrating, resulting in fewer shades of grey

ANSWER c. Hardening the quality of the x-ray primary beam to make it more penetrating. This makes it easier to pass through large patients or dense tissue like contrast or bone. Too high a kV may over-penetrate contrast agents and result in gray angiograms. kV chiefly affects penetration and film contrast. The mA and exposure time (sec) chiefly affects film density and blackness. The terms "film" contrast and "film" density may be dated because many labs are now cineless. Thus, we prefer the terms "Image" contrast and "Image" density. These same principles apply to digital imaging.
BE ABLE TO MATCH ALL ANSWERS BELOW:
  1. **Increase kilovoltage (kV)** - Hardening the quality of the x-ray primary beam to make it more penetrating (can also increase density).
  2. **Decreasing kilovoltage (kV)** - Softening the quality of the x-ray beam to make it less penetrating (can also reduce film density).
  3. **Increase milli Amperage (mAs)** - Increasing the quantity of radiation in the primary beam, resulting in increased film blackness
  4. **Decreasing milli Amperage (mAs)** - Decreasing the quantity of radiation in the primary beam, resulting in decreased film blackness

Bushong says,
  "Low kVp results in high subject contrast, sometimes called short-scale contrast, since the radiographic image will appear either black or white with few shades of grey. On the other hand, high kVp results in low subject contrast, or long-scale contrast." (many shades of grey)

Although the main effect of kV is on image contrast, a 15% increase in kV will double the image density. So kV actually affects both image contrast and density. Note that the product of mA and seconds is termed mAs. The mAs determines the number of x-ray photons produced at the target and in the primary beam hitting the patients skin, and thus, the blackness of the radiograph. Doubling the mAs doubles the film density or blackness. See: Bushong, chapter on "Concepts of Radiation" Keywords: x-ray kV primarily determines film contrast, mAs primarily determines density

916. X-ray photon strength is most affected by:
a. Pulse width
b. Frame rate
c. Kilovoltage
d. Milliamperage

Answer: c. Kilovoltage. X-rays come out of the tube with different energy levels. An 80 kVp tube will generate it's highest energy X-rays at 80 kV, but there will be a range of lower energy rays termed the "Bremsstrahlung x-ray spectrum." The lower energy X-rays are usually filtered out by aluminum, as they tend to be absorbed by the skin and cause burns. Bushong says, "kVp is the primary control of beam quality and therefore beam penetrability.... Perhaps most importantly, kilovoltage controls the scale of contrast on the finished radiograph." See: Bushong, chapter on "Radiographic Technique" Keywords: X-Ray photon strength = kVp

917. In X-ray technique, inadequate mA results in:
a. Inadequate contrast
b. Inadequate beam penetration
c. Inadequate x-ray photons being generated
d. More radiation exposure due too long exposure time

Answer: c. Inadequate photons are generated. MA determines how many X-rays are generated and thus the density of a film. kVp determines the energy of those X-rays, their penetration and resulting contrast. Bushong says, "kVp is the primary control of beam quality and therefore beam penetrability.... Perhaps most importantly, kilovoltage controls the scale of contrast on the finished radiograph." See: Bushong, chapter on "Radiographic Technique" Keywords: low mA = Inadequate number of photons generated

918. The degree of blackness on an area of X-ray film is termed it's:
a. Resolution
b. Radiolucence
c. Contrast
d. Density

ANSWER d. Density. The degree of blackness on a film is termed radiographic density. It is chiefly regulated by mAs - the quantity of x-ray photons created at the tube target in one cine pulse. The more x-ray photons exposing a section of film, the blacker the film will be. Density can be measured in Hounsfield (HU) units. See: Bushong, chapter on "Concepts of Radiation" Keywords: Film density = blackness

919. You are doing coronary angiography on a large individual in steeply angulated views. The primary change made by automatic cine exposure systems to maintain adequate cine film blackening in these patients is to increase:
a. Increase mA
b. Increase kV
c. Increase mSec exposure time
d. Increase camera "f" stop

ANSWER b. Increase kV. All of the above will increase film blackening, but kV is the most efficient. Baim and Grossman say:
"Film blackening could also be increased by widening the pulse width (exposure time) but doubling the msec would cause significant motion blurring and double patient dose. The primary change made by the automatic exposure system to maintain optimal film blackening is thus alteration in the kV. This is not without its price, however, since optimal imaging of iodine-based contrast agents is best achieved with comparatively low photon energies (70 to 80 kV). These relatively low photon energies provide the best contrast between water and iodine (whose x-ray absorption is greatest at 33 keV, . . .) An underpowered generator or cine pulse system that tries to compensate by using high (100 to 120 kV) energies thus tends to produce grainy, low-contrast angiographic images in which both water and iodine look grey."
See: Baim and Grossman, chapter on "Angiography..." Keywords: optimal film blackness

920. A major advantage of using high "mA" settings during, angiography is:
a. Reduced patient dose
b. Decreased cine run time
c. Decreased pulse width duration
d. Decreased heat load on the X-ray tube

ANSWER: c. Decreased pulse width duration reduces motion blurring by shortening the exposure time. This is termed better "temporal resolution."
   The product of mA and time is mAs. It is the mAs that determine the total number of x rays in a single cine frame exposure. Increasing mA allows one to reduce the milli-seconds of exposure, and reduce motion blurring. This is analogous to letting more light into a regular camera by changing the f-stop or diaphragm opening. More light/photons allows you to shorten the exposure time and reduce motion blurring in an exposure.
See: Bushong, chapter on "Radiographic Technique" Keywords: short pulse width freezes motion

921. Which of the following controls affects both the QUALITY and QUANTITY of the primary X-ray beam?
a. kVp
b. mA
c. mAs
d. Exposure time

ANSWER a. kVp or kilo-Voltage potential changes both the quality (hardness and penetration) and quantity (number of x-ray photons) in the primary beam. We think of kV as primarily affecting the quality (grey scale) of the image while mA primarily effects the brightness of the image. Using the analogy of a black and white TV, the kV knob would control contrast whereas the mA knob would control brightness. Bushong says:

"*An increase in kVp results in a shift of the x-ray emission spectrum toward the high-energy side, causing an increase in the effective energy of the beam, thus making it more penetrable.*"

See: Bushong, chapter on "Concepts of Radiation" Keywords: kV determines x-ray quality

922. In general, low contrast angiographic films shot with _____ kV can recover more diagnostic information and more anatomic detail, because their greater latitude allows distinction of _____ between extremes of black and white.
   a. Lower, more shades of grey
   b. Lower, fewer shades of grey
   c. Higher, more shades of grey
   d. Higher, fewer shades of grey

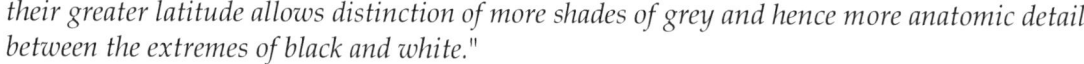

ANSWER a. Lower, more shades of grey. Baim and Grossman say,

"*In general, films with lower contrast can recover more diagnostic information because their greater latitude allows distinction of more shades of grey and hence more anatomic detail between the extremes of black and white.*"

A lab can use films of low, medium, or high contrast. Low contrast films have an inherent wide latitude and are more "forgiving." I.e., they let you select a wider variety of techniques before the images become too "black and white" and "contrasty." Too "contrasty" is analogous to turning up your black and white TV contrast control until parts of the image appear either pure black or pure white. See: Baim and Grossman, chapter on "Angiography..." Keywords: Low contrast = more shades of grey

INTERACTION WITH MATTER
Penetration, kV, MA

923. In coronary cine angiography, the mA setting has the greatest influence over:
   a. Image resolution
   b. Beam penetration and quality
   c. Ultimate density of the image
   d. Overall contrast of the image

ANSWER: c. Ultimate density of the film or the blackness of the image. MA is the current through the filament that generates electrons and hence more X-ray photons. More photons increase the blackness (density) of the film or image. Bushong says, "the mAs determines the number of x rays in the primary beam and therefore principally controls the radiation quantity. It has little influence over radiation quality. The mAs is the key factor in the control of density on the radiograph." mAs is the product of mA and exposure time in seconds. mAs is rather like a garden hose, more flow (mA) and more time (pulse width) gives the total amount of water on your garden (quantity of radiation in one exposure). See: Bushong, chapter on "Radiographic Technique" Keywords: x ray mA = film density

924. In chest radiography high kilo-voltage technique on the X-ray generator tends to increase the:
a. Umbra (edge distortion)
b. Penumbra (central image blur)
c. Short scale contrast (more contrast fewer grey tones)
d. Long scale contrast (less contrast with more grey tones)

ANSWER d. Long scale contrast (more grey tones). Increasing kV gives better penetration of the body with higher energy X-rays. It increases image density. But if the mAs (Milliamp x seconds) are turned down as the kV goes up, more grey scale results, termed long scale contrast, or decreased contrast. Understand the relationships between density, mA, exposure time, kV, and contrast. Note that angiography is different from radiography. In angiography the contrast is best seen at low kV. High kV technique may over-penetrate it making it seem grey and washed out. See: Bushong, chapter on "Special X-ray Equipment and procedures." Keywords: Long scale contrast (more grey tones)

925. The best way to reduce blurring due to heart motion artifact is:
a. Increasing mA and density
b. Increasing kV and penetration
c. Decreasing cine pulse width
d. Decreasing focal spot size
e. Have patient hold his breath

ANSWER c. Decreasing cine pulse width lowers the mSec exposure time. This will expose the film faster and stop-frame the motion. Normally this requires admitting more light by opening the camera iris (f stop setting). In our case it will require increasing the mA and /or kV to increase the intensity of x-rays and hence the density or darkness of X-ray films.

This is similar to action photography where the shutter speed is reduced. Photographers usually turn the exposure time down from 1/60 sec to 1/500 sec to take stop motion sports photographs. Making faster exposures requires that more light be admitted by opening the camera iris (f stop setting). The kV is usually kept about 70 for cardiac Fluoroscopy. See: Bushong, chapter on "Radiographic Quality"

926. In coronary cine angiography a long pulse width (exposure time) may cause:
a. Blurring
b. Quantum mottle
c. Inadequate contrast
d. Inadequate photon production

Answer: a. Blurring due to motion. Just as in sports photography, you need a short exposure time to "freeze frame" rapid motions. Short pulse widths are needed in cardiac cineangiography. Otherwise, blurring occurs in individual frames as the arteries move across the screen. See: Bushong, chapter on "Radiographic Technique" Keywords: short pulse width needed in cine

927. **What kV range should be used for cardiac angiography, because radiopaque dye absorbs best in this range?**
a. 40-50 kV
b. 70-90 kV
c. 100-150 kV
d. 200-300 kV

ANSWER b. 70-90 kV. These lower kV settings provide the best visualization of contrast. *Baim and Grossman say,*
> "optimal imaging of iodine-based contrast agents is best achieved with comparatively low photon energies (70 to 80 kV). These relatively low photon energies provide the best contrast between water and iodine (whose x-ray absorption is greatest at 33 keV, . . .) An underpowered generator or cine pulse system that tries to compensate by using high (100 to 120 kV) energies thus tends to produce grainy, low-contrast angiographic images in which both water and iodine look grey."

Although Baim recommends 70-80 kV other authors say the best kV range is 80-90 kVp. See: Baim and Grossman, chapter on "Angiography..." contrast angiography

928. **Angiographic images may deteriorate on a large patient shot at extreme angulation. What type of images result if the kVp must be increased from 80 to 120 kVp?**
a. Reduced film blackening (under-exposure)
b. Increased film blackening (over-exposure)
c. Black-and-white, shorter scale contrast (high contrasty)
d. Grainy, flat, washed out, long scale contrast (low contrast)

ANSWER d. Grainy, flat, washed out, long scale contrast. To maintain film blackness, the x-ray generator may be forced to increase the kV if the tube cannot generate enough mA. This is especially true in steep views on large patients. Increased kV over-penetrates the dye and reduces the contrast between it and soft tissue. Baim and Grossman say,
> "An underpowered generator or cine pulse system that tries to compensate by using high (100 to 120 kV) energies thus tends to produce grainy, low-contrast angiographic images in which both water and iodine look grey."

Although long scale contrast with many shades of grey is good for chest radiography, cine-angiography requires optimum contrast between dye and the heart muscle. Most labs want the coronary arteries black and the rest of the heart white, although some labs like reversed images resembling cine angiograms - where the arteries appear white (since contrast absorbs X-rays). Since contrast best absorbs low kV x-rays, optimal angiography is done in the 70-90 kV range.
See: Baim and Grossman, chapter on "Angiography..." Keywords: High kV cine angiography = grainy, flat, long scale contrast

929. In chest radiography, changing the X-ray technique setting labeled #1 (increasing kV) affects the X-ray production by _____ beam quality, and _____ beam quantity.

*1. Increasing kV
2. Decreasing kV
3. Increasing mAs
4. Decreasing mAs

a. Making no change in quality, Decreasing quantity
b. Making no change in quality, Increasing quantity
c. Hardening quality, Increasing quantity
d. Softening quality, Decreasing quantity

ANSWER c. Hardening quality, Increasing quantity. Increased kV increases the penetrating energy and frequency of the x-rays. These are termed hard x-rays, as opposed to the soft low-energy x-rays. The softest low-energy rays should be filtered out before they reach the patient by an aluminum filter. This is because soft X-rays are too easily absorbed by tissue and thus contribute little to the X-ray image. Although the main effect of kV is on contrast, a 15% increase in kV will double the number of x-rays produced and the film density. So kV changes affect both X-ray quality and quantity. MA and exposure time (mAs) strictly regulate the quantity of x-rays produced and film density. They have no effect on x-ray quality. Be able to match all answers below.
BE ABLE TO MATCH ALL ANSWERS BELOW:

1. Increasing kV   - Hardens X-ray quality,   Increasing X-ray quantity
2. Decreasing kV   - Softens X-ray quality,   Decreasing X-ray quantity
3. Increasing mAs   -No change in quality,   Increases X-ray quantity
4. Decreasing mAs   -No change in quality,   Decreases X-ray quantity

See: Baim and Grossman, chapter on "Angiography..." Keywords: Increasing kV = beam hardening quality, Increasing quantity

IMAGE PRODUCTION
IMAGE

930. From the list below, which 3 are related to recorded detail, resolution, and sharpness on the CINE image? (Select 3 below)
a. kVp
b. Film speed
c. Focal spot size
d. Source to image distance
e. Speed of X-radiation

ANSWERS: b, c, & d.
a. kVp - NO
b. Film speed - YES
c. Focal spot size - YES
d. Source to image distance - YES
e. Speed of X-radiation is fixed at light speed - NO
Although kVp increases penetration and contrast, it does not improve image sharpness. The higher the film speed, the grainier the film, and the less fine its resolution. What

increases resolution is using smaller focal-spots, increasing the distance between focal-spot and film/image, and optimizing film speed and graininess. All X-rays travel at one speed - light speed. **See:** Bushong, chapter on "Radiographic Quality." **Keywords:** film detail, resolution, and sharpness all improved by slower film speed, smaller focal-spot size, and longer focal film distance

931. During fluoroscopy lowering the image intensifier closer to the patient increases the image:
a. Magnification
b. Density
c. Sharpness
d. Contrast

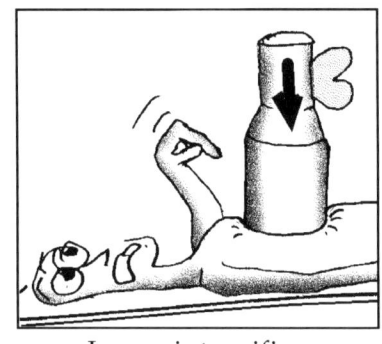

Image intensifier close to chest

ANSWER c. Sharpness. Consider a shadow of your hand on the wall. As you move away from the wall the shadow becomes hazy and poorly defined. The closer the object is to the image intensifier (short object-film distance) the finer the clarity and resolution. Kern says,

> "When the image intensifier is close to the chest wall and the heart, the image obtained is sharp. . . . When the heart lies further from the image intensifier and closer to the x-ray source, the image is magnified but poorly defined and hazy. Increased x-ray source-to-image distances require more kilovoltage, also degrading the image. . . . The image intensifier should be as close to the patient's chest as possible. This optimizes the image and decreases the scatter radiation."

Placing the image intensifier close to the patient's chest also reduces radiation scatter and resulting exposure to the patient and staff.

See: Kern, chapter on "Angiographic Data." Keywords: moving image intensifier down gives sharper image

932. Your X-ray tube has two focal spots: a 1.2 mm focal-spot and a 0.6 mm focal-spot. The smaller focal-spot (0.6 mm) is most commonly used on _____ cine angiography cases, because it _____ image resolution .
a. Pediatric, Improves
b. Adult, Improves
c. All, Improves
d. Adult, Reduces
e. Pediatric, Reduces

ANSWER a. Pediatric, Improves. Although the smaller focal spot provides better resolution for children, it may overheat on the angulated views needed for adult coronary cases. Thus, the small focal spot tube is usually only used for pediatric angiography - not adult. Baim and Grossman say,

> "Two focal spots are included in most catheterization laboratory x-ray tubes. . . . Whereas the small focal spot (usually 0.6 mm) more closely resembles a "point source" and thus provides potentially better geometric sharpness, the small focal spot in most x-ray tubes is quite limited in terms of its power handling capacity (35 kW). This forces the automatic exposure control to

resort to a low mA-high kV technique, which provides adequate film blackening only at the expense of poor image contrast. The small focal spot thus usually is used only for fluoroscopy or cineangiography in pediatric patients. Routine cineangiography in adult patients, particularly when performed in extreme angulation, are better performed using the larger (usually 1.0 mm) focal spot."

See: Baim and Grossman, chapter on "Angiography...")." Keywords: small focal spot has theoretically better resolution but easily overheats, so is used on pediatric angiography only

933. An X-ray with many shades of grey is described as having:
a. High density
b. Low density
c. Long-scale contrast
d. Short-scale contrast

ANSWER c. Long-scale contrast. Radiographic contrast is the difference between the densities seen on the x-ray.

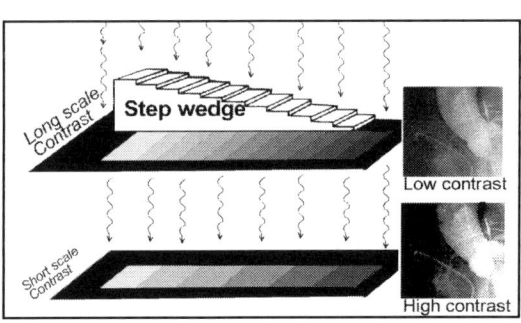

If there are many shades of grey between black and white the x-ray is said to have "long-scale contrast" or "low contrast." Note how smoothly the greys blend together. If there are few shades of grey it is "short-scale contrast" or "high contrast." These images tend to look black and white. These same terms are used in digital radiography. See: Bushong, chapter on "Radiographic Quality." Keywords: Long scale contrast = low contrast = many shades of grey

934. In coronary fluorography what effect will decreasing X-ray pulse duration (exposure time) have on the final image?
a. Increased density with motion blurring
b. Increased density with reduced motion artifact
c. Reduced density with motion blurring
d. Reduced density with reduced motion artifact

ANSWER d. Reduced density with reduced motion artifact. Decreasing cine pulse width lowers the mSec exposure time. This will expose the film faster and stop frame the motion. Normally this requires admitting more light by opening the camera iris (f stop setting). In our case it will require increasing the mA and/or kV to increase the intensity of x-rays and hence the density or darkness of X-ray films.

This is similar to action photography where the shutter speed is reduced. Photographers usually turn the exposure time down from 1/60 sec to 1/500 sec to take stop motion sports photographs. The kV is usually kept about 70 for cardiac Fluoroscopy. **See**: Bushong, chapter on "Radiographic Quality" **Keywords**: Reduced cine pulse width reduces exposure time, motion artifact, and film density

GRIDS & SCATTER

935. In the cath lab most harmful scatter radiation comes from the:
a. Lead shielding
b. Fluoroscope screen
c. X-ray tube
d. Patient

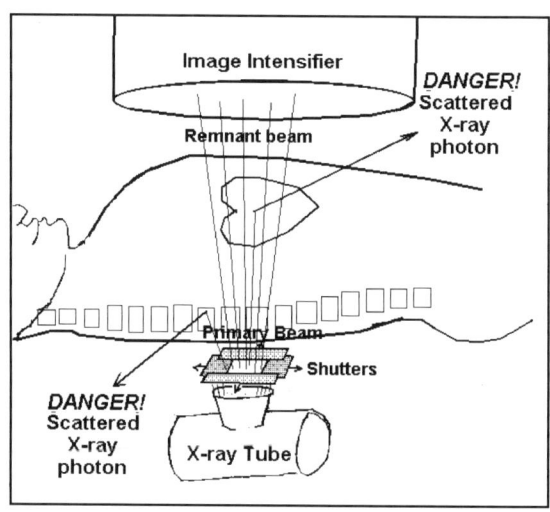

ANSWER d. Patient. Imagine the patient "glowing" when he/she is being x-rayed. His "glow" is secondary scatter radiation that can expose you. Bushong says,
> "*the scattering object can be considered as a new source of radiation. During both radiography and fluoroscopy, the patient is the single most important scattering object.*"

Kern says,
> "*Scatter from this beam (primary beam) exposes all subjects to radiation in a dose geometrically inverse to the distance from the source. Radiation scatter is increased when the angle of the tube is set obliquely. . . . Acrylic shields and table-mounted lead aprons should be used to reduce the amount of scatter.*"

See: Kern, chapter on "Angiographic Data." **Keywords**: scatter radiation from patient exposes personnel to secondary radiation

936. The primary purpose in using a grid in radiography is to:
a. Change the radiographic contrast scale
b. Decrease the patient exposure
c. Filter scatter radiation
d. Penetrate bony and obese patients better

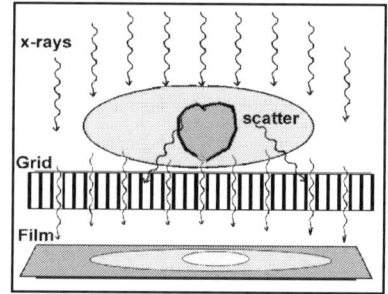

ANSWER c. Filter scatter radiation. A grid is made by alternating radiopaque lead strips and radiolucent spacing material. It is placed between the patient and the film to trap scatter radiation before it reaches the film. Scatter radiation tends to fog the film. A grid is rather like a Venetian blind that only lets light through in one direction. Note on the diagram how the scatter radiation in the diagram is absorbed into the parallel plates of the grid. Many image intensifiers are fitted with a grid to improve image clarity. **See**: Bushong, chapter on "The Grid."
Keywords: function of Grid = absorb scatter radiation

937. In angiography X-ray grids are positioned between the patient and the:
   a. X-ray tube, to reduce scatter radiation fog
   b. X-ray tube, to filter out dangerous high energy radiation
   c. Detector. to reduce scatter radiation fog
   d. Detector, to filter out dangerous high energy radiation

ANSWER c. Image intensifier, to reduce scatter radiation fog. X-rays that interact with the patient's tissues may give off scatter radiation in all directions. The scatter radiation going into the room poses a hazard to the staff. Scatter radiation going into the film fogs the film. Placing a grid between the patient and the film reduces most of the scatter heading toward the film and helps clarify it. The only problem with grids is they leave little stripes in the film. But, the grid may be moved during exposure to blur these stripes. A moving grid is termed a "Bucky" after its inventor. Grids are commonly used with cut film and may be built into a fluoroscopic image intensifier. **See**: Bushong, chapter on "Filtration."
Keywords: Grids placed between source and the patient

938. At cath, if the physician asks you to "collimate," he wants you to:
   a. Change the magnification mode
   b. Lower the image intensifier
   c. Move in the lead shutters
   d. Pan the table during injection

ANSWER c. Move in the lead shutters. "Coning down" or "collimating" adjusts the lead shutters to cut the field of view down. These controls are usually readily available on or near the catheterization table. You want keep the shutters open enough to view all the important anatomy on the screen, yet keep them closed enough to clarify the image by reducing scatter radiation. These lead shutters absorb the unnecessary radiation, reduce patient exposure, scatter to the staff, and film fog due to scatter radiation.
See: Bushong, chapter on "Filtration." **Keywords**: collimation = coning down = moving in the lead shutters

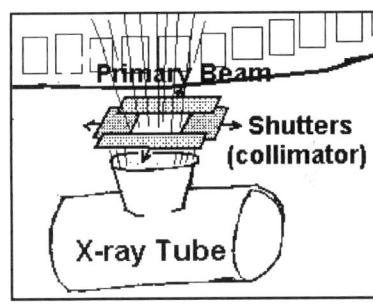

FILTRATION

939. Aluminum or copper filtration of primary X-ray beams is required by law to selectively filter out harmful?
   a. Soft - low energy X-rays
   b. Soft - high energy X-rays
   c. Hard - low energy X-rays
   d. Hard - high energy X-rays

ANSWER a. Soft - low energy X-rays. The most damaging X-rays are low frequency and low energy because they are easily absorbed by the skin and soft tissues. Another reason to eliminate these soft low energy rays is that they do not contribute to the x-ray image. Very few have enough energy to penetrate the tissues and get to the film. As shown in the diagram aluminum filters the softest and lowest energy rays out before they can irradiate the patient. For cine-angiography we want the bell curve to peak out around 70 -90 kV. **See**: Bushong, chapter on "The Grid."
Keywords: Grids placed between patient and film.

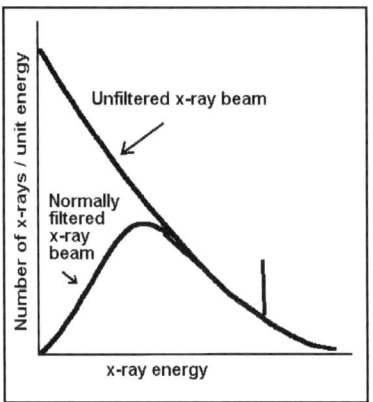

Filtration selectively removes low-energy x-rays
(after Bushong 10.4)

QUALITY CONTROL

940. Image "noise" appears as graininess on a fluoroscopic image. Image noise _____ as the patient X-ray dose increases. How much noise is allowed on a coronary floro image?
a. Increases, None
b. Increases, small amounts
c. Decreases, None
d. Decreases, small amounts

ANSWER d. Decreases, small amounts of noise are allowed to reduce patient dose. Good images are a balance between KV, Ma, for adequate contrast, density and noise to keep patient dose down. Fluoro is a low-dose X-ray for catheter advance, not for final images.

SCAI standards say, "Noise increases as the X-ray dose decreases. Noise should be readily apparent in fluoroscopic imaging in order to minimize patient dose. Most current digital image algorithms decrease noise by image smoothing without increasing dose." **See:** SCAI standards, Radiation Safety In the Cardiac Catheterization Laboratory, 2015

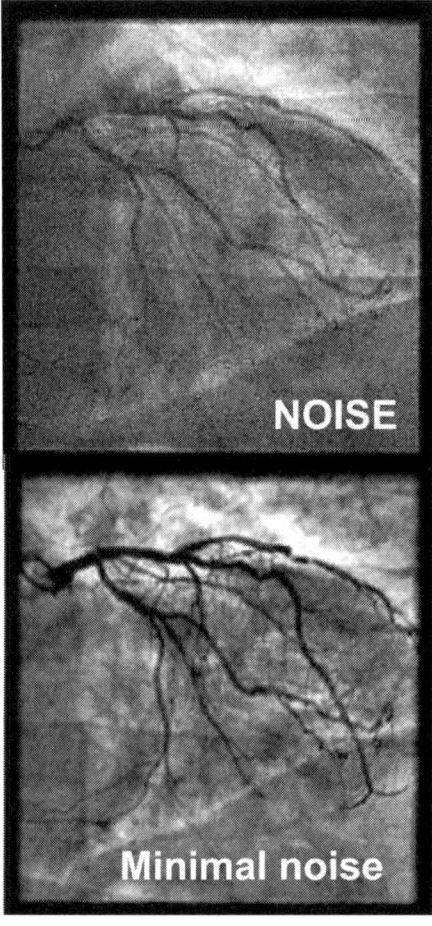

941. What instruments are used in X-ray quality control testing to measure the intensity of various film exposures?
a. Step wedge & sensitometer
b. Step wedge & densitometer
c. Spinning top & sensitometer
d. Spinning top & densitometer

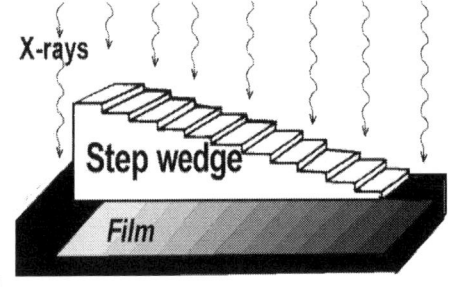

ANSWER b. Step wedge & densitometer. Bushong says,

"The principal measurements involved in sensitometry are exposure to the film and the percentage of light transmitted through the processed film. Such measurements are used to describe the relationship between density, the degree of blackness on the film, and exposure. This relationship is called a characteristic curve, ... Two pieces of apparatus are needed to construct a characteristic curve: an aluminum step wedge, sometimes called a penetrometer, and a densitometer."

See: Bushong, chapter on "Radiographic Quality" **Keywords**: sensitometry, densitometer, step wedge (penetrometer), characteristic curve

942. What does the "line-pair" test evaluate?
a. Timer accuracy
b. Film speed factors
c. Resolution
d. Log-relative exposure

ANSWER c. Resolution. A systems resolution can be measured as the minimal distance at which individual wires can be distinguished from one another. The smaller the wires and the closer together they can be clearly imaged the better the systems resolution. Bushong says,

Filmed Line Pairs

"The resolution of the screen (or X-ray system) is its ability to produce an accurate and clear image. Resolution is usually measured by the minimum line spacing that can be detected and imaged. . . . The number of line pairs per unit length is called the spacial frequency, and for a CT scanner it is expressed in line pairs per centimeter. . . . Increasing spatial frequency means better resolution of small objects."

Image intensifiers are available with input diameters of up to 45 cm, and a resolution of approximately 2-3 line pairs / mm. Flat panel detectors offer increased sensitivity to X-rays, and therefore have the potential to reduce patient radiation dose. Temporal resolution is also improved over image intensifiers, reducing motion blurring. Spatial resolution is approximately equal, although an image intensifier operating in 'magnification' mode may be slightly better than a flat panel.
See: Bushong, chapter on "Intensifying screens" and "Computed Tomography." Keywords: line pairs

Radiation Safety

Biological Effects

943. Identify 3 major damaging <u>somatic</u> effects of ionizing radiation overexposure. (Select 3 answers below.)
  a. Genetic mutation
  b. Erythema
  c. Cancer
  d. Cataracts
  e. Viral disease

ANSWERS: b, c, & d.
a. Genetic mutation - NO. It is not a somatic risk.
b. Erythema - YES
c. Cancer - YES
d. Cataracts - YES
e. Viral disease - No
Somatic refers to the body tissue damage, as opposed to genetic or cancer risks. Baim and Grossman say,

> "**Genetic damage** may lead to mutations in the offspring of an exposed individual. Bear in mind, however, that such mutations occur spontaneously and that laboratory studies suggest that very large exposures (nearly 100,000 mRem) are required to double the baseline risk of mutation. This means that the major danger of radiation exposure is the **somatic risk**, which may include either **direct tissue** injury (by a nonstochastic mechanism that has a defined threshold dose, such as cataracts) or **carcinogenesis** (a stochastic risk whose probability is proportional to dose at any level, such as thyroid cancer or leukemia)."

See: Baim and Grossman, chapter on "Angiography...")." **Keywords**: radiation somatic damage = cancer or tissue damage, genetic damage = mutations

944. Cath lab personnel are at increased risk of radiation-induced cancer. What are the 3 organs most sensitive to radiation-induced cancer? (Select 3 below.)
  a. Bone marrow (leukemia)
  b. Female breast (breast cancer)
  c. Thyroid (Thyroid cancer)
  d. Eyes (cataracts)
  e. Hands (arthritis)

ANSWERS: a, b, & c.
a. Bone marrow (leukemia) - YES
b. Female breast (breast cancer) - YES
c. Thyroid (thyroid cancer) - YES
d. Eyes (cataracts) - NO
e. Hands (arthritis) - NO
The eyes are at increased risk of developing cataracts and protective leaded glass should be worn by all exposed personnel. However, cataracts are not a carcinogenic pathology. Baim

and Grossman say,
> "The issue of stochastic risks (carcinogenesis) is clearly also of concern for catheterization personnel. The organs most sensitive to radiation-induced cancer are the bone marrow, female breast, and the thyroid."

See: Baim and Grossman, chapter on "Angiography...")." **Keywords**: radiation induced cancers are leukemia, breast, thyroid, (cataracts are not cancer caused)

945. During what period of pregnancy is the fetus most radiosensitive?
a. Egg prior to fertilization
b. First trimester
c. Second trimester
d. Third trimester

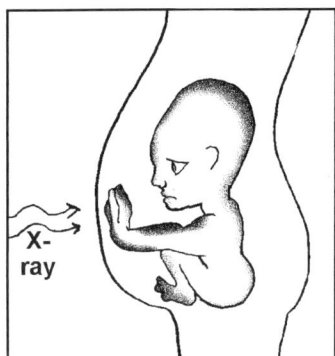

Fetus sensitive to radiation

ANSWER b. First trimester. The first months after conception are the most dangerous. Radiation selectively damages the fastest growing cells. That's why it is used to destroy fast growing cancer cells. The first 3 months are when radiation can most adversely effect the fetus. Pregnant lab staff should be moved out of the lab during the entire pregnancy period. If it is necessary for a pregnant staff member to be in the lab, most labs require women to use extra precautions like: acrylic lead shields, double film badges, and maximum distance from the patient.

See: Bushong, chapter on "Radiation Protection Procedures" **Keywords**: First trimester of pregnancy fetus is most radiosensitive

946. Pregnant cath lab staff members should receive special radiation protection. What is the upper allowed radiation limit to the fetus during the entire gestation period?
a. 0.1 rem
b. 0.5 Rem
c. 1.0 Rem
d. 5.0 Rem

ANSWER b. 0.5 Rem. Note that this is 1/10th of the maximum permissible dose to adult radiation workers. Johnson says,
> "The total whole body dose equivalent to the fetus should be limited to 0.5 Rem for the entire pregnancy. This is best achieved if the monthly fetal EDE is limited to 0.05 Rem. This roughly corresponds to an abdominal skin dose to the mother of about 1 Rem. While it is a good idea to monitor all workers at waist level under the lead apron, this should be mandatory for potentially pregnant individuals. . . . Every hospital should have an established pregnancy policy for female employees exposed to radiation."

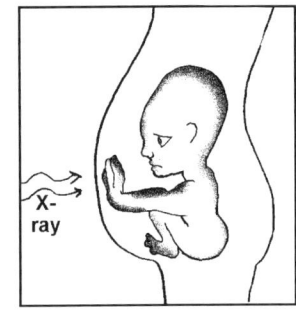

Although it is impossible to measure the actual dose the fetus receives, the best monitoring method is to have the mother wear a

two film badges, one on her collar and another under her apron.
See: Johnson, et. all, Review of Radiation Safety in the Cardiac Catheterization Laboratory." in *Catheterization and Cardiovascular Diagnosis* 1992. **Keywords:** pregnancy allowable dose = one tenth of usual MPD or 0.5 Rem

947. What is the likelihood of any adverse radiation effects on cath lab personnel whose dose is kept below recommended guidelines?
a. Zero
b. Remote
c. Probable
d. Inevitable

ANSWER b. Remote. Although your likelihood of radiation effects is remote, you must not become complacent about radiation safety. It could lead to an accidental overexposure. It has been estimated that 1% of all leukemia cases in the general population results from diagnostic radiography. Bushong says,

> "Radiology is now considered a completely safe occupation... Current studies suggest that even the low doses of x-radiation employed in routine diagnostic procedures may result in a small incidence of latent harmful effects. It is also well established that the human fetus is highly sensitive to x-radiation early in pregnancy. This sensitivity decreases as the age of the fetus increases.... At radiation doses below the MPD, neither somatic nor genetic responses should occur. At doses at the level of the MPD, the risk is not zero, but it is small and consistent with the risks associated with other occupations and reasonable in light of the benefits derived."

See: Bushong, chapter on "Concepts of Radiation"

RADIATION PROTECTION

948. The X-ray dose per frame of cine fluorography approximately _____:
a. 2-5 times greater than fluoroscopy
b. 10-15 times greater than fluoroscopy
c. 2-5 times less than fluoroscopy.
d. 10-15 times less than fluoroscopy

ANSWER: b. 15 times greater than fluoroscopy. Grossman says, "cinefluoroscophic units are calibrated such that the per-frame dose for acquisition is approximately 15 times greater than for fluoroscopy. A single frame acquired in acquisition mode thus delivers about the same patient dose as one second of pulsed fluoroscopy at 15 fps....Fluoroscopy thus involves <10% [7%= 1/15] of the x-ray beam intensity that is used for permanent image recording (cine-angiography). However, because fluoroscopic times are much longer than cine times, fluoroscopy typically provides more than half of the patient's total dose." Digital fluorographic imaging is still 10 times greater exposure than fluoro.
See, Grossman, chapter on Cineangiographic Imaging. Keywords: Cine =15x fluoro

949. For safety purposes the maximum Occupational Dose Limit (ODL) of whole body X-radiation that radiologic personnel are allowed to accumulate IN ANY ONE YEAR period is:
a. 0.5 Rem/yr.
b. 2.5 Rem/yr.
c. 5.0 Rem/yr
d. 10.0 Rem/yr.

ANSWER c. 5.0 Rem/yr. This Occupational Dose Limit (ODL) was previously termed the MPD (Maximum Permissible Dose). NCRP = National Council of Radiation Protection and Measurements recommends a maximum accumulation of 5 Rem (5000 mRem) in any one-year period. More than this, and you may be asked to stay out of X-ray for a year. The two important dose limits to remember are an accumulated dose limit of 1 Rem per year of age, or 5 Rems in any one year (see next question). Occupational dose limits are:

Pregnant Worker	0.5 REM/gestation period
Cumulated Dose Lifetime (DDE)	1 REM/year of age
Deep Dose Equivalent (DDE)	5 REM/year
Lens of Eye Dose Equivalent (EDE)	15 REM/year
Shallow Dose Equivalent (SDE)	50 REM/year

Although these are the absolute maximum limits most states require notification and corrective actions when a worker's dose limit reaches 1/10th of any of these maximum numbers. **See**: Johnson, et. all, Review of Radiation Safety in the Cardiac Catheterization Laboratory." in *Catheterization and Cardiovascular Diagnosis* 1992.

950. The maximum accumulated Occupational Dose Limit of deep whole body X-radiation that radiologic personnel are allowed to accumulate in his/her lifetime is:
a. 0.5 Rem/yr. x age
b. 2.5 Rem/yr. x age
c. 1.0 Rem/yr x age
d. 5.0 Rem/yr. x age

ANSWER c. 1.0 Rem/yr x age. This is the amount allowed to accumulate in a radiation worker in his/her lifetime (Cumulative dose lifetime). This is important because the effects of radiation damage accumulate throughout your life. That is why your film badge reports both monthly, quarterly, and life-time accumulated radiation doses, and why you must transfer your radiation records whenever you move to another hospital or monitoring service. This number is easy to remember, if you are 21 years old, your accumulated life-time dose limit is 21 Rem (21,000 MRem).

NCRP = National Council of Radiation Protection and Measurements. Note, that the maximum lifetime accumulated dose limit has recently changed. It used to start at age 18 instead of at birth. Since the lifetime accumulated dose has recently been reduced by 18 Rems, there is concern that young interventionalists may quickly exceed this life-time accumulated dose recommendation. **See**: Johnson, et. all, Review of Radiation Safety in the Cardiac Catheterization Laboratory." in *Catheterization and Cardiovascular Diagnosis* 1992. **Keywords:** life-time permissible dose, accumulated dose = 1 Rem x age

951. Which of the following reduces patient X-radiation exposure during cardiac catheterization? (Select 3.)
   a. Use cones and lead apertures to collimate
   b. Put lead drape with a hole in it over the patient
   c. Use grids and buckys in secondary beam
   d. Use a digital flat plate detector instead of II
   e. Reduce cine film rate from 30 to 15/sec

ANSWERS: a, d & e.
a. Use cones and lead apertures to collimate - YES.
b. Protect the patient with a lead apron outside the area of study - YES.
c. Use grids and buckys in secondary beam - NO.
d. Digital flat plate detector- YES. Better resolution than image intensifier and no distortion.
e. Reducing film rate from 30 to 15/sec YES, will cut patient exposure in half.
Grids reduce fog to the film. But they may actually **increase** the needed exposure, because some of the remnant beam is blocked by the lead strips in the grid. A bucky is a motorized vibrating grid that reduces the stripes commonly seen in grid collimated films. Grids are most often used in cut film angiography. **See:** Bushong, chapter on "Radiographic Quality"

952. The cath lab operator gets the most scatter radiation when shooting the _____ angiographic view?
   a. LAO caudal
   b. RAO caudal
   c. LAO cranial
   d. RAO cranial

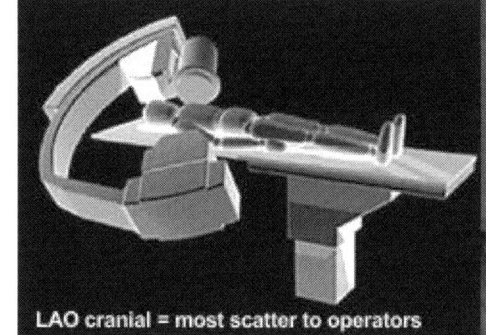

Answer: c. LAO cranial. The worst Xrays for staff come from scatter radiation from the patient where Xrays enter the chest. So, keep away from the X-ray tube. Remember, the II or flat plate detector is opposite the tube. So, in LAO views the tube will be on the patients right, near the operator - bad scatter. In cranial views the tube is even closer to the operator who stands to the right of the patient. During C-arm procedures standing on the side of the image intensifier is safest because there is more scatter produced at the entrance surface side of the patient.

Grossman says, "These duties can occur in a potentially high radiation zone... This is particularly important during angulated shots such as the left lateral or left anterior oblique cranial projections, which place the operator in close proximity to the beam entry point." See: Grossman, chapter on Cinangiographic Imaging, Radiation Safety, and Contrast Agents

953. When only one film badge is worn by cath lab personnel, it should be worn:
a. On the collar outside the lead apron
b. On the waist outside the lead apron
c. On the waist inside the lead apron
d. On the finger whenever scrubbed in

ANSWER a. On the collar outside the lead apron.
Bushong says:
> "if the technologist participates in fluoroscopy and wears a protective apron, as recommended, then the personnel monitor should be positioned on the collar above the protective apron. . . . It has been shown that during fluoroscopy, when a protective apron is worn, exposure to the collar region is 10 to 20 times greater than that to the trunk of the body beneath the protective apron. So if the personnel monitor is worn beneath the protective apron, it will record a falsely low exposure and will not indicate what could be hazardous exposure to unprotected body parts."

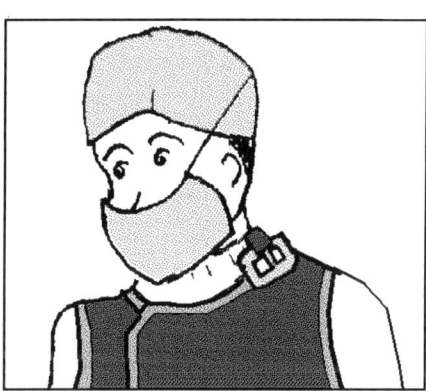
Collar film badge

See: Bushong, chapter on "Radiation Protection Procedures" **Keywords**: Wear badge on collar outside of lead apron

954. Current recommendations are for all cath lab operators (cardiologist) to wear two film badges located, one on the collar ____ and one on the ___ .
a. *Inside* the lead apron, belt *inside* the lead apron
b. *Inside* the lead apron, belt *outside* the lead apron
c. *Outside* the lead apron, belt *inside* the lead apron
d. *Outside* the lead apron, belt *outside* the lead apron

ANSWER c. One on collar outside the lead apron and one on the belt inside the lead apron. These should both face outward, toward the radiation source. Baim and Grossman say,
> "If a single "collar" badge is worn , it should be worn on the left shirt collar outside the lead apron, to give a maximal view of head and neck exposure. Current recommendations also call for a second "waist" badge, which is worn on the operator's belt just beneath the lead apron."

Note that this same recommendation also applies to pregnant staff members.
See: Baim and Grossman, chapter on "Angiography...")." **Keywords**: 2 radiation badges worn outside collar (facing outward) and on belt inside apron

955. A lead apron should be equivalent to ____ mm of lead, which will filter out ____ % of the X-rays.
a. 0.5 mm, 40%
b. 0.5 mm, 80%
c. 1.0 mm, 40%
d. 1.0 mm, 80%

ANSWER b. 0.5 mm, 80%. Kern says,
  "*Lead aprons should contain 0.5-mm thick lead lining. . . . lead aprons (preferably wraparound): >=0.5 mm thickness provides 80% protection.*"
  One advantage of a wrap around lead apron is that where it crosses in front actually doubles the protection where you need it most.
  See: Kern, chapter on "Introduction to the Catheterization Laboratory." **Keywords**: lead aprons 0.5 mm lead filters out 80% of x-rays

956. Leaded eyeglasses are primarily designed to protect you from:
  a. Laser and ultraviolet radiation
  b. Eye cancer
  c. Retinal damage
  d. Cataract formation

ANSWER d. Cataract formation. Kern says,
  "*It has been known that a single x-ray exposure of 200 R can produce cataract formation in humans. Eyeglasses made of 0.5 to 0.75-mm lead-equivalent glass should be worn by personnel exposed to radiation on a daily basis. . . . Plastic lenses offer no eye protection from radiation.*"
  See: Kern, chapter on "Introduction to the Cath Lab."

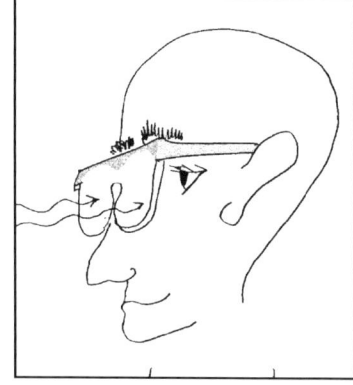
Leaded eye glasses

957. According to the "inverse square law" your most effective protection from damaging X-radiation is:
  a. A lead barrier between you and patient (apron)
  b. Increased space between you and the patient (distance)
  c. Aluminum filtration of primary beam (filtration)
  d. Digital imaging (DSA)

ANSWER b. Increased space between you and the patient (distance). Getting distance between you and the patient greatly reduces your exposure to scatter radiation. The patient is the source of virtually all of the scatter radiation in the room. Distance follows the inverse square law. Doubling your distance from the patient will *decrease* your exposure by a factor of 2^2 or 4. Tripling the distance between you and the patient will *decrease* your exposure by a factor of 3^2 or 9. **See**: Bushong, chapter on "Radiographic Quality" **Keywords**: Reduce staff exposure by getting away from the X-ray tube.

958. If you stand 4 feet away from a radiation source, instead of 2 feet away, you will reduce your total body radiation exposure by:
  a. ½ or 50%
  b. 3/4 or 75%
  c. 7/8 or 88%
  d. 15/16 or 94%

ANSWER b. 3/4 or 75%. Since you are doubling the distance, and the "Inverse square law" says that when radiation is emitted from a point source, the intensity decreases rapidly with the square of the distance from the source. $I_1/I_2 = D_2^2/D_1^2$. Assuming the initial radiation intensity is one and solving for I_2 gives:

$I_2 = I_1 (D_1^2/D_2^2) = 1 (2^2/4^2) = 1 (4/16) = 1/4$.

Doubling the distance from a radiation source reduces the intensity of the radiation to 1/4. Thus, doubling the Focal Film distance (ffd) will *decrease* the film density by a factor of 2^2 or 4. Thus, it is reduced 3/4 or 75%. **See**: Bushong, chapter on "Electromagnetic Radiation" **Keywords**: Inverse square law $I_1/I_2 = D_2^2/D_1^2$

959. Identify the 3 cardinal principles that the cath lab nurse should use to minimize X-ray exposure in the cath lab. (Select 3 answers below)
a. Time
b. Distance
c. Shielding
d. Beam filtration
e. Avoid Angulated views

ANSWERS: a, b, & c.
a. Time - YES
b. Distance - YES
c. Shielding - YES
d. Beam filtration is usually permanently set up un the X-ray housing - NO
e. Angulated views do yield more scattered radiation, but these are unavoidable.
These settings do effect the primary x-ray beam, which does produce dangerous scatter radiation, but, these settings are required to get high quality x-ray images, and nursing staff have no control over them. Bushong says, "basic radiation-control principles in diagnostic radiology: Understand and apply the cardinal principles of radiation control: time, distance and shielding."
    1. Minimize the time you are exposed to radiation
    2. Get as far away from the scatter radiation as possible
    3. Shield yourself with lead
See: Bushong, chapter on 'Concepts of Radiation' **Keywords**: time, distance and shielding

960. What happens when you take your foot off of the fluoroscopic foot pedal?
a. The production of primary and scattered radiation immediately stops.
b. The amount of radiation from the source decays with a half-life of 1-2 minutes
c. A lead shutter immediately blocks the X-ray beam to prevent the emission of primary radiation.
d. Low levels of radiation continue to be generated to keep the tube up to temperature

Answer a. The production of primary and scattered radiation immediately stops, because the electron filament and cathode (mA) shut off. Since X-rays travel at the speed of light and cannot be stored, shutdown is immediate. See: Bushong, chapter on "X-Ray Tube" Keyword: off fluoro pedal = 0 output

961. Which indicator provides the best estimate of the risk of a radiation skin injury?
   a. Fluoroscopic time
   b. Kerma area-product
   c. Air dose at the skin level
   d. Milliamp seconds (MAS)

Answer: b. Kerma area-product or Dose Area Product (DA. Dose area product (DAP), also called Kerma area product (KAP) is a quantity that reflects not only the dose but also the area of tissue irradiated. Therefore, it may be a better indicator of risk than dose. The DAP is expressed in Sievert square centimeters or (Gy*cm^2). Coronary angiography exposes patients to an average DAP in the range of 20 to 106 Gy*cm^2. DAP for PCI is about double that. If a radiation dose is spread out over a large skin area, there is less chance of a burn. Fluoro time alone does not account for: gantry motion, patient size, fluoro mode or CINE.

To reduce the risk of skin burns, the monitoring tech should alert the operator at 4000, 5000 mGy (same as for contrast alerts). When a significant dose threshold is exceeded it should be noted in the patient's medical record.

To avoid skin burns in radiation therapy, shaped radiation beams are aimed from several angles of exposure to intersect at a tumor, providing a much larger absorbed dose on the tumor than in the surrounding healthy tissue [and skin]. Brachytherapy, in which a radiation source is placed in an expanded artery to reduce restenosis minimizes exposure to healthy tissue and skin.

962. Skin burns from X-radiation:
   a. May take a year to evolve and heal
   b. Are clinically similar to thermal burns.
   c. May show up in low doses of X-radiation (<1 Gy)
   d. May not show up with high doses of X-radiation (>10 Gy)

Answer: a. May take a year to evolve and heal.

Bushong says, "After a single dose of 3 to 10 Gy an initial mild erythema may occur within the first or second day. This first wave of erythema then subsides, only to be followed by a second wave that reaches maximum intensity in about 2 weeks. At

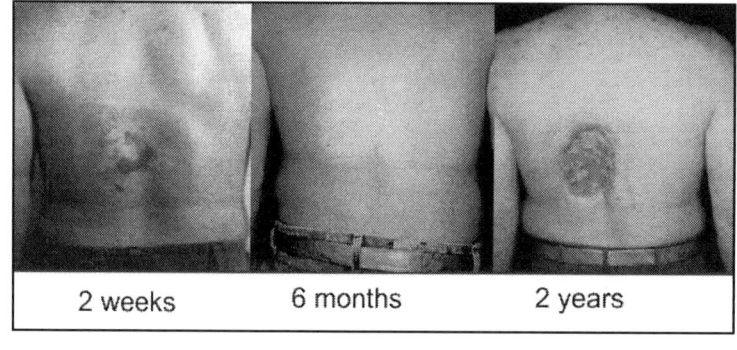

2 weeks   6 months   2 years

higher doses, this second wave of erythema is followed by a moist desqaumation, which in turn may lead to a dry desquamation. These skin effects follow a nonlinear, threshold radiation-induced relationship.... Small doses of x-radiation do not cause erythema. Extremely high doses of x-radiation cause erythema in all persons so irradiated." This may take months to years to heal. Note the picture showing the time progression of an x-radiation burn from a PCI. This patient received over 20 Gy of radiation. See: Bushong, chapter on "X-Ray Tube" Keyword: Radiation burns heal slowly

963. For cath lab staff the recommended safe level of X-ray radiation exposure is:
a. <5 MSv/year
b. <5 Rem/year
c. There is NO safe level
d. Current levels of fluoroscopy in industry is safe

ANSWER: c. There is NO safe level
    Braunwald says, "The main guiding principle of x-ray exposure is ALARA (As Low As Reasonably Achievable). This implies that no level of radiation is completely safe to patients or providers....The basic principles of minimizing radiation exposure include minimizing fluoroscopic beam time for fluoroscopy, using beam collimation, positioning the x-ray source and image reception optimally, using the least magnification possible, changing the radiographic projection in long procedures to minimize entrance port skin exposure, recording the estimated patient dose, and selecting equipment with dose reduction features including low fluoroscopy mode." See: Braunwald, chapter on Cardiac Cath
    Braunwald says, "Stochastic effects are related to probability and not proportional to dose, although the likelihood of an effect is related to dose. Examples of this effect include neoplasms and genetic defects. The estimated dose range for cardiac catheterization is 1 to 10 millisievert (mSv), which is the equivalent of 2 to 3 years of natural background radiation. The typical dose is 3 to 5 mSv" See: Braunwald, chapter on "Technical Aspects of Cardiac Catheterization"

DIGITAL RADIOGRAPHY

964. What is the basic visible unit (dot) comprising a "digital" cardiac image?
a. Byte
b. Bit
c. Pixel
d. Raster line

ANSWER c. Pixel. The smaller the pixel size the finer the resolution of the screen. In a standard 512 by 512 digital scanner the product is 262,144 cells of information. Each pixel or cell can have depth in terms of how many bits of grey it can display. A raster line is one horizontal line on the screen - usually 512 pixels long. Higher resolutions are available. **See:** Bushong, chapter on "Computed Tomography" **Keywords:** pixel = 1 cell on a display screen containing grey scale information

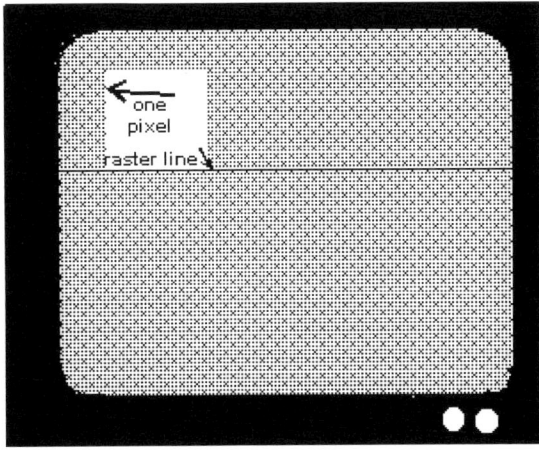

965. In flat panel detectors each pixel in the image comes from:
a. An MRI detector cell
b. Image intensifier xy matrix
c. One X-ray photon's impact
d. One photodiode in the detector

Answer. d. One photodiode in the detector that accumulates all the X-ray photons hitting one Cesium Iodide needle crystal. The crystal scintilates (phosphoreses) and caries the light to a photodiode beneath it. The density on each pixel in the image may result from hundreds or thousands of X-ray photons hitting that crystal and being converted into an electrical signal by the photodiode.

Konica minolta says, "a CsI scintillator is made to contact directly over a TFT 1 sensor panel without any protective layer in between them. This technology has made it possible to guide the light emitted from the scintillator to the photodiode without causing the light to be dispersed at the interface with the TFT sensor. " See: https://www.konicaminolta.com/healthcare/products/dr/aerodr/feature.html

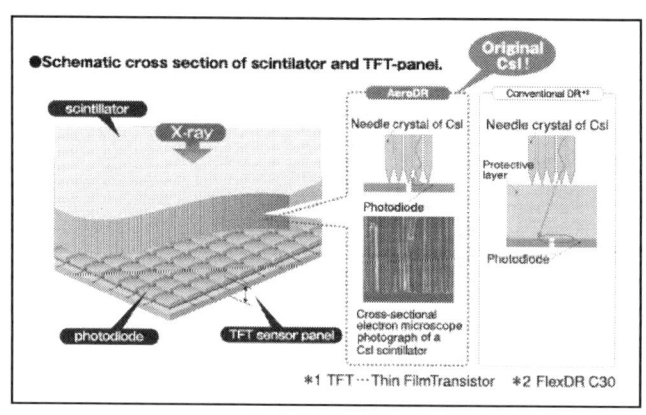

966. When making a subtraction cine-angiogram the mask is made from the:
a. Cut film negative
b. Scout film (just prior to injection)
c. Angiogram (post injection)
d. Subtraction (prior - post injection)

ANSWER b. Scout film is shown at #1. A mask is made from the scout film just before the angiogram is shot. This mask film is then inverted (black to white and white to black) to get its negative image.
BE ABLE TO MATCH ALL ANSWERS BELOW:
  1. **Mask:** is made from the scout film before the angiogram is shot
  2. **Inverted mask:** Inverting reverses the colors, making all the blacks white and all the whites black
  3. **Angiogram:** shows contrast superimposed on the bones and dense structure.
  4. **Subtracted image:** is the sum of films #2 and

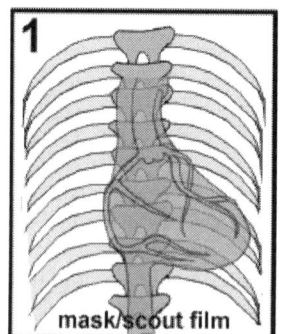
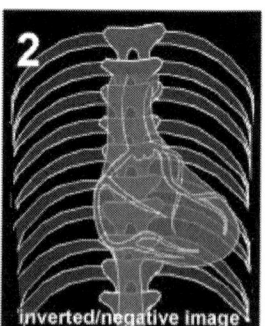
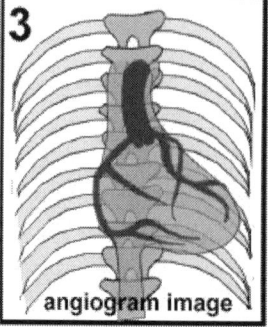
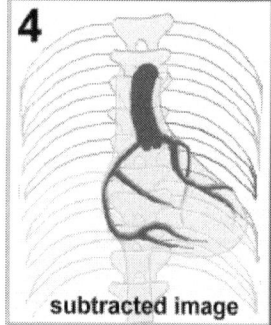

#3.
When perfect alignment of the occurs between the 2 images, the bones and surrounding anatomic structures are canceled out leaving only the contrast in the coronary arteries. This is termed the digital "subtracted" angiogram or DSA. **See**: Bushong, chapter on "Concepts of Radiation" **Keywords**: DSA, scout film = negative of scout film

967. In digital subtraction angiography (DSA) what two films are merged to give the final subtracted image?
a. Scout film & angiogram
b. Inverted scout film & angiogram
c. High contrast scout film & edge enhanced angiogram
d. Low contrast scout film & high contrast angiogram

ANSWER b. Inverted scout film & angiogram. These two images are shown in the diagram as #2 and #3. When these two films are put on top of each other and enhanced, the result is #4 the subtracted image where all the bones fade seem to away. Bushong describes the temporal subtraction method using a mask as follows:

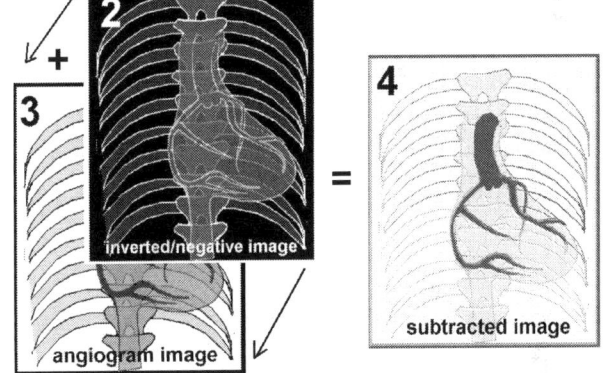

"Before the bolus of contrast medium reaches the anatomic site, an initial x-ray pulse exposure is made. The image obtained is stored in primary memory and displayed on video monitor A. This is the **mask image.**

This mask image is followed by a series of additional images that are stored in adjacent memory locations. While these subsequent images are being acquired, the mask image is subtracted from each and the result is either stored in primary memory, ... or dumped to a secondary memory (disc)."

A mask is made from the scout film before the angiogram is shot (shown at #1). Before the subtraction can occur this mask must be "inverted." Inverting makes all the blacks white and all the whites black (Shown at #2). This is termed the "negative" or "inverted" image. Subtracting images really means adding a positive to a negative to end up with a grey color. When the angiogram is added to the negative (shown at #4) the bones all disappear leaving the contrast in the arteries. This subtraction process can be expressed mathematically as: Image #4 (subtracted) = Image #3 (angiogram) - image #1 (mask)
See: Bushong, chapter on "Concepts of Radiation"

Did you review basic X-ray interpretation online, mostly chest films at - http://www.radiologyassistant.nl/en/p497b2a265d96d/chest-x-ray-basic-interpretation.html
a. Yes
b. No

Did you review the 50 online RT questions - multiple choice at: https://www.nde-ed.org/EducationResources/CommunityCollege/Radiography/Quizzes/rtquiz50.htm
a. Yes
b. No

REFERENCES:

Bushong, Steward C., *Radiologic Science for Technologists, Physics, Biology, and Protection*, 9th Ed., Mosby-Elsevier, 2008

Baim, D. S. and Grossman W., *Cardiac Catheterization, Angiography, and Intervention*, 6th Ed., Lea and Febiger, 2006

Braunwald, et. al. Ed., *Heart Disease, a Textbook of CV Medicine*, 8th Ed., Saunders, 2008

Peterson, K.L, and Nicod, P., Cardiac Catheterization, Methods, Diagnosis, and Therapy, 1st Ed., W.B. Saunders Co., 1997

Pepine, J. C., and Hill, J. A., et. al., *Diagnostic and Therapeutic Cardiac Catheterization*, 2nd Ed., Williams and Wilkins, 1994

Kern, M. J., Ed., *The Cardiac Catheterization Handbook*, 6th Ed., Mosby-Year Book, Inc., 2016

Johnson, Moore, and Baltar, *Review of Radiation Safety in the Cardiac Catheterization Laboratory*, in Catheterization and Cardiovascular Diagnosis - Journal, 1992

Saia, D.A., *Appleton & Lange's Review for the RADIOGRAPHY EXAMINATION*, 1st Ed., Appleton & Lange, 1995

X-ray Outline

1. Introduction to X-ray
    a. Roentgen
    b. Crooke
    c. Edison
    d. Radiolucent/opaque
    e. Phosphor
2. X-Ray Equipment
    a. Tube
        i. Anode (rotating)
        ii. Cathode
        iii. Target
        iv. Filament
        v. Focusing cup
        vi. focal spot
        vii. source image distance
        viii. electron beam
        ix. Filament temperature
    b. Generation
        i. X=ray produced when an Electron is suddenly slowed
    c. Image Intensifier
        i. Light Amplification
        ii. Input Phosphor
        iii. Photocathode
        iv. Electrostatic lenses
        v. Anode
        vi. Output Phosphor
        vii. mag modes
    d. Video
        i. Standard US broadcast
        ii. Raster lines
        iii. Progressive scanning

iv. Digital recording
v. DICOM standard
vi. Video tape
vii. Direct video monitoring
viii. Cine angiogram
ix. Digital frame grabber
x. CD Rom
xi. DVD
3. Interaction with Matter
    a. Measures of Radiation
        i. Dosimetry
        ii. REM
        iii. RAD
        iv. Roentgen
        v. Curie
        vi. Rem
        vii. Sievert (Sv)
        viii. Rad (rad)
        ix. Roentgen (R)
        x. Film badges in Milli-REM
    b. Radiation Physics
        i. Characteristics of X-rays
            (1) Attenuation
            (2) Absorption
            (3) Scatter
            (4) Reflection
            (5) penetrates tissue
            (6) speed of light
            (7) electromagnetic radiation
    c. Radiation Quality and Quantity
        i. Ionizing radiation- injury
        ii. Photon = quantum EM radiation
    d. kV and Ma
        i. Increasing kilovoltage (kV)
        ii. Decreasing kilovoltage (kV)
        iii. Increasing milli- Amp-sec (mAs)
        iv. Decreasing milli-Amp-sec (mAs)
        v. Density
        vi. Penetration
            (1) Hard/soft X-rays
        vii. Contrast/shades of grey
        viii. kV
        ix. mA
        x. Exposure time
4. Image Production
    a. Image
        i. Resolution (line pairs)
        ii. Sharpness
        iii. Contrast
        iv. Increased mA used for cine
        v. Increased dose = less noise
    b. Grids and Scatter Radiation
        i. Grid construction
        ii. Radiation fog
        iii. Use of grids
        iv. Collimation
        v. Lead shutters
        vi. Advantages of "coning down"
    c. Filtration
        i. Aluminum filters
        ii. soft - low energy X-rays
        iii. Reducing Patient absorbed dose
    d. Quality Control
        i. Step wedge
        ii. densitometer
    e. Focal spot size
    f. Long-scale contrast
5. Radiation Effects
    a. Biological Effects
        i. Somatic
            (1) Erythema
            (2) Cataracts
        ii. Genetic
            (1) Genetic mutation
            (2) Cancer
            (3) Bone marrow (leukemia)
            (4) Female breast (breast cancer)Thyroid (Thyroid cancer)
    b. Radiation Protection
        i. Fetus most sensitive
            (1) First trimester
        ii. Dose limits
        iii. Pregnant Worker
        iv. 0.5 REM/gestation pd.
        v. Cumulated Dose Lifetime (DDE) = 1 REM/year of age
        vi. Deep Dose Equivalent (DDE) = 5 REM/year
        vii. Lens of Eye Dose Equivalent (EDE) = 15 REM/year
        viii. Shallow Dose Equivalent (SDE) = 50 REM/year
    c. Film badges
    d. Lead aprons
    e. Leaded glasses
    f. Thyroid shields
    g. Distance
        i. Inverse square law
6. Digital Radiography
    a. Cineless Lab
        i. Equipment
        ii. Flat plate detector
        iii. Thin Film Transistor (TFT)
        iv. Photodiode
        v. No focusing optics
        vi.
    b. Pixel
    c. Digital Subtraction Angiography (DSA)
        i. Cut film negative
        ii. Scout film (prior to injection)
        iii. Angiogram (post injection)
        iv. Subtraction (prior - post injection)

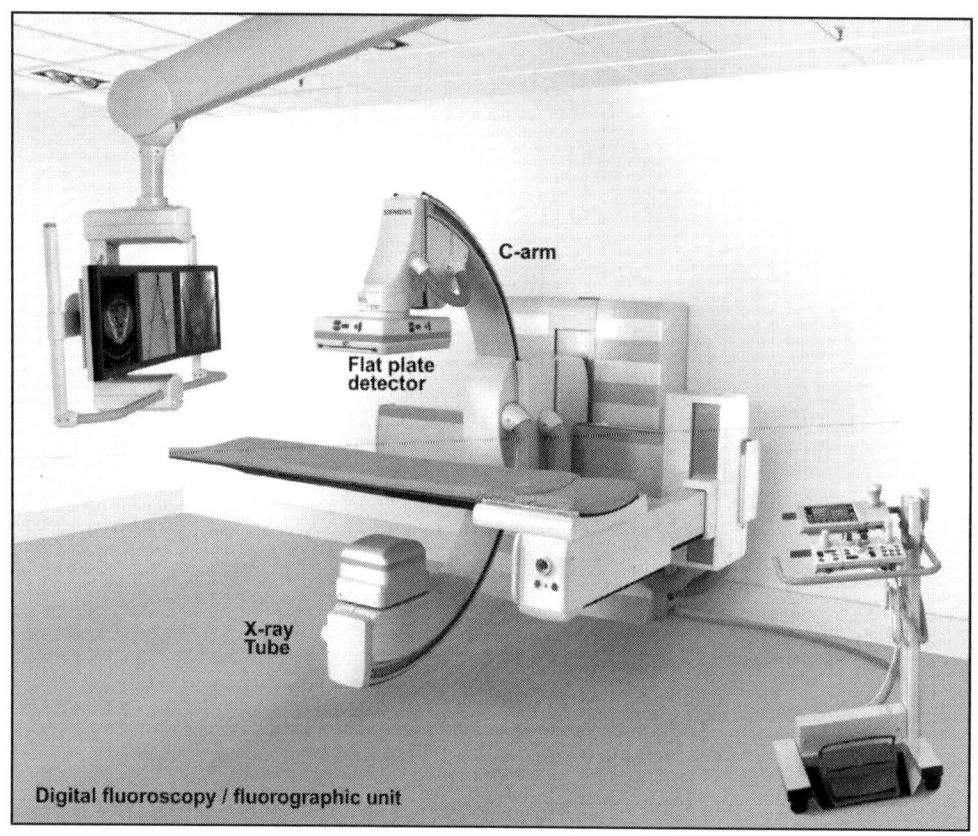

BASIC CV - FORMULAS

MEASUREMENTS/ CONVERSION
*Linear (length)   :   1 in = 2.54 cm
*Mass (Weight)   :   1 Kg = 2.2 lb
 Volume   :   1 L = 1000 ml = 1.05 qt.
*Pressure   :   1 atmosphere = 760 mmHg or Torr = 15 psi

PHYSICS FORMULAS   *(Vol. 1, Chapter A3)*
*Velocity   :   V = d / t   =distance / time
 Force   :   F = m x a   = Mass x Acceleration
 Work   :   W = F x d   = Force x distance
 Power   : P_w = F x d / t = Force x distance / time
*Pressure   :   P = F / A   = Force / Area
*Density   :   D = wt/vol.
 Acceleration   :   a =V / t   = Velocity / time
*Area (square)   :   b x w = base x width
 Area (triangle)   :   ½ b x h = ½ base x height
 Volume (rectangular):   b x w x h = base x width x height
*Temperature   :   F = [(9/5) C] + 32
   F = degrees Fahrenheit, C = degrees Celsius

PHYSICAL PRINCIPLES   *(Vol. 1, Chapter A3)*
*Distance   :   D = V x t
   Distance = Velocity x time
 Acceleration   :   A = V / t = Velocity / time = D / t^2

Graham's Law Diffusion: $$D = \frac{\Delta P \times A \times S}{d \times \sqrt{MW}}$$

D = rate of diffusion, ΔP = Pressure gradient
A = Area, S = Solubility, d = density, MW = Molecular Weight

Henry's Law Gases   :S = C x P / t =Sol. coef. x Partial Pr. / temp.
Dalton's Law Gases: P_t = P_1 + P_2 +... P_n = Sum of partial pressures

ULTRASOUND   :   *(Vol. 1 Chapter A3)*
*Period = 1/ frequency
*Wavelength = propagation speed / frequency
   Wavelength = propagation speed x Period
      *(note: in soft tissue propogation speed = 1540 M/sec)

PHYSIOLOGY   (Vol. 1, Chapter A3)

Ohm's Law (fluid) : $R = (P_i - P_o) / Q$ = Pressure drop/blood flow
Continuity Eqn. : $Q = V \times A$ = Velocity x Area
Poisieulle's Law :

$$Q = \frac{\pi(P_i - P_o)r^4}{8\eta l}$$

Q = flow, P_i = Pressure in, r = radius, η = viscosity, l = length
or since $R = (P_i - P_o) / Q$

Poiseuille's Resistance: $R = 8(\text{Viscosity})(\text{Length}) / (\pi)(\text{radius})^4$
= (revised Ohm's law)

Laplace Law : $T = P \times R$ Tension = Pressure x radius
Kinetic Energy : $\frac{1}{2}mv^2$ = 1/2 mass x velocity^2
Potential Energy : mgh = mass x gravity x height
Bernoulli Eqn. : $K = 1/2 mv^2 + mgh$
Starling's Eqn. : Fluid Movement = $k(P_c + \pi_i) - (P_i + \pi_p)$.
where k = constant
π_p = plasma protein oncotic pressure
P_c = hydrostatic capillary pressure

HEMODYNAMICS   (See: Review Book Vol. III)

*Heart Rate : HR = 60/RR interval = 60 x paper speed/mm. RR int.
*Stroke Volume : SV = EDV - ESV
SV = End Systolic LV vol - End Diast. LV Vol.
*Ejection Fraction : EF = SV/EDV x 100%
SV = End Systolic LV vol - End Diast. LV Vol.
*Regurgitant Fraction   Regurg./min/ LVMF x 100%

*Cardiac Output : CO = SV x HR
This CO also termed LVMF (LV minute Flow)
*Cardiac Index : CI = CO/BSA
CO = Cardiac Output; BSA = Body Surface Area
*Arterial Pulse Pressure: pp = s - d   = systolic - diastolic
*Mean Blood Pressure :mean BP = (s + 2 d)/3 = (systolic + 2 x diastolic) / 3
*Systemic Vasc. Resistance: SVR = (mean BP - mean CVP) / CO
usually SVR = (mean AO - mean RA) / CO
mean BP : mean BP = CO x SVR
*Compliance : $\Delta V / \Delta P$ = change in Volume / change in Press.

PHARMACOLOGY (Vol. IV, F6 & F7)
*Concentration : C = wt/vol.   = solute/solvent
*Amount : Amount = C x V   = Conc. x Volume
*Administration rate: Amount/min = C x V/t   = Conc. x Vol./time

Appendix: INVASIVE BASICS FORMULAS — -539-

RCIS exam will require you to learn additional formulas.
See, Vol 3 Hemodynamics

ACID BASE & O2   *(Review Book, Vol. I, ch. B2)*

pH : $pH = \log[1/H^+]$ where H^+ = Hydrogen ion conc.

*Hgb. O2 Content :   **CaO2 = 1.39 x Hgb x O2 Sat/100**

Plasma O2 Content: Physically dissolved O2 = .004 X PO_2 = CpO_2 in vol%.
Total O2 Cont C_tO_2 = Hgb O2 + Plasma O2 content in vol. %
      = 1.39 x O2 Sat x Hgb + .004 X PO_2
Hgb. O2 Capacity :   O2 Cap. = 1.39 x 100% Sat x Hgb

*% O2 Saturation :   **CaO2 / O2 Capacity**

ELECTRICITY   *(Vol. 1, Chapter A3)*

Series Resistance : $R_{eff} = R_1 + R_2 \ldots + R_n$
   Effective total Resistance = Sum Res.

Parallel Resistance :
$$\frac{1}{R_{eff}} = \frac{1}{R_1} + \frac{1}{R_2} + \ldots \frac{1}{R_n}$$

Ohm's Law : $V = I \times R$
Voltage = Current x Resistance
Power   :   Watts = V x I   = Voltage x Current
Energy   :   Energy = Power x time = V x I x t   = Watt Sec or Joules

*Indicates an **important formula** worth **memorizing**. Understand the relationships described by each equation, and how to solve for each variable.

Cardiovascular Review Books

PERFECT TO:
Self Study at home or in the cath lab.
Help staff pass the Cath Lab Registry Exams.
Resource for in-service educators.
Assess your cath lab knowledge and skills.
Text to accompany CV Review CD

TODD's CV REVIEW BOOKS

- Vol. I: Invasive Basics
    Includes Pt. Care, A&P, Pathology
- Vol. II: Cath Lab Diagnostic Techniques
- Vol. III: Cath Lab Hemodynamics
- Vol. IV: Cath Lab Interventions
- Vol. V, Practice Exams, Includes 7 Invasive Mock Exams

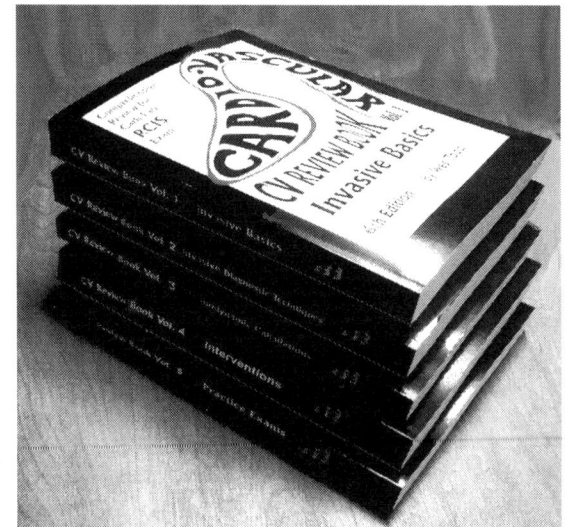

5 Vol. Book Set

Recommended for all cath lab staff,
    Invasive students, Cath lab nurses
    & Technicians.

We recommend that your prepare for your exam with all our instructional materials.

Together they complement each other.

Order from www.Amazon.com Or www.westodd.com

More information at http://www.westodd.com
Or Email info@westodd.com

Made in the USA
Columbia, SC
16 July 2022